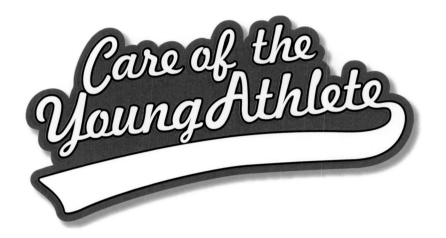

AMERICAN ACADEMY OF ORTHOPAEDIC SURGEONS

AMERICAN ACADEMY OF PEDIATRICS

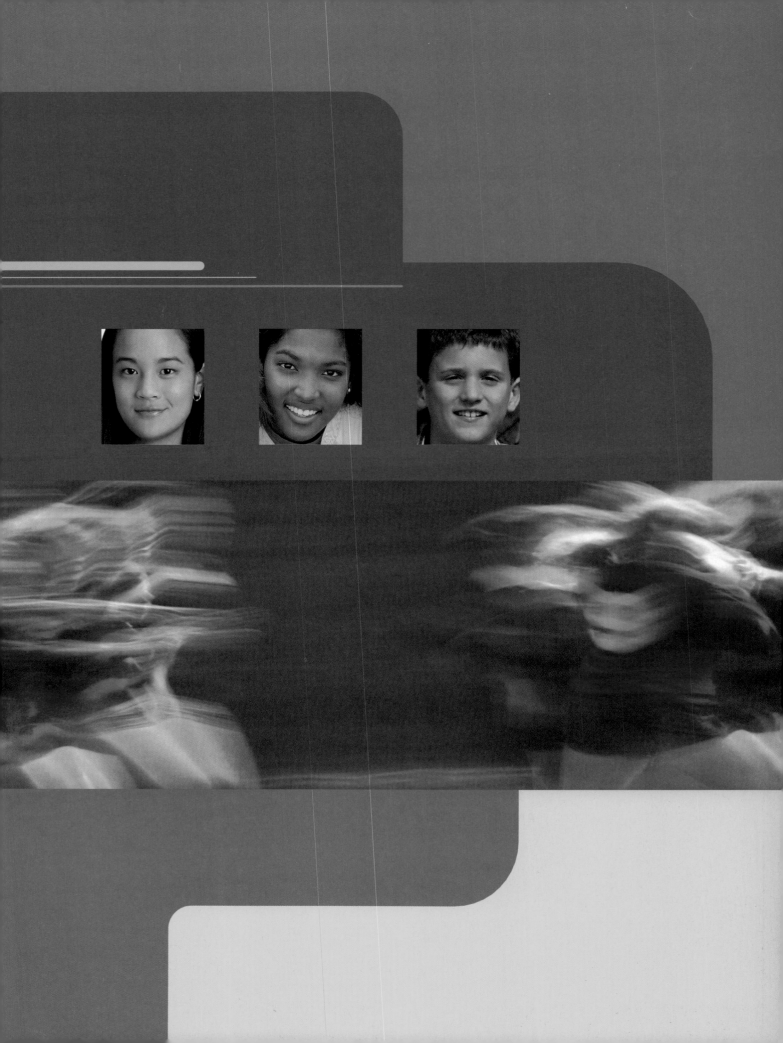

Care of the Young Athlete

J. Andy Sullivan, MD
Steven J. Anderson, MD
EDITORS

American Academy
of Orthopaedic Surgeons

American Academy
of Pediatrics

The material presented in *Care of the Young Athlete* has been made available by the American Academy of Orthopaedic Surgeons (AAOS) and the American Academy of Pediatrics (AAP) for educational purposes only. This material is not intended to present the only, or necessarily best, methods or procedures for the medical situations discussed, but rather is intended to represent an approach, view, statement, or opinion of the author(s) or producer(s), which may be helpful to others who face similar situations. The recommendations in this publication do not indicate an exclusive course of treatment or serve as a standard of medical care. Variations, taking into account individual circumstances, may be appropriate.

Some drugs or medical devices demonstrated in AAOS courses or described in AAOS print or electronic publications have not been cleared by the Food and Drug Administration (FDA) or have been cleared for specific uses only.

The FDA has stated that it is the responsibility of the physician to determine the FDA clearance status of each drug or device he or she wishes to use in clinical practice.

Furthermore, any statements about commercial products are solely the opinion(s) of the author(s) and do not represent an AAOS or AAP endorsement or evaluation of these products. These statements may not be used in advertising or for any commercial purpose.

ISBN 0-89203-214-6 AAOS

ISBN 1-58110-050-7 AAP

Library of Congress Cataloging-in-Publication Data:

Care of the young athlete/edited by Steven J. Anderson, J. Andy Sullivan.
p. cm.
Developed by the American Academy of Pediatrics and the American Academy of Orthopaedic Surgeons.
Includes bibliographical references and index.
ISBN 0-89203-214-6 (hc)
1. Pediatric sports medicine. I. Anderson, Steven J. II. Sullivan, J. Andy. III. American Academy of Pediatrics.
IV. American Academy of Orthopaedic Surgeons.

RC1218.C45 C37 2000
617.1'027'083—dc21

99-086578

Acknowledgments

American Academy of Orthopaedic Surgeons Editorial Board

J. Andy Sullivan, MD
Don H. O'Donoghue Professor and Endowed Chair
Department of Orthopedic Surgery
University of Oklahoma College of Medicine
Oklahoma City, Oklahoma

William Herndon, MD
Oklahoma Sports Center and Orthopedics
Oklahoma City, Oklahoma

Donald W. McGinnis, MD
Assistant Professor
Director, Division of Sports Medicine
Department of Orthopedic Surgery and Rehabilitation
University of Oklahoma Health Sciences Center
Oklahoma City, Oklahoma

American Academy of Pediatrics Editorial Board

Steven J. Anderson, MD
Clinical Professor, Pediatrics
University of Washington
Seattle, Washington

Gregory L. Landry, MD
Professor of Pediatrics
Head Medical Team Physician,
    UW Madison Athletic Teams
University of Wisconsin Medical School
Madison, Wisconsin

Oded Bar-Or, MD
Professor of Pediatrics
Director, Children's Exercise and Nutrition Centre
McMaster University
Hamilton, Ontario, Canada

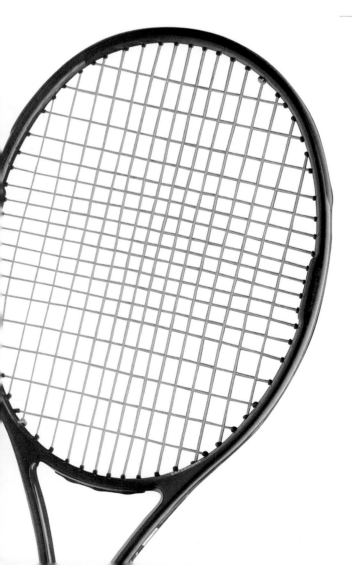

Contributors

Steven J. Anderson, MD
Clinical Professor, Pediatrics
University of Washington
Seattle, Washington

William R. Barfield, PhD
Adjunct Assistant Professor
Department of Orthopaedic Surgery
Medical University of South Carolina
Charleston, South Carolina

Oded Bar-Or, MD
Professor of Pediatrics
Director, Children's Exercise & Nutrition Centre
McMaster University
Hamilton, Ontario, Canada

James Richard Barrett, MD
Associate Professor of Family Medicine
Director, Primary Care Sports Medicine
    Fellowship Program
Department of Family Medicine
University of Oklahoma Health Sciences Center
Oklahoma City, Oklahoma

Rodney S.W. Basler, MD
Past Chair, Taskforce on Sportsmedicine,
    American Academy of Dermatology
Assistant Professor of Internal Medicine
University of Nebraska Medical Center
Lincoln, Nebraska

James H. Beaty, MD
Professor
University of Tennessee, Campbell Clinic
Department of Orthopaedic Surgery
Memphis, Tennessee

David T. Bernhardt, MD
Associate Professor
Pediatrics and Sports Medicine
University of Wisconsin
Madison, Wisconsin

Frank M. Chang, MD
Director, Orthopaedic Surgery, The Children's Hospital
Associate Professor, University of Colorado Health
    Sciences Center
University of Colorado
Denver, Colorado

John F. Coyle, MD
Clinical Professor of Medicine
The University of Oklahoma
College of Medicine, Tulsa
Tulsa, Oklahoma

John A. Fox, MD
Assistant Professor of Orthopaedics
Vanderbilt Pediatric Orthopaedics
Vanderbilt University Medical Center
Nashville, Tennessee

Carlos A. Garcia-Moral, MD
Clinical Professor, Department of Orthopaedic
    Surgery and Rehabilitation
University of Oklahoma
Oklahoma City, Oklahoma

Jorge E. Gomez, MS, MD
Assistant Professor, Department of Pediatrics
University of Texas Health Center at San Antonio
San Antonio, Texas

Daniel Gould, PhD
Professor
Exercise and Sport Science
Greensboro, North Carolina

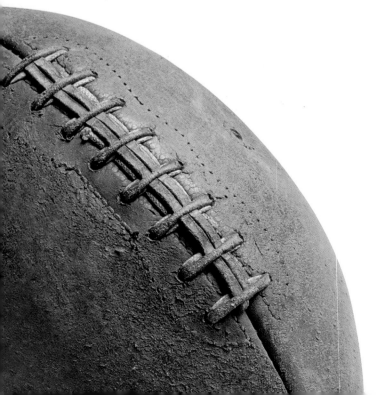

Neil E. Green, MD
Professor of Orthopaedics
Vanderbilt Pediatric Orthopaedics
Vanderbilt University Medical Center
Nashville, Tennessee

Bernard A. Griesemer, MD
Director, HealthTracks Center
St. John's Health System
Springfield, Missouri

Richard H. Gross, MD
Professor, Departments of Orthopaedic Surgery
    and Pediatrics
Medical University of South Carolina
Charleston, South Carolina

Curtis R. Gruel, MD
Associate Professor
Department of Orthopaedic Surgery
    and Rehabilitation
University of Oklahoma Health Sciences Center
Oklahoma City, Oklahoma

Sally S. Harris, MD, MPH
Sports Medicine and Pediatrics
Palo Alto Medical Clinic
Palo Alto, California

Helge Hebestreit, MD
Pediatric Hospital
University of Würzburg
Würzburg, Germany

William A. Herndon, MD
Oklahoma Sports Science and Orthopaedics
Oklahoma City, Oklahoma

John B. Jeffers, DVM, MD
Director of Emergency Department
Director of Resident Education
Department of Ophthalmology
Wills Eye Hospital
Philadelphia, Pennsylvania

Geoffrey Stephen Kuhlman, MD
Sports Medicine Fellow
Department of Family Medicine
University of Oklahoma Health Sciences Center
Oklahoma City, Oklahoma

Gregory L. Landry, MD
Professor of Pediatrics
Head Medical Team Physician
University of Wisconsin-Madison
University of Wisconsin Medical School
Madison, Wisconsin

Mervyn Letts, MD, FRCSC
Head, Division of Pediatric Orthopaedics
University of Ottawa
Children's Hospital Eastern Ontario
Ottawa, Ontario, Canada

Barbara J. Long, MD, MPH
Assistant Professor of Pediatrics
University of Pittsburgh School of Medicine
Adolescent Medicine
Children's Hospital of Pittsburgh
Pittsburgh, Pennsylvania

P. Cameron Mantor, MD
Associate Professor of Surgery, Pediatric Surgery
University of Oklahoma Health Sciences Center
Oklahoma City, Oklahoma

Donald W. McGinnis, MD
Assistant Professor
Director, Division of Sports Medicine
Department of Orthopedic Surgery and Rehabilitation
University of Oklahoma Health Sciences Center
Oklahoma City, Oklahoma

Larry G. McLain, MD
Director, Inpatient Pediatrics
Department of Pediatrics
University of Illinois College of Medicine
Chicago, Illinois

Russel Medbery
Doctoral Student
Central Michigan University
Mount Pleasant, Michigan

David M. Orenstein, MD
Professor of Pediatrics
University of Pittsburgh School of Medicine
Pittsburgh, Pennsylvania

Charles B. Pasque, MD
Assistant Professor
Sports Medicine Division
Department of Orthopaedic Surgery
    and Rehabilitation
University of Oklahoma Health Sciences Center
Oklahoma City, Oklahoma

Peter D. Pizzutillo, MD
Director, Department of Orthopaedic Surgery
McP Hahneman School of Medicine
St. Christopher's Hospital for Children
Philadelphia, Pennsylvania

Frederick E. Reed, Jr, MD
Clinical Associate Professor
MUSC Department of Orthopaedics
Medical University of South Carolina
Charleston, South Carolina

Stephen G. Rice, MD, PhD, MPH
Program Director, Primary Care Sports
    Medicine Fellowship
Co-Director, Jersey Shore Sports Medicine Center
Department of Pediatrics
Jersey Shore Medical Center
Neptune, New Jersey

William L. Risser, MD, PhD
Professor of Pediatrics
Department of Pediatrics
University of Texas-Houston Medical School
Houston, Texas

Thomas W. Rowland, MD
Director of Pediatric Cardiology
Baystate Medical Center
Springfield, Massachusetts

John F. Sarwark, MD
Interim Division Head
Pediatric Orthopaedic Surgery
Children's Memorial Hospital
Chicago, Illinois

Brock E. Schnebel, MD
Associate Clinical Professor and Head Physician
University of Oklahoma Department of Athletics
Department of Orthopaedic Surgery
    and Rehabilitation
University of Oklahoma Health Sciences Center
Oklahoma City, Oklahoma

George Sortiropoulous, MD
Student Health Center
University of Missouri
Columbia, Missouri

Eric Small, MD
Pediatric Sports Medicine, Clinical Instructor
    in Pediatrics
Department of Pediatrics
Mount Sinai Medical Center
New York, New York

Bryan W. Smith, MD, PhD
Clinical Assistant Professor of Pediatrics
    and Orthopaedics
Head Athletic Team Physician
James A. Taylor Student Health Service
University of North Carolina
Chapel Hill, North Carolina

Carl L. Stanitski, MD
Professor, Department of Orthopaedics
Medical University of South Carolina
Charleston, North Carolina

Suzanne Nelson Steen, DSc, RD
Sports Nutritionist
Department of Intercollegiate Athletics
The University of Washington
Seattle, Washington

Paul R. Stricker, MD
Assistant Professor, Department of Orthopaedics
Assistant Professor, Department of Pediatrics
Team Physician, Vanderbilt Athletics
Vanderbilt Sports Medicine Center
Vanderbilt University Medical Center
Nashville, Tennessee

J. Andy Sullivan, MD
Don H. O'Donoghue Professor and Endowed Chair
Department of Orthopedic Surgery
University of Oklahoma College of Medicine
Oklahoma City, Oklahoma

Steven M. Sullivan, DDS
Professor and Chairman
Department of Oral and Maxillofacial Surgery
University of Oklahoma
Oklahoma City, Oklahoma

Weyton Tam, MD
Clinical Assistant Professor
Department of Radiology
Oklahoma University Health Science Center
Oklahoma City, Oklahoma

David Tuggle, MD
Professor and Chief
Section of Pediatric Surgery
Children's Hospital of Oklahoma
University of Oklahoma College of Medicine
Oklahoma City, Oklahoma

Reginald Washington, MD
Chairman, Department of Pediatrics
Infant and Children's Hospital
Presbyterian/St. Luke's Medical Center
Denver, Colorado

David A. Yngve, MD
Associate Professor
Department of Orthopaedics and Rehabilitation
Universtiy of Texas Medical Branch
Galveston, Texas

Letha Yurko-Griffin, MD, PhD
Team Physician
Georgia State University
Peachtree Orthopaedic Clinic
Atlanta, Georgia

Reviewers

Erik Adams, MD, PhD
Sports Medicine Program
The Monroe Clinic
Monroe, Wisconsin

Mark A. Anderson PhD, PT, ATC
Associate Professor and Director of Graduate Studies
Department of Rehabilitation Sciences
University of Oklahoma Health Sciences Center
Oklahoma City, Oklahoma

James Richard Barrett, MD
Associate Professor of Family Medicine
Director, Primary Care Sports Medicine
   Fellowship Program
Department of Family Medicine
University of Oklahoma
Oklahoma City, Oklahoma

Tom Coniglione, MD
Clinical Professor of Medicine
Oklahoma University College of Medicine
Oklahoma City, Oklahoma

E. Randy Eichner, MD
Professor of Medicine
Team Internist, University of Oklahoma
   Varsity Athletics
University of Oklahoma Health Sciences Center
Oklahoma City, Oklahoma

Michael K. Eshleman, MD
Director, Primary Care Sports Medicine Fellowship
Department of Family Medicine
University of Washington
Seattle, Washington

Karl B. Fields, MD
Professor of Family Medicine
Residency and Sports Medicine Director
The Moses H. Cone Hospital Family Practice
   Residency Program
Greensboro, North Carolina

William A. Grana, MD, MPH
Chairman
Department of Orthopedics
University of Arizona
Tucson, Arizona

Robert E. Hannemann, MD
Past President
American Academy of Pediatrics
Visiting Professor
Child Psychology and Biomedical Engineering
Purdue University
Lafayette, Indiana

Walter W. Huurman, MD
Director of Pediatric Orthopaedics
Professor, Orthopaedics and Pediatrics
Departments of Orthopaedic Surgery and Pediatrics
University of Nebraska
Omaha, Nebraska

Thomas M. Jinguji, MD
University of Washington Physicians Network
Kent, Washington

Mimi D. Johnson, MD
Clinical Associate Professor
Department of Pediatrics
University of Washington
Seattle, Washington

Daniel E. Kraft, MD
Methodist Sports Medicine
Indianapolis, Indiana

Carl F. Krein, MA, AT, PT
Professor Emeritus
Department of Physical Education and Health Fitness
Central Connecticut State University
New Britain, Connecticut

Claire M.A. LeBlanc, MD, FRCP(C)
Assistant Professor
University of Ottawa
Department of Rheumatology
Children's Hospital of Eastern Ontario
Ottawa, Ontario Canada

Thomas J. Martin, MD
Team Physician
Associate Professor
Orthopaedics
Pennsylvania State University
State College, Pennsylvania

William A. Primos, MD
Director, Primary Care Sports Medicine
Metrolina Orthopaedics and Sports Medicine
Charlotte, North Carolina

Kathy Reilly, MD, MPH
Assistant Professor, Vice Chair
Division of Family Medicine
University of Oklahoma Health Sciences Center
Oklahoma City, Oklahoma

Paul R. Stricker, MD
Assistant Professor, Departments of
Pediatrics and Orthopaedics
Team Physician, Vanderbilt University
Vanderbilt Sports Medicine Center
Vanderbilt University Medical Center
Nashville, Tennessee

Edward P. Tyson, MD
Assistant Professor of Pediatrics
Director, Adolescent Clinics
Children's Hospital of Oklahoma
Oklahoma City, Oklahoma

Andrew P. Winterstein, PhD, ATC
Assistant Faculty Associate/Staff Athletic Trainer
Department of Kinesiology/Division of
Intercollegiate Athletics
University of Wisconsin—Madison
Madison, Wisconsin

Table of Contents

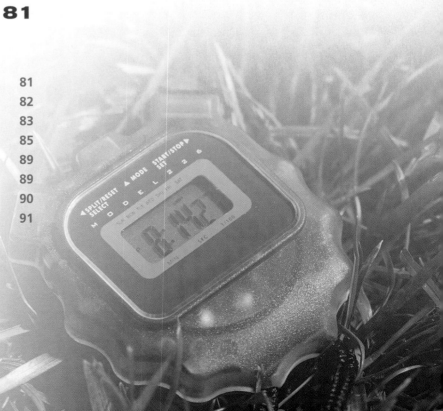

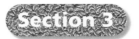

Every child and adolescent should have an opportunity to participate in sports and regular physical activity. Participation can be associated with both health benefits and health risks. To ensure safe participation, physicians caring for children and adolescents must be able to provide advice on appropriate activity and be prepared to care for an injury or illness that jeopardizes health or continued participation. With healthy activity as a goal for everyone, restricting participation within reason as a means to limit risk is no more acceptable than promoting participation without regard to safety.

Care of the Young Athlete has been written as a practical guide to help physicians optimize the benefit-to-risk ratio of sports and physical activity for their patients. The topics have been selected and organized to reflect the health and safety issues most likely to be addressed and managed by primary care practitioners. Section 1 addresses the risks and benefits of physical activity and sports. Readiness is addressed from a developmental and health perspective. Section 2 discusses the effects of training, along with nutritional requirements, performance-enhancing substances, and psychological issues. Section 3 focuses on concerns specific to female athletes, physically challenged athletes, as well as sideline care, injury prevention, and general issues about the ability to play following injury or illness.

The final two sections focus on medical and musculoskeletal problems commonly seen in young athletes. Each chapter begins with a review of anatomy and physiology, followed by the essentials: clinical evaluation, treatment, and return to play. The information provided in both sections is intended to expand the range of conditions that can be comfortably and competently managed without specialty referral. When appropriate, recommendations for specialty referral are given. Finally, an appendix provides frequently used forms and policy statements from the American Academy of Pediatrics and the American Academy of Orthopaedic Surgeons.

We would like to thank the members of the Editorial Board, Greg Landry, MD; Oded Bar-Or, MD; Richard Herndon, MD; and Don McGinnis, MD, for all the hours of work and the time spent away from home necessary to bring this project to fruition. We also thank all of the authors for generously donating their time, expertise, and lunch hours on behalf of this collaborative effort. The reviewers were key to this project, as their careful scrutiny of this work made the finished product more clear and relevant. Thanks and recognition must also be extended to Lynne Roby Shindoll of the AAOS and Allison Rand of the AAP for their spirited efforts to keep this project on track and on time. Finally, we would like to thank you, the reader, for your interest in providing the best possible care of the young athlete.

Steven J. Anderson, MD
American Academy of Pediatrics

J. Andy Sullivan, MD
American Academy of Orthopaedic Surgeons

1

General Health and Fitness

Section Editor
Gregory L. Landry, MD

Chapter 1

Benefits of Sports Participation

GREGORY L. LANDRY, MD

Like most books on sports medicine, this text is written to assist physicians in managing a variety of problems associated with sports participation. The discussion includes a wide range of medical problems, psychological problems, and various types of injuries. In the United States, large sums of money and time are spent managing injuries in children sustained during sports participation. An analysis of the cost of injuries in the United States revealed that over 800 million dollars were spent on childhood sports injuries in 1987, second only to the 1.2 billion spent on falls. Sometimes, young athletes are encouraged to remain in sports activities even after they have been injured. Despite the risk of injury, record numbers of youngsters are participating in sports. So why are sports so popular? What is it about sports that is so important to our society, and why should we as physicians encourage our young patients to participate in sports?

The benefits of sports participation are discussed in this chapter in an attempt to answer these questions. Physicians and others would not spend so much time caring for athletes if there were not something desirable about participation in sports. This chapter emphasizes the psychosocial benefits of participation in sports, because the physical benefits are discussed in other chapters.

Definitions

Many of the benefits of participation in sports occur because most sports include physical activity. Physical activity is defined as any body movement produced by skeletal muscle that results in energy expenditure. Physical fitness is a set of attributes that are related to health, skills, or both. Sports participation usually involves physical activity but may not improve physical fitness. Children are said to "play" sports, which implies that there is physical activity or action by way of amusement or recreation.

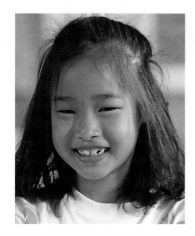

When children play, their behavior is free, spontaneous, and expressive. Sports are often thought of as highly competitive and organized. For the purpose of the following discussion, the broadest definition of sport is intended without implying that the benefits of participation must occur in a competitive activity.

Psychosocial Benefits

The most important benefits of sports participation for children are psychosocial. From early in infancy, humans engage in play activities, which have an important function during development in that it helps children learn about objects and events. Between the ages of 2 and 7 years, children spend most of their waking hours in play. They experiment with various kinds of social interactions through cooperation, sharing, or competition. They also engage in a lot of make-believe play, testing skills that they are unable to do in the real world, such as driving a car or cooking.

By age 6 years, most children understand rules and if a particular activity has no rules, they will create them. Children also tend to exert pressure on their peers to follow the rules. This process teaches children that social systems depend on rules and that society depends on individuals following the rules. A child's interest in rules is very compatible with the introduction of sports where rules are an important part of the game.

When children begin elementary school, the number of significant people in their lives expands to include school-mates and teachers. This is an important time for children as they begin to discover and judge their own abilities and to form a stable self-concept and feelings of self-worth. Many children enter organized sports programs at this time.

Self-concept and Self-esteem

Self-concept and self-esteem develop based on how children interpret others' responses to them and on how children compare their skills and characteristics with those of others. Comparison and competition in a variety of activities begin around age 5 years and increase throughout the time the child is in elementary school, which is a great time to test motor skills in sports activities. Children should begin sports at a relatively young age so that they will learn to understand that their physical, cognitive, musical, and artistic talents differ compared with those of their peers. Although physically talented youngsters may acquire new skills faster than those who are less physically talented, virtually all children can acquire motor skills and have fun by participating in sports activities. Because no single sport tests all motor skills, a variety of sports activities should be offered to young children. Successful acquisition of these skills helps children to feel competent and proud that they have mastered a skill. Children who

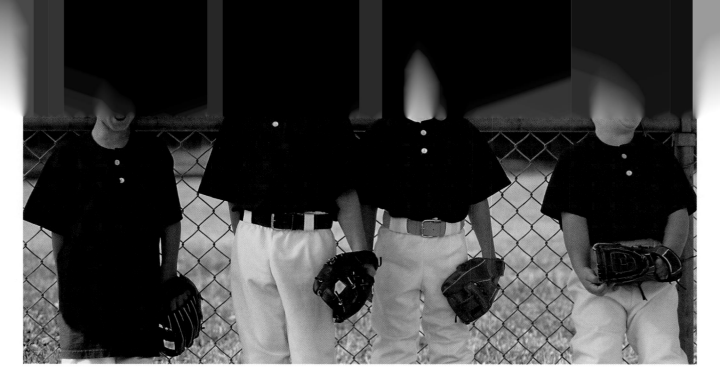

perceive themselves to be competent, in control, and successful will want to play that same game or sports activity the very next day. Known as competence motivation, this process demonstrates that a child is motivated to achieve competence at performing a task.

Motivational Factors and Competence

Factors that motivate children to play sports provide some insight into the benefits of sports participation. These factors are traditionally termed intrinsic and extrinsic factors. Competence motivation, the process described above, is a powerful intrinsic factor. As a child acquires new skills, the approval of important adults such as parents and coaches is an important extrinsic factor. Children rely on the comments of important adults to help them judge their competency. Peer approval is another extrinsic factor that acquires increasing importance as the child becomes an adolescent. Ribbons and trophies are also extrinsic motivators, but they are not as powerful or sustained as other factors.

Children are attracted to activities that they consider to be fun. Research from both the United States and Canada confirm that children participate in sports principally to have fun. Boys and girls report that they want to improve their skills, obtain physical fitness, spend time with existing friends and sometimes make new friends (**Table 1.1**). As children get older, they report that they like to test their abilities against others and participate for the excitement of the game. Adolescents enjoy being competitive, winning, and achieving goals. Girls tend to be more goal oriented, particularly with personal goals, while boys tend to be motivated to win. When asked about why they try to play well, children between ages 9 and 14 all reported that the most important

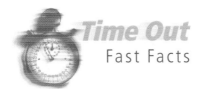

Table 1.1	Reasons Children Want to Play Sports
• To have fun	• To make new friends
• To improve their skills	• To succeed or win
• To learn new skills	• To become physically fit
• To be with their friends	

Table 1.2 *Reasons for Trying to Perform Well in Sports*

	Order of importance	
Reason for trying to play well	9–11 years old	12–14 years old
1. Feeling good about how you played	1	1
2. Making sure you won't blame yourself for losing	2	2
3. Being praised by your parents for playing well	6	4
4. Making sure your parents won't be displeased with your play	3	8
5. Making your coach proud of you	4	3
6. Making sure your coach won't be displeased with you	5	6
7. Making the other kids like you more	8	7
8. Making sure the other kids don't get upset with you	7	5

Reproduced with permission from National Association for Sport and Physical Education (NASPE): *Parents' Complete Guide to Youth Sports.* Reston, VA, National Association for Sport and Physical Education, 1989, p 39.

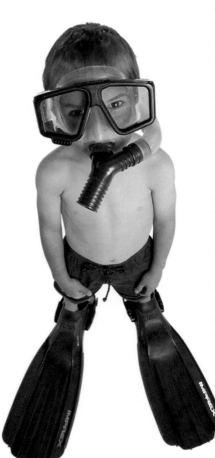

reason was "feeling good about how you played" (**Table 1.2**). Of note is that extrinsic rewards appear at the bottom of the list.

Not all children benefit from continued participation in certain sports. Some children discover that some motor skills are more difficult for them to master when compared with their peers. Self-selection begins to occur among school-age children as they participate in a variety of sports. Children who find a particular sports activity difficult will rarely feel competent when participating. Therefore, they will be more attracted to another activity. For example, a child who is physically less capable at sports that require cardiopulmonary endurance is not likely to enjoy distance running or swimming because these sports seem so much easier for his or her peers. It is hoped that this child will feel competent in a sport that requires a different physical skill.

Participation in sports does not offer the same psychosocial benefits for all children. Sports participation tends to attract the most physically talented children because they tend to benefit the most from these activities. Because they acquire motor skills more easily than other children, participation improves their sense of self-esteem and self-worth. For them, participation in sports activities builds self-confidence.

Sports participation does not necessarily prepare children for everyday life, but it does provide an activity that is separate from the rest of their lives that allows them to experiment with their own physical skills. Sports participation also allows children to experience success and failure in an activity that is unrelated to school and family. Sports activities are safer because the consequences of their successes and failures are much less significant than real-life endeavors. For example, failing to learn the rules of a sport is lower risk than failing to learn the rules of the road for a young bicyclist, where the results may be catastrophic.

The Importance of Adult Involvement

Children benefit from the presence of adults in sports activities, particularly when the involved adults focus on teaching skills and exhibiting a positive "sportsman-like" attitude. Adults typically organize games and ensure that the rules are followed. They may also teach children how to choose teams and how to keep score. With the help of adults, children feel a sense of accomplishment when they have learned something new, and they may learn more skills and fundamentals of the sport with adult involvement.

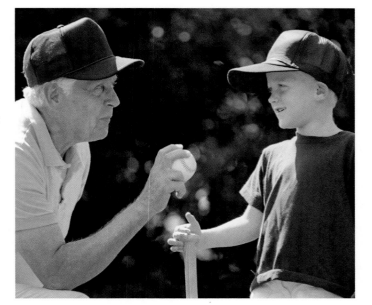

When given an opportunity for free play without adult supervision, children learn different skills, such as negotiating and cooperating with their peers. They learn to be creative in choosing teams, and they often modify the rules to make the game more fun. One of the most common modifications is the well-known "do-overs" in which rulings are disputed. Children want the score of games to be close, so if it becomes dramatically one-sided, they may stop and chose teams again or trade players to make the score closer. They may increase the size of the team when other children arrive to allow everyone a chance to play. Children may also actually help one another learn new skills and may modify the rules to give children with less talent a chance to learn. For example, a younger child might get an extra strike in baseball to give him or her a better chance at hitting the ball. Clearly, children can benefit from participating in sports activities without adult involvement.

Competition

Older children value competition more than their younger counterparts, but children of all ages tend to enjoy team sports. Team sports offer an opportunity for camaraderie, a chance to be with friends outside of school, and a chance to work with peers toward a common goal (winning the game.) Children may participate to compete or learn about competition during sports participation. Children younger than age 10 years rarely appreciate competition in the same way as adolescents and adults. They enjoy participating in sports for fun and to show off their new skills. Competition would be more desirable for younger children if it was controlled better and designed for children instead of the involved adults.

An outstanding example of controlled competition that includes younger children is the Special Olympics program. In this program, the emphasis is on individual effort, the ability to finish a competition, and the view that everyone who participates is a winner. All participants receive a medal or a ribbon. In this environment, competition results in joy and compassion because individual development and achievement are emphasized. Individuals tend to be judged on their own improvement instead of what type of ribbon they won. Participants in the Special Olympics have fun and almost always seem proud of what they can do during the competition. The environment fostered by the Special Olympics should be modeled by adults who manage sports programs for able-bodied and able-minded children. When managed properly, controlled competition would increase the psychosocial benefit of many youth sports.

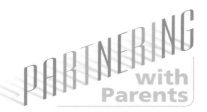

Is it safe for my child to play sports without adult supervision?

In most cases, children will learn as much without adults as with adult involvement. Children learn important skills that would not be learned with adult supervision.

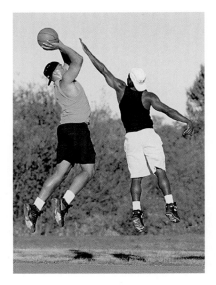

Other Benefits

Sports participation offers many other benefits for children as they enter adolescence and high school. Habitual physical activity, such as adolescents' experience in most organized sports, is positively correlated with academic performance. Studies have also shown that school dropout rates, teen pregnancy rates, and involvement in risk behaviors such as smoking and substance use are decreased in adolescents who participate in sports. Organized basketball programs have reduced unlawful behavior by inner-city boys. With these known benefits, it may be even more important to keep children involved in sports during adolescence.

In most communities, participation in sports is highly valued and elevates a child's social status. Playing on a team may mean wearing clothing with a team logo and having the opportunity to travel to new places. A young athlete who plays well in high school may receive financial aid for his or her college education.

Physical Benefits

Sports participation helps in the development of a child's motor skills. Studies have suggested that certain motor skills will not develop well unless they are performed during the appropriate time in childhood. For example, a child may have trouble hitting a ball with a bat if he or she is not encouraged to do so early in the school-age years. If eye-hand coordination is not developed at the proper time, the child may struggle to master this skill as an adolescent. Critical periods for learning particular skills are part of normal brain development; the younger the child, the more plastic the brain is at acquiring new skills. Note, however, that the importance of a critical learning period in neurologic development does not apply to all motor skills, but probably only to the most complex motor skills.

Certain skills should not be taught before a child is developmentally ready. Therefore, parents must be cautioned that children who are pushed to do "too much too soon" may become frustrated, which may lower their self-esteem. For example, tracking and picking up the velocity of a ball are rarely developed before the age of 8 years, so T-ball is a good way for a 6-year-old child to learn to hit a ball with a bat. Asking a 5-year-old child to hit a thrown ball will not accelerate his or her development and does not offer any long-term advantage to the young athlete.

Physical Growth and Maturation

Many studies have shown that physical activity is important in promoting growth and development of children. Although it is difficult to separate the genetic determinants of growth and maturation, most researchers would agree that, in the presence of good nutrition, exercise is good for growing children. Children who are physically active probably do not alter genetically programmed growth and maturation processes, but the activity helps them develop their full genetic potential. Sports participation that includes physical activity improves the body composition of the young athletes. Studies of school-age children have shown that participants in organized sports had greater total daily energy expenditure than those who did not participate.

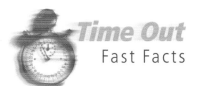

Time Out
Fast Facts

Children who are pushed to do too much too soon can become frustrated, which ultimately lowers self-esteem.

The most active children have less fat and lower body weight than their less active counterparts. This is the most important physical characteristic that can be altered by exercise in children.

Training and Fitness

Despite the great interest in determining whether aerobic and/or anaerobic power is increased in children through training and sports participation, there seems to be too little training effect to give a child any sense of mastery. Adolescents, however, can achieve significant improvement, which may help motivate them to continue training. Chapter 7 provides detailed information on the effects of training on a child's body.

Despite the long-standing belief that strength training was not beneficial to young athletes and was too risky, studies have shown a benefit. Although few young children will enroll in a strength program for the sheer joy of lifting, if the program focuses on sport-specific tasks, they may experience improved sports performance as a result. This benefit is most relevant to children participating in any sport that involves power.

Health-Related Benefits

Children of all ages should be taught that physical activity is an important part of everyday life. Cardiovascular fitness is key in preventing coronary artery disease, hypertension, obesity, and non-insulin-dependent diabetes mellitus. Less intense physical activity has even been shown to benefit health. In fact, the greatest reduction in relative risk of all-cause mortality in adults occurs between the lowest level of fitness and the next lowest level. The effects of exercise on cardiovascular risk factors in children has not been studied extensively, but experts agree that regular exercise habits begin in childhood, establishing patterns that may persist through life. More recent studies on all-cause mortality in adults strongly indicate that any physical activity is better than none at all; therefore, any type of sports participation is better than none at all. Fortunately, children and adolescents will be likely to continue participating in sports activities that they enjoy and may reap the health benefits later in life.

Most children prefer to perform physical activities with other people, preferably with others their same age. Most sports activities are good for children because sports motivate them to be physically active. Habitual exercise begins in childhood, and children who participate in sports activities are more likely to be active as adults.

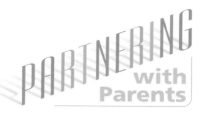

Why should my child participate in sports?

Participation in sports helps children enjoy physical activity and often leads to increased physical fitness. Participating in physical activity is important for a child's health.

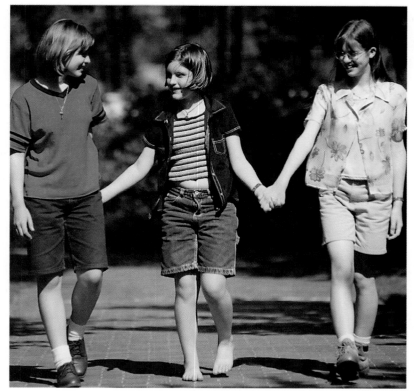

FINISH LINE

Many of the benefits of sports participation in children and adolescents are psychosocial, increasing self-confidence and self-esteem in children as they master new skills and improve their bodies with increased aerobic capacity and strength. Children participate because they perceive the activity as fun and will continue if they have more positive than negative experiences. If young athletes continue to participate in sports, they may develop regular exercise habits that will prevent the adult diseases associated with inactivity.

For More Information

1. Blair SN, Kohl HW III, Paffenbarger RS Jr, Clark DG, Cooper KH, Gibbons LW: Physical fitness and all-cause mortality: A prospective study of healthy men and women. *JAMA* 1989;262:2395–2401.

2. Coakley JJ (ed): *Sport in Society: Issues and Controversies,* ed 4. St. Louis, MO, Times Mirror/Mosby College Pub, 1990.

3. Smith RE, Smoll FL, Smith NJ (eds): *Parents' Complete Guide to Youth Sports.* Costa Mesa, CA, HDL Publishing Co, 1989.

4. U.S. Department of Health and Human Services: *Physical Activity and Health: A Report of the Surgeon General.* Atlanta, GA, U.S. Department of Health and Human Services, 1996.

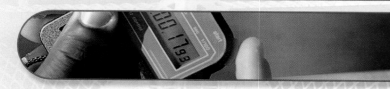

Chapter 2

Risks of Injury During Sports Participation

STEPHEN G. RICE, MD, PhD, MPH

Virtually all physical activities and sports carry some risk of injury or even catastrophic outcome. If prevention of all injuries were the goal, the only appropriate solution would be to eliminate sports and recreational activities. Injuries are an inevitable outcome of challenging competition; striving to push the body to its limit entails the risk of exceeding that limit. Loss of control or facing forces greater than the body or a specific body part can withstand often results in traumatic injury. Similarly, excessive training may result in an overuse injury rather than the desired conditioning or performance outcome.

Today, increasing numbers of athletes are engaging in intense training for a single sport at very young ages on a year-round basis or participating in multiple sports during a single season. Both of these behaviors increase the risk of overuse injuries. Summer sports camps have grown in popularity recently, but pose the risk of both acute and overuse injuries if the athlete has not undertaken appropriate sport-specific physical conditioning in the weeks prior to attending camp.

Physicians seek to provide guidance to parents who ask, "Is this activity safe for my child?" or "Is this activity appropriate for my child?" Data from epidemiologic studies can identify the risk of injury in various sports activities. If a parent believes that the benefits clearly outweigh the risks, the activity is worthwhile; if the risks exceed the benefits, it may be concluded that the activity is too dangerous to justify participation. This analysis varies among families, depending on their values and relative comfort with risk in sports activities.

Initial key steps toward the prevention and management of injuries include the recognition and acceptance by athletes, coaches, and parents that some risk is always present during physical activity. Managing or controlling risk associated with sports activity requires identifying and quantifying such risks and then using methods and techniques to minimize them. Risk is assessed,

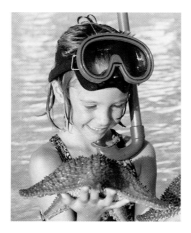

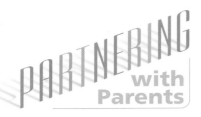

Is there a significant risk of injury to very young children from sports participation?

Although participation in any sport entails some risk, children younger than 10 years of age are more at risk of injury from recreational activities than from organized team sports.

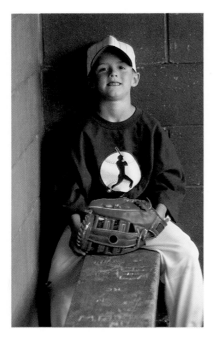

predicted, or measured through careful injury surveillance studies that note the frequency of injury in a given sport, as well as factors leading to or associated with such injury.

When similar definitions and methodologies are used, meaningful comparisons of risk within sports and among sports becomes feasible. Through analysis of the injury data, trends or patterns of related variables may emerge that lead to the development of specific strategies and interventions designed to reduce the frequency of future injuries. In this chapter, the relative frequency of injuries in various sport activities is presented, as are data regarding catastrophic injuries.

Definitions

An athletic injury is a medical condition, resulting from athletic activity, that causes a limitation or restriction on participation in that activity or for which medical treatment was received. The two most common procedures for developing a definition of injury in the context of sports activity are either an accurate, specific diagnosis and/or time lost from participation. Days of time lost are counted until the athlete returns to full, unrestricted participation.

To establish injury rates, information regarding the total number of participants or the total number of athletic exposures is also required. An athletic exposure, a unit of risk, is defined as one athlete participating in one practice or contest in which he or she is exposed to the possibility of an athletic injury (an opportunity to become injured through participation).

Data about the number of injuries give numerator information; data about the population at risk give denominator information. Injury rate data are usually expressed in terms of injuries per unit of participation or risk, such as injuries per 100 athletes per season or injuries per 1,000 athletic exposures. The quality of the denominator often determines the accuracy and power of the data, making injury rate per 1,000 athletic exposures a more accurate method of reporting than injuries per 100 athletes per season.

Results of Injury Surveillance Studies

Reliable data about the risks of participation are generally lacking in recreational youth sports, including organized, competitive, and team sports. The consensus among studies that do exist indicates that injury rates are low in all organized sports at the youth level because prepubertal athletes do not often generate sufficient force during collisions or falls to cause tissue damage. Injury rates rise dramatically when participants reach puberty because athletes get bigger, stronger, faster, and more aggressive with age. Because the kinetic energy of a collision is related to both mass and velocity, the adolescent generates and receives considerably more force than the prepubertal child.

Among children younger than age 10 years, fractures and catastrophic injuries occur more frequently from individual recreational activities than from organized sports. Such injuries often occur from falls or collisions while riding bicycles or horses, using skateboards or in-line skates, while on trampolines or sleds, climbing trees and fences, and general "rough-housing." A substantial percentage of these injuries occur while the child is learning the activity (during the first week), before full acquisition of the skills has been achieved.

Among organized high school sports, several large ongoing injury surveillance and epidemiologic studies have been undertaken and reveal consistent patterns of data. The National Athletic Trainers Association (NATA) gathers injury data and disseminates its findings each year on 10 sports from over 200 high schools nationwide that employ certified athletic trainers. The Athletic Health Care System (AHCS) has studied injuries in 18 sports among 20 high schools in the Seattle area since 1979, using specifically trained coaches and their student athletic trainers as reporters. The AHCS database has over 60,000 athletes who have participated in over 2.5 million days of athletic activity.

Results of NATA and AHCS Studies

Both NATA and AHCS studies reveal, for example, that 35% of football players sustain at least one time-loss injury per season, the highest among the sports surveyed. About 70% to 80% of reportable injuries in all sports are minor, causing the athlete to miss fewer than 5 to 7 days of participation. From 4% to 8% of injuries entail a time loss of greater than 3 weeks. More than 60% of injuries in all high school sports (including football) occur in practice, reflecting the greater number of practices compared to games and the participation of all athletes throughout practice compared to a small number on the field at the same time during games. On a minute-by-minute basis, however, game action produces more football injuries than practice.

Wrestling, football, and gymnastics are high on the list of injury frequency and severity in every injury study. Girls' cross-country has the highest reported rate of injury among all high school sports (injuries/1,000 athletic exposures), with boys' cross-country in fifth place (**Table 2.1**). Girls' soccer (fourth place) and boys' soccer (seventh place) were also in this top tier.

The NATA high school injury data reveal that girls in soccer and softball have statistically significantly higher injury rates than boys in soccer and baseball, while rates in basketball are equal. Although overall surgeries and knee sprains are higher for girls than boys in basketball, soccer,

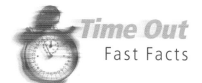

Time Out
Fast Facts

More than 60% of injuries in all high school sports occur in practice.

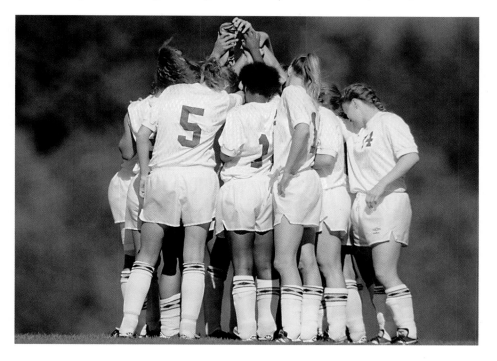

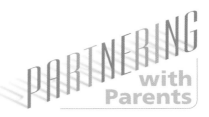

What can be done to ensure that children are safe when participating in organized sports?

Ensure that children are well coached and supervised, that the playing surface is safe, and that protective equipment is well fitted and in good condition.

and softball/baseball, these differences have not attained statistical significance. Anterior cruciate ligament injuries in soccer, for both boys and girls, occur significantly more frequently than in basketball.

Different sports stress different body parts, resulting in a variable distribution of injuries among different sports. For example, the NATA data show that 75% of injuries in girls' soccer occur to the lower extremity compared with 60% to 65% for girls' basketball, volleyball, and field hockey. The AHCS data show that in cross-country running 94% of injuries involved the lower extremities, compared with 80% to 85% for soccer and 70% to 74% for basketball. Swimmers, tennis players, and baseball pitchers tend to have higher percentages of upper extremity injuries, whereas gymnasts tend to have an equal distribution between upper and lower extremity injuries. Most injuries in cross-country running are caused by overuse, while most injuries in wrestling are caused by acute trauma.

The most commonly injured body parts vary with age and sports activity. The youngest athletes often sustain upper extremity injuries from falling on an outstretched arm, especially fractures to the wrist, forearm, and clavicle.

Table 2.1 *All Sports Injury Data Analysis: Fall 1979 through Spring 1992*

*Rank	Sport	Season	Total Athletes	Injury Rate/100 Athletes/Season
1	Girls' cross-country	Fall	1,299	61.4
2	Football	Fall	8,560	58.8
3	Wrestling	Winter	3,624	49.7
4	Girls' soccer	Fall	3,186	43.7
5	Boys' cross-country	Fall	2,481	38.7
6	Girls' gymnastics	Winter	1,082	38.9
7	Boys' soccer	Spring	3,848	36.4
8	Girls' basketball	Winter	3,634	34.5
9	Girls' track	Spring	3,543	24.8
10	Boys' basketball	Winter	3,874	29.2
11	Volleyball	Fall	3,444	19.9
12	Softball	Spring	2,957	18.3
13	Boys' track	Spring	4,425	17.3
14	Baseball	Spring	3,397	17.1
15	Fast pitch	Spring	134	11.9
16	Coed swimming	Winter	4,004	8.3
17	Coed tennis	Fall/Spring	4,096	7.0
18	Coed golf	Fall/Spring	2,170	1.4
	Combined totals		**59,758**	**30.6**

*Ranking based on Injury Rate/1,000 Athletic Exposures
© *Stephen G. Rice, MD, 1993*

Among older children and adolescents, the lower extremity is more likely to be injured.

The AHCS data on body part distribution of 8,479 injuries among all 18 high school sports over an 8-year period indicated that 55% of injuries were to the lower leg (knee and below); 12.6% to the upper leg (thigh, groin, and hip); 13% to the back, neck, and head; and 19.4% to the upper extremity (**Table 2.2**). More specifically in the lower extremity, ankle injuries were 22.8%, knee injuries 16.7%, shin/calf 9.8%, and foot 5.7%. The length of time loss from (or severity of) knee injuries exceeds that of ankle injuries, with 13% of athletes with knee injuries missing more than 3 weeks versus 7% of athletes with ankle injuries.

Catastrophic Injury Studies

The National Center for Catastrophic Sports Injury Research at the University of North Carolina-Chapel Hill tracks and reports annually on catastrophic injuries and sports-related deaths among high school and college athletes. Catastrophic injury is defined as any severe spinal, spinal cord, or cerebral injury. Three categories of outcomes are identified: fatal; nonfatal with permanent disability;

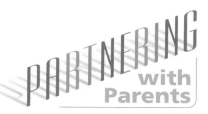

Which sport has the highest rate of injury?

High school boys have the highest rate of injury per athletic exposure in football. The highest injury rate for girls occurs in cross-country.

Injury Rate/1,000 Athletic Exposures	**Significant Injury Rate/1,000 Athletic Exposures	***Major Injury Rate/1,000 Athletic Exposures	Percent of Different Athletes Injured
17.3	3.3	0.9	33.1%
12.7	3.1	0.9	36.7%
11.8	2.6	1.0	32.1%
11.6	2.9	0.7	31.6%
10.5	2.3	0.5	24.6%
10.0	2.3	0.7	26.2%
9.5	2.1	0.4	25.2%
7.1	1.7	0.5	24.2%
6.2	1.6	0.3	18.0%
5.5	1.3	0.3	22.9%
5.4	1.1	0.3	16.1%
4.8	1.2	0.3	14.8%
4.4	1.1	0.3	13.6%
4.2	1.0	0.3	14.4%
2.4	1.2	0.6	11.9%
2.2	0.5	0.0	6.4%
1.9	0.4	0.1	5.8%
0.8	0.0	0.0	1.3%
7.6	**1.8**	**0.5**	**21.1%**

** Significant injuries are defined as five or more consecutive games and/or practices in which the athlete was not at full participation.

***Major injuries are defined as 15 or more consecutive games and/or practices in which the athlete was not at full participation.

Note: Injury implies time loss with no participation and/or limited participation. With a typical high school schedule of participating 5 days per week, this means essentially a "1-week" injury for a significant injury and a "3-week" injury for a major injury.

Table 2.2 *Injuries by Body Part. All Injuries—All Sports in Percentages*

Body Part	Number	Percentage	Game	Practice	1 day	2-4 days	5-15 days	>15 days
					Length of Injury			
Ankle	1,937	22.8	30.8	69.2	31.5	37.4	24.3	6.8
Knee	1,415	16.7	26.6	73.4	31.7	31.8	23.8	12.7
Hand, wrist, elbow	1,126	13.3	29.5	70.5	43.9	27.7	19.7	8.7
Shin, calf	829	9.8	20.3	79.7	33.5	36.3	21.1	9.0
Thigh, groin	623	7.3	15.6	84.4	32.6	43.2	22.0	2.2
Head, neck, collarbone	618	7.3	42.4	57.6	51.3	31.9	12.9	3.9
Shoulder	517	6.1	31.8	68.2	33.7	35.2	22.4	8.7
Foot	485	5.7	17.8	82.2	36.1	36.2	21.9	5.8
Back	484	5.7	25.3	74.7	32.0	38.4	20.5	9.1
Hip	234	2.8	24.2	75.8	37.6	37.2	18.8	6.4
Hamstring	211	2.5	22.4	77.6	27.5	40.3	25.1	7.1
Totals	**8,479**	**100**	**27.2**	**72.8**	**35.4**	**35.0**	**21.7**	**7.9**

© Stephen G. Rice, MD, 1993

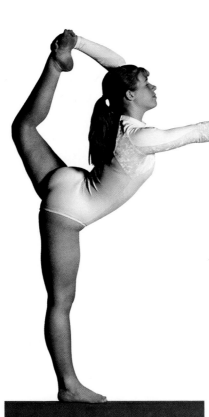

and serious with no permanent functional disability, such as a fractured cervical vertebra with complete recovery. Each year approximately 175 cases of paraplegia and 75 cases of quadriplegia are related to a sports injury.

Types of Catastrophic Injuries

Catastrophic injuries are also divided into two etiologic categories: direct and indirect. Direct injuries are those resulting directly from participation in the skills of the sport, such as tackling in football or making a save in hockey. Trauma is the cause of these injuries. Indirect injuries are caused by a systemic failure as the result of exertion while participating in a sport or activity or by a complication secondary to a nonfatal injury. These injuries are nontraumatic. Sudden cardiac death and dehydration/hyperthermia death are examples of indirect catastrophic injury.

Catastrophic injury data from the fall of 1982 through the spring of 1997 are reported in Tables 2.3 and 2.4, expressing the injury rate per 100,000 participants per year. The data are separated by gender, by cause, and by outcome. Among boys, gymnasts had the highest rates for direct traumatic fatalities and permanent injuries; ice hockey was second in both categories. Football was fourth in direct fatalities, and third in both permanent and serious injuries. Wrestling was eighth in fatalities, and fourth in both permanent and serious injuries. Among high school girls, only track-and-field experienced a single direct fatality during the 15-year time span. Gymnastics was the only girls' sport with rates comparable to boys' sports for nonfatal permanent injuries or serious injuries.

Indirect fatalities

Indirect (nontraumatic) fatalities in high school male athletes are also shown in **Table 2.3**. The sports with the highest estimated death rates per 100,000 athletes per year were lacrosse, basketball, ice hockey, soccer, football, cross-country, and wrestling, respectively. Among girls, indirect fatalities were reported in basketball, swimming, track, volleyball, cross-country, and soccer. The estimated indirect fatality rate for boys is more than five times greater than that for girls (**Table 2.4**).

The etiology of indirect sports fatalities among high school and college athletes was cardiovascular in 74%, noncardiovascular in 22%, and undetermined in the remaining 4%. Among cardiovascular deaths, hypertrophic cardiomyopathy (HCM) or probable HCM was implicated in 56%, coronary artery anomalies in 16%, myocarditis in 7%, aortic stenosis in 6%, and cardiomyopathies in 5%, with miscellaneous diagnoses making up the remaining 10%.

Among noncardiovascular conditions (22%) that caused fatalities, hyperthermia was implicated in 43%, rhabdomyolysis and sickle cell trait in 23%, status asthmaticus in 13%, and electrocution caused by lightning in 10%. One death each was the result of exercise-induced anaphylaxis, aspiration/gastrointestinal bleeding, and an Arnold-Chiari type II malformation.

Direct fatalities

Direct (traumatic) fatalities in high school football have been reduced dramatically since 1976, when spearing (or using the head as the first point of contact) was banned. The death rate decreased by more than 50%

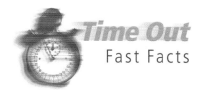

Time Out
Fast Facts

The highest rates of direct traumatic fatalities and permanent injuries among boys' and girls' sports occur in gymnastics.

Table 2.3 *High School Direct and Indirect Injuries—Fatal, Nonfatal, and Serious Injuries 1982–1983 to 1996–1997**

BOYS

Sport	Season	Direct			Indirect		
		Fatal	Nonfatal	Serious	Fatal	Nonfatal	Serious
Cross-country	Fall	0.00	0.04	0.00	0.38	0.00	0.00
Football	Fall	0.29	0.70	0.78	0.41	0.00	0.01
Soccer	Fall/Spring	0.12	0.06	0.18	0.45	0.00	0.00
Basketball	Winter	0.00	0.03	0.04	0.60	0.00	0.00
Gymnastics	Winter	1.42	1.42	1.42	0.00	0.00	0.00
Ice hockey	Winter	0.57	1.15	1.43	0.57	0.00	0.00
Swimming	Winter	0.00	0.17	0.25	0.00	0.00	0.00
Wrestling	Winter	0.06	0.56	0.31	0.37	0.00	0.00
Baseball	Spring	0.10	0.18	0.18	0.11	0.00	0.00
Lacrosse	Spring	0.34	0.00	0.00	0.69	0.00	0.00
Tennis	Fall/Spring	0.00	0.00	0.00	0.05	0.00	0.00
Track	Spring	0.21	0.14	0.14	0.21	0.00	0.00

Source: National Center for Catastrophic Sports Injury Research, Fifteenth Annual Report, 1998
* Injury rates per 100,000 participants
Direct: Injuries resulting directly from participation in the skills of the sport; caused by trauma
Indirect: Injuries caused by a systemic failure as the result of exertion while participating in a sport or activity or by a complication secondary to a nonfatal injury
Fatal: Athlete died
Nonfatal: Athlete left with permanent disability
Serious: Severe injury, but athlete recovered to be left with no permanent functional disability

Table 2.4 *High School Direct and Indirect Injuries—Fatal, Nonfatal, and Serious Injuries 1982–1983 to 1996–1997**

GIRLS

Sport	Season	Direct			Indirect		
		Fatal	Nonfatal	Serious	Fatal	Nonfatal	Serious
Cross-country	Fall	0.00	0.00	0.00	0.06	0.00	0.00
Football	Fall	0.00	0.00	0.00	0.00	0.00	0.00
Soccer	Fall	0.00	0.00	0.00	0.05	0.00	0.00
Volleyball	Fall	0.00	0.09	0.00	0.09	0.00	0.00
Basketball	Winter	0.00	0.02	0.03	0.12	0.00	0.02
Gymnastics	Winter	0.00	1.44	0.72	0.00	0.00	0.00
Ice hockey	Winter	0.00	0.00	0.00	0.00	0.00	0.00
Swimming	Winter	0.00	0.15	0.00	0.29	0.00	0.07
Wrestling	Winter	0.00	0.00	0.00	0.00	0.00	0.00
Softball	Spring	0.05	0.00	0.00	0.00	0.00	0.00
Lacrosse	Spring	0.00	0.00	0.00	0.00	0.00	0.00
Tennis	Spring	0.00	0.00	0.00	0.00	0.00	0.00
Track	Spring	0.02	0.00	0.04	0.07	0.00	0.00

Source: National Center for Catastrophic Sports Injury Research, Fifteenth Annual Report, 1998
* Injury rates per 100,000 participants
Direct: Injuries resulting directly from participation in the skills of the sport; caused by trauma
Indirect: Injuries caused by a systemic failure as the result of exertion while participating in a sport or activity or by a complication secondary to a nonfatal injury
Fatal: Athlete died
Nonfatal: Athlete left with permanent disability
Serious: Severe injury, but athlete recovered to be left with no permanent functional disability

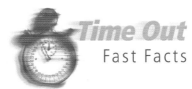

Time Out
Fast Facts

Young children usually sustain upper extremity injuries, whereas older children and adolescents incur more injuries to the lower extremities.

immediately and continued to decline steadily during the 1980s and from 1990 through 1994 (0 to 3 annually in these 5 years). Four such deaths occurred in 1995, five in 1996, and six in 1997. Among high school athletes, 90% of the direct deaths between 1960 and 1992 involved the head, neck, and brainstem. Injuries to the heart, kidney, and abdominal organs accounted for the remaining 10% of direct football deaths. The direct fatality rate per 100,000 participants in football over the 15-year time span was 0.29.

Catastrophic cervical spine injuries in football (in which there is incomplete recovery) continue to occur annually, ranging from four to 18 injuries per year in the 15-year time span. The direct permanent catastrophic injury rate per 100,000 athletes per year in football is 0.70.

Head injuries have attracted increasing attention in this past decade with the recognition of the catastrophic second-impact syndrome and the cumulative effects of multiple episodes of closed head trauma. At the professional sports level, especially in the collision sports of football and hockey, the effects of repetitive concussive events have been evident among athletes who have been forced into retirement.

The frequencies of these closed head traumatic brain injuries vary widely among various studies. When athletes are questioned directly about prior head injury, the rate is about 20 head injuries per 100 athletes per season in football. When head injuries are tabulated as one part of an injury surveillance reporting system, however, the reported rates are about half or less of that obtained through direct interviews.

Through the use of various diagnostic imaging techniques and neuropsychologic testing, the tools available to the physician to assess and manage both mild brain trauma and more severe forms of head injury continue to improve each year. Additional information about head injuries is presented in chapter 18.

Recreational Activities Studies

Injury data from organized and unorganized activities are obtained through the Consumer Product Safety Commission (CPSC) and its National Electronic Injury Surveillance System (NEISS). A selected number of emergency departments in all regions of the country and of varying population densities participate. These facilities record injuries which are then tabulated and projected to generate national totals. Significant injury is associated each year with bicycling (falling, collision with a stationary object, hit by a moving vehicle), skateboarding, in-line skating, jumping on a trampoline, snowboarding, skiing, and sledding—all activities done at high speed or with high energy transfer.

Several examples of the clinical applications of epidemiologic research to recreational injuries can be found in bicycling, skateboarding, and all-terrain vehicles (ATVs). The benefit of wearing bicycle helmets to prevent or minimize head injuries is the most obvious case. Skateboarders and in-line skaters who wear protective devices on the head, elbows, wrists, and knees substantially reduce their risk of injury. The most common skating injuries occur to the wrist and forearm; therefore, the most important piece of equipment, other than a helmet, is wrist guards.

When the CPSC detected significant numbers of serious injuries from ATV accidents through its NEISS reporting system, the CPSC and the manufacturers embarked on a series of interventions. These included modifications to the vehicles, recommending a minimum age for drivers, and educational courses or requirements for all drivers.

Clinical Applications and Examples

Athletic equipment is often used for safety and injury prevention. Batting helmets in baseball, shin guards in soccer, headgear in wrestling to protect ears, and football and hockey helmets and pads are common examples.

When injury surveillance identifies previously unrecognized injuries, questions arise as to whether new equipment or modifications of existing equipment could prevent or reduce the severity of such injuries. Only by knowing the mechanism and frequency of such injuries and the efficacy and costs of the new equipment can it be reasonably determined if such changes are indicated and appropriate.

Several examples currently under consideration include chest protectors for young baseball players to prevent commotio cordis, a fatal cardiac arrhythmia produced by blunt trauma to the chest by a batted or thrown ball. Some experts believe the ice hockey helmet should be altered to provide protection to the carotid arteries to prevent skate blade lacerations and to provide protection to the ears to prevent ruptured eardrums. Protective helmets are being considered for soccer goalies, and helmets and face shields are being considered for women's lacrosse.

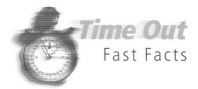

Time Out
Fast Facts

The often-fatal second impact syndrome occurs when a second, seemingly insignificant, head injury takes place before total resolution of symptoms of a previous head injury.

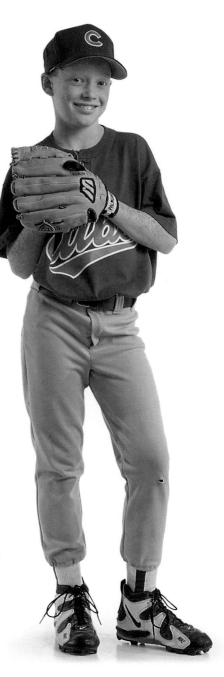

FINISH LINE

> Injury surveillance studies consistently show high injury rates in football, gymnastics, wrestling, and cross-country. Catastrophic injuries are most likely to occur in gymnastics, ice hockey, and lacrosse. Injury data may help physicians to advise parents on the risks of sports participation, but more importantly, it leads to improvements in rules and protective equipment to prevent injuries.

For More Information

1. Caine DJ, Caine CG, Lindner KJ (eds): *Epidemiology of Sports Injuries.* Champaign, IL, Human Kinetics, 1996.

2. Mueller FO, Cantu RC: National Center for Catastrophic Sports Injury Research. Fifteenth Annual Report, Fall 1982–Spring 1997. Chapel Hill, NC, 1998.

3. Mueller FO, Cantu RC, Van Camp SP (eds): *Catastrophic Injuries in High School and College Sports.* Champaign, IL, Human Kinetics, 1996, vol 8.

4. Powell JW: Epidemiological research for injury prevention programs in sports, in Mueller FO, Ryan AJ (eds): *Prevention of Athletic Injuries: The Role of the Sports Medicine Team.* Philadelphia, PA, FA Davis Company, 1991, pp 11–25.

5. Rice SG: Epidemiology and mechanisms of sports injuries, in Teitz CC (ed): *Scientific Foundations of Sports Medicine.* Toronto, Canada, BC Decker, 1989, pp 3–23.

Injury Data Resources

1. Athletic Health Care System, Department of Pediatrics, Jersey Shore Medical Center, Neptune, New Jersey.

2. National Center for Catastrophic Sports Injury Research, University of North Carolina, Chapel Hill, North Carolina.

3. National High School Sports Injury Surveillance System, National Athletic Trainers Association. Dallas, Texas.

4. NEISS Data Highlight: National Electronic Injury/Illness Surveillance System (NEISS). Bureau of Epidemiology, US Consumer Products Safety Commission. Bethesda, Maryland.

Chapter 3

Readiness to Participate in Sports

S A L L Y   S .   H A R R I S ,   M D ,   M P H

Assessing "sports readiness" is a process in which an individual child's cognitive, social, and motor development is evaluated to determine whether the child can meet the demands of the sport. An attempt to play a sport that is at a developmental level beyond the child is frustrating and the result unsuccessful. The structure of organized sports may destroy the flexibility for children to play at their own developmental level. Recognizing the developmental appropriateness of an individual child's participation in sports can enable health care providers to advocate appropriate sports activities and to appropriately advise parents, coaches, and community sports programs.

The Role of Physical and Cognitive Growth

The dramatic changes of physical growth are quite apparent during childhood, but children also develop in other less obvious ways that have important implications for appropriate sports activities. Children should not be expected to respond to coaching, interact with teammates, or understand strategies the same way as adults would.

One example of the developmental limitations of children in sports is described by the term "beehive soccer" (**Figure 3.1**). This term describes the way children between ages 6 and 8 years play soccer. The children follow the ball like a swarm of bees, not necessarily heading toward the goal. Coaches and parents can often be observed shouting directions about players' field positions and the execution of plays. These children fail to follow the adults' instructions because they lack the social and cognitive skills for competition, teamwork, rapid decision making, and appropriate positioning. Children at this age do not really understand the game; rather, they demonstrate physical skills and the ability to imitate. Individuals who coach children at this level should accept a little chaos and emphasize learning basic skills rather

Figure 3.1 Children between the ages 6 and 8 years commonly play "beehive soccer" because their social and cognitive skills have yet to fully develop.

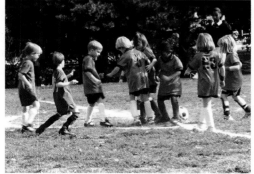

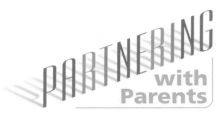

At what age have children attained the necessary motor development to participate in organized sports?

Many children acquire the motor skills necessary to participate in sports by age 6 years.

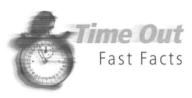

When given the opportunity, children naturally select and modify activities so that they can participate successfully and have fun.

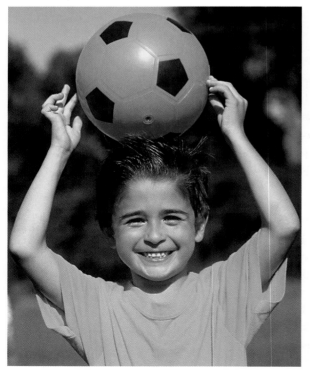

than condition children to play at a level that they are cognitively and socially not capable of understanding. Coaching that attempts to avoid "beehive soccer" may result in decreased interest and boredom, and can undermine much of the spontaneous action and personal involvement that makes the experience fun for children.

Motor Development

Because sports readiness requires that motor development match the demands of the sport, it is important to understand how children acquire motor skills. The fundamental skills include throwing, kicking, running, jumping, catching, striking, hopping, and skipping. By preschool age, children have acquired some of these skills, but it is not until early elementary school age that most children have acquired the majority of them. Therefore, age 6 years is thought to be appropriate for most children to begin organized sports activities that require performing these skills in various combinations. Prior to this age, most children do not have the necessary motor skills to perform the skills required for organized sports.

Sequence of Development

Like the developmental milestones of infancy, such as rolling over, sitting up, crawling, and walking, the fundamental motor skills required for organized sports develop in a certain sequence. At the most basic levels, acquisition of motor skills seems to be an innate process, independent of gender, disabilities, or stage of physical maturity. Like other childhood developmental milestones, the rate at which children master motor skills varies widely. It cannot be predicted by the age, size, weight, or strength of an individual child. Although it may be possible to accelerate the acquisition and refinement of fundamental motor skills by early instruction and practice, children are unlikely to respond until they are ready developmentally. Children will respond to instruction and repetitive practice only after they reach the relevant level of motor development. There is no scientific evidence to support the notion that it is possible to groom a toddler to become a future champion athlete by intensive instruction and practice at a young age. Such experiences have not been shown to accelerate motor development or lead to better sports performance later on.

While most children acquire the fundamental motor skills at a basic level naturally through play experiences, instruction and practice are necessary to fully develop fundamental motor skills to their most mature level. Each fundamental skill is composed of a series of stages of development of that skill. The sequence for developing the motor skill of kicking is shown in **Table 3.1**. A child who fails to progress through all the stages may not be as proficient in sports activities as one who has fully developed motor skills. "Throwing like a girl" is a common example of failure to progress to the fully developed stage of throwing and can limit a child's proficiency in a variety of physical activities that require a throwing or serving motion.

Table 3.1 *The Developmental Sequence of Kicking*

Stage 1

With no leg windup, the child pushes the ball with his foot from a stationary position. He usually steps back afterward to regain his balance. Most boys and girls reach this stage at about age 2.

Stage 2

The child again begins from a stationary position, but in preparing to kick, there is both leg windup to the rear as well as some opposition of the arms and legs. Balance is recovered by stepping backwards or to the side. Most boys reach this stage by age 3½; most girls reach it by age 4.

Stage 3

The child takes one or more steps to approach the ball. The kicking foot stays close to the ground until the moment of contact. After the kick, the child steps forward or to the side to regain balance. Most boys achieve this stage by age 4½, compared with age 6 for most girls.

Stage 4

The child approaches the ball with several rapid steps, leaps before the kick and usually hops on the support leg afterward. The body generally inclines backward during the windup. Most boys reach this stage by age 7, most girls by age 8.

© 1992 by the New York Times Co. Reprinted by permission.

Poor Motor Development

Few children have difficulty achieving the expected level of motor development, but those who do are often considered clumsy or uncoordinated. These children should be evaluated to determine whether their poor motor skills are simply the result of a delay in motor development or whether they have some underlying physical abnormality that may be limiting motor skill performance. In some children, poor motor skill development is caused by a learning disability regarding motor skill development, called developmental coordination disorder. Children with this disorder often have problems learning both gross and fine motor skills and are most often identified because they have difficulty with fine motor skills, such as handwriting and tying their shoes. Interventions such as appropriate selection of physical activities and physical therapy help these childen; however, evidence suggests that children with this disorder simply do not outgrow the problem.

Predicting Sports Readiness

If sports readiness cannot be predicted on the basis of age or other specific parameters, how is a child's readiness to learn certain skills or participate in certain sports activities determined? There is no scientific answer to this question from a neurodevelopmental standpoint. When given the opportunity, children naturally select and modify activities so that they can participate successfully and have fun. Simple modifications, such as the use of smaller balls, smaller fields, shorter games and practices, fewer participants playing at the same time, frequent changing of positions, and not keeping score, can be used to tailor sports activities to the developmental level of the child.

Selection of appropriate sports activities for children can be guided by an understanding of the developmental skills and limitations of specific age groups. This information is summarized in **Table 3.2** and discussed in more detail on page 22.

Early Childhood (2 to 5 years)

Attempts to master the basic skills consume most of the focus of children's sports activities. Balance is limited because the children are just starting to

The Bill of Rights of Young Athletes

- The right to participate in sports
- The right to participate at a level commensurate with each child's developmental level
- The right to have qualified adult leadership
- The right to participate in safe and healthy environments
- The right of children to share in the leadership and decision-making of their sports participation
- The right to play as a child and not as an adult
- The right to proper preparation for participation in sports
- The right for equal opportunity to strive for success
- The right to be treated with dignity
- The right to have fun in sports

Reprinted with permission from Martens R, Seefeldt V (eds): *Guidelines in Children's Sports.* Reston, VA, National Association for Sport and Physical Education (NASPE), 1979, p 15.

Table 3.2 *Developmental Skills for Sports and Sports Recommendations During Childhood*

Early Childhood (2 to 5 years)

Motor Skills
- Limited fundamental skills
- Limited balance skills

Learning
- Extremely short attention span
- Poor selective attention
- Egocentric learning—trial and error
- Visual and auditory cues are important

Vision
- Not fully mature before ages 6 to 7 (farsighted)
- Difficulty tracking and judging velocity of moving objects

Sports Recommendations
- Emphasize fundamental skills with minimal variation and limited instruction
- Emphasize fun, playfulness, exploration, and experimentation rather than competition
- *Activities:* Running, swimming, tumbling, throwing, catching

Middle Childhood (6 to 9 years)

Motor Skills
- Continued improvement in fundamental skills
- Posture and balance become more automatic
- Improved reaction times
- Beginning transitional skills

Learning
- Short attention span
- Limited development of memory and rapid decision making

Vision
- Improved tracking
- Limited directionality

Sports Recommendations
- Emphasize fundamental skills and beginning transitional skills
- Flexible rules of sports
- Allow free time in practices
- Short instruction time
- Minimal competition
- *Activities:* entry-level soccer and baseball

Late Childhood (10 to 12 years)

Motor Skills
- Improved transitional skills
- Ability to master complex motor skills
- Temporary decline in balance control at puberty

Learning
- Selective attention
- Able to use memory strategies for sports such as football and basketball

Vision
- Adult patterns

Sports Recommendations
- Emphasis on skill development
- Increasing emphasis on tactics and strategy
- Emphasize factors promoting continued participation
- *Activities:* entry level for complex skill sports (football, basketball)

Adapted with permission from Nelson MA: Developmental skills and children's sports. *Physician Sportsmed* 1991;19:67–79. McGraw-Hill, Inc.

integrate visual, vestibular, and proprioceptive cues. Children younger than ages 6 or 7 years are farsighted. Imprecise eye movements limit their ability to track and judge the speed of moving objects and should not be misinterpreted as a lack of coordination. Appropriate sports activities include running, swimming, tumbling, throwing, and catching. Instruction should be limited and follow a show-and-tell format. Competition should be avoided; it does not add anything of value to the experience and may detract.

Middle Childhood (6 to 9 years)

At this age, children are beginning to master transitional skills, which are fundamental skills performed in various combinations and with variations, such as throwing for distance or accuracy. These skills are required for participation in an organized sports activity. Vision is almost mature, but children in this age group still have difficulty determining the direction in which a moving object is traveling. Entry-level baseball and soccer are more appropriate than sports such as football that cannot as easily be adapted to a more basic level. Rules should be flexible to promote success, action, and participation. Prior to puberty, there are no significant differences between boys and girls in height, weight, strength, endurance, or motor skill development; therefore, children in this age group can participate equally on a coed basis.

Late Childhood (10 to 12 years)

Children at this age have the cognitive ability to understand and remember strategies for sports such as football and basketball. Their vision is fully mature. They are generally ready to participate in most sports activities that require more complex motor and cognitive skills. Coaches can begin to incorporate instruction on tactics and strategy. However, most experts believe that skill development, fun, and participation should take priority over competition.

Some children in this age group may be beginning their pubertal growth spurt during which there may be a temporary decline in coordination and balance. A child's resulting inability to perform a skill as effectively as in the previous sports season can be a frustrating experience if it is misinterpreted as a lack of talent or effort.

During the pubertal growth spurt, the physical differences between children, particularly boys of the same age, can be dramatic and have implications for choice of appropriate sports activities. Pubertal weight gain in both sexes is caused by a gain in fat and fat-free mass, but fat mass increases more in girls and fat-free mass increases more in boys. Therefore, after puberty, girls are generally no longer able to compete equally in a coed setting. Boys who begin their pubertal growth spurt ahead of other boys their age will be temporarily taller, heavier, and stronger. However, this should not be misconstrued as superior ability or talent. Success due to advanced physical maturity can lead to unrealistic expectations that these boys will continue to be outstanding athletes. Attempts should be made for these boys to participate and compete with boys of similar maturational status. Similarly, boys who mature later may experience a temporary physical disadvantage in sports that should not be misinterpreted as a lack of talent or ability. These boys should be encouraged to participate initially in sports with less emphasis on physical size, such as racquet sports, soccer, martial arts, wrestling, and certain track events.

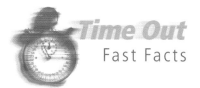

Time Out
Fast Facts

Success due to advanced physical maturity often leads to unrealistic expectations that children will continue to be outstanding athletes.

The structure of organized sports often impedes the ability of children to play at their own developmental level.

By age 15 years, 75% of children who have been involved in organized sports have dropped out.

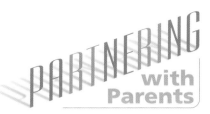

PARTNERING with Parents

Is it appropriate for boys and girls to practice and compete together?

Prior to the onset of puberty, there are no significant differences in size, strength, endurance, or motor skills that would preclude boys and girls from competing together or against one another.

Does involvement in sports at a very early age improve a child's chances of excelling in athletics?

Children will not necessarily benefit from practice or repetition of skills until they have reached their motor "milestones." There is no evidence to suggest that they achieve these milestones any sooner as a result of training.

FINISH LINE

It is estimated that by age 15 years, 75% of children who had been involved in organized sports have dropped out. This suggests that many youth sports programs are organized in ways that do not promote the interests of the children, but rather those of the adults involved. Game structures and adults' expectations for performance should be revised to match the interests and developmental capabilities of the children to provide positive sports experiences during childhood as a basis for lifelong involvement. The key principles governing appropriate sports activities for children are eloquently summarized in "The Bill of Rights of Young Athletes."

For More Information

1. Branta C, Haubenstricker J, Seefeldt V: Age changes in motor skills during childhood and adolescence. *Exerc Sport Sci Rev* 1984;12:467–520.

2. Gould D, Weiss MR (eds): *Advances in Pediatric Sport Sciences.* Champaign, IL, Human Kinetics, 1987, vol 2, pp 61–86.

3. Nelson MA: Developmental skills and children's sports. *Physician Sportsmed* 1991;19:67–79.

4. Seefeldt V, Haubenstricker J: Patterns, phases, or stages: An analytical model for the study of developmental movement, in Kelso JAS, Clark JE (eds): *The Development of Movement Control and Coordination.* Chichester, NY, John Wiley, 1982, pp 309–318.

5. Willoughby C, Polatajko HJ: Motor problems in children with developmental coordination disorder: Review of the literature. *Am J Occup Ther* 1995;49:787–794.

Chapter 4

Growth and Maturation

JORGE E. GÓMEZ, MS, MD

Parents often have questions about sports preparedness, training capabilities, and skill development, all of which are directly related to age-specific changes in the neuromotor, cardiovascular, and cognitive/integrative systems. To best answer these questions, the physician must understand the normal development of these systems as they relate to sports participation.

Infancy (Birth to 2 years)

Many parents are concerned about whether real or perceived aberrancies in neuromotor or musculoskeletal development during their child's first year of life will have bearing on later sports competencies.

The mean age at which infants begin to walk independently is about age 13 months, with a range of between ages 9 and 17 months. Late walking is probably not related to neuromotor retardation, but may be the result of an inherited dependent behavioral style or a lack of parental emphasis on gross motor skills. Conversely, genetics may explain why African-American, Mexican, East Indian, and Middle Eastern infants achieve gross motor milestones earlier than white North American infants. Cultural customs of infant swaddling or carrying, which limit movement, appear to have no effect on the age of walking.

An infant's natural curiosity and drive to attain self-sufficiency provide the impetus for trying increasingly complex patterns of movement. Attainment of gross and fine motor milestones in infancy follows a predictable pattern that is largely predetermined.

Encouragement and training of motor skills at this age in an attempt to produce early development appears to have no effect on the age of walking. For example, the use of infant walkers has no effect on the age of walking, and may even cause a delay in walking. Early age of walking has not been shown to predict earlier achievement of complex sports-related skills. Similarly, the arm and leg movements demonstrated by infants placed in water are purely reflexive and do not predict swimming aptitude. Relying on an infant's apparent swimming ability is potentially dangerous.

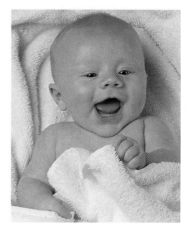

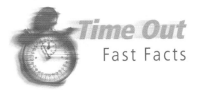

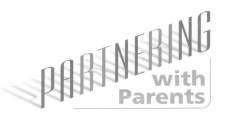

Is it acceptable for a young child to play a single sport year round?

During middle childhood, it is important that children experience a variety of activities to master motor skills that are more difficult to acquire later. There is also a concern over the risk of overuse injuries in young athletes who play a single sport year round.

Early Childhood (2 to 5 years)

The preschool years are most notable for the dramatic change in body composition and the improvement in gait and specific motor skills.

Both fat mass and fat-free mass increase gradually with body size between ages 2 and 6 years. The percentage of fat, however, declines between the ages of 3 and 6 years, more so for boys than for girls, coinciding with decreased caloric intake and increased energy expenditure.

Between ages 2 and 3 years, the child's normal bow legs will slowly evolve into a nearly straight quadriceps angle on its way to a maximum average valgus angle of 12° by around age 3 years (**Figure 4.1**). Persistence or worsening of the bow legs beyond age 2 years warrants investigation for pathologic causes such as epiphyseal dysplasia (eg, Blount's disease) (**Figure 4.2**).

Increases in limb and stride length between ages 2 and 4 years parallel the refinement in walking skill. As walking proficiency develops, the base of support is narrowed, and arm movements become more synchronous with the stride. By age 4 years, most children achieve an adult walking pattern. The arms can now be used for increasingly complex tasks.

Handedness is usually established by about age 2 years, but is often not firmly established until ages 3 or 4 years. Handedness is largely predetermined, and, left-handedness has not prevented notable athletes from achieving high levels of success.

Gross motor development during the preschool years is fairly uniform in boys and girls, but there are some differences in development of sport-specific skills. The age at which 60% of boys achieve a mature running pattern is about age 4 years, 2 months, while for girls it is about age 5 years. Most boys achieve a mature throwing pattern by age 6 years, whereas girls this age still tend to throw with the feet fixed and with little trunk rotation. Jumping and catching develop at the same rate in boys and girls. Girls tend to be proficient in skipping and hopping earlier than boys, and by age 6 years, kicking and striking are more advanced in boys.

New skills are learned by application of fundamental movements to new situations. The freedom to try new things, to move, and to explore is essential for motor development. Observation of toddler play reveals the fundamental conflict of dependence versus independence when involved in exploration.

Figure 4.1 Normal progression from bow legs of infancy through slow evolution to a physiologic valgus angle of about 12° at age 3 (toddler).

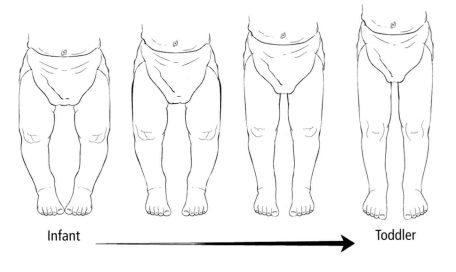

Infant ⟶ Toddler

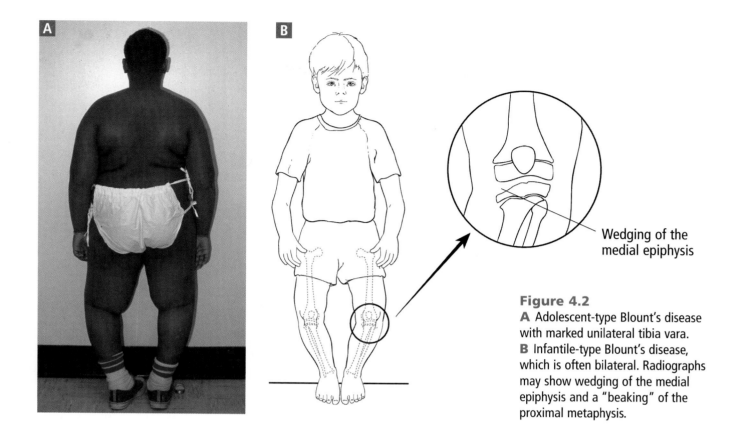

Wedging of the
medial epiphysis

Figure 4.2
A Adolescent-type Blount's disease
with marked unilateral tibia vara.
B Infantile-type Blount's disease,
which is often bilateral. Radiographs
may show wedging of the medial
epiphysis and a "beaking" of the
proximal metaphysis.

The child moves away from the parent, tries something new, returns to the
parent for approval and reassurance, and the cycle is repeated. For this cycle
to lead to successful motor learning, the parent must be willing to both reassure and to give up control. Excessive parental guidance and monitoring
squelches the child's sense of self-discovery, making learning or mastering
new skills boring and unrewarding. Criticism or ridicule over mistakes in the
performance of motor skills will surely deter future willing participation in
these skills.

The leg aches referred to as "growing pains"
are most common in early childhood. The
etiology of this condition is not known, and
growing pains remains a diagnosis of exclusion. However, these pains typically occur at
rest, usually at night, never during activity,
and are confined to the thighs, knees, or
calves in a child who has a normal musculoskeletal examination and no signs or symptoms of systemic disease. Children with these
pains find massage comforting, and parents
often give acetaminophen or ibuprofen,
which may or may not help. Passive stretching of the quadriceps, hamstrings, and calves
at bedtime may benefit some children.
Parents can be reassured about the benign
and self-limited nature of this condition.

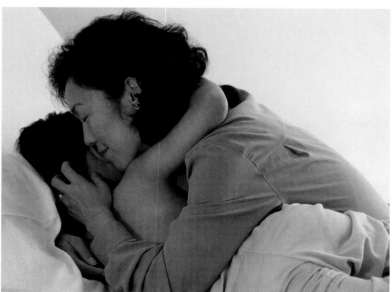

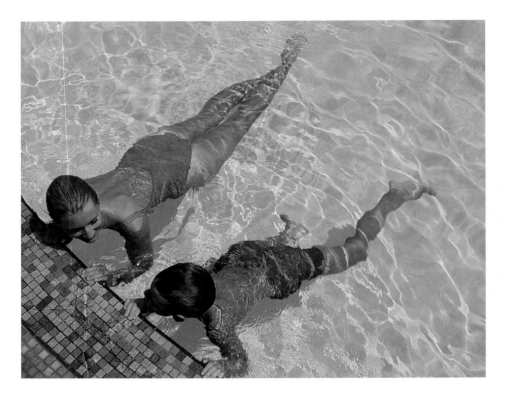

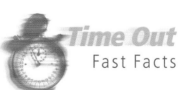

If athletes were matched according to their level of physical maturity, wouldn't there be less risk for injury?

Although it would probably more closely match their physical abilities and therefore "level the playing field," there is little evidence to suggest that it would lower the incidence of injuries.

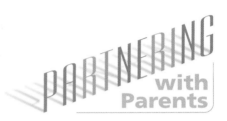

Time Out
Fast Facts

Choice of sport or the intensity of training is unlikely to cause either premature or delayed onset of puberty.

The strongest predictor of aerobic capacity during adolescence is the stage of maturity.

Middle to Late Childhood (6 to 12 years)

Growth is fairly steady during the elementary school years. Toward the end of this period, it is common for girls to become temporarily taller and heavier than boys of the same age because of the earlier onset of puberty. Percent fat mass actually declines or remains steady, with girls always having a slightly higher percent. Flexibility may be increased. The incidence of generalized joint hypermobility, defined as the ability to extend the hands and thumbs parallel to the forearm, hyperextension of the knees and elbows, and ability to touch the palms to the floor, is highest in school-age children (5% to 7%). Children with hypermobility may be at increased risk of glenohumeral and patellar subluxation or dislocation, but the risk of other injuries is not increased.

Grip, arm, shoulder, and quadriceps strength begin to diverge in boys and girls between ages 6 to 12 years, but these differences are small compared with those seen in adolescence. Tasks that depend on explosive power, such as the vertical jump, long jump, and throw for distance, also diverge slowly, with boys always having a slight edge. Running speed is nearly equal between boys and girls between ages 9 and 11 years, and girls tend to have better balance than boys of the same age. Although children at this age tend to have same gender playmates, boys and girls are able to compete quite evenly.

Most children achieve mature patterns of fundamental motor skills during elementary school. Most girls achieve a mature throwing technique by age 8 years; 60% of children achieve mature kicking and striking patterns at about age 7 years for boys and age 8 years for girls. Mature hopping and catching patterns are achieved between ages 7 and 8 years for most boys and girls.

Capacities for aerobic and anaerobic exercise increase slowly during the middle childhood, but are quite limited in comparison with adolescent capacities. This limitation probably has minimal impact on play and sports activities because most play during early and middle childhood is at submaximal cardiorespiratory function. Analysis of movement patterns during free play of young children indicates that they are active in short bursts, with 95% of high-intensity bursts lasting less than 15 seconds. Most of their activities, however, are in the low to moderate intensity range.

Mastering new skills becomes more significant during middle childhood, when success and mastery become closely linked with the child's sense of self-worth. The drive to achieve self-efficacy and to acquire social acceptance explains why children at this age are able to immerse themselves in academic, artistic, and athletic activities with great energy and for prolonged periods. Sports and dance may provide opportunities for mastery of neuromotor skills and for social recognition and interaction, which build self-efficacy.

There appear to be critical periods between ages 10 to 12 years and early adolescence during which acquisition of some specific skills is easiest, and after which acquisition of those skills to the same degree is either extremely difficult or impossible. Such skills include hitting a baseball or tennis ball and shooting a basketball. The precise ages for this window and the time frame of such a window has not been studied. Therefore, active time for the school-age child is theoretically better spent in learning and refining sport-specific skills.

Early Adolescence (13 to 15 years)

The increases in muscle mass, muscle strength, and cardiopulmonary endurance that occur during puberty are greater than those that occur at any other age.

Both fat mass and fat-free mass continue to increase in both boys and girls during early and midadolescence. With the onset of puberty, girls tend to accumulate fat mass at a greater rate than boys. By the end of high school, most girls have nearly twice the percent body fat as boys.

Muscle strength accelerates dramatically in boys during puberty. Girls continue to increase their muscle strength during this time, but the increase is more gradual. These differences in muscle strength gains are reflected in differences in performance of tasks requiring muscle power, defined as the product of strength and velocity of contraction. During puberty, boys have a sharp increase in the performance of vertical or horizontal jumping, throwing, and sprinting, whereas girls show gradual improvement or reach a plateau in their performance of these skills.

Increased tightness of the hamstrings and ankle dorsiflexors occurs during puberty and is greatest during the height spurt around age 12 years in girls and age 14 years in boys. Dancers and gymnasts may be most sensitive to the loss of flexibility associated with the height spurt. Hamstring tightness may contribute to

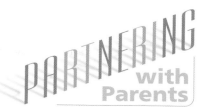

Is it safe for an 8-year-old child to participate in endurance activities?

Children at this age are physiologically more suited for activities that are intermittent in nature. They usually prefer activities of low to moderate intensity, with occasional "bursts" of high-intensity activity.

Figure 4.3
A Muscle groups that tend to lose flexibility during adolescent growth spurt. **B** The loss of flexibility increases stress to the patellofemoral joint, which may produce pain.

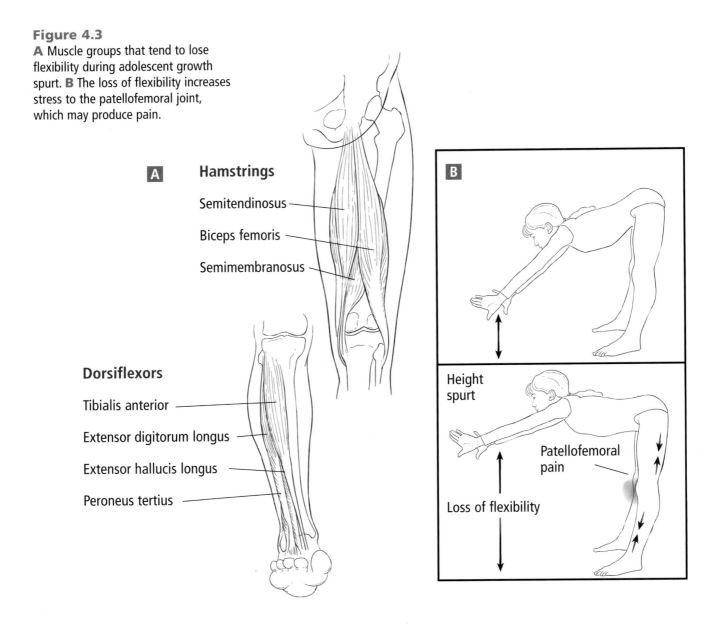

A Hamstrings

Semitendinosus

Biceps femoris

Semimembranosus

Dorsiflexors

Tibialis anterior

Extensor digitorum longus

Extensor hallucis longus

Peroneus tertius

B

Height spurt

Loss of flexibility

Patellofemoral pain

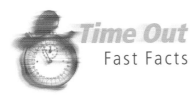

Skill acquisition is easiest during middle childhood and early adolescence.

increased stress at the patellofemoral joint, leading to patellofemoral pain, which becomes increasingly common during this age (**Figure 4.3**).

Differences in physical performance early in adolescence are more strongly influenced by the age at onset of puberty than by chronologic age. Boys who mature early tend to be taller, have greater muscle mass and fat mass, and have greater arm, grip, and explosive strength (jumping and sprinting) than boys who mature later. Girls who mature early tend to be taller, have greater fat mass and fat-free mass than average- or late-maturing girls, but have only a modest advantage in strength. Girls who mature later perform better on tests of upper extremity strength than average-maturing girls, perhaps because of a lower ratio of fat to fat-free mass, and they generally perform better on tasks requiring balance.

The strongest predictor of changes in aerobic capacity (maximal oxygen uptake or VO_{2max}) during early adolescence is stage of maturity. Increases in

Vo_{2max} result from the development of pulmonary ventilation, cardiac output, muscular oxygen extraction, and oxidative metabolism, which are strongly related to physical maturity. The increase in Vo_{2max} during adolescence, in comparison with the lack of change in Vo_{2max} per kg body weight, indicates that the increase in aerobic power is directly related to dimensional changes in the oxygen delivery and muscular systems. Levels of physical activity and fatness correlate much less strongly with increasing aerobic power during puberty than do visceral and muscular growth. The capacity for anaerobic (intense, short burst) exercise increases more gradually than does aerobic capacity.

Questions often arise about whether early- versus late-maturing boys and girls are better suited to certain sports. Data from cross-sectional studies of pubertal athletes have generally shown that early-maturing boys tend to excel in sports requiring speed and strength; in one study, elite-level male track and field performers ages 10 to 15 years were more mature for their age than average. Elite female track and field athletes had average skeletal maturity for their age, but throwers (eg, shot, discus) were more mature than average. In contrast, elite female gymnasts have later onset of menarche and narrower hips and shoulders than average girls. It is unlikely that the choice of sport or the intensity of training cause either premature or delayed onset of puberty in either male or female athletes.

Mismatching children by maturity status during early adolescence results in an unfair competitive advantage to those who are more mature; however, there is little evidence that such mismatching increases the risk of injury to those who are less mature. The incidence of musculoskeletal injury is lower during early adolescence than during middle or late adolescence.

Late Adolescence (16 to 20 years)

Boys continue to increase in strength, speed, and size during late adolescence, although the rate of increase is not nearly as great as during puberty. Girls do not have significant increases in fat-free mass during late adolescence, but continue to accumulate fat mass, which often has an adverse effect on

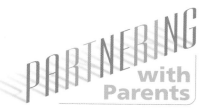

Will a late-maturing adolescent ever catch up with his peers?

Although children with growth delay often "catch up" in terms of stature, boys who mature early usually continue to be heavier and exhibit greater upper body strength.

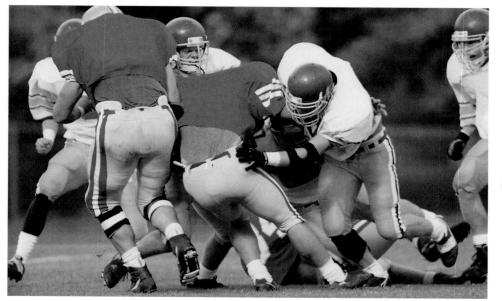

Time Out
Fast Facts

Increases in strength, muscle mass, and cardiopulmonary endurance are greater during puberty than at any other time.

performance. In general, both muscular strength and aerobic capacity continue to increase into adulthood, but the rate of increase is much more gradual than during puberty.

Differences in boys' stature associated with differences in the age of onset of puberty will vanish by late adolescence. Children with familial late maturation or constitutional growth delay can be reassured that they will "catch up" with their peers by high school. However, some functional differences will persist. Even in late adolescence, early-maturing boys will continue to be heavier and continue to outperform average- or late-maturing boys on tests of arm strength.

Whether an adolescent remains active in sports into young adulthood may depend on how he or she chooses to confront the developmental tasks of adolescence, and whether athletics fits into his or her personal scheme for dealing with these tasks. The processes of emancipating from the family, forming a sexual identity, identifying with a peer group, developing the capacity for intimacy, and preparing for adult education or employment place great demands on physical and emotional energy. Adolescents at this age should be encouraged to view athletics as a means for relieving stress, maintaining vigor, and providing social interactions.

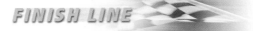

FINISH LINE

Physicians must help parents and youth coaches understand the range of attainment of developmental milestones in young athletes. Normal growth and maturation influences the timing of acquisition of an athlete's skills and influences the risk of various injuries at different ages.

For More Information

1. Bailey RC, Olson J, Pepper SL, Porszasz J, Barstow TJ, Cooper DM: The level and tempo of children's physical activities: An observational study. *Med Sci Sports Exerc* 1995;27:1033–1041.

2. Dixon SD, Stein MT (eds): *Encounters With Children: Pediatric Behavior and Development,* ed 2. St. Louis, MO, Mosby Year Book, 1992.

3. Malina RM, Bouchard C (eds): *Growth, Maturation, and Physical Activity.* Champaign, IL, Human Kinetics, 1991.

4. Morrissy RT (ed): *Lovell and Winter's Pediatric Orthopaedics,* ed 3. Philadelphia, PA, JB Lippincott, 1990.

5. Rowland TW (ed): *Developmental Exercise Physiology.* Champaign, IL, Human Kinetics, 1996.

Chapter 5

Promoting Physical Activity

BARBARA J. LONG, MD, MPH

Physicians and other primary care providers who work with children and adolescents traditionally have been responsible for providing a broad range of anticipatory guidance in areas such as child growth and development, accident/injury prevention, dietary counseling, and parenting issues. Because there is sufficient evidence that the processes of cardiovascular disease begin in childhood, prevention has become another important counseling area for physicians. Despite the recognized importance of lipid screening, nutrition counseling, obesity treatment, and regular exercise, it is not at all clear to what degree or how effectively physicians address these areas. Issues surrounding the promotion of regular physical activity are discussed herein and an outline for a behaviorally oriented approach intended to help physicians effectively promote physical activity among youths is presented.

Defining Physical Activity

Physical activity is any body movement produced by skeletal musculature that results in energy expenditure; *physical fitness* is the ability to perform physical activity, and exercise is planned, structured, and repetitive body movement done to improve or maintain physical fitness. Physical fitness is a physiologic trait, while physical activity is a behavior. Physical activity can occur during exercise, during the routine activities of daily living (walking, stair climbing, occupational work), and during the free play of children and youths. Physicians should counsel children and their parents to promote or increase physical activity. The goal is to involve all children in a variety of activities that will enhance their current physical and psychological well-being and to promote active lifestyle choices that will continue into adulthood.

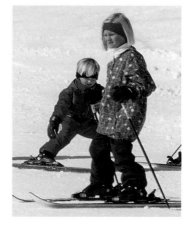

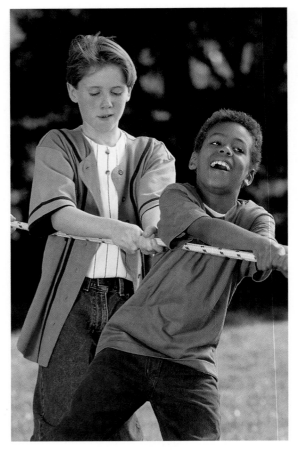

Epidemiology of Physical Activity

Two large US population-based studies, the National Children and Youth Fitness Study (NCYFS) and the Youth Risk Behavior Survey (YRBS), have helped delineate patterns of physical activity among youths. In the mid-1980s, the NCYFS measured the physical fitness and physical activity habits of a national sample of children ages 10 to 18 years. Results showed that students between the grades 7 and 12 reported spending an average of 1.8 hours per day on activity outside of physical education classes. The YRBS, sponsored by the Centers for Disease Control and Prevention (CDC), was first administered in 1990 and has been repeated in 1991, 1993, 1995, and 1997. The 1995 YRBS showed that 52% of girls and 74% of boys in grades 9 through 12 reported involvement in vigorous activity (**Table 5.1**). Vigorous activity was defined as activity lasting for at least 20 minutes that made the students breathe hard and sweat during 3 or more of the 7 days preceding the survey. A total of 61% of girls and 81% of boys in grade 9 reported involvement in vigorous activity, but by grade 12, only 41% and 67% of girls and boys, respectively, remained involved in vigorous activity.

The number of girls participating in organized team sports has increased fivefold since the passage of Title IX in 1972. Even though more girls are involved in sports, the YRBS data showed that their participation in team sports decreased from grades 9 to 12. Reviewing these surveys reveals several important trends.

Although children are active, especially when compared with adults, physical activity decreases significantly during adolescence. This decline is consistent across participation in physical education classes, involvement in vigorous or moderate activity, and participation in team sports. Boys are more active than girls across all ages, and the decline in activity across adolescence is more marked for girls than for boys, particularly minority girls. Because this decline continues into adulthood, physical activity promotion should begin during childhood and adolescence.

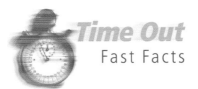

Time Out
Fast Facts

Many physicians perceive that they are ineffective at changing patient behavior with regard to regular physical activity.

Physician Behavior

The counseling behaviors of physicians in terms of the frequency and quality of physical activity counseling are related to their training, perceived effectiveness at changing patient behavior, practice settings, and their own personal physical activity practices. There appears to be a significant gap between physicians' recognition of the importance of promoting regular activity and the perception of their effectiveness at changing patient behavior. In previous studies of physician counseling behaviors with adults, frequently cited barriers to counseling included: lack of time, lack of training, lack of standardized recommendations and counseling techniques, lack of reimbursement, and lack of effectiveness at changing patient behavior. These barriers need to be addressed to facilitate adequate counseling about physical activity within the clinical setting. The sections below review current physical activity guidelines for youths and strategies that can be used to address some of these known barriers to counseling.

Table 5.1 *Percentage of Young People Involved in Vigorous Physical Activity**

Demographic group	1992 NHIS-YRBS**		1995 YRBS†	
	Percent	95% confidence interval	Percent	95% confidence interval
Overall	**53.7**	**(52.5, 54.9)**	**63.7**	**(60.4, 66.9)**
Sex				
Males	60.2	(58.6, 61.8)	74.4	(72.1, 76.6)
Females	47.2	(45.6, 48.8)	52.1	(47.5, 56.8)
Race/Ethnicity				
White, non-Hispanic	54.6	(53.2, 56.0)	67.0	(62.6, 71.4)
Males	60.2	(58.4, 62.0)	76.0	(73.0, 78.9)
Females	49.0	(46.8, 51.2)	56.7	(50.0, 63.4)
Black, non-Hispanic	52.6	(49.9, 55.3)	53.2	(49.6, 56.8)
Males	62.7	(58.8, 66.6)	68.1	(62.8, 73.4)
Females	42.3	(38.6, 46.0)	41.3	(35.5, 42.1)
Hispanic	49.5	(46.6, 52.4)	57.3	(53.7, 60.9)
Males	56.7	(52.6, 60.8)	69.7	(64.9, 74.5)
Females	41.7	(38.2, 45.2)	45.2	(39.9, 50.6)

Age (years)—males			**Grade in school—males**		
12	70.8	(66.7, 74.9)			
13	73.7	(69.4, 78.0)			
14	76.1	(72.2, 80.0)			
15	82.6	(68.1. 71.1)	9	80.8	(75.9, 85.6)
16	65.6	(60.3, 70.9)	10	75.9	(72.5, 79.3)
17	60.2	(54.7, 65.7)	11	70.2	(67.5, 72.9)
18	48.4	(43.1, 53.7)	12	66.9	(63.0, 70.7)
19	44.1	(38.4, 49.8)			
20	43.4	(38.5, 48.3)			
21	42.2	(37.1, 47.3)			

Age (years)—females			**Grade in school—females**		
12	66.2	(62.1, 70.3)			
13	63.1	(58.0, 68.2)			
14	63.1	(58.4, 67.8)			
15	56.6	(51.9, 61.3)	9	60.9	(54.8, 67.0)
16	50.9	(45.6, 56.2)	10	54.4	(47.6, 61.3)
17	43.6	(38.1, 49.1)	11	44.7	(40.6, 48.9)
18	37.5	(32.2, 42.8)	12	41.0	(34.6, 47.5)
19	32.6	(27.3, 37.9)			
20	28.2	(23.9, 32.5)			
21	30.2	(25.5, 34.9)			

Annual family income		
<$10,000	46.7	(43.2, 50.2)
$10,000-19,999	48.5	(46.0, 51.1)
$20,000-34,999	55.0	(52.5, 57.6)
$35,000-49,999	58.4	(55.5, 61.3)
$50,000+	60.2	(57.9, 62.6)

*Data represent percentage of young people reporting participation in vigorous physical activity during 3 or more of the 7 days preceding the survey, by demographic group, 1992 National Health Interview Survey-Youth Risk Behavior Survey (NHIS-YRBS) and 1995 Youth Risk Behavior Survey (YRBS), United States.

** A national household-based survey of youths aged 12-21 years.

† A national school-based survey of students in grades 9-12.

Source: Centers for Disease Control and Prevention, National Center for Health Statistics, NHIS-YRBS, 1992 machine readable data file and documentation, 1993; Centers for Disease Control and Prevention, National Center for Chronic Disease Prevention and Health Promotion, YRBS 1995 data tape (in press).

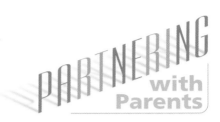

My child has never enjoyed organized or team sports. How can I encourage her to increase her activity level?

Limit sedentary activities, such as watching television and playing video games, and encourage a more active lifestyle, including stair climbing, walking, and riding a bicycle. Exercising with a friend or family member may help. Perhaps most important, however, is for a parent to teach by example and be an active role model.

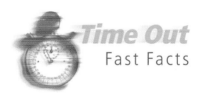

Physicians should promote a variety of activities that are fun and can be easily incorporated into the lifestyle of their young patients.

Basic Recommendations for Promoting Activity

Several sets of recommendations or guidelines have been developed to establish parameters for promoting physical activity among youth. These guidelines define the quantity and quality of activity needed to optimize physical fitness and to identify the health-related benefits of physical activity. All of these guidelines have incorporated the input of experts and the current scientific literature, yet acknowledge the gaps in research.

Both sets of recommendations emphasize daily physical activity. It is believed that participating in regular physical activity is probably more important for obtaining health-related benefits than is the intensity of the activity. Although obtaining physical fitness is a desirable goal, youth are inherently fit. Therefore, the recommendations focus on maintaining activity levels that will help to maintain fitness levels and to avoid a decline in activity levels through the adolescent years. Recommendations for youth should focus on promoting a variety of activities that are fun and can be easily incorporated into their lifestyle. These activities can include team sports, individual sports, and recreational or lifetime activities, such as walking, bicycling, and swimming. Any form of physical activity that is regular, enjoyable, and sustainable is the desired endpoint. However, parents and youth coaches should avoid the use of exercise as punishment for bad behavior. This implies that exercise is not fun, just the opposite of what should be promoted.

The Challenges of Providing Activity Counseling

Because of its many short- and long-term benefits, promoting physical activity should be a priority in every physician setting. Unfortunately, fitting this type of counseling into the list of tasks that need to be addressed during a well-child visit is often difficult, especially when limited reimbursement and time are allocated for health-promotion counseling.

Assessment of Current Activity

The patient's level of physical activity should be assessed at every well-child visit. This can be part of a standard health assessment form completed by the patient or parent in the waiting room, part of the nursing assessment, or part of the physician interview. Additional assessment can be made by the physician or office staff if the initial assessment identifies a child or adolescent who is sedentary or only intermittently active. As part of the problem identification, it is important to determine the child's readiness to make a behavior change, as well as to identify potential barriers to change. Inactive youth can be asked if they are interested in becoming more active. Those who are active can be asked how likely it is they will continue their activity over the next 3 to 6 months. Then, a counseling approach based on current activity and readiness to change or maintain behavior can be used. Creating solutions is a joint effort between the physician and child and should include the parents whenever possible.

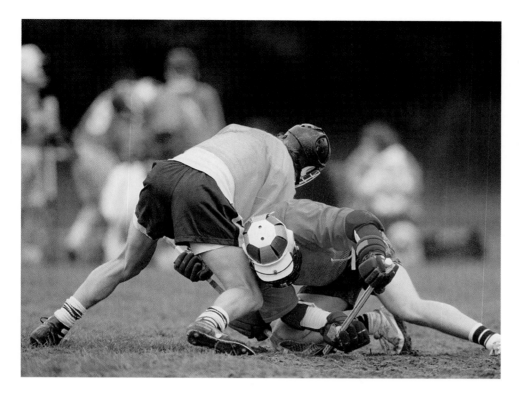

1993 International
Consensus Conference
on Physical Activity
Guidelines for Adolescents

1. All adolescents should be
   physically active daily, or nearly
   every day, as part of play,
   games, sports, work, transportation, recreation, physical
   education, or planned exercise
   in the context of family, school,
   and community activities.

2. Adolescents should engage in
   three or more sessions per
   week of activities that last 20
   minutes or more at a time and
   that require moderate to vigorous levels of exertion.

Interventions

Most physicians are familiar with and quite skilled at problem identification. Providing useful solutions or effective health promotion interventions within the confines of a busy clinical setting is more difficult. Some restraints, such as time and reimbursement, will not be changed until practice styles and reimbursement patterns are redefined. Therefore, efforts need to be focused on brief, yet effective interventions that easily can be incorporated into current practice patterns.

Promoting physical activity starts with providing magazines or other educational materials that promote healthy lifestyles and physical activity in the waiting room. Posters or pictures showing different types of activities, both vigorous and moderate, being done by a variety of children and adolescents with and without adults send a healthy message to patients and their families.

Readiness and behavior modification

Successful models in adult physical activity counseling have incorporated concepts from stages of change theory, social cognitive theory, and behavior modification techniques. These include identifying the patient's readiness to make a behavioral change, goal setting, creating contracts, addressing barriers, and enlisting social support. These concepts can easily be incorporated into brief clinical counseling interventions and can be adapted to a variety of health behaviors.

The key point is that a physical activity prescription is needed only for those patients who are ready to make a change. Youngsters who meet the recommended levels of activity should receive brief reinforcement about

Guidelines of the Health
Education Authority
of England for
Youth Participation in
Regular Health-Enhancing
Physical Activity

1. All young people should participate in physical activity of
   at least moderate intensity for
   1 hour per day.

2. Young people who currently
   do little activity should participate in physical activity of at
   least moderate intensity for at
   least 30 minutes per day.

3. At least twice a week, some of
   these activities should help to
   enhance and maintain muscular strength and flexibility and
   bone health.

Vern Seefeldt, 1973

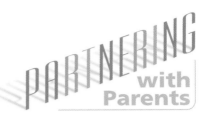

How much exercise do children need?

Ideally, children should participate in moderately strenuous activity for at least 30 minutes a day. The effects of exercise are cumulative, and multiple sessions of short duration result in most of the health benefits compared with single episodes of longer duration.

their healthy lifestyle and encouragement about continuing their activity. This approach is more satisfying for patients and physicians, is a much better use of valuable counseling minutes, and allows physicians to spend the most time with patients who are ready to make positive changes.

For inactive children or adolescents who are not ready to change, identifying potential benefits and current barriers to activity can be an important first step. Often physical activity can be recommended for a medical reason, such as an increase in weight disproportionate to an increase in height, borderline blood pressure for age, or a strong family history of cardiovascular disease and/or diabetes. Because young people are much more focused on the present than on potential long-term benefits of physical activity, emphasizing current benefits can be a more effective motivation than the prevention of distant chronic diseases. Common patient barriers to physical activity include lack of time, lack of access to facilities, unsafe neighborhoods, and dislike of exercise. For this group, identifying salient benefits and addressing the barriers can be the first step toward getting the individual or family to think about becoming more physically active.

Physical activity prescription

Presenting recommendations as a "physical activity prescription" is a useful concept. Writing a patient a prescription uses a medical model with which both physicians and patients are familiar. It also takes advantage of the "white coat effect" and reinforces to patients that physical activity is as important to their health as any medication that might be prescribed. Allowing the patient, and parent when appropriate, to participate in setting the physical activity goal will enhance compliance with the prescription. For many children, parents play an important role in any behavioral change; therefore, counseling needs to target both the child and the parent. Adapting simple behavioral change concepts into counseling will help make the limited time available for counseling more effective.

For inactive or intermittently active youngsters who are interested in increasing their activity level, counseling should include an actual activity plan or physical activity prescription. Because these patients are ready to change, any counseling or direction provided is much more likely to translate into a behavior change. Focus should be placed on increasing moderate physical activity to between 30 and 60 minutes per day. This can be accomplished by accumulating several bouts of 10 to 15 minutes of activity. It is important to have the child be as clear as possible regarding the plan, including type of activity and intensity, location, when he or she is going to be active, and for how long. In order to make the plan detailed, the child will need to anticipate barriers and create solutions. The more detailed the plan, the more likely the child is to meet his or her goal.

Creating a social climate for physical activity

Physical activity needs to be fun and accessible for the individual if it is to be continued. It is important to help children choose an activity routine that is fun, developmentally appropriate, and realistic given his or her individual, family, and community resources. One method that has been used frequently in exercise prescription for adults incorporates the mnemonic FITT, which stands for frequency, intensity, time (duration), and type of activity. This can be useful for creating a physical activity prescription, and it can be used as a simple way to record recommendations in the medical record.

Suggestions for increasing physical activity can include walking or bicycling for transportation and planning physically active rather than sedentary activities with friends. Many adolescents, especially girls, may not be active because they think organized sports is the only type of exercise that "counts." Therefore, it is important to help adolescents identify the physical activity they may already be getting (eg, walking), as well as to reinforce the benefits of other lifetime activities such as bicycling, dancing, skating, and swimming.

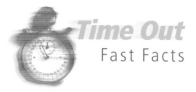

Time Out
Fast Facts

Identifying a social support system or an exercise partner is an important component in making a successful behavior change.

FITT Method

Frequency: The goal should be to include some type of physical activity daily. It is important to educate your patients that activities of daily living (ie, walking/bicycling for transportation) count as physical activity.

Intensity: The goal should be for the daily activity to be of at least moderate intensity, with ideally several bouts of more vigorous activity over the week. Vigorous activity is often defined as activity that makes you breathe hard and sweat. As mentioned above, the intensity is felt to be less important than establishing and maintaining the regular activity.

Time: The goal should be the accumulation of between 30 and 60 minutes of activity daily. Acknowledge that accumulation of activity in 10- to 15-minute bouts provides nearly all the health benefits of longer bouts of sustained activity. This can be a great way to encourage physical activity in individuals less inclined to participate in more organized team sports or longer bouts of sustained activity. This concept may also lead to the incorporation of lifestyle activities that may be more easily maintained over time.

Type: The activities can include a variety of team sports, individual sports, recreational activities, family activities, and lifestyle activities such as walking or bicycling for transportation, household chores, and taking the stairs when-ever possible. Several bouts a week of weightbearing activities that promote muscle strength, flexibility, and bone health are desirable. Involvement in a variety of activities may help by decreasing burn out and overuse syndromes, and increasing the enjoyment factor and promoting maintenance of the activities. Injuries and lack of enjoyment are frequently cited as reasons adolescents quit participating in activities.

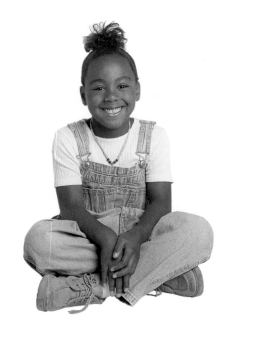

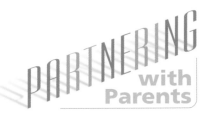

What are the best activities or sports to promote for children?

Although team and individual sports are beneficial for a variety of reasons, it may be at least as important to encourage lifetime activities such as walking, dancing, and bicycling. These activities can be enjoyed later in life and may be more acceptable to children who lack the motor skills to excel at sports.

Identifying ways to incorporate increased physical activity into the activities of daily living can also be useful. Examples include taking the stairs whenever possible, getting off the bus a stop earlier, taking walks with friends rather than talking on the telephone, and walking at least one lap of the mall before shopping.

Identifying a social support or physical activity buddy has been identified as an important component in making a successful behavior change. Parents of younger children should plan active times or vacations with their children. This increases their children's activity and provides an excellent role model for their children.

Safety Concerns

When neighborhood safety is a barrier, activities that can be done indoors, such as exercise to videos and dancing to popular music, should be recommended. Decreasing the amount of time spent in sedentary behaviors, such as watching television, talking on the telephone, playing computer or video games, especially in the late afternoon and early evening, will translate into more accumulated daily activity. Stretching while watching television or using some type of exercise equipment such as a stationary bicycle can increase activity during an otherwise sedentary time. Although the link between physical activity and television watching is not clear, increased watching has been linked to obesity. It makes intuitive sense that one way to increase activity is to decrease the amount of sedentary behavior.

Reinforcement

The behavior of the child or adolescent who is appropriately active should be reinforced. Often it is helpful to identify the health benefits of regular activity, such as maintenance of appropriate weight, increased energy, improved sense of well-being, and self-esteem. It can also be useful to assess how confident a patient is that he or she will remain active and to provide solutions for any identified potential barriers to maintaining that activity.

Physicians and other health care providers need to be good role models for their patients and their families. This includes a personal plan for incorporating physical activity within their own busy schedules. Studies with internists show that physicians who are regular exercisers are more likely to provide more frequent and more aggressive physical activity counseling for their patients.

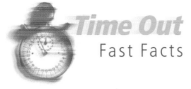

The decline in activity during adolescence is more marked for girls than for boys.

Community and Schools

Physicians can play an important role in promoting physical activity by being good role models for an active lifestyle and being advocates for physical activity in other arenas. Children and adolescents spend most of their time attending school. Physicians need to advocate for more health education and physical education that includes aerobic lifestyle activities (ie, walking, jogging, dancing), as well as teaching sport-specific skills. In addition, physicians can become more involved with teachers and coaching staffs. This communication improves the care of the young athlete and increases the effectiveness of the physicians, teachers, and coaching staffs. Changes in school policy potentially reach larger numbers of children than the promotion of physical activity with individuals in the office. Guidelines exist for the establishment of appropriate health education and physical education curricula. Physicians can be valuable advocates for promoting these guidelines.

Physicians are also important advocates for the availability of safe and accessible places for physical activity to occur within the community. This advocacy ranges from promoting the availability of open spaces, parks, recreation centers, and community centers to promoting the availability of schools and school playgrounds after hours. The CDC has published a set of guidelines for promoting physical activity within the community.

The American Academy of Pediatrics has developed a list of recommendations for assessing physical activity and fitness in the office setting. The following checklist incorporates many of those recommendations, but focuses on ways physicians can promote the behavior of regular physical activity (**Table 5.2**).

Table 5.2 *Keys to Promoting Physical Fitness and Activity*

In the Clinic

1. Ensure that the clinical setting is "physical activity friendly" by including posters, videos, pictures, magazines, and other patient education materials that promote physical activity and healthy lifestyle choices.

2. Be a good role model. Incorporate 30 minutes of moderate activity into your daily routine on most days of the week. You will be a better counselor and a healthier individual.

3. Assess and record the level of physical activity in all your well-child visits.

4. If a patient is inactive and not interested in changing, give the patient some reasons to reconsider and address any identified barriers to activity.

5. If a patient is inactive and ready to change, help the patient create an activity plan that is fun, developmentally appropriate, and realistic.

6. As part of any activity plan, identify the FITT.

7. Identify a social support or "activity buddy" for your patient. This could be a friend or a family member.

8. Record your recommendations in the medical chart and follow-up with patients at subsequent visits.

9. Advocate for physical activity counseling to be part of your managed care service requirements and thus reimbursable.

In the Community

1. Be an advocate in your community schools for more physical education and health education classes; classes that encourage lifetime activities as well as competitive sports.

2. Be an advocate in your community for more safe and convenient venues for activity, including parks, recreation centers, bicycle lanes, access to school facilities, and playgrounds for after school activities.

3. Become familiar with resources in your community, including the YMCA, community recreation departments, community sports programs, and other youth programs.

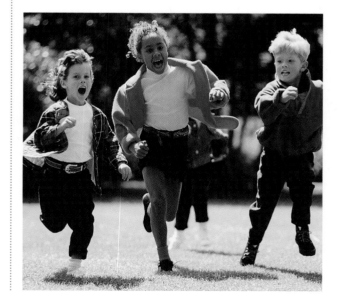

FINISH LINE

Physicians and other health care providers are an important part of a national effort to increase physical activity among the population. Levels of physical activity should be assessed in the office and inactive youth should be encouraged to increase their activity. A written physical activity prescription is helpful to those patients who demonstrate a willingness to change their behavior. Involvement with schools and communities to create policies that promote physical activity is an effective way to promote physical activity in large numbers of children. By promoting lifetime activities as well as organized sports and athletics, physicians can positively impact the current health and well-being of youth and potentially make an impact on the prevention of chronic diseases in adulthood.

For More Information

1. American Academy of Pediatrics, Committee on Sports Medicine and Fitness: Assessing physical activity and fitness in the office setting. *Pediatrics* 1994;93:686–688.

2. Elster AB, Kuznets NJ (eds): *Guidelines for Adolescent Preventive Services (GAPS): Recommendations and Rationale.* Baltimore, MD, Williams and Wilkins, 1994.

3. Green M (ed): *Bright Futures: Guidelines for Health Supervision of Infants, Children, and Adolescents.* Arlington, VA, National Center for Education in Maternal and Child Health, 1994.

4. Centers for Disease Control and Prevention: Guidelines for school and community programs to promote lifelong physical activity among young people. *Morb Mortal Wkly Rep* 1997;46:1–36.

5. National Centers for Chronic Disease Prevention and Health Promotion: Physical Activity and Health: A Report of the Surgeon General. Atlanta, GA, US Department of Health and Human Services, Centers for Disease Control and Prevention, 1996.

6. Sallis JF, Patrick K: Physical activity guidelines for adolescents: Consensus statement. *Pediatr Exerc Sci* 1994;6:434–447.

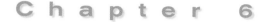

Chapter 6

The Preparticipation Physical Evaluation

JAMES R. BARRETT, MD
GEOFFREY S. KUHLMAN, MD
CARL L. STANITSKI, MD
ERIC SMALL, MD

Over six million high school students participate in sports each year. With this many participants, the preparticipation physical evaluation (PPE) is one of the most commonly performed examinations. Many physicians dread the tediousness of these exams, given the lack of consistent guidelines for performing them in the past. However, over the past decade, the PPE has evolved to allow physicians to provide quality examinations nationwide. In the early 1990s, the American Academy of Family Physicians, the American Academy of Pediatrics, the American Medical Society for Sports Medicine, the American Orthopaedic Society for Sports Medicine, and the American Osteopathic Academy of Sports Medicine formed the Preparticipation Examination Task Force to standardize the conduct and content of these examinations. In 1992, the Task Force published recommendations for the PPE based on the consensus of the current literature. These guidelines were updated in 1997 and serve as the basis for the current PPE.

Goals of the PPE

The purpose of the PPE is not to disqualify athletes; less than 2% are actually disqualified based on the results of the evaluation. Rather, the primary goals of the PPE are to detect conditions that might predispose the athlete to injury, to detect conditions that might be life threatening or disabling, and to meet legal or insurance requirements. The secondary goals are to determine general health, to counsel athletes on health-related issues, and to assess fitness level.

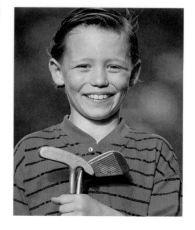

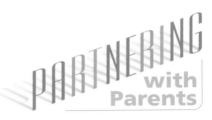

*My son had a physical exam-
ination for participation in
football last year. Does he
still need to see his physician
this year?*

While the PPE is often quite comprehensive, it was never designed
to take the place of a regular
physician visit. The setting or time
allocation for the PPE is often not
conducive to discussions of health
issues that are of primary importance during the adolescent years,
such as drug and alcohol use,
smoking, sexual activity education,
safety issues, and diagnosis of
depression.

*When should my child have a
PPE, relative to the beginning
of an athletic season?*

The best time for the PPE is about
4 to 6 weeks before the beginning of the athletic season. This
allows enough time for thorough
evaluations, consultations, and
rehabilitation of any identified
musculoskeletal injuries.

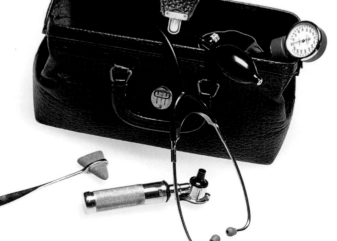

Identifying athletes who may need
further diagnostic testing, counseling,
and/or rehabilitation is the primary
goal of the PPE, but there are a
number of other expectations.
Sometimes, parents expect the PPE to
be a comprehensive evaluation of the
athlete's health, including areas that
may be considered unrelated to sports
participation, such as teenage sexu-
ality, substance abuse, immunizations,
behavioral counseling, and others.
Parents frequently use the PPE as
the only medical evaluation for their
child or adolescent, expecting it to be
comprehensive. In contrast, many
physicians view the PPE as a cursory

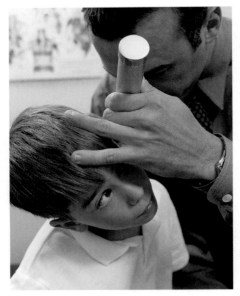

examination, intended only to detect conditions that might limit or impair
athletic endeavors. Because parents and physicians view the evaluation differently, it is critical that parents be clearly advised about the intent of the PPE to
clarify its scope and purpose.

Methods of Conducting the PPE

The PPE is typically conducted in one of three ways: the locker room method,
the station method, and the office-based method.

In the locker room method, athletes traditionally are lined up single file
while the physician examines each athlete individually. One benefit of this
method is that it requires few personnel and can be done with little preparation. However, it affords little privacy for the athlete, is usually noisy so that
the physician has a difficult time auscultating the heart and lungs, and is
often too brief.

The station method divides the examination into several components with
physicians, nurses, athletic trainers, and coaches each assigned one task. This
method is ideally suited for screening large numbers of athletes. Two benefits
of this method are its relative efficiency and its high yield in identifying
abnormalities. However, this method affords less rapport with athletes and a
lack of privacy.

The individual office-based method has the advantages of
an established physician-patient relationship in which the
past medical history is known and continuity of care is fostered. The disadvantages can include a lack of consistency
among physicians, potential unfamiliarity with the sport
and disqualifying conditions by the physician, and the lack
of cost-effectiveness.

Timing

Ideally, the PPE is performed early enough in the preseason to ensure that athletes who have medical problems can be thoroughly evaluated and treated, but not so early that intervening injuries are likely to occur. Most sources recommend that the evaluation take place at least 4 to 6 weeks before the first scheduled practice.

The American Academy of Pediatrics recommends yearly health supervisions for adolescents, but most sports medicine physicians feel that athletes do not need a complete evaluation every year. Most sources recommend that the PPE be conducted before the beginning of each new level of competition (ie, middle school or junior high, high school, and college) with annual updates of the history and targeted physical examinations of areas of concern. Despite these recommendations, most state high school athletic associations require annual evaluations. A recent survey of all 50 states and the District of Columbia found that 65% of states require annual examination of all athletes competing in high school sports.

History

As with any health evaluation, the history identifies most potential problems for young athletes. The key to identifying these problems is the questionnaire that systematically screens for conditions that frequently cause problems in athletes or that could lead to sudden death during athletic activity. **Table 6.1** lists some of the most important questions to ask in the examination. Note that the PPE forms provided by state high school athletic associations do not incorporate all of the screening questions recommended by the Preparticipation Examination Task Force. Some states encourage use of the forms written by the Task Force.

Most experts agree that despite the best screening of athletes for sudden death, only a few who die could have been detected through the screening history and physical examination.

Athletes typically complete their history forms without input from their parents. One study showed that only 40% of PPE forms matched when filled out independently by parent and child. It is essential that both the athlete and the parents complete the form together, so that a thorough and accurate history is obtained.

Physical Examination

Two key components of the physical examination identify most athletes who warrant further evaluation or disqualification. The history and musculoskeletal examinations detect most of the problems noted on the evaluation and should be the focus of any preparticipation screening. The medical evaluation form recommended by the Preparticipation Examination Task Force is shown in **Figure 6.1**.

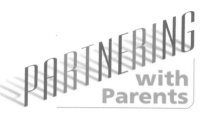

Do I need to attend the PPE with my child?

Although you may not be asked to attend the PPE with your child, it is very important that you review the accuracy and completeness of the past medical history and family history that is given. Your child may not know or remember some of the history. Most of the important information obtained in the PPE is obtained from the history.

Table 6.1 — *Medical History Questions*

Question	Reason
1. Injury or illness since last checkup?	Targets potential physical examination concerns
2. Chronic illnesses, hospitalizations, or surgeries?	Identifies potential counseling or rehabilitation issues
3. Any medications or supplements of any type?	Identifies drugs that may inhibit or interfere with sports participation
4. Allergies to medications, insects, food?	Alerts physicians and trainers for potential allergic reactions
5. Dizziness, passed out, chest pain with exercise; history of sudden death in a close relative < 50 years old?	Identifies potential causes of sudden death due to cardiovascular problems
6. History of hypertension or murmur?	Targets cardiovascular concerns
7. Ever been restricted from sports by physician?	Identifies potential disqualifying problems
8. Any skin problems?	Identifies potential transmittable disease during contact
9. Concussion, "knocked out", unconsciousness, or memory loss, seizure, or severe/frequent headache?	Targets neurologic concerns
10. Stinger, burner, pinched nerve, numbness/tingling in extremities?	Targets neurologic concerns
11. Problems while exercising in the heat?	Targets heat illness concerns
12. Asthma, allergies, wheezing, difficulty breathing, chest pain?	Identifies potential for exercise-induced asthma
13. Special equipment or devices not usually used in your sport?	Identifies potential concerns for physician follow-up
14. Glasses, contacts, or vision or eye problems?	Identifies ophthalmologic concerns
15. Strain, sprain, fracture, joint pain or swelling?	Identifies potential musculoskeletal problems
16. Concerns about weight, do you lose weight regularly for your sport?	Identifies potential disordered eating
17. Feel stressed out?	Clue to ask follow up questions regarding drug use, eating problems, sexuality, home/school problems
18. Recent immunizations (tetanus, measles, hepatitis B, chickenpox)	Health maintenance issues
19. Female only: Menstrual history	Identifies oligomenorrhea and amenorrhea and potential risk for poor nutrition, stress fractures

Adapted with permission from the American Academy of Family Physicians, American Academy of Pediatrics, American Medical Society for Sports Medicine, American Orthopaedic Society for Sports Medicine, Osteopathic Academy of Sports Medicine: The PPE physical examination, in *Preparticipation Physical Examination*, ed 2. Minneapolis, MN, McGraw-Hill, 1997, pp 17–27.

PHYSICAL EXAMINATION

Name _____   Date of birth _____

Height _____ Weight_____% Body fat (optional) _____ Pulse _____ BP ___ / ___(___/___, ___/ ___)

Vision R 20/ _____ L 20/ _____ Corrected: Y N Pupils: Equal_____ Unequal_____

	Normal	Abnormal Findings	Initials*
MEDICAL			
Appearance			
Eyes/Ears/Nose/Throat			
Lymph Nodes			
Heart			
Pulses			
Lungs			
Abdomen			
Genitalia (males only)			
Skin			
MUSCULOSKELETAL			
Neck			
Back			
Shoulder/arm			
Elbow/forearm			
Wrist/hand			
Hip/thigh			
Knee			
Leg/ankle			
Foot			

*Station-based examination only

CLEARANCE

❑ Cleared

❑ Cleared after completing evaluation/rehabilitation for: _____

_____

_____

_____

❑ Not cleared for:_____ Reason: _____

Recommendations:_____

_____

_____

_____

Name of physician (print/type _____ Date_____

Address _____ Phone _____

Signature of physician _____, MD or DO

Adapted with permission from the American Academy of Family Physicians, American Academy of Pediatrics, American Medical Society for Sports Medicine, American Orthopaedic Society for Sports Medicine, Osteopathic Academy of Sports Medicine: The PPE physical examination, in *Preparticipation Physical Examination*, ed 2. Minneapolis, MN, McGraw-Hill, 1997, pp 17-27.

Figure 6.1 Medical evaluation form

Table 6.2	*Cardiovascular Screening in Athletes*	
Condition	**Cardiovascular Examination**	**Abnormality**
Hypertension	Blood pressure	Varies with age—general guideline is >135/85 mm Hg in adolescents
Coarctation of aorta	Femoral pulses	Decreased intensity of pulse
Hypertrophic cardiomyopathy	Auscultation with provocative maneuvers (standing, supine, valsalva	Systolic ejection murmur that intensifies with standing or Valsalva's maneuver)
Marfan's symdrome	Auscultation	Aortic (decrescendo diastolic murmur) or mitral insufficiency (holosystolic murmur)

Adapted with permission from Maron BJ, Thompson PO, Puffer JC: Cardiovascular preparticipation screening of competitive athletes: A Statement from the Sudden Death Committee [clinical cardiology] and Congenital Cardiac Defects Committee [cardiovascular disease in the young] American Heart Association. *Circulation* 1996;94:850–856.

Special Considerations for the Examination of Injured or Symptomatic Joints

- Inspect for visual deformity, muscle mass, asymmetry, and swelling.

- Palpate for localized areas of tenderness, warmth, and effusion.

- Assess range of motion (eg, an athlete with hip pain should be tested for loss of internal rotation and abduction, which can be seen in slipped capital femoral epiphysis and Legg-Calvé-Perthes disease).

- Test neurovascular status by evaluating muscle strength, sensation, reflexes, and pulses of the involved limb (eg, an athlete with a history of burners should undergo complete neurovascular testing of the neck and upper extremities).

- Test joint stability (eg, an athlete with knee pain should undergo tests for valgus and varus stress, the Lachman's test, and the posterior drawer test) as discussed in Chapter 36.

Cardiovascular Examination

The cardiovascular examination should include evaluation of peripheral pulses, murmurs, and blood pressure. **Table 6.2** summarizes important aspects of the screening cardiovascular examination. Note that all diastolic murmurs and grade 3/6 systolic murmurs warrant further evaluation. Hypertrophic cardiomyopathy (HCM) may produce a systolic murmur that cannot be distinguished from an innocent murmur. The murmur of HCM increases in intensity with a Valsalva maneuver (decreased ventricular filling, increased obstruction) and decreases with squatting (increased ventricular filling, decreased obstruction). Note that it will also increase in intensity when the athlete moves from a squatting to standing position.

Blood pressures obtained during the PPE are often elevated; sometimes, this is due to the use of a blood pressure cuff that is too small, particularly in large adolescents. However, at times the athlete's blood pressure is truly elevated, given that a table with age-based norms is used. Hypertension is rarely severe enough to disqualify an athlete from participation, but it needs to be identified and followed by the athlete's regular physician.

Musculoskeletal Examination

The musculoskeletal examination is of particular importance because it typically accounts for 50% of the abnormal physical findings identified on the PPE. The examination should focus on areas previously injured or on areas that are symptomatic. Ninety-two percent of orthopaedic injuries are detected on the basis of the history alone. The 2-minute orthopaedic screening examination is a quick screening for detecting musculoskeletal problems in asymptomatic individuals. **Figure 6.2** shows how to conduct this examination.

Some authorities recommend a sport-specific approach to the physical examination. This method emphasizes those areas that are most commonly injured or diseased in each specific sport. For example, a swimmer's examination would focus on the shoulders and ears (otitis externa), whereas a wrestler's examination would emphasize the skin, body fat composition, and shoulder.

Figure 6.2 The general musculoskeletal screening examination.

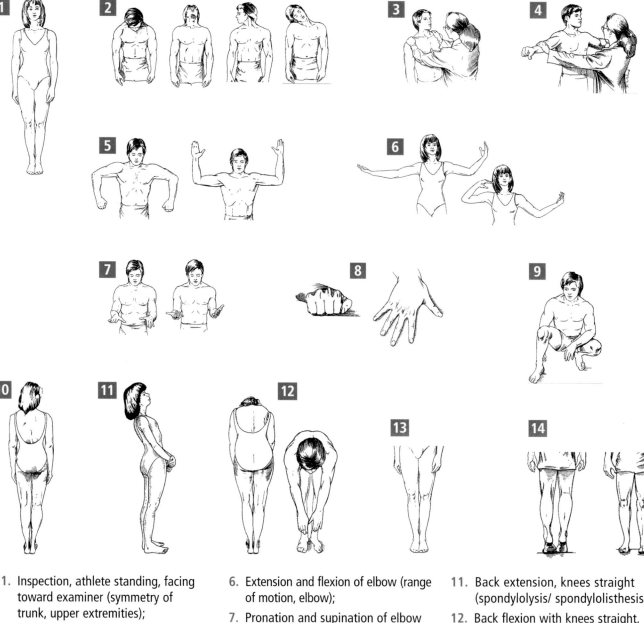

1. Inspection, athlete standing, facing toward examiner (symmetry of trunk, upper extremities);

2. Forward flexion, extension, rotation, lateral flexion of neck (range of motion, cervical spine);

3. Resisted shoulder shrug (strength, trapezius);

4. Resisted shoulder abduction (strength, deltoid);

5. Internal and external rotation of shoulder (range of motion, glenohumeral joint);

6. Extension and flexion of elbow (range of motion, elbow);

7. Pronation and supination of elbow (range of motion, elbow and wrist);

8. Clench fist, then spread fingers (range of motion, hand and fingers);

9. "Duck walk" four steps (motion of hip, knee, and ankle; strength; balance);

10. Inspection, athlete facing away from examiner (symmetry of trunk, upper extremities);

11. Back extension, knees straight (spondylolysis/ spondylolisthesis);

12. Back flexion with knees straight, facing toward and away from examiner (range of motion, thoracic and lumbosacral spine; spine curvature; hamstring flexibility);

13. Inspection of lower extremities, contraction of quadriceps muscles (alignment, symmetry);

14. Standing on toes, then on heels (symmetry, calf; strength; balance).

Figures 2.1-2.9 and 2.11-2.14 © 1997 Rebekah Dodson; Figure 2.10 © Terry Boles.

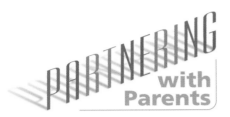

How often will my son or daughter need a preparticipation physical evaluation (PPE)?

The frequency of required evaluations varies by state. Most commonly, a physical evaluation is required every year. To determine the requirements of your state, check with the school district or the state high school athletic association.

Laboratory Studies

Laboratory studies have not been shown to be cost-effective or warranted in young athletes who are asymptomatic. Obtaining a routine urinalysis and hematocrit on all athletes has been largely abandoned, as these tests do not identify athletes who require disqualification and have a high rate of false-positive results. Similarly, electrocardiogram, echocardiogram, and stress testing are not recommended as screening tests for asymptomatic individuals because of the high rate of false-positive tests and their high costs.

Sports Classification

Sports are classified based on the likelihood of collision injury and on the strenuousness of exercise. These classifications are used to guide physicians on the risk of injury and the degree of cardiopulmonary fitness required. The American Academy of Pediatrics has established classification guidelines that can be found in **Tables 6.3** and **6.4**.

Table 6.3 *Sport Classification by Contact*

Contact/Collision	Limited Contact	Noncontact
Basketball	Baseball	Archery
Boxing	Bicycling	Badminton
Diving	Cheerleading	Body building
Field hockey	Canoeing/Kayaking (white water)	Canoeing/Kayaking (flat water)
Football (flag, tackle)	Fencing	Crew/Rowing
Ice hockey	Field (high jump, pole vault)	Curling
Lacrosse	Floor hockey	Dancing
Martial arts	Gymnastics	Field events (discus, javelin, shot put)
Rodeo	Handball	Golf
Rugby	Horseback riding	Orienteering
Ski jumping	Racquetball	Power lifting
Soccer	Skating (ice, in-line, roller)	Race walking
Team handball	Skiing (downhill, water)	Riflery
Water polo	Softball	Rope jumping
Wrestling	Squash	Running
	Ultimate frisbee	Sailing
	Volleyball	Scuba diving
	Windsurfing/Surfing	Strength training
		Swimming
		Table tennis
		Tennis
		Track
		Weight lifting

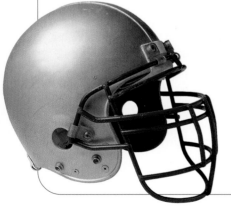

Adapted with permission from American Academy of Pediatrics Committee on Sports Medicine and Fitness: Medical conditions affecting sports participation. *Pediatrics* 1994;94:757–760.

Table 6.4 *Sports Classification by Intensity*

High to Moderate Intensity	High to Moderate Intensity	High to Moderate Static Intensity	Low Dynamic and Low Intensity
Boxing	Badminton	Archery	Bowling
Crew/Rowing	Baseball	Auto racing	Cricket
Cross-country skiing	Basketball	Diving	Curling
Cycling	Field hockey	Equestrian	Golf
Downhill skiing	Lacrosse	Field events (jumping)	Riflery
Fencing	Orienteering	Field events (throwing)	
Football	Ping-pong	Gymnastics	
Ice hockey	Race walking	Karate or judo	
Rugby	Racquetball	Motorcycling	
Running (sprint)	Soccer	Rodeoing	
Speed skating	Squash	Sailing	
Water polo	Swimming	Ski jumping	
Wrestling	Tennis	Water skiing	
	Volleyball	Weight lifting	

Adapted with permission from American Academy of Pediatrics Committee on Sports Medicine and Fitness: Medical conditions affecting sports participation. *Pediatrics* 1994;94:757–760.

Clearance to Play

Few athletes are disqualified from activity based on conditions identified during the PPE. **Table 6.5** lists the most current recommendations regarding medical conditions and contraindications to participation. This table is designed to be understood by medical and nonmedical personnel. In the "Explanation" section below, "needs evaluation" means that a physician with appropriate knowledge and experience should assess the safety of a given sport for an athlete with the listed medical condition. Unless otherwise noted, this is because of the variability of the severity of the disease or of the risk of injury among the specific sports, or both. It is important to work with athletes to find safe, enjoyable sports in which they can participate and not eliminate all sports participation, depending on the condition that is detected. For specific cardiac conditions, refer to the proceedings of the 26th Bethesda Conference on cardiovascular abnormalities and participation in sports and in Chapter 17. **Figure 6.3** is a sample Clearance to Return to Play form.

Occasionally, an athlete will disagree with a physician's recommendation for restricting participation in a particular sport. In these cases, it is important to fully explain the reasons for the recommendation and consider having the athlete and parent sign a document acknowledging that this discussion occurred and that they were informed of the risks. Athletes who request a second opinion should be encouraged to do so. Ultimately, the team physician is responsible for ensuring that athletes are able to participate safely and without undue risk of injury.

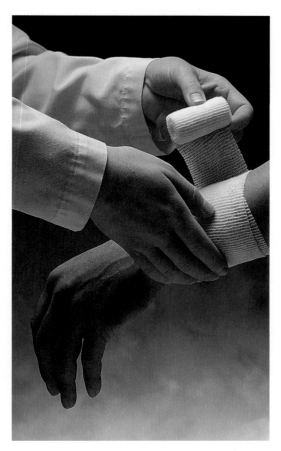

Table 6.5 *Medical Conditions and Sports Participation*

Condition	Participate?	Explanation
Atlantoaxial instability (instability of the joint between cervical vertebrae 1 and 2)	Qualified Yes	Athlete needs evaluation to assess risk of spinal cord injury during sports partipation.
Bleeding disorder	Qualified Yes	Athlete needs evaluation
Cardiovascular diseases Carditis (inflammation of the heart)	No	Carditis may result in sudden death with exertion.
Hypertension (high blood pressure)	Qualified Yes	Those with significant essential (unexplained) hypertension should avoid weight and power lifting, body building, and strength training. Those with secondary hypertension (hypertension caused by a previously identified disease), or severe essential hypertension, need evaluation.[1]
Congenital heart disease (structural heart defects present at birth)	Qualified Yes	Those with mild forms may participate fully; those with moderate or severe forms, or who have undergone surgery, need evaluation.[2]
Dysrhythmia (irregular heart rhythm)	Qualified Yes	Athlete needs evaluation because some types require therapy or make certain sports dangerous, or both.
Mitral valve prolapse (abnormal heart valve)	Qualified Yes	Those with symptoms (chest pain, symptoms of possible dysrhythmia) or evidence of mitral regurgitation (leaking) on physical examination need evaluation. All others may participate fully.
Heart murmur	Qualified Yes	If the murmur is innocent (does not indicate heart disease), full participation is permitted. Otherwise the athlete needs evaluation (see "Congenital heart disease" and "Mitral valve prolapse" above).
Cerebral palsy	Qualified Yes	Athlete needs evaluation.
Diabetes mellitus	Yes	All sports can be played with proper attention to diet, hydration, and insulin therapy. Particular attention is needed for activities that last 30 minutes or more.
Diarrhea	Qualified No	Unless disease is mild, no participation is permitted, because diarrhea may increase the risk of dehydration and heat illness. See "Fever" below.
Eating disorders Anorexia nervosa Bulimia nervosa	Qualified Yes	These patients need both medical and psychiatric assessment before participation.
Eyes Functionally one-eyed athlete Loss of an eye Detached retina Previous eye surgery or serious eye injury	Qualified Yes	A functionally one-eyed athlete has a best corrected visual acuity of <20/40 in the worse eye. These athletes would suffer significant disability if the better eye was seriously injured as would those with loss of an eye. Some athletes who have previously undergone eye surgery or had a serious eye injury may have an increased risk of injury because of weakened eye tissue. Availability of eye guards approved by the American Society of Testing Materials (ASTM) and other protective equipment may allow participation in most sports, but this must be judged on an individual basis.

[1] for details see *Pediatrics* 1987;79:1–25
[2] for details see *Med Sci Sports Exerc* 1994;26(suppl 10):S246–S253.

Continued.

Table 6.5 *Medical Conditions and Sports Participation—cont'd.*

Condition	Participate?	Explanation
Fever	No	Fever can increase cardiopulmonary effort, reduce maximum exercise capacity, make heat illness more likely, and increase orthostatic hypotension during exercise. Fever may rarely accompany myocarditis or other infections that may make exercise dangerous.
Heat illness, history of	Qualified Yes	Because of the increased likelihood of recurrence, the athlete needs individual assessment to determine the presence of predisposing conditions and to arrange a prevention strategy.
HIV infection	Yes	Because of the apparent minimal risk to others, all sports may be played that the state of health allows. In all athletes, skin lesions should be properly covered, and athletic personnel should use universal precautions when handling blood or body fluids with visible blood.
Kidney: absence of one	Qualified Yes	Athlete needs individual assessment for contact/collision and limited contact sports.
Liver: enlarged	Qualified Yes	If the liver is acutely enlarged, participation should be avoided because of risk of rupture. If the liver is chronically enlarged, individual assessment is needed before collision/contact or limited contact sports are played.
Malignancy	Qualified Yes	Athlete needs individual assessment.
Musculoskeletal disorders	Qualified Yes	Athlete needs individual assessment.
Neurologic		
History of serious head or spine trauma, severe or repeated, concussions, or craniotomy.	Qualified Yes	Athlete needs individual assessment for collision/ contact or limited contact sports, and also for noncontact sports if there are deficits in judgment or cognition. Recent research supports a conservative approach to management of concussions. Risk of convulsion during participation is minimal.
Convulsive disorder, well controlled	Yes	
Convulsive disorder, poorly controlled	Qualified Yes	Athlete needs individual assessment for collision/contact or limited contact sports. Avoid the following noncontact sports: archery, riflery, swimming, weight or power lifting, strength training, or sports involving heights. In these sports, occurrence of a convulsion may be a risk to self or others.
Obesity	Qualified Yes	Because of the risk of heat illness, obese persons need careful acclimatization and hydration.
Organ transplant recipient	Qualified Yes	Athlete needs individual assessment.
Ovary: absence		Risk of severe injury to the remaining ovary is minimal.

Continued.

Table 6.5 *Medical Conditions and Sports Participation—cont'd.*

Condition	Participate?	Explanation
Respiratory Pulmonary compromise including cystic fibrosis		Athlete needs individual assessment, but generally all sports may be played if oxygenation remains satisfactory during a graded exercise test. Patients with cystic fibrosis need acclimatization and good hydration to reduce the risk of heat illness.
Asthma	Yes	With proper medication and education, only athletes with the most severe asthma will have to modify their participation.
Acute upper respiratory infection	Qualified Yes	Upper respiratory obstruction may affect pulmonary function. Athlete needs individual assessment for all but mild diseases. See "Fever" above.
Sickle cell disease	Qualified Yes	Athlete needs individual assessment. In general if status of the illness permits, all but high exertion, collision/contact sports may be played. Overheating, dehydration, and chilling must be avoided.
Sickle cell trait	Yes	It is unlikely that individuals with sickle cell trait (AS) have an increased risk of sudden death or other medical problems during athletic participation except under the most extreme condition of heat, humidity, and possibly increased altitude. These individuals, like all athletes, should be carefully conditioned, acclimatized, and hydrated to reduce any possible risk.
Skin: boils, herpes simplex, impetigo, scabies, molluscum contagiosum	Qualified Yes	While the patient is contagious, participation in gymnastics with mats, martial arts, wrestling, or other collision/contact or limited contact sports is not allowed. Herpes simplex virus probably is not transmitted via mats.
Spleen, enlarged	Qualified Yes	Patients with acutely enlarged spleens should avoid all sports because of risk of rupture. Those with chronically enlarged spleens need individual assessment before playing collision/contact or limited contact sports.
Testicle: absent or undescended	Yes	Certain sports may require a protective cup.

Adapted with permission from American Academy of Pediatrics Committee on Sports Medicine and Fitness: Medical conditions affecting sports participation. *Pediatrics* 1994;94:757–760.

Figure 6.3 Sample Clearance to Return to Play form.

Clearance to Return to Play

Name_____ Date _____

Diagnosis _____

May return to: ❑ Full participation in _____ on _____
                                                    (sport or activity)   (date)

                ❑ Limited participation (with the following restrictions):

                _____

                ❑ Not cleared to participate until_____

Special Instructions:

General conditioning exercises that can be continued during recovery:

_____

Rehabilitation exercises: _____

Recommendation for taping, pads, and/or protective equipment:

_____

Medications (or other treatments) that may need to be taken during school or available at practice/games:

_____

Suggested number of practices to complete before returning to games or competition:_____

Medical follow-up with: _____ Date:_____

_____

Physician name _____ Phone _____

Address _____

Signature _____

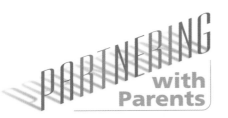

Will my child need to undergo any laboratory or radiographic studies at the PPE?

Routine laboratory studies and radiographs are not generally indicated. Based on information obtained during the history and physical examination, however, your physician may feel that further studies are indicated.

FINISH LINE

Over the past decade, the format of the PPE has changed significantly. Thanks in large part to the work of the Preparticipation Examination Task Force, more standardized recommendations for screening athletes prior to sports participation have been developed. The next step is to implement these changes on a local level to ensure more consistency in the evaluation process. By doing so, young athletes will be safer when participating in sporting events.

For More Information

1. Fahrenbach MC, Thompson PD: The preparticipation sports examination: Cardiovascular considerations for screening. *Cardiol Clin* 1992;10:319–328.

2. Glover DW, Maron BJ: Profile of preparticipation cardiovascular screening for high school athletes. *JAMA* 1998;279:1817–1819.

3. Grafe MW, Paul GR, Foster TE: The preparticipation sports examination. for high school and college athletes. *Clin Sports Med* 1997;16:569–591.

4. Maron BJ, Mitchell JH: Revised eligibility recommendations for competitive athletes with cardiovascular abnormalities: *J Am Coll Cardiol* 1994;24:848–850.

5. Smith DM, Kovan JR, Rich BSE, Tanner SM (eds): *Preparticipation Physical Evaluation,* ed 2. Minneapolis, MN, McGraw-Hill, 1997.

Chapter 7

Effects of Training on a Child's Body

THOMAS W. ROWLAND, MD

By its nature, exercise is designed to place stress on body systems. The goal of repeated bouts of exercise during training is to stimulate adaptive physiologic responses that will enhance performance. For example, when an individual performs regular resistance training, it is anticipated that the response to stress placed on skeletal muscle will be improved strength. Similarly, when an athlete runs 5 miles a day, stresses are placed on the heart, lungs, and skeletal muscles. Adaptive changes in these systems increase the ability of muscles to use oxygen and, therefore, improve performance in distance running events.

The stresses of training, when applied within certain limits, are beneficial to sports performance. Excessive training places an undue amount of stress on the body, leading to tissue breakdown and injury. Therefore, scheduling training that remains within the bounds of positive adaptation is necessary.

The concept of adaptive response to applied demand is relevant for young athletes, as well as adults. Children are growing, and the body systems under stress from training are immature. This fact raises two important questions about the training of young athletes: first, might their responses to training dictate different training regimens than those used for adults; second, how do the growing tissues of young athletes respond to the stresses of early intense training?

Because children are becoming increasingly involved in training programs that once would have been considered intense even for elite adult athletes, understanding the child's response to training becomes increasingly relevant. Such knowledge is far from complete, and many questions remain unanswered. The result is a gap between what is known and what needs to be known when counseling young athletes, parents, and coaches. Additional research is needed to narrow this gap over time.

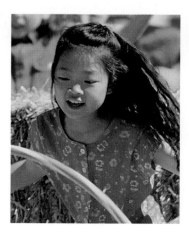

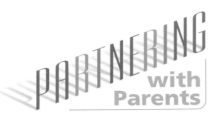

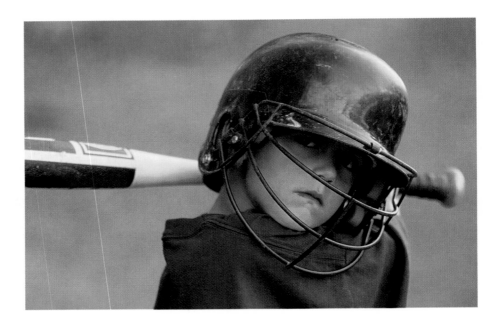

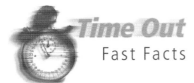

The Young Athlete's Response to Training

Measuring the physiologic and performance responses to physical training in children is difficult. Speed, endurance, and strength normally improve as a result of natural growth and development. Therefore, it is difficult to differentiate the effects of exercise from the normal improvement in motor performance with growth.

Nonetheless, there is a growing body of information about how children respond to endurance, short-burst, and resistance training. And there is evidence that in certain areas, specifically in aerobic training, prepubertal children may differ from adults in their adaptations to training.

Aerobic Training

An adult who participates in a program of regular endurance exercise typically demonstrates a set of physiologic changes called the "fitness effect." This includes a lower resting heart rate and greater maximal stroke volume and cardiac output. These changes result in greater ability of the body to use oxygen for aerobic metabolism, indicated by measurement of maximal oxygen uptake ($V_{O_{2max}}$) on bicycle or treadmill testing. A previously sedentary adult can be expected to improve $V_{O_{2max}}$ by 15% to 30% given a program of adequate intensity, frequency, and duration (three 30-minute sessions a week for 8 weeks in which the heart works at 75% of maximum).

Studies in children that have followed the same program design as those in adults have generally indicated a rise of $V_{O_{2max}}$ of only 5% to 10% in both boys and girls. Moreover, a significant percentage of children in these studies demonstrate no increase in maximal oxygen uptake with a level of training that leads to predictable gains in adults.

Other evidence that children have a diminished response to aerobic training comes from a comparison of values of $V_{O_{2max}}$ in child and adult endurance athletes. Boys who are distance runners usually have a $V_{O_{2max}}$ of about 65 mL/kg/min, compared with 52 mL/kg/min in the average nontraining boy. Young adult male distance runners often have a $V_{O_{2max}}$ of 75 mL/kg/min, while the nonathletic man has a VO_{2max} of 45 mL/kg/min. This has suggested to some researchers that a "ceiling" exists for VO_{2max} before puberty, and the hormonal influences surrounding adolescence enhance aerobic trainability.

The reason that children show a diminished response of VO_{2max} to training compared with adults is unclear. Some believe that the higher daily physical activity levels of children might have a training effect; therefore, further structured training programs do not significantly increase activity levels. Others argue that a training benefit from daily activity is unlikely because of the following: 1) the spontaneous activity of children is typically short-burst rather than sustained, and 2) children who are deprived of daily activities (ie, prolonged bed rest) do not experience a large decrease in VO_{2max}. Moreover, there does not appear to be a strong relationship between VO_{2max} and the amount of habitual physical activity.

Biologic differences probably are responsible for the blunted VO_{2max} response to endurance training in children. This issue is difficult to address, because the physiologic mechanisms responsible for increases in VO_{2max} in individuals of any age are not well understood. However, increases in maximal cardiac stroke volume mediated by augmented plasma volume and/or improved oxygen extraction by muscles may be greater after puberty.

The diminished changes in VO_{2max} with endurance training in children may mean that improvement in actual performance in endurance events (ie, distance running) is also limited. VO_{2max} is generally linked to an athlete's ability in such events; however, factors such as motivation, body physique, and enhanced efficiency of movement may contribute to any improvement in endurance performance with training in children. Studies that longitudinally compare endurance performance in training child athletes with that in non-training children are needed to determine the trainability of endurance athletes who have not reached puberty.

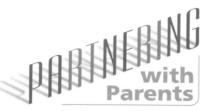

Is it possible for prepubertal children to increase their strength through a weight-training program?

Yes. Several studies have shown strength gains of 20% to 30% for both boys and girls involved in strength training programs. However, these gains are not accompanied by increased muscle size. It is unclear as to how these strength gains affect performance.

Anaerobic Training

Short-burst sports activities, such as sprints, jumping events, and downhill skiing, are anaerobic in nature, meaning that these events do not rely on oxygen for release of energy for muscular contraction. The mechanisms underlying the physiologic and performance responses to training in these events are poorly understood, but almost certainly are different than those involved in endurance or aerobic training.

Assessing adaptations to anaerobic training is difficult because there is no established standard regimen of activity intensity and duration for anaerobic training, and there is no simple laboratory marker for anaerobic fitness as VO_{2max} is for aerobic fitness. The two most common means of assessing the level of anaerobic fitness are performance on field tests (eg, 50-yd sprint times) and maximal and mean power measured in the laboratory during a 30-second bout of all-out bicycling (eg, the Wingate test).

Training programs of short-duration, high-intensity exercise improve markers of anaerobic performance in adults. This experience has generally indicated that to be effective, such training needs to be of high intensity and performed to near exhaustion.

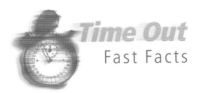

Training during childhood does not seem to affect measures of pulmonary function.

Very little information, however, is available on the responses of children to anaerobic training. Three studies have indicated that children's performance on Wingate tests can be improved with anaerobic training, but limited data have suggested failure of such training to improve sprint time. It is unclear, then, whether the qualitative or quantitative responses to anaerobic training differ in children and adults. Similarly, the most effective training regimens that might increase abilities in short-burst activities in children are unknown.

Strength Training

As recently as 30 years ago, children were considered to be incapable of improving muscle strength through resistance training. This conclusion was based on the assumption that circulating levels of testosterone are necessary for such responses.

Abundant research has subsequently proven this concept false. Since 1980, a series of resistance training studies using free weights over an 8- to 20-week training regimen have shown significant improvement in strength (about 20% to 30%). The magnitude of increased strength observed in these studies has been equivalent to that seen in studies involving adults. Moreover, strength improvements have been similar in boys and girls.

Interestingly, the increased strength observed when prepubertal children undergo resistance training is not accompanied by an increase in muscle size. Thus, weight training to improve the appearance of "muscle bulk" in young boys will not be effective. This observation leads to some intriguing questions about the mechanism for strength improvement in children. Strength has been considered a close reflection of muscle fiber size. Given that improvements in strength with resistance training in children occur without concomitant changes in fiber size, other factors, such as neural adaptations or enhanced intrinsic force-producing capacity of muscle, must be involved.

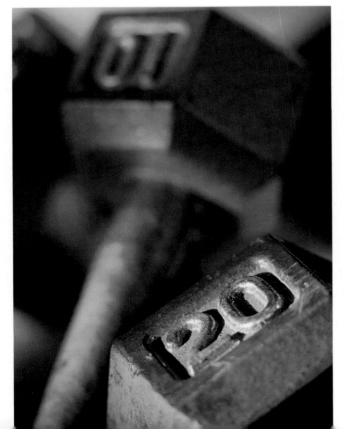

Studies that examine strength training programs for children have dispelled concerns that such activities may be unsafe for children if they have proper technique and strict supervision. Musculoskeletal injuries and loss of flexibility have not been observed as a result of these programs. Although acute injuries have been reported, these injuries involved children in unsupervised programs performing inappropriate resistance exercise, often in the home or in an unstructured setting.

Based on this information, properly designed resistance training programs are appropriate for children who want to gain strength and are involved in sports. This is especially true for young athletes who are motivated and can accept coaching instruction and who have attained proficiency in the skills of their sport. Strength training may help protect against injury and enhance performance. Moreover, such training may increase bone mineral content and help protect against future osteoporosis.

Training Effects on Specific Body Systems

Physical exercise requires coordinated functional responses of body systems that not only produce muscular propulsion, but also maintain the body's fluid, acid-base, and temperature homeostasis. Repetitive bouts of such exercise stimulate anatomic and physiologic adaptations in these systems. Research suggests that children and adults may differ in some of these responses.

Cardiovascular System

Adult athletes, particularly those involved in endurance sports, have a greater cardiac functional capacity than nonathletes. In addition, they typically have a constellation of findings identified as an "athlete's heart." Such findings include heart murmurs, significant resting bradycardia, electrocardiographic changes (eg, left ventricular hypertrophy, conduction delays), and echocardiograms showing left ventricular enlargement and/or hypertrophy.

Young endurance athletes also have a higher maximal cardiac output than nonathletic youngsters, although values (relative to body size) are less than those of their adult counterparts. Prepubertal endurance athletes, even those who are highly trained, do not usually have signs of the athlete's heart. This is particularly true of young distance runners, whose physical examinations, electrocardiograms, and echocardiograms have not been shown to differ from those of nonathletic children. Some studies in young swimmers, however, have demonstrated larger left ventricular dimensions on echocardiograms than in nonswimmers.

Biologic characteristics of pre- and postpubertal athletes may be responsible for the cardiac differences associated with endurance. However, the findings of the athlete's heart probably occur from sustained endurance training, which generally is lacking in the young athlete. Left ventricular size is not significantly determined by genetic factors, implying that differences in heart dimensions in older athletes and nonathletes are a manifestation of extended endurance training rather than genetic preselection.

Physicians caring for adults are aware that findings of the athlete's heart are normal physiologic responses to intensive endurance training, and that these athletes should not be falsely labeled as having heart disease. Because the young athlete does not typically exhibit such findings, features of the athlete's heart observed in a prepubertal athlete deserve a more thorough investigation into possible underlying heart disease.

Pulmonary System

Optimal lung function is obviously important for oxygen use and athletic performance, particularly in endurance events. Yet differences in measures of pulmonary function between young endurance athletes and nonathletes are not consistently observed. Young endurance athletes often have a greater maximal minute ventilation during exercise than nonathletic children, but these differences are less impressive and more variable than differences in VO_{2max}.

Training programs in nonathletic children do, however, typically lead to improvements in maximal ventilation that are of similar magnitude to increases in VO_{2max}. Such increases are the result of improved maximal tidal volume because maximal breathing rates do not change with training.

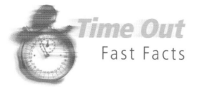

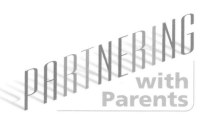

PARTNERING with Parents

Is strength training safe for prepubertal children?

Well-designed and supervised strength training programs are safe for prepubertal children. By definition, weight training involves repetitive lifts of submaximal weight. But weight training differs from weightlifting. Weightlifting, which is a competitive event involving single lifts of maximal weight, is not appropriate for prepubertal children.

Like $V_{O_{2max}}$, maximal ventilation ($V_{E_{2max}}$) does not typically change in young athletes as they train. This observation is consistent with the recognized negative relationship between a pretraining level of aerobic fitness and the magnitude response of $V_{O_{2max}}$ and $V_{E_{2max}}$ to a period of endurance training.

Reproductive System

Girls involved in exercise typically exhibit a later age of onset of menses (menarche) compared with nonathletes. The average age of menarche in these athletes is ages 13 to 14 years, compared with ages 12.3 to 12.8 years in healthy American nonathletes. Various explanations of this phenomenon include a true "delayed" onset of menses, a direct training effect that is linked to low body fat, the "energy drain" of training, psychological stress, and nutritional deficiencies.

Others have considered the later age of menarche in athletes as simply reflecting preselection; that is, girls with later menarche are more likely to stay involved in sports. This occurs because body features linked to later menarche (slender physique, long legs, low body fat) are also associated with successful athletic performance.

Delayed menarche should be distinguished from secondary amenorrhea, or cessation of menses following menarche. Secondary amenorrhea can result from intensive physical training, particularly in endurance sports. This effect often is linked to inadequate nutritional intake, because either a decrease in training volume or improvement in dietary habits may cause a resumption of regular menses. Although this "sports amenorrhea" has been viewed as benign, recent concerns have been raised regarding the effects of prolonged hypoestrogenemia on bone mineralization. Thus, extended amenorrhea from sports training in the teenage years may predispose these girls to later osteoporosis. More information on amenorrhea is provided in chapter 15 on female athletes.

Evidence also exists that exercise in children and adolescents, particularly in weightbearing sports, may improve bone mineralization. Although extended periods of amenorrhea and low estrogen should be avoided, participation in sports may be important for long-term bone health.

Little information is available about the effects of exercise on reproductive function in boys. High school cross-country athletes often mature later, but there is no evidence that cross-country training alters serum testosterone levels or delays secondary sexual characteristics in young male athletes.

Immune Function

Abundant research data indicate that exercise is associated with immunologic responses, including leukocytosis, elevations in T cell and B cell concentrations, and higher natural killer cell counts. However, the degree to which these changes influence clinical susceptibility to infection is uncertain. Studies in mice indicate that the risk of developing severe viral infections (myocarditis, poliomyelitis) is greater with Coxsackie infection and forced swimming.

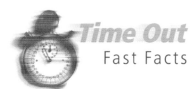

Time Out
Fast Facts

Extended periods of amenorrhea during the teenage years may predispose girls to osteoporosis.

In addition, other studies have suggested a greater incidence of viral respiratory infections in adult athletes than in nonathletes.

Few studies of immune function and exercise exist in the pediatric population. The alterations in immune function seen in children with acute bouts of exercise mimic those in adults. The nature and magnitude of these changes in athletic children do not differ from those of their nonathletic peers. Aerobic training in children has been shown to decrease resting leukocyte counts.

The clinical implications of these findings in children are unknown. A study of 12-year-old swimmers, hockey players, and gymnasts showed no differences in incidence of respiratory infections compared with nonathletes.

FINISH LINE

Aerobic and anaerobic training has only a modest effect on children. However, children can benefit significantly from strength training. In adults, training alters heart and lung function, but these changes have not been observed in children. Alterations in immune function occur with exercise in both children and adults. In girls, exercise may delay menarche and/or produce secondary amenorrhea, which increases the risk of decreased bone mineralization. More research is needed on the effects of various training methods on young athletes.

For More Information

1. Cahill BR, Misner JE, Boileau RA: The clinical importance of the anaerobic energy system and its assessment in human performance. *Am J Sports Med* 1997;25:863–872.

2. Malina RM: Menarche in athletes: A synthesis and hypothesis. *Ann Hum Biol* 1983;10:1–24.

3. Rowland TW (ed): *Developmental Exercise Physiology.* Champaign, IL, Human Kinetics, 1996, pp 97–116.

4. Rowland TW (ed): *Exercise and Children's Health.* Champaign, IL, Human Kinetics, 1990, pp 85–95.

5. Rowland TW: The physiological impact of intensive training on the prepubertal athlete, in Cahill BR, Pearl AJ (eds): *Intensive Participation in Children's Sports.* Champaign, IL, Human Kinetics, 1993, pp 167–193.

Section Editor
Oded Bar-Or, MD

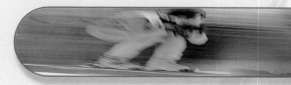

Chapter 8

Thermoregulation

JOHN F. COYLE, MD

Heatstroke is the third most common cause of exercise-related death in US high school athletes, following head injuries and cardiac disorders. Exercise-related heat illnesses also precipitate thousands of visits to the emergency department annually by young athletes. But these dramatic events are just a small fraction of the damage caused by the effects of heat during exercise. Untold harm comes from poor athletic performance and athlete dropout because of excessive thermal stress.

Basics of Thermoregulation

Heat storage in the exercising athlete is determined by the balance between heat generation and heat dissipation. Less than 25% of the energy expended during play is transformed into movement. The rest becomes heat. The more vigorous the athlete's efforts, the greater the amount of heat that will be generated. Besides endogenous heat production, four heat transfer processes complete the thermoregulation picture.

Evaporation of Sweat

As the athlete produces heat during exercise, blood warmed by the muscles stimulates temperature receptors in the deep core. These receptors plus peripheral thermal sensors stimulate the thermoregulatory center in the hypothalamus, which in turn inhibits cutaneous vasomotor tone and initiates sweating. Evaporation of sweat is the most powerful of the heat loss mechanisms in hot conditions. As the water in sweat evaporates, the phase change from liquid to gas consumes about 580 kcal of heat/liter of sweat evaporated. Dripping sweat affords no benefit; only sweat that evaporates provides cooling.

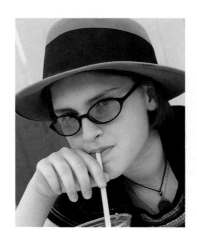

Convection

The transfer of heat by circulation of a liquid or gas, this is the mechanism by which hot air warms and frigid air cools the athlete. Convection is also the means by which heat is transferred by the blood.

Radiation

Direct sunlight may raise air temperature by 15°F. Infrared waves from thermal reservoirs such as buildings, streets, tennis courts, and the ground can heat the athlete. Alternatively, a warm athlete will radiate heat into a cold environment.

Conduction

When two solids or liquids are in contact, heat equilibrium will be established. This mechanism plays a minor role in warm-weather athletics, although it can be important in cold-weather sports. This process is extremely important in the water.

Ambient Temperature and Wind

Air temperature plays a critical role in determining the mechanism of heat dissipation (**Figure 8.1**). As temperature increases, the opportunity for heat loss via convection and radiation falls progressively. At an air temperature of 95°F, heat begins to flow passively into the athlete, and evaporation of sweat becomes the only avenue for body cooling. If high relative humidity is present, evaporation is suppressed. Both temperature and humidity must be measured to accurately assess heat stress.

The thermal effect of wind is variable. At temperatures below 95°F and relative humidity below 100%, air movement always produces cooling. When the air temperature is above 95°F, wind provides cooling only at certain levels of humidity. Paradoxically, a hot, dry wind is actually worse for the athlete. In view of these findings, ideal conditions for endurance events consist of an air temperature of about 50°F, moderate relative humidity, and an overcast sky with a gentle breeze. The converse is also true. At a temperature of 95°F with a relative humidity of 60%, a world-record marathon is no longer possible, due simply to heat balance considerations.

Figure 8.1 Heat loss by a vigorously exercising athlete at various air temperatures.

Adapted with permission from Nielsen B: Olympics in Atlanta: A fight against physics. *Med Sci Sports Exerc* 1996;28:665–668.

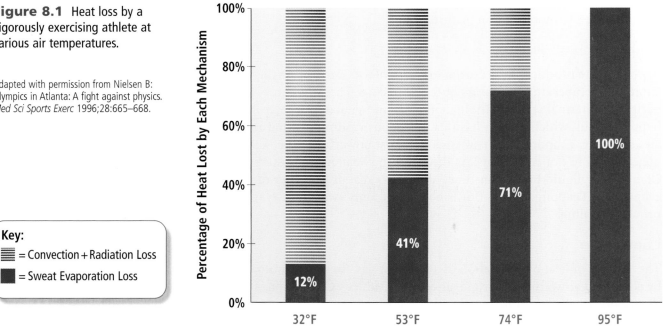

Key:
≡ = Convection + Radiation Loss
■ = Sweat Evaporation Loss

Measuring Environmental Heat Stress

The normal heat stress conditions for a specific time and place can be obtained by referring to local weather archives or to an Internet source. Consulting these resources will help to avoid heat stress catastrophes, but the only method that affords a high degree of safety is on-site monitoring of temperature, radiant heat, and relative humidity. Reports from local airports are of limited applicability, since they may substantially underestimate heat conditions at the sports site.

The gold standard measurement of heat stress is the Wet Bulb Globe Temperature (WBGT), a composite index that is derived from a weighted average of dry bulb, wet bulb, and black globe temperatures. Dry bulb (DB) temperature is a simple air temperature, usually shielded from direct sunlight; wet bulb (WB) temperature is measured by putting a wetted cotton sleeve over the bulb of a thermometer, thus allowing evaporative cooling; black globe temperature, which reflects radiation, is measured by placing the bulb of a thermometer inside a black sphere.

Devices that measure WBGT directly are expensive. A far more practical approach is use of a sling psychrometer, an inexpensive compact instrument that allows for immediate, on-the-field measurement of dry bulb and wet bulb temperatures. In fact, WBGT can be closely approximated with a sling psychrometer by simply averaging the dry bulb and wet bulb temperatures: Estimated WBGT = [DB + WB]/2. Once on-site temperature and humidity conditions have been determined, several different sets of heat stress standards can be applied (**Tables 8.1** to **8.4**).

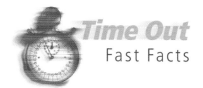

Time Out
Fast Facts

Both temperature and humidity must be measured to accurately assess environmental heat stress.

Table 8.1 *Restraints on Activities at Different Levels of Heat Stress*

| Wet Bulb Globe Temperature | | Restraints on Activities |
°C	°F	
<24	<75	All activities allowed, but be alert for prodromes of heat-related illness in prolonged events
24.0–25.9	75.0–78.6	Longer rest periods in the shade. Enforce drinking every 15 minutes
26–29	79–84	Stop activity of unacclimatized and other persons with high risk. Limit activities of all others (disallow long-distance races, cut down further duration of other activities)
>29	>84	Cancel all athletic activities

Adapted with permission from American Academy of Pediatrics Committee on Sports Medicine and Fitness: Athletics in hot and cold environments, in Dyment PG (ed): *Sports Medicine: Health Care for Young Athletes,* ed 2. Elk Grove Village, IL, American Academy of Pediatrics, 1991, pp 84–98.

Table 8.2 *Wet Bulb Globe Temperature Guide to Activity*

Under 60° F	Safe, but always observe athletes
61–65°	Observe players carefully
66–70°	Caution
71–75°	Shorter practice sessions; more frequent water and rest breaks
75°+	Danger level and extreme caution

Adapted with permission from Fox EL, Mathews DK (eds): *The Physiological Basis of Physical Education and Athletics,* ed 3. Philadelphia, PA, Saunders College Publishing, 1981, pp 454–485, McGraw-Hill, Inc.

Table 8.3 *Weather Guide for Activities Lasting 30 Minutes or More*

	Relative Humidity	
Air Temperature (°F)	Danger Zone	Critical Zone
70	80%	100%
75	70%	100%
80	50%	80%
85	40%	68%
90	20%	40%
100	10%	30%

Adapted with permission from Fox EL, Mathews DK (eds): *The Physiological Basis of Physical Education and Athletics,* ed 3. Philadelphia, PA, Saunders College Publishing, 1981, pp 454–485.

Table 8.4 *Football Practice: Wet Bulb Temperature Recommendations*

WBT°F	WBT°C	Duration of Practice	Attire	Fluid Consumption
<60	<15.5	2 hours	Full gear	No precautions
61-66	15.6-18.9	2 hours	Full gear	16 oz per hour plain water, at least 1 break per hour
67-74	19-23.3	2 hours	Full gear	24 oz per hour, at least 1 break per hour
75-77	23.4-25	2 hours: 45 min work 15 min rest	Shorts, shoulder pads, remove helmet when possible	24 oz per hour, at least 1 break every 15 minutes, 6 oz per break
78-79	25.1-26.1	2 hours: 45 min work, 15 min rest	Shirt, shorts only. No helmets	32 oz per hour, at least 1 break every 15 minutes, 8 oz per break
>80	>26.1	No practice	No practice	Normal consumption

Adapted with permission from Fairfax County (VA) Public Schools: Weather guidelines wet bulb temperature recommendations, in *Athletic Training Program Policies and Procedures Manual,* ed 2. 1994, p 8-1.

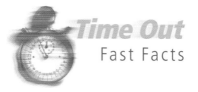

Time Out
Fast Facts

Several days of repeated heat stress may increase the risk of heat injury.

Special Heat Illness Concerns

Thermoregulation in children has several unique features:

- *Surface area-to-mass ratio (S/M).* This ratio is much higher in children than in adults. A high S/M is useful at moderate temperatures, since an increase in convective surface promotes cooling. Conversely, in most extreme conditions (ie, air temperature greater than 95°F, in cold climates, and in water), high S/M becomes a liability, as heat flow between the environment and the child increases.

- *Blood volume in children.* Even when blood volume is indexed for body weight, it is less than in adults. Since exercise shifts blood volume peripherally and sweating tends to produce relative hypovolemia, the risk of reduced cardiac filling is increased.

- *Sweat gland function.* The number of sweat glands in an individual becomes fixed by about age 3 years. Since total body surface area in early childhood is much less than in the adult, this would seem to give the child a heat dissipation advantage, with a very high density of sweat glands. Unfortunately, young children's sweat glands show diminished sensitivity to thermal stress stimulation, a condition that persists until about age 14 years. Onset of sweating is delayed and sweating rate is lower in prepubertal children.

- *Mechanical efficiency of motion.* The endearing waddling gait of the toddler is terribly inefficient. As children grow, mechanical efficiency improves, but does not reach adult levels until adolescence. As a result, children use more energy, and consequently generate more heat to move.

- *The rate of heat acclimatization.* The rate of acclimatization in children is significantly slower than in adults. The degree of acclimatization achieved in 6 days by young men requires 12 days for 8-to 10-year-old boys.

At moderate temperatures, thermoregulation is similar in children and adults. In extreme conditions, children are at a distinct disadvantage because of these differences.

Heat-Related Illnesses

Heat Cramps

The term "heat cramps" is a misnomer; the condition should actually be termed exercise cramps. Muscle cramping in the context of vigorous exercise appears to be related to alterations in spinal neural reflex activity activated by muscle fatigue and can occur at any air temperature. Prolonged exercise in hot weather can make cramping more likely, probably due in part to fluid and electrolyte shifts associated with copious sweating. Since cramping is believed to be largely the result of muscle fatigue, one approach to treatment would be to establish better overall fitness. Although no universal solution to this problem is available, experts have recommended analysis of sodium balance in affected athletes, with some responding dramatically to small increases in dietary sodium. This dietary change may be something as simple as drinking tomato juice for breakfast. Anecdotally, drinking a small quantity of a brine solution (½ teaspoonful of salt in 16 oz of water) at the first sign of cramps has been shown to successfully abort some cramping episodes.

Heat Syncope

This condition is characterized by an abrupt loss of consciousness in a heat-exposed athlete whose core temperature is normal or only mildly elevated. As skin and core temperatures increase during exercise, there is reflex vasodilatation of the skin vasculature to promote heat release. Dilation of the blood vessels that supply active muscles further increases the vascular space. As long as the athlete keeps moving, this relative hypovolemia is compensated by the effect of peripheral muscle contraction. However, once the athlete stops moving, there is abrupt development of reduced cardiac return, reduced cardiac output, and postural hypotension. Cerebral hypoperfusion occurs, resulting in syncope. The severity of this condition varies significantly, depending on the individual, and vasovagal tendencies may play a role in syncope in some athletes.

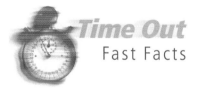
Time Out
Fast Facts

Heat syncope tends to occur during the first 5 days of heat exposure.

The onset of sweating is delayed and sweating rates are lower in prepubertal children than in adults or postpubertal adolescents.

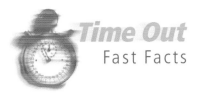

Time Out
Fast Facts

Oral and tympanic temperature measurements should not be used when assessing athletes experiencing a suspected heat illness.

Heat syncope tends to occur during the first 5 days of heat exposure, before full volume expansion has occurred, and its incidence decreases dramatically as heat acclimatization is achieved. The first step in treatment is to carefully move the player to a cool place, check rectal temperature to exclude heatstroke, and then evaluate the athlete for injuries that may have occurred with falling after loss of consciousness. Barring other injuries, treatment should consist of support and fluids as necessary. The athlete should be instructed in safe heat acclimatization methods, since acclimatization is known to markedly reduce the likelihood of heat syncope.

Remember that all methods for measuring body temperature in the field are approximations of measuring the body's core temperature. The usual gold standard in research is to use an esophageal probe and thermister. However, the most practical method in the field is a rectal thermometer. Oral and aural measurements are not accurate and should not be used to assess athletes. Even in a busy medical tent, an athlete can be covered with a towel to discreetly measure a rectal temperature.

Heat Exhaustion

Defined as an inability to continue activity because of fatigue in the context of an elevated core temperature, heat exhaustion is often marked by collapse. In acclimatized athletes, heat exhaustion occurs at a rectal temperature of between 100.4°F and 104°F. Severe muscle cramping sometimes follows. Other symptoms

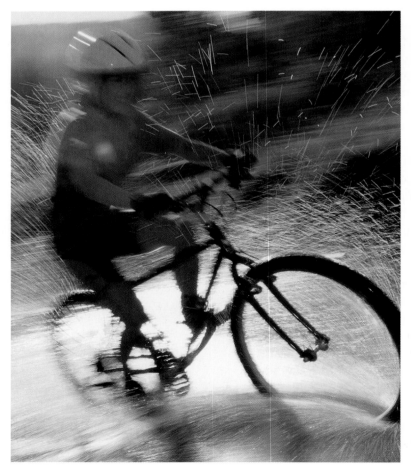

can include mild confusion, headache, dizziness, chills, and nausea. Heat exhaustion is also characterized by severe muscle fatigue and moderate elevation of rectal temperature. Some degree of hypovolemia because of sweat loss is usually present. Electrolyte imbalance caused by sodium loss may coexist.

Management should begin with immediately moving the athlete to a cool, shaded place. All unnecessary clothing should be removed, and the athlete's rectal temperature should be checked. If the patient is oriented and able to drink, he or she should be given cold water or cold glucose-electrolyte fluid. Athletes who have a rectal temperature of greater than 104°F should be seriously considered for cold water immersion. If intravenous rehydration is felt to be necessary, EMS should be contacted. However, every attempt should be made to begin cooling and rehydration prior to their arrival.

Once the athlete has been sufficiently cooled, he or she should receive detailed instructions in techniques to prevent another episode, including proper acclimatization, adequate hydration, and exercising at realistic levels of exertion. Acclimatization results in a 50% fall in the rate of heat exhaustion. Heat exhaustion occurs earlier in exercise in those who are volume depleted and may be linked to exercise performed at an unrealistically high effort level. Athletes who have experienced one episode of heat injury are at higher than average risk for another.

Heatstroke

A true medical emergency, in the same category as drowning or cardiac arrest, heatstroke is always associated with a core temperature (if measured immediately) in excess of 104°F and abnormal mental status. The athlete may or may not be sweating. Blood pressure is often (but not always) low, and tachycardia is usually present. Heatstroke results from inability of the athlete's heat dissipation system to cope with a heat load, allowing the core temperature to rise to the point of severe multi-system malfunction. Since the brain is exquisitely sensitive to temperature elevation, the first sign of heatstroke is usually confusion, with subsequent seizure or coma. If the athlete's core temperature is not lowered promptly, multi-system injury (renal failure, rhabdomyolysis, liver failure, disseminated intravascular coagulation, brain injury, myocardial depression) can develop, followed by permanent disability or death. Animal models and human observations have revealed significant individual variation in susceptibility to heatstroke. It has been clearly shown that both severity and duration of core temperature elevation determine the outcome of heatstroke. What has been learned about treatment is simple: Time and cooling are everything.

Organizers of road races have recognized that most heatstroke collapse occurs within view of the finish line, a finding that suggests that cumulative heat buildup plus the motivation for finishing at maximum performance are the main contributors to the crisis. In light of this fact, 50-gallon tubs filled to a depth of about 8 inches with water and ice are kept in an area near the finish line. Plastic wading pools also work well for this purpose. Athletes who show signs of severe staggering, confusion, seizure, or collapse are immediately plunged into the ice water bath. The tub or pool is small enough for the athlete's trunk to fit in the water, but the arms, legs, and head dangle outside. This immersion is very briefly delayed by a temperature check. Thereafter, rectal temperature is measured every 5 to 10 minutes. When rectal temperature has fallen to 102°F, the runner is removed from the bath to avoid "overshoot hypothermia." As a result of this technique, these critically ill runners rarely require hospitalization.

This level of expert treatment is clearly not possible at all athletic venues. A more practical approach is to ensure that coaches and officials understand the fundamentals of heatstroke management, as do EMTs and emergency physicians. Any previously healthy athlete who collapses abruptly in the context of vigorous exercise (without head trauma) must be checked immediately for cardiac arrhythmia. If no arrhythmia is detected, heatstroke should be assumed to be present. The nearest emergency department should be advised about the patient, and personnel there should prepare a cold water bath. During transport, the athlete's rectal temperature should be checked, and an intravenous line and cooling measures initiated. Upon arrival at the emergency department, the athlete should be placed in the cold water bath.

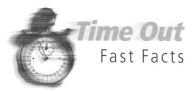

Time Out
Fast Facts

Once an athlete has experienced an episode of heat illness, he or she is at greater than average risk of a second heat injury.

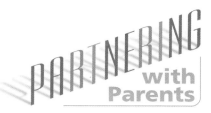

PARTNERING with Parents

Is salt supplementation necessary for exercise in the heat?

Although small amounts of salt are lost through perspiration, the major component of sweat is water. For very warm conditions or exercise lasting more than 60 to 90 minutes, a dilute glucose/electrolyte solution may be beneficial. Small amounts of salt added to food at meals should adequately replenish salt loses. Salt tablets should never be used.

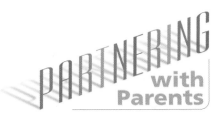

Time from collapse to bath should be 20 minutes or less. Treatment of heatstroke is complicated by obesity, which impairs heat transfer, making cold water immersion an even more desirable form of therapy. Complex diagnostic tests such as CT scans should be postponed until the athlete's core temperature has been lowered.

Prevention of Heat Injury

In the general population of youth sport participants, several risk factors account for the most heat-related injuries.

Environmental Conditions

The first step in preventing heat illness is thoughtful scheduling. In the United States, the incidence of heat stress illnesses peaks in the period midway between April 15 and October 15. Sports organizers should be aware of weather conditions *likely* to develop during active exercise. This information can be obtained from local weather archives or from Internet sources. Moreover, the shape of the diurnal heat stress curve must be appreciated. For example, during the summer in the south central United States, the hottest moment of the day is 3:45 PM DST. The period between 12:30 PM to 6 PM represents a virtual "heat stress plateau" in which temperatures will usually show little change (**Figure 8.2**). Coaches looking for "the cool of the afternoon" will need to wait until sunset. A more rational plan is used by the US Marines at their Parris Island, SC, recruit training center. Vigorous physical training is scheduled from 7 AM to 9 AM. However, even with optimal scheduling, exercise-related heat injury can still occur. Heatstroke has been recorded at an air temperature of 66°F with a relative humidity of 96% (WBGT 65°F). To minimize the risk of heat injury, sling psychrometer temperatures should be measured at regular intervals during games or practices held in hot weather. Exercise programs should then be modified as outlined in Tables 8.1 to 8.4.

Dehydration

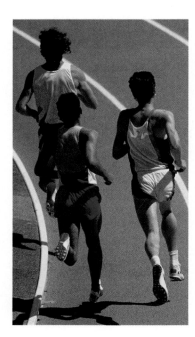

An athlete's initial volume status is critically important. Sweating begins when core temperature reaches approximately 99.5°F, and total body water may decline progressively from that point. Even mild initial dehydration has been shown to significantly impair endurance performance. To best prevent dehydration, athletes should begin competition with urine that is dilute (colorless) and should drink at regular intervals, regardless of thirst. Events lasting less than 30 minutes are not usually affected by oral fluid intake during the event. For medium-length (30 to 60 minutes) events, plain cool water is a reasonable choice. Longer events (more than 60 minutes) associated with copious sweating should include fluid replacement with a dilute glucose-electrolyte drink.

One of the main benefits of sports drinks is their greater palatability. One study has shown that children will consume nearly twice as much sports drink as water. How much to drink depends on the athlete's size and sweat rate. Ordinarily, athletes should drink something every 15 to 20 minutes, even if they are not thirsty. Unfortunately, a few cases of profound hyponatremia with seizure have been associated with too-vigorous hydration with plain water. Drinking from a cup results in greater fluid intake than use of fountain or spigot devices.

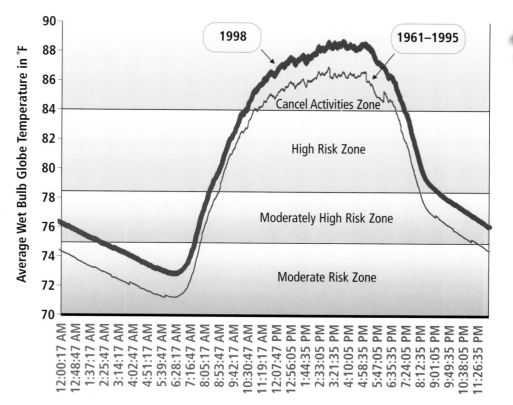

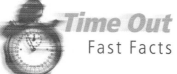

The rate of acclimatization in children is significantly slower than it is in adults.

Adapted with permission from Fox EL, Mathews DK, Kaufman WS, Bowers RW: Effects of football equipment on thermal balance and energy cost during exercise. *Res Q Exerc Sport* 1966;37:332–339. © by the American Alliance for Health, Physical Education, Recreation and Dance, Reston, VA.

Figure 8.2 Wet bulb globe temperature: average values for July and August 1998, recorded on a tennis court in the mid-southern United States. American Academy of Pediatrics heat risk standards.

Lack of Acclimatization

Athletes who normally exercise in a moderate climate will experience reduced performance when they arrive in conditions of high heat stress. Adapting to exercise in hot weather, termed *acclimatization*, results in a lower resting core temperature, expanded intravascular volume, sweating earlier and more profusely during exercise, and production of sweat with a lower concentration of sodium. Acclimatization can be accomplished within 10 to 12 days of heat exposure, employing daily hot weather exercise at 50% to 70% of maximum effort for 1.5 to 2 hours per day. Upon returning to cooler conditions, heat tolerance will be maintained for 1 to 4 weeks.

Acclimatization concerns are especially important in the following situations: during the spring-to-summer weather transition period; for athletes who are returning to play after inactivity, illness, or injury; and for the unusual athlete who is traveling to competition in a different climatic zone. Young children acclimatize more slowly than do adolescents and adults.

Deconditioning and Fatigue

Athletes who are highly conditioned have already achieved a certain level of heat tolerance, since core temperature will rise to some extent with vigorous exercise even in cool temperatures. Those who have low cardiovascular fitness will show increased susceptibility to heat illness. The effects of several days of heat exposure appear to be cumulative, and repetitive heat stress may increase the risk of heat injury.

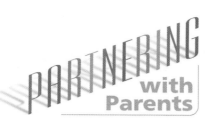

What is the best fluid for hydration during exercise?

For bouts of exercise lasting less than 1 hour, chilled water is adequate. For longer events, a dilute glucose/electrolyte solution is best. Glucose content of about 6% provides fuel for exercise and helps facilitate the absorption of electrolytes and water. Much higher glucose concentrations create an osmotic effect and draw water from the vascular space into the abdomen.

Case Study | Football

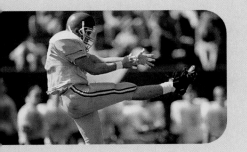

In the United States, football is the team sport that has the greatest number of participants, estimated at 1.5 million players per year. Unlike other sports, it is a rare year when one or more heatstroke deaths do not occur in conjunction with football practice. The reasons for this are numerous, and an examination of football may shed light on the general problem of exercise-related heat illness.

Most football players are not properly conditioned before the beginning of practice in the late summer. The ritual of "going out for the team" may be the first sustained exercise that some players have had in the 2 months since classes ended in the previous spring. There is a widespread tendency to downplay the need for aerobic conditioning, which requires a minimum of 6 weeks of regular exercise at 50% to 70% of maximum oxygen uptake to achieve.

Because of the structure of American football, many body types are necessary for a successful team. In general, wide receivers are slender sprinters; running backs are muscular and quick, and interior linemen are heavy and strong. It is vitally important to note that virtually all heatstroke deaths in American football players occur within the first 2 weeks of practice, and nearly all of the victims are interior linemen. This telling statistic reflects much of the above discussion of heat illness risk factors. Practice tends to be held after noon, in the most severe heat stress conditions, and many of the players have not achieved heat acclimatization. The interior linemen are usually the largest players, and many are obese and have low overall aerobic fitness, despite great strength. If the afternoon practice is the second part of a "two-a-day" schedule, many of the players will have had a severely depressed appetite after the first session and will be unable or unwilling to eat or drink much before the second session, markedly increasing the risk of dehydration.

The role of the football uniform is of critical importance in the development of heat illness. Because the uniform has many thick elements and a great deal of totally impermeable plastic, the amount of skin surface available for heat

Figure 8.3
Exercise in a football uniform vs exercise in shorts: rectal temperature during and after running at 6 mph.

Adapted with permission from Mathews DK, Fox EL, Tanzi D: Physiological responses during exercise and recovery in a football uniform. *J Appl Physiol* 1969;26:611–615 (Figure 1).

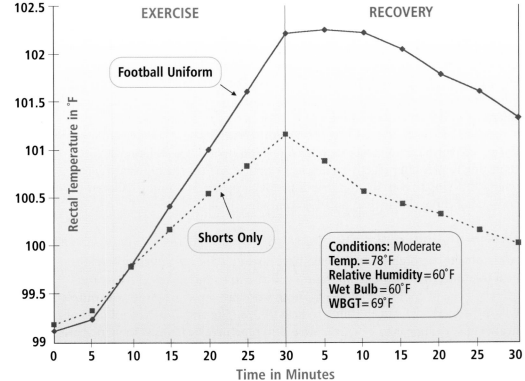

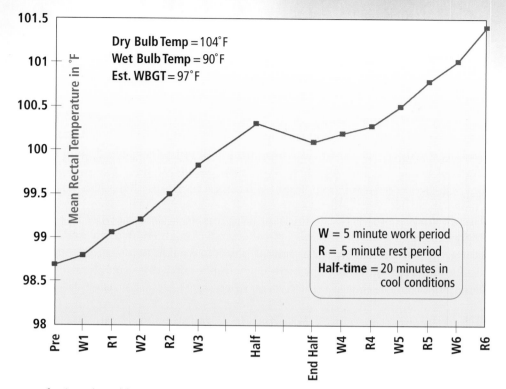

Dry Bulb Temp = 104°F
Wet Bulb Temp = 90°F
Est. WBGT = 97°F

W = 5 minute work period
R = 5 minute rest period
Half-time = 20 minutes in
                cool conditions

Figure 8.4
Exercise in a football uniform in
very hot conditions: rectal temperature during a simulated "game."

Adapted with permission from Van Handel P,
Blosser P, Butts N: A method of heat stress
prevention for football players. *Am Correct
Ther J* 1973;27:180–183.

transfer is reduced by 50% or more. In obese interior linemen, this reduction of
evaporative surface occurs in addition to an already-reduced surface-to-mass ratio.
Core temperature rises significantly more during exercise in a football uniform
than in shorts alone or in shorts plus a backpack that weighs the same amount as
a football uniform (**Figure 8.3**). Furthermore, hot weather exercise during a simulated "game" while wearing a football uniform results in a continuously rising
core temperature in a stair-step pattern throughout the entire event (**Figure 8.4**).
Significant cooling does not occur during "time-outs" or, surprisingly, even during
the 20-minute "halftime" break. Add to this the almost universal pattern of ending a practice session with "wind sprints," which applies to the already overheat-
ed and dehydrated interior linemen a final burst of strongly encouraged energy
production. When this ritual is played out over a population of 1.5 million participants, a few heatstroke disasters are likely to occur.

An accurate description of a complex problem will often contain its solution. In
an ideal football program, all players would undergo a preliminary physical examination to reveal exclusionary illness and document use of medications and drugs.
Players would be strongly advised to begin diligent physical conditioning preparation, starting 6 weeks before the first practice. The first day of practice would
include height and weight determination, and those with a BMI of greater than
26 would be given special conditioning attention. A qualifying physical fitness
examination would follow, and those of low fitness would begin a remedial program specially designed to safely bring them up to the requirements of the sport.
Shorts and shirts only (no helmets) should be worn in practices for the first 10
days, as heat acclimatization was being established. All vigorous physical exercise
would be scheduled for the early morning hours. Players would be weighed
before and after practice, and players who were losing weight (suggesting dehydration) would be held out of practice. Regular fluid intake would be enforced.
Players would be monitored, and those showing signs of illness would be cooled
and rested. Practices would not end with wind sprints. If estimated WBGT exceeded 80°F, practice would be moved into an air-conditioned gym. These recommendations are realistic. Most of these methods are already used by successful college
and professional football programs.

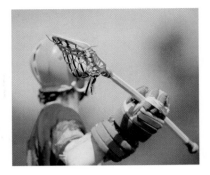

Obesity

Obesity can have various definitions, but for older adolescents, the Marine Corps has found a Body Mass Index [BMI = (weight in kg)/(height in m)^2] of greater than 26 to be associated with increased risk of exercise-related heat injury. The overweight athlete has two principal disadvantages in hot weather. First, the need to move a large body mass will require generation of more heat, regardless of body composition. Second, adipose tissue is "dead weight" and has a reduced ability to store heat. Although not universally present, low levels of overall fitness frequently accompany obesity.

Recent Febrile Illness

Febrile illness changes the hypothalamic temperature control center to a higher "set point" level. Athletes with a fever start at an abnormally high core temperature, leaving less room for physiologic gain before problems occur. For reasons that are not completely understood, abnormalities of hypo-thalamic thermoregulatory function may persist for up to 12 weeks after a febrile illness, rendering the athlete more vulnerable to heat stress illness.

Sleep Deprivation

The circadian cycle of body temperature is intimately linked to the indi-vidual's sleep-waking routine. Disruption of that routine can be linked to temperature control alteration, raising susceptibility to heat illness.

Sunburn

Sunburn reduces the ability of the skin to transfer heat and to sweat.

Drugs and Medications

A number of drugs can promote exercise-related heat injury, either by impair-ing thermoregulation or by increasing heat production (**Table 8.5**). Parents of children taking medications should be made aware of their potential side effects, and they must alert coaches and administrators about the child's increased risk for heat-related problems.

The Rules of the Game

The rules of most sports, practice sessions, and games are completely arbi-trary, dictated more by tradition than common sense. The patterns that gov-ern specific practice sessions are as well. There is no reason that coaches or

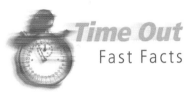

Time Out
Fast Facts

Thermoregulatory dysfunction may persist for up to 12 weeks after a febrile illness.

Table 8.5 *Drugs Associated With Heat Intolerance*

Phenothiazines (haloperidol, perphenazine, thioridazine, chlorpromazine)	Amphetamines
Anticholinergic agents (benztropine, atropine, belladonna extracts)	Lithium plus fluoxetine (Prozac)
Beta-blockers, diuretics, laxatives, antihistamines, methyldopa, MAO inhibitors, tricyclic antidepressants, vasoconstrictors	Miscellaneous agents (cannabinoids, phenycyclidine [PCP], phentermine, Ecstasy, alcohol, cocaine, LSD, opiates [withdrawal])

Adapted with permission from Epstein Y: Heat intolerance: Predisposing factor or residual injury? *Med Sci Sports Exerc* 1990;22:29–35.

Figure 8.5
Wind chill factor chart.

Air Temperature	Estimated Wind Speed			
	0 mph	10 mph	20 mph	30 mph
30°F	30°F	16°F	4°F	-2°F Little Risk
20°F	20°F	4°F	-10°F	-18°F
10°F	10°F	-9°F	-25°F	-33F Increased Risk
0°F	0°F	-24°F	-39°F	-48°F
-10°F	-10°F	-33°F	-53°F	-63°F
-20°F	-20°F	-46°F	-67°F	-79°F Great Risk

Wind Chill and the Risk of Freezing Exposed Flesh

officials cannot adjust practice and play routines in response to unpredictable conditions that impose increased risk of heat injury. For example, at a WBGT of 80°F, a soccer match that usually consists of two 20-minute halves with a 10-minute halftime could be reformatted as four 8-minute quarters with 5 minutes between quarters and a 10-minute halftime. Adjustments like these are routinely made by military and industrial planners to minimize injury, with good results.

Special Cold Illness Concerns

Few studies have dealt with the response of young people to exercise in cold conditions, but this limited body of research underscores the interaction of anatomy, physiology, and weather conditions.

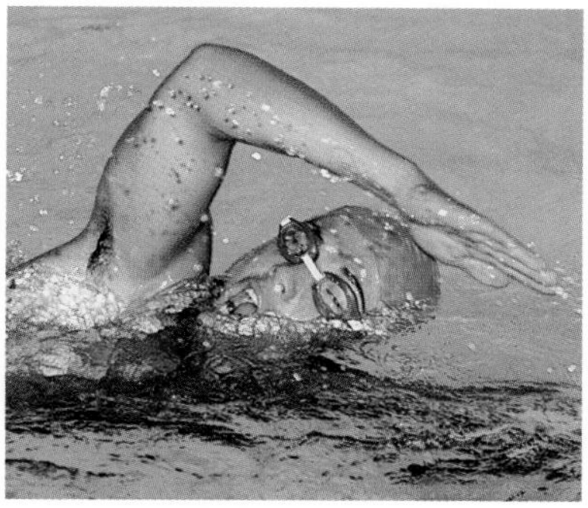

Anatomy and Physiology

Children have physical characteristics that enhance heat loss in cold conditions, particularly their higher body surface area-to-mass ratio (as much as 190% of that found in adults). Children also typically have a smaller mass and less subcutaneous fat thickness than adults. These characteristics facilitate passive heat loss by convection and radiation, the processes that account for 90% of heat dissipation when the air temperature is 32°F. Passive heat loss is further increased by air movement, and wind chill factor is of critical importance in determining cold stress risk (**Figure 8.5**).

One hypothermia problem that occurs, albeit infrequently, concerns maintaining adequate core temperature in small children swimming in cold water. Since water has 25 to 30 times the conductivity of air, heat transfer from the child to the water is very efficient. Because children usually become very uncomfortable and leave the water before serious injury has occurred, this problem rarely occurs in swimmers. However, lake swimmers in long-distance competitions can experience this problem.

Acclimatization to cold conditions is limited. Studies in adults have shown that repeated exposure to cold results in a higher shivering threshold, increased vasoconstriction, increased blood flow to frequently exposed extremities, and an elevated basal metabolic rate. Initial cold acclimatization

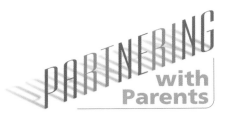

How much fluid should a child drink before and during exercise?

Athletes need to pay close attention to fluid intake throughout the day as well as prior to and during exercise. During hotter conditions and more vigorous workouts, greater amounts of fluids should be consumed. A practical guideline is to drink enough fluid to cause the urine to be clear prior to beginning a workout and to consume some fluid every 15-20 minutes during exercise.

takes about 10 days, but humoral changes (eg, increased secretion of thyroid hormone) may take much longer. It is not known whether children show similar adaptation. Still, it is clear that young people exercising in cold conditions can maintain core temperature as well as adults, offsetting their tendency to increased passive heat loss by more intense vasoconstriction and a higher metabolic rate. Children have greater difficulty in maintaining core temperature at rest in cold conditions.

Thermoregulation in cold weather differs from warm-weather conditions in three principal ways. First, shivering generates additional muscular heat, further lowering the efficiency of energy expenditure. Second, substantial respiratory heat loss occurs in cold weather. Finally, adding or removing additional clothing efficiently aids in the thermoregulatory process. The latter is especially important in the head and neck regions which, because of high blood flow, can act as points of rapid heat transfer.

Successful thermoregulation in cold weather hinges on the balance between the generation and dissipation of heat. Even in extremely cold conditions, properly clothed young athletes can exercise sufficiently to raise their core temperature. Overheating becomes a problem if clothing is excessive for the climatic conditions and level of exertion. If the athlete is forced to markedly reduce his or her level of exercise or remove clothing, excessive cooling can occur. Of note, the mechanical inefficiency associated with movement in children actually generates more heat than similar activity would produce in an adult and may offer a temporary advantage in very cold conditions. Cold-weather athletes must be able to add and remove layers of clothing as conditions change during competition.

Evaporation of sweat makes a minor contribution to heat dissipation during cold-weather exercise, but fluid losses can be substantial if exercise is prolonged, especially if relative humidity is low. Fluid replacement is an essential part of maintaining cold-weather athletes, and use of carbohydrate-electrolyte drinks in Nordic competitions has been associated with improved fluid balance compared with that associated with consuming plain water.

Weather Conditions

Defining the upper thermal boundary of "cold weather" is not always easy. The American College of Sports Medicine has listed a WBGT of 50°F or below, which corresponds to an air temperature of 55°F with a relative humidity of 44%. Cases of hypothermia have been reported with air temperatures as high as 65°F in marathon runners competing in wet, windy conditions. Conversely, the ideal conditions for a record-setting marathon probably consist of an air temperature of 50°F, an overcast sky, a gentle breeze, and a light mist. It must be remembered that thermogenesis can be exhausted, and very prolonged exercise in cool conditions (more than 4 hours) may promote hypothermia.

The hazard of truly frigid conditions must also be considered. Nordic competitions are routinely postponed if air temperature is ⁻4°F or less. This is because of the increased risk of frostbite associated with race pace. Since air movement augments passive heat loss, wind effects expressed as wind chill factor must be understood to properly assess the hazard of a cold air temperature.

Cold-Related Illnesses

Two major illnesses are associated with excessive exposure to cold during exercise:

Hypothermia

Hypothermia is defined as a lowering of core temperature to less than 97°F. Stages of hypothermia include mild (93°F to 97°F), moderate (86°F to 93°F) and severe (less than 86°F). Mild hypothermia can often be treated locally with rewarming, but moderate and severe hypothermia entail serious risks and require immediate hospitalization.

- Mild hypothermia is characterized by shivering and foot stamping. Blood vessels are constricted, breathing is rapid, and the athlete may become withdrawn.

- Moderate hypothermia is characterized by muscle stiffness and loss of coordination. Respirations slow, the pulse rate decreases, and confusion, lethargy, and sleepiness may develop.

- Severe hypothermia leads to a weak pulse, arrhythmias, very slow respirations, and possibly a coma. This condition is a medical emergency.

Treatment of hypothermia focuses on controlled rewarming. The athlete should be taken from outdoor exposure, wet clothing should be removed, and rewarming begun with warm blankets, radiant heat, and hot air. Hot objects should not be placed directly on the skin. Care must be taken to limit tissue damage, and the athlete should not be allowed to walk.

Frostbite

Localized complications of cold exposure include frostnip and frostbite. Frostnip is defined as severe chilling of exposed body parts without tissue freezing. The fingers, nose, ears, and face are especially prone to this condition, which is treated by rewarming.

Frostbite is crystallization of fluids in the skin or subcutaneous tissue after exposure to temperatures of less than 31°F. Frostbite can appear within minutes at wind chill values of less than -67°F, conditions produced by an air temperature of -20°F and a 20 mph wind. Frostbite can cause permanent injury to tissue, but this risk is greatly increased if initial rewarming is followed by repeat tissue freezing. For that reason, assiduous attention must be paid to continuous warming after the rewarming process has begun.

The treatment of frostbite can be complex. Initial measures include removing the athlete from the cold environment and removing wet or restrictive clothing. Great care should be taken to avoid further injury of tissue that has already been damaged. The athlete should not be allowed to stand on a frostbitten foot, and the skin should not be rubbed nor should blisters be opened. Warm water (100°F to 112°F) can be used to rewarm a frostbitten extremity, but this is best done in the emergency department. Surgical debridement may be needed in severe cases.

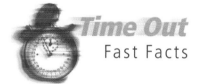

Time Out
Fast Facts

Do not rub or open blisters on frostbitten areas.

Prevention of Cold Injury

An intriguing scheduling issue has emerged from cold-weather youth sports. In our society, cold weather tends to be seen as a phenomenon that can quickly cause illness and death, while heat is often regarded as a minor inconvenience. This attitude is maintained by coaches and event organizers despite the fact that the number of deaths and severe illnesses caused by heatstroke vastly outnumbers hypothermia injuries. Summertime athletic events are routinely scheduled for dates and places known to be associated with dangerously hot weather conditions, and heat stress measurements are rarely made at the time of those competitions. Conversely, as a result of frostbite in Nordic events, scrupulous attention is paid to climatic conditions in cold weather, with postponement of Nordic competition when air temperature is less than -4°F. If similar respect were shown for a WBGT of 90°F (the US Marine Corps policy during recruit training) a great deal of heat-related illness could be avoided.

FINISH LINE

Thermoregulation is a key element in the success of the young athlete. Careful attention to factors that contribute to maintenance of an appropriate core temperature will minimize injuries, enhance performance, and maximize individual participation. Physicians and coaches should work together to promote this vitally important aspect of sport.

For More Information

1. Armstrong LE, De Luca JP, Hubbard RW: Time course of recovery and heat acclimation ability of prior exertional heatstroke patients. *Med Sci Sports Exerc* 1990;22:36–48.

2. American Academy of Pediatrics, Committee on Sports Medicine and Fitness: Athletics in hot and cold environments, in Dyment PG (ed): *Sports Medicine: Health Care for Young Athletes*, ed 2. Elk Grove Village, IL, American Academy of Pediatrics, 1991, pp 84–98.

3. Coyle JF: *The Zunis Foundation. http://www.zunis.org*

4. Falk B: Effects of thermal stress during rest and exercise in the paediatric population. *Sports Med* 1998;25:221–240.

5. Fox EL, Mathews DK (eds): *The Physiological Basis of Physical Education and Athletics*, ed 3. Philadelphia, PA, Saunders College Publishing, 1981, pp 454–485.

6. Shapiro Y, Seidman DS: Field and clinical observations of exertional heat stroke patients. *Med Sci Sports Exerc* 1990;22:6–14.

7. Smolander J, Bar-Or O, Korhonen O, Ilmarinen J: Thermoregulation during rest and exercise in the cold in pre- and early pubescent boys and in young men. *J Appl Physiol* 1992;72:1589–1594.

Chapter 9

Nutrition and Weight Control

S U Z A N N E   N E L S O N   S T E E N ,   D S c ,   R D
D A V I D   T .   B E R N H A R D T ,   M D

Athletes at all levels of competition often search for an edge in hopes of improving performance. While improvements in equipment, coaching, training environment, and specific sport techniques have resulted in improved performance, individual athletes may look to weight management as a means to improve their performance. Depending on the sport, weight loss or gain may be beneficial; however, when taken to extremes, these strategies may have adverse effects on the young athlete.

This chapter provides guidelines to help ensure that young athletes receive appropriate nutrition and follow weight control practices that are compatible with optimal needs for growth and development.

Physical Growth

All children should have their weight, height, weight in relation to height, and standard height for age evaluated and assessed by a qualified health professional using, for example, the National Center for Health Statistics growth charts. Routine plotting of weight and height is essential for tracking normal growth and identifying patterns that indicate growth abnormalities related to nutrition or underlying disease. Although individual children differ in their rates of growth, when either height or weight deviates from the child's usual growth percentiles, the etiology of the change should be investigated.

Assessment of weight in relation to height enables assessment of current nutrition status and growth that is specific to the child's body size. At a single point in time, weight-for-height is a more sensitive index of appropriate growth than weight-for-age, since appropriateness of body weight is dependent on total body size, not on age (**Figure 9.1**). In contrast to the weight-for-height assessment, height-for-age comparison is an index of previous nutrition and growth status. A reduction in height velocity is slower to develop in the presence of

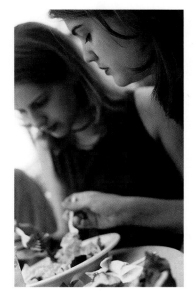

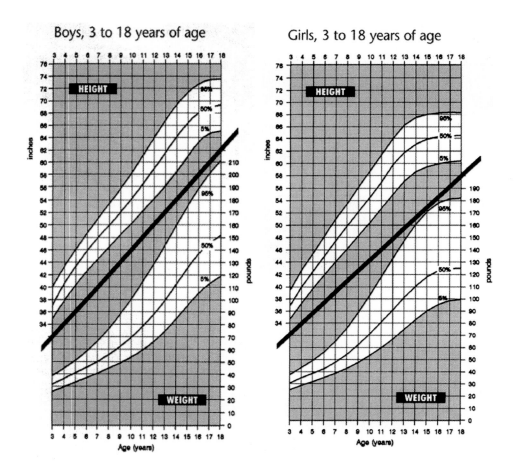

Figure 9.1
Weight-for-height charts.

Courtesy of the Agency for Healthcare Research and Quality.

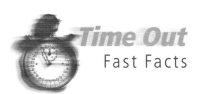

Body composition equations derived from adult samples are not appropriate for use with children.

under-nutrition than a decrease in weight velocity. Therefore, height-for-age can be an index of chronic malnutrition.

The actual increments in height and weight during the school-age years are small when compared with those of infancy and adolescence. Weight increases an average of 5 to 7 lb each year until the child is age 9 or 10 years. The rate of weight gain then increases and is considered an initial sign of approaching puberty. Height increments average 2″ to 2½″ per year from age 2 years until puberty, when children undergo hormonal changes that mark the beginning of adolescence. Nutritional needs prior to and during this period of rapid growth increase significantly.

Assessment of Body Composition

Body composition assessment has important implications for health, fitness, and performance. In the young athlete, evaluation is challenging because of several factors that affect the conceptual basis for estimating fat and lean tissue. First, children have higher body water content and lower bone mineral content; therefore, they have a lower body density than adults. Equations that use conversion constants derived from adult samples are not appropriate for children because they may overestimate body fatness by 3% to 6% and underestimate lean body weight.

Another limitation when estimating fat and lean tissue in the young athlete is that the chemical composition of the fat-free mass changes as the child passes through puberty. There are significant changes in the relation of skinfolds to

Table 9.1	*Estimated Average Calories and Protein Needs for Children and Adolescents (per kg of body weight)*				
Age (years)	Kcal (per kg)	Kcal (per day)	Protein (g/kg)	Protein (g/day)
4 to 6	90	1,800	1.2	24
7 to 10	70	2,000	1.0	28
11 to 14 (m)	55	2,500	1.0	45
11 to 14 (f)	47	2,200	1.0	46
15 to 18 (m)	45	3,000	0.9	59
15 to 18 (f)	40	2,200	0.8	44

Adapted with permission from National Research Council: *Recommended Dietary Allowances,* ed 10. Washington, DC, National Academy Press, 1989.

density from prepubescence to puberty and from puberty to postpubescence. As a result, estimates of body fatness by skinfolds, body widths, and circumferences may reflect alterations in the composition of the fat-free body components, which include water, minerals, and protein, rather than alterations in actual fat content.

From a practical standpoint, body composition measurements, in combination with growth charts and sound clinical judgment, can be used by a trained health professional to monitor changes in fat and lean tissue during training, and to determine a range of weights for the young athlete based on optimal health. Although helpful in evaluating the fitness and performance of mature athletes, body composition measurements should not be used to manipulate body fat for sports participation or to set stringent weight loss guidelines in the prepubertal athlete. Doing so may adversely affect normal growth and development.

Calorie Requirements

Before puberty, a child's nutritional needs are modest compared with those during adolescence, which is characterized by rapid growth and high nutritional demands. **Table 9.1** shows how the Recommended Dietary Allowance (RDA) can be used to estimate caloric needs for normal growth and development per kilogram of body weight.

Estimated calories should consider current dietary intake, rate of growth, age, gender, weight, and energy demands of the sport. Although data on adult athletes have shown that differences in daily energy requirements depend on the volume of training and the energy cost of the specific sport, there is no similar data on young children. The energy needs of children differ because of lower body mass, lower skill level, and the decrease in metabolic cost per kilogram of body mass that occurs with age. Energy "wastefulness" in children's movement is caused by a lack of adequate co-contraction of antagonist muscles during walking and running. Calories expended per kilogram of body weight for young athletes can be estimated using **Table 9.2.**

Although the exact energy needs of young athletes have not been determined, on average, active teenagers require 1,500 to 3,000 kcal/day more energy than the RDA. However, no energy balance studies have been done to verify this suggestion. Although studies have shown that adolescent female athletes have

Table 9.2	Calorie Equivalents of Children's Activities*

Activity	Body weight (in kg)									
	20	25	30	35	40	45	50	55	60	65
Basketball	34	43	51	60	68	77	85	94	102	110
Calisthenics	13	17	20	23	26	30	33	36	40	43
Bicycling										
10 km/h	15	17	20	23	26	29	33	36	39	42
15 km/h	22	27	32	36	41	46	50	55	60	65
Figure skating	40	50	60	70	80	90	100	110	120	130
Ice hockey (on-ice time)	52	65	78	91	104	117	130	143	156	168
Running										
8 km/h	37	45	52	60	66	72	78	84	90	95
10 km/h	48	55	64	73	79	85	92	100	107	113
Soccer (game)	36	45	54	63	72	81	90	99	108	117
Swimming (30 m/min)										
Breast	19	24	29	34	38	43	48	53	58	62
Front crawl	25	31	37	43	49	56	62	68	74	80
Back	17	21	25	30	34	38	42	47	51	55
Tennis	22	28	33	39	44	50	55	61	66	72
Walking										
4 km/h	17	19	21	23	26	28	30	32	34	36
6 km/h	24	26	28	30	32	34	37	40	43	48

*kcal per 10 minutes of activity

Adapted with permission from: Bar-Or O: *Pediatric Sports Medicine for the Practitioner*, Appendix IV. New York, NY, Springer Verlag, 1983.

reported energy intakes well above recommended levels, many report marginal or inadequate energy intakes. While the average energy intakes of young male athletes appear to be adequate, certain male athletes, such as those trying to restrict energy to make weight (wrestlers, lightweight crew) report low energy intakes.

Several factors may affect the young athlete's food intake, including socioeconomic status, the individual responsible for food purchase and preparation, access to sufficient calories, intentional weight loss, body image disturbance, peer pressure, and health problems.

To meet nutrition needs for physical activity and health, the training diet should provide about 55% to 60% of total energy from carbohydrates, 12% to 15% from protein, and 25% to 30% from fat. The key messages of variety, balance, and moderation in food choices should be promoted. Planning intake around the Food Guide Pyramid encourages daily consumption of a variety of foods (**Figure 9.2**). The number of calories that the Food Guide Pyramid provides varies depending on the selection of foods within the groups and the number of servings eaten. The minimum number of servings from the Food Guide Pyramid provides about 1,600 calories when low-fat, lean foods from the five groups are consumed, and fats and sweets are used sparingly.

Consuming the maximum number of servings, with a limited use of fats and sweets, provides about 2,800 calories per day.

Macronutrient Requirements

Carbohydrates During Exercise

How much and what type of fuel is used depends on the intensity and duration of activity. Intermittent sports such as football or basketball rely primarily on glucose from stored glycogen in the muscles for fuel. Endurance sports such as long-distance running or bicycling use glycogen stores first and then turn to fat as the preferred fuel for energy. For any activity, the body prefers to use carbohydrates for energy, however, the muscles and liver can store only a limited amount of glycogen.

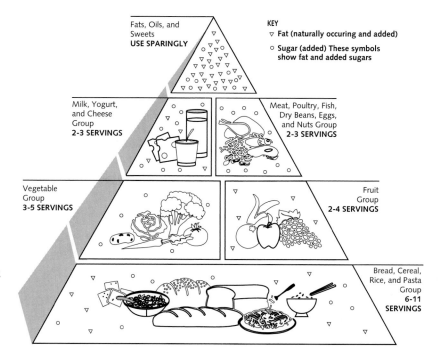

Figure 9.2
The Food Guide Pyramid.

Adapted from United States Department of Agriculture.

When young athletes report that they have difficulty maintaining their usual exercise intensity and that their performance has deteriorated, the reason is usually inadequate consumption of carbohydrates and/or calories. Consuming a carbohydrate-rich diet and resting on intermittent days to permit adequate muscle glycogen synthesis can prevent glycogen depletion.

Carbohydrates are the cornerstone of the athlete's diet. For very young children, additional carbohydrates can be encouraged by including more servings from the following groups: the bread, cereal, rice, and pasta group; the milk, yogurt, and cheese group; the vegetable group; and the fruit group.

For adolescents, carbohydrate needs can be calculated using 6 to 8 g carbohydrate/kg body weight. A list of high-carbohydrate foods as shown in **Table 9.3,** in addition to the Food Guide Pyramid, can help adolescents incorporate high-carbohydrate foods into their diet.

Based on studies in adult athletes, consuming high-carbohydrate fluids and foods immediately after training increases muscle glycogen storage and improves recovery time. Current guidelines based on studies in adult athletes suggest that 1.5 g carbohydrate/kg body weight should be consumed 30 minutes after exercise, followed by an additional 1.5 g/kg 2 hours later. This regimen is particularly beneficial for an adolescent athlete who trains twice a day.

Because of the energy demands of training, some adolescents may have difficulty consuming sufficient amounts of carbohydrates from food. In this case, commercial high-carbohydrate beverages, such as Gatorlode (70 g carbohydrate, 280 calories), may be needed to boost carbohydrate calories. These products provide supplemental carbohydrates and calories, but should not be used to replace regular food.

Fasting, dieting, or chronically omitting carbohydrate-rich foods will decrease muscle glycogen levels. Fad diets, (such as "The Zone" and "Atkins Diet)" that restrict carbohydrates and calories, do not provide young growing athletes with adequate energy and micronutrients.

Table 9.3 *Common High-Carbohydrate Foods*

Food	Amount	Grams of carbohydrate	Food	Amount	Grams of carbohydrate
Beans			*Fruits*		
Navy beans	½ cup	24	Apple	1 medium	21
Kidney beans	½ cup	20	Dried apricot	½ cup	40
Garbanzo beans (chickpeas)	½ cup	22	Banana	1 medium	27
Pinto beans	½ cup	22	Cantaloupe	½ cup	7
Breads, Cereals, Grains			Cranberry juice	½ cup	19
Rice	1 cup cooked	50	Orange	1 medium	16
Spaghetti	1 cup cooked	34	Orange juice	½ cup	12
Flour tortilla	1	15	Peach	1 medium	10
Waffle	2	17	Pear	1 medium	30
Bagel	2 oz	31	Raisins	1/2 cup	57
Breadsticks	4 sticks	30	*Vegetables*		
Whole wheat bread	2 slices	24	Baked potato	Large	50
Fig bar	1	10	Corn	½ cup	21
Cheerios	½ cup	8	Carrot	1 medium	8
Oatmeal	½ cup	13	*Dairy*		
Shredded wheat	1 biscuit	18	Yogurt (fruit)	1 cup	42
English muffin	1	30	Yogurt (frozen, low-fat)	1 cup	34
Graham crackers	2 squares	11			
Oatmeal raisin cookie	1	9			
Popcorn	1 cup	6			
Pretzels	1 oz	21			

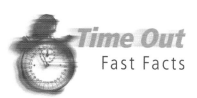

Children should receive no more than 30% of their total calories from fat sources.

Fat During Exercise

Even though maximal performance is impossible without muscle glycogen, fat also provides energy for exercise. As described earlier, blood glucose and muscle glycogen provide working muscles with most of their energy, and duration and intensity of activity determine how much fat the body contributes as fuel. In general, exercise must be performed for 30 to 60 minutes before fatty acids are available for energy. As the intensity of the exercise increases, working muscles have less oxygen available to them, and fat cannot be used as fuel. The muscle will shift to glycogen utilization. Sports with short bursts of activity such as a 50-yd swim, a gymnastics routine, or a baseball game, use very little fat for energy.

Interestingly, children use relatively more fat and less carbohydrate when compared with adults. The cause for this difference is not clear. The greater use of fat as a fuel by children does not increase the dietary recommendation for fat, however.

How much fat should a young athlete consume? Fat is an essential nutrient for the growing athlete and should be consumed in *moderation*. Of course, children who eat a large amount of fried foods, desserts, or fast foods are most likely consuming too much fat and not enough carbohydrates and other important nutrients. The American Dietetic Association, the American Academy of Pediatrics, and the American Heart Association support the following guidelines for fat consumption in children:

- Total fat—no more than 30% total calories/day

- Saturated fat—no more than 10% of total calories/day

- Cholesterol—less than 30 mg/day

High-fat diets have been promoted to improve endurance performance. The claim is that "fat loading" enables athletes to burn fat, rather than glycogen, as the major fuel source. Because fat stores are plentiful and glycogen stores are limited, fat loading supposedly improves endurance. However, there is no convincing evidence that a high-fat diet increases endurance. In fact, just the opposite is likely to occur. Eating too much fat will decrease the intake of carbohydrates, fiber, and other important nutrients. Muscle glycogen stores cannot be adequately maintained on a high-fat diet, and performance will be impaired. In addition, high-fat diets have been associated with sudden death and heart rhythm disturbances because of protein and potassium losses.

Protein During Exercise

When muscle glycogen stores are low as the result of prolonged exercise or a low-carbohydrate diet, protein may contribute as much as 10% of the energy needed for exercise. However, when muscle glycogen stores are high, the contribution of protein for energy is no more than about 5%. Athletes also use more protein for fuel when they do not eat enough calories. Consuming a high-carbohydrate diet during repeated days of heavy training helps to maintain muscle glycogen stores and reduces the use of protein as fuel.

The RDAs for protein/kg/body weight are shown in Table 9.1. Additional protein requirements for athletes in this age group have not been specifically evaluated. However, young athletes may need more protein based on the following:

- Athletes who are just beginning a training program should consume 1.0–1.5 g/kg/d and adequate calories to reduce the loss associated with increased protein turnover and nitrogen loss.

- Endurance athletes need 1.2–1.4 g/kg/d.

- Resistance training athletes need 1.6–1.7 g/kg/d.

- Athletes who chronically restrict calories require higher intakes of protein to allow for adequate synthesis and repair of muscle tissue.

- Young athletes who consume most of their proteins from plant sources should consume sufficient calories and a wide variety of grains and vegetables to obtain adequate protein.

Protein needs can be met by including more servings from the following foods: meat, poultry, fish, dry beans and peas, eggs, and nuts group; milk, yogurt, and cheese group; bread, cereal, rice, and pasta group; and the vegetable group. The protein content of some common foods is shown in **Table 9.4.**

Protein supplements

Protein supplements have not been shown to enhance muscle development, strength, or endurance. In addition, supplementation with specific amino acids will not increase muscle mass, decrease body fat, or improve endurance. Many

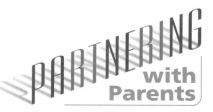

Is there an increased protein requirement for athletes who are involved in weight training?

While there is an increased need for protein, it rarely exceeds 2 g/kg/body weight.

Table 9.4 *Protein Content in Common Foods*

Food	Amount	Grams of Protein	Food	Amount	Grams of Protein
Meat, Fish, Poultry			**Breads, Cereals, Grains**		
Lean beef	1 oz	8	Macaroni and cheese	½ cup	9
Chicken	1 oz	8	Spaghetti	1 cup cooked	8
Turkey breast	1 oz	8	Bagel	2 oz	6
Fish	1 oz	7	Raisin bran	1 oz (⅔ cup)	3
Eggs	1	6	Rice	1 cup cooked	3
Beans, Nuts			Bread	1 slice	2
Kidney beans	½ cup	9	**Vegetables**		
Navy beans	½ cup	7	Baked potato	1 large	4
Garbanzo beans (chickpeas)	½ cup	6	Peas, green	½ cup	4
Tofu	2 oz	5	Corn	½ cup	2
Peanut butter	1 tbsp	4	Lettuce	¼ head	1
Dairy			Carrot	1 large	1
Low-fat cottage cheese	½ cup	13	**Fruits**		
Milk, whole, skim	1 cup	8	Banana	1 medium	1
Yogurt	1 cup	8	Orange	1 medium	1
Cheddar cheese	1 oz	7	Apple	1 medium	1
Ice cream	½ cup	4			
Frozen yogurt	½ cup	4			
American cheese	1 oz	3			

athletes do not realize that excess protein is either burned for energy or converted to fat. Consuming too much protein, whether from food or supplements, can lead to dehydration, weight gain, and increased calcium loss from the body. High-protein diets are also usually high in fat. Consuming a high-protein, high-fat diet after heavy training does not allow for complete replacement of muscle glycogen and may impair performance. This type of diet also takes a long time to digest and can cause the athlete to feel sluggish. By comparison, a high-carbohydrate diet is easily digested and quickly restores muscle glycogen.

Commercial weight gain supplements may contain unproven additives like chromium picolinate, and dangerous compounds such as ephedrine. Nonfat dry milk can be used as an alternative to boost protein, as it is a high-quality, inexpensive protein supplement (¹/₄ cup provides 11 g protein).

Vegetarian diet

When carefully planned, a diet that derives its protein from vegetable sources can provide adequate protein, carbohydrates, and vitamins and minerals that the young athlete needs to sustain growth and prolonged workouts. Protein intake on a lacto-ovo vegetarian diet or a semi-vegetarian diet should provide adequate calories and high-quality protein from eggs and dairy products. However, athletes on a strict vegetarian diet may have difficulty obtaining calories, necessary protein, and other nutrients such as calcium, vitamins D and B12, zinc, and iron. Eliminating foods that contain important vitamins and minerals can be risky unless the young athlete is prepared to assume the additional responsibility necessary to maintain good health and proper growth.

Eating Before Exercise

The pre-exercise meal serves two principal functions: 1) to prevent athletes from feeling hungry before or during activity; and 2) to supply fuel to the muscles during training and competition. A carbohydrate-rich meal should be consumed 1 to 4 hours before exercise. To avoid potential gastrointestinal distress, the size of the meal should be reduced the closer to exercise it is consumed. For example, a small meal of 300 to 400 calories is appropriate 1 hour before exercise, whereas a large meal of 700 to 800 calories can be consumed 4 hours before exercise. Examples of high-carbohydrate foods and fluids to include in the preexercise meal are listed in **Table 9.5.**

In contrast to carbohydrates that are rapidly digested to provide a readily available source of energy, fatty foods should be limited because they delay gastric emptying and can contribute to a sluggish, heavy feeling. Many high-protein foods such as eggs, cheese, and meat are also high in fat and should also be limited before exercise.

High-fiber foods (especially those high in bran) should be avoided prior to activity as they can cause abdominal cramping and necessitate a bathroom break during exercise. Gas-forming foods such as beans, broccoli, cauliflower, and onions should be minimized, as should extremely salty foods that can cause fluid retention and a bloated feeling.

Macronutrients

Adolescent athletes are at increased risk of iron deficiency because of increased growth demands, lower energy intake, inadequate dietary intake, and exercise-related loss. Adolescent girls have additional losses through menstruation; therefore, iron stores must be monitored in female athletes. By focusing on prevention and intervening when iron stores are low, athletes can avoid iron-deficiency anemia and the accompanying decline in athletic performance.

On average, an adolescent's calcium intake is reported to be one half to two thirds of the RDA. Inadequate consumption may place the female athlete at

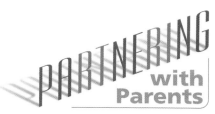

How important is the pre-event meal?

Pre-event meals are principally important to avoid hunger during the event and to provide some additional fuel for exercise. Ideally, this meal should consist of something that is easily digested and quickly emptied from the stomach (ie, low in fat and protein and high in carbohydrates).

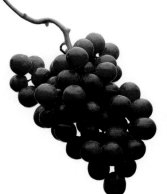

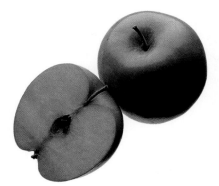

Table 9.5 *Pre-exercise Meal Guidelines*

1 to 2 hours before	2 to 3 hours before	3 or more hours before
Fruit or vegetable juices, sports drinks	Fruit or vegetable juices, sports drinks	Fruit or vegetable juices, sports drinks
Fresh fruit (low fiber)	Fresh fruit	Fresh fruit
	Breads, bagels, crackers, English muffins	Breads, bagels, crackers, English muffins
		Peanut butter, lean meat, low-fat cheese
		Low-fat yogurt (regular or frozen)
		Pasta with tomato sauce
		Cereal with low-fat milk

risk for stress fractures and osteoporosis. These complications are most relevant for female adolescents (especially those who have the female athlete triad: disordered eating, menstrual dysfunction, and bone mineral disorders). These issues are described in more detail in chapter 15.

Research is lacking regarding the use of dietary supplements and ergogenic aids by young athletes, as discussed in chapter 10. Because athletes are looking for a competitive edge, they may consume a variety of substances, including vitamins and minerals that they believe have performance enhancing properties. Although vitamin and mineral supplementation may improve the nutritional status of individuals with deficiencies, no scientific evidence supports the general use of supplements to improve athletic performance. Especially in young athletes, the unsupervised, indiscriminate use of vitamins and minerals raises health concerns and cost issues.

Special Fluid Needs of Children

Compared with adults and even adolescents, preadolescent children must be especially careful to drink enough before and during exercise. Preadolescent children do not tolerate temperature extremes as well as adults. They produce less sweat, yet generate more heat during exercise and are less able to transfer this heat from muscles to the skin. The relative surface area of the skin is greater for a child compared with an adult, and results in greater heat gain in extreme heat and greater heat loss in cold weather.

Fluid Requirements

With a disproportionate risk of dehydration in children, fluids play a critical role in maintaining the health and performance of the young athlete. Thus, fluid restriction should never be used as a disciplinary measure. Water or some type of beverage should be available at all times of training and competition, and in all climates, not only in hot, humid environments. Because a substantial level of dehydration can be reached before an athlete ever feels "thirsty," special emphasis should be placed on ensuring adequate fluid intake, via "fluid breaks" for children and adolescents before, during, and after physical activity.

Fluid Guidelines

Athletes should be provided with their own bottle and encouraged to drink 4 to 8 oz every 15 to 20 minutes during physical activity, even when they do not feel thirsty. Monitoring fluid intake is essential, particularly for children, because they do not instinctively drink enough fluid to replace water losses. If the young athlete tires easily and repeatedly in practice, appears irritable, and performance suddenly declines, dehydration and/or inadequate caloric intake may be the cause. Therefore, frequent fluid and rest breaks in the shade should be scheduled. All athletes should drink something before they return to practice or play. After exercise, young athletes need to replace fluid lost during exercise by drinking 16 to 24 oz for each pound of weight lost. Chapter 8 addresses fluid requirements in hot, humid environments in more detail.

Choosing the Right Fluids

Although plain water is the most economical source of fluid to hydrate the body, children may be more likely to drink sufficient amounts if they are given flavored fluids. To enhance the athlete's willingness to drink, beverages consumed

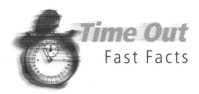

Fast Facts

Dehydration or inadequate caloric intake may contribute to early fatigue, irritability, or a sudden decline in performance.

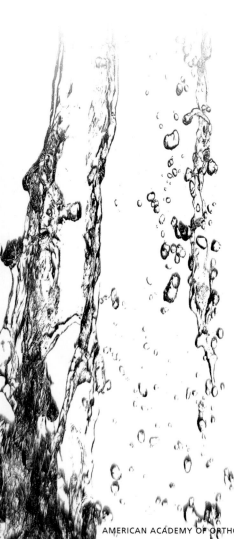

during exercise should be palatable and stimulate thirst. Flavor preference varies widely. It is best to identify the specific flavor(s) that athletes prefer and then provide fluids accordingly. In a recent study, 9- to 12-year-old boys performed three 3-hour intermittent sessions of moderate exercise in a warm climate. Children voluntarily consumed more when they drank sports drinks (38 oz) than when they drank plain water (20 oz) or flavored water (30 oz). The authors concluded that while flavoring of water reduces children's voluntary dehydration, the addition of 6% carbohydrates and 18 mmol/L sodium chloride prevents it altogether.

Juice or carbonated soda should not be used for fluid replacement during activity because these beverages contain too much carbohydrate (10% to 12%) and may cause gastric discomfort, delayed gastric emptying, and delayed intestinal absorption because of their high osmolarity. It is also best to avoid caffeinated beverages (iced tea, certain soft drinks) because they promote diuresis. The potential side effects of agitation, nausea, muscle tremors, palpitations, and headaches after consuming caffeine are not conducive to optimal performance, particularly for children.

Weight Control Practices

The concept of ideal body weight for purposes of sports performance is frequently misunderstood, particularly concerning how dietary changes can help an athlete achieve a desired weight. Some parents and coaches encourage their children to eat excessively, with the erroneous belief that this will build strength and endurance more quickly. However, indiscriminate consumption, in which food intake exceeds the child's caloric requirement, may be the start of a lifelong struggle with excess body fat. At the other extreme, a restrictive diet and/or dehydration practices, instituted for purposes of weight loss, performance, or esthetics, may endanger the health of a child.

Weight Loss Issues

For some sports, parents or coaches may place sudden and extreme weight control demands on young athletes, such as running laps during hot weather to eliminate excess body fat. Food intake may also be chronically restricted in an effort to enhance performance. Fatigue, heat exhaustion, and illness can be the result. Nutritional needs for growth and development must be placed before athletic considerations.

Some athletes resort to unhealthy techniques to lose weight. Although traditionally thought to occur in sport such as figure skating and gymnastics, where image or appearance contributes to success, or wrestling to "make weight," all sports can be affected. Whether a long-distance runner thinks that weight loss will contribute to faster times on the cross-country course or a parent believes that his or her child will compete better at a lower weight in weight-class football, athletes from every sport have resorted to ill-advised weight loss techniques. These weight loss behaviors include caloric restriction, anorectic drugs, vomiting, diuretic and laxative use, excessive exercise, and the use of rubber suits, steam rooms, saunas, and spitting in an attempt to lose water weight. Rapid dehydration or water loss behavior is more popular in sports with strict weight classes such as wrestling and lightweight crew.

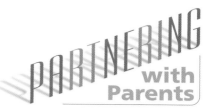

Are liquid meals a safe and effective alternative for athletes who have difficulty eating prior to competition?

Yes. They are also advantageous because they are high in fluid content, easily digestible, and emptied quickly from the stomach.

Table 9.6 *Dehydration and Starvation Effects on Health and Performance*

Organ System	Effect	Organ System	Effect
Endocrine	Growth retardation	Psychological	Decrease in school performance
	Decrease in testosterone		Depression and mood swings
	Amenorrhea	Fluid and electrolytes	Decrease in plasma volume and renal blood flow
	Osteoporosis		
Neuromuscular	Decrease in strength and power		Electrolyte abnormalities → cardiac dysfunction
	Decrease in endurance		
	Decrease in isometric endurance and short-term sprinting	Thermoregulation	Increased susceptibility to hyperthermia

Adapted with permission from Perriello VA Jr, Almquist J, Conkwright D Jr, et al: Health and weight control management among wrestlers: A proposed program for high school athletes. *Va Med Quart* 1995;122:179–183.

Consequences of extreme weight loss

The consequences of extreme weight loss are well known and include a significant morbidity rate. Research and the recent tragic deaths of three collegiate wrestlers have raised awareness among athletes, coaches, administrators, athletic trainers, and physicians that fluid restriction can have serious consequences. In 1997, three wrestlers died while engaged in a rapid weight loss program in an attempt to qualify for competition. All three were involved in similar programs that promoted dehydration through perspiration and resulted in hyperthermia. **Table 9.6** lists the negative effects that starvation and fluid restriction may have on the performance and health of the athlete.

A six-part program developed by the American College of Sports Medicine to educate wrestlers about the dangers of cyclical weight control through starvation and fluid restriction is shown in **Table 9.7.**

Following the deaths in 1997, the NCAA established new guidelines that included adding a 7-lb weight allowance to each weight class, prohibiting the use of tools (drugs and environmental conditions) used to dehydrate, establishing a weigh-in time 2 hours prior to competition, and establishing a permanent healthy weight class for each wrestler early in the season.

These same guidelines could easily be implemented at the high school level and used in other weight-restricted sports such as lightweight crew. It is important to note that education only solves part of the problem. Active implementation of the recommendations and rule changes are more likely to make sports such as wrestling and lightweight crew safer and healthier.

Disordered eating

Eating disorders are characterized by gross disturbances in eating behavior that can result in serious medical problems and can even be fatal. These include anorexia nervosa, bulimia nervosa, and eating disorders not otherwise specified (NOS). Data on the prevalence of eating disorders in athletic populations are limited and equivocal. While most studies have used surveys to evaluate preoccupation with food and weight, use of pathogenic weight control methods, or disturbed body image, only a few studies have examined clinical eating disorders.

Existing studies suggest that eating problems are more common among athletes than nonathletes, and even more prevalent among those athletes where weight and appearance are considered important to performance. It is important to recognize that many athletes using unhealthy weight loss methods may

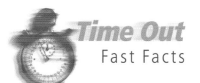

Time Out
Fast Facts

Forty-five percent of high school wrestlers exhibit at least two of the diagnostic criteria for bulimia nervosa.

Table 9.7 *Components of the American College of Sports Medicine Weight Control Program for Wrestlers*

1. Educate coaches and wrestlers about adverse consequences of prolonged fasting and dehydration on physical performance and health.
2. Discourage the use of rubber suits, steam rooms, hot boxes, saunas, laxatives, and diuretics for making weight.
3. Adopt new state or national governing body legislation that schedules weigh-ins immediately prior to competition.
4. Schedule daily weigh-ins before and after practice to monitor weight loss and dehydration.
5. Assess body composition: Boys age 16 years and younger with a body fat of less than 7% or those older than age 16 years with a body fat of less than 5% need medical clearance before being allowed to compete.
6. Emphasize proper nutrition on a daily basis.

Adapted with permission from Oppliger RA, Case HS, Horswill CA, Landry GL, Shelter AC: American College of Sports Medicine position stand: Weight loss in wrestlers. *Med Sci Sports Exerc* 1996;28:ix–xii.

show significant symptoms of eating disorders but do not meet all of the *Diagnostic and Statistical Manual of Mental Disorders, ed 4 (DSM-IV)* criteria. Even when a few symptoms are present, intervention is needed because both health and performance may be compromised. Early identification may prevent the development of the full disorder.

Psychological, biological, and social factors are implicated in the development of eating disorders. For the athlete, specific factors within the athletic environment may act as triggers for the development of eating disorders, such as prolonged periods of dieting and exercise, frequent weight fluctuations, a sudden increase in training volume, pressure from coaches to reduce weight for performance, or traumatic events such as loss of a coach or an injury.

Treatment of eating disorders requires a team of health care professionals that includes a physician, psychologist, and nutritionist. For athletes who have a significant disordered eating pattern, the same team of professionals may help prevent progression to a more severe problem. The success of the treatment plan is based on establishing a trusting relationship between the athlete and the health care team. Education of coaches, athletes, parents, and administrators is a key aspect of prevention.

Weight Gain Issues

Many young athletes are encouraged to gain weight in hopes of improving their strength through increased muscle mass. Power lifting, bodybuilding, football, and other power sports are frequently cited as sports where gains in muscle mass and weight lead to better performance. Unfortunately, many well-meaning (but misinformed) parents and coaches also advise children to take supplements in an effort to promote early athletic development, improve performance, and as "nutrition insurance." However, eventual maturity and athletic ability do not depend on how early children begin adolescence.

Ergogenic aids

Advertisements of commercially available ergogenic aids make hundreds of claims about improved performance. Some commonly available supplements include amino acids, androstenedione, boron, carnitine, choline, chromium, creatine, dibercozide, ferulic acid, gamma oryzanol, medium-chain triglycerides, weight gain powders, and yohimbine.

With this vast array of supplements to choose from, young athletes must be educated to view manufacturer's claims with a critical eye. For many of these

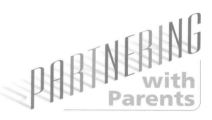

Is there any benefit to a postevent meal?

Yes. Consuming carbohydrates within 30 minutes after vigorous exercise followed by additional carbohydrates 2 hours later enhances muscle glycogen stores. This glycogen build-up exceeds that which would occur by consuming the same amount of nutrients later in the day.

supplements, there is no regulation regarding their purity, safety, dosing, benefits, or side effects, and there is very little research to support their marketing claims. While manufacturers may conduct blind placebo-controlled trials to support the benefits or risks of these substances, in many cases, research findings on small study populations are extrapolated to inappropriate conclusions.

Aside from being potentially harmful, performance enhancing supplements can give athletes a false sense of security. They may assume that their "morning dose" of supplements is a proper substitute for healthy food and fluid choices throughout the day. In addition, they may erroneously associate improvements in performance with whatever supplements they happened to be taking and may be less likely to attribute progress to training, hard work, and nutrition.

Performance enhancing substances are discussed in more detail in chapter 10.

Combating "supplement insurance"

To move away from this reliance on "supplement insurance," young athletes need to feel confident about eating ordinary foods. Parents, coaches, and physicians must emphasize how ordinary foods promote muscle growth and optimal performance. From a practical standpoint, this is yet another important reason to encourage young athletes to keep records of what they eat, how they train, and how their performance improves. These records can be used to illustrate the importance of good dietary and training habits as the cause of improvement, rather than allowing an athlete to erroneously associate his or her athletic accomplishments with a pill or powder.

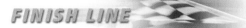

FINISH LINE

More research is needed on the nutritional intake and needs of young athletes. The key to health and performance cannot be found in any one food or supplement. Rather, the combination of proper exercise, strength training, and nutrition is the best strategy to achieve improved performance.

For More Information

1. American Psychiatric Association: *Diagnostic and Statistical Manual of Mental Disorders,* ed 4. Washington, DC, American Psychiatric Association, 1994.

2. Bar-Or O: Children's responses to exercise in hot climates: Implications for performance and health. *Gatorade Sports Science Exchange* 1994;7:49.

3. Coleman E, Steen SN, (eds): *The Ultimate Sports Nutrition Handbook,* Palo Alto, CA, Bull Publishing Co, 1996.

4. Lohman TG (ed): *Advances in Body Composition Assessment,* Champaign, IL, Human Kinetics, 1992.

5. Sundgot-Borgen J: Risk and trigger factors for the development of eating disorders in female elite athletes. *Med Sci Sports Exerc* 1994;26:414–419. Check also: Eating Disorders, in Berning JR, Steen SN (eds): *Nutrition for Sport and Exercise,* ed 2. Gaithersburg, MD, Aspen Publishing, 1998, pp 187–204.

Chapter 10

Performance Enhancing Substances

BERNARD A. GRIESEMER, MD

Young athletes today are participating in increasingly competitive sports at much earlier ages. The societal rewards for success in sports also continue to increase with no apparent end in sight. These two factors have increased the incentives for young athletes to consider the use of ergogenic substances to enhance their athletic performance.

The term "ergogenic" derives from Greek roots meaning "to make work." For young athletes, performance enhancing substances are considered to be "ergogenic" if they can be proven, in controlled studies, to increase power and/or endurance. While some of the substances and techniques used by young athletes are used exclusively for ergogenic effects, other substances, including many common nonprescription drugs, produce ergogenic effects that are secondary to the substance's intended use.

Physicians need to be familiar with the substances used for performance enhancement so that they can effectively counsel their patients regarding the effects and side effects of these substances. Athletes, coaches, and medical support staff are encouraged to contact their sport's governing body directly in order to determine the status of any of the substances used to enhance performance.

Ergogenic Drugs
Anabolic Steroids

The use of anabolic-androgenic steroids for sports performance enhancement has been reported in medical literature for more than 40 years. When used in conjunction with an adequate strength-training program and diet, steroids will contribute to gains in muscle size and strength. However, steroids have not been shown to enhance aerobic capacity, and there is little evidence that they enhance overall athletic performance, unless the sport depends primarily on strength (eg, weight lifting).

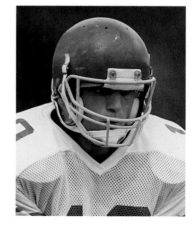

Table 10.1 *Patterns of Usage for Anabolic-Androgenic Steroids*

Investigator/ Year of Report	Number of Athletes	Grade Level	Male (percent)	Female (percent)	Percent of Total Using Steroids
Corder et al, 1975	1,393 total				0.7%
	208 athletes	—			4.0%
Newman,1986	5,029	8			3.0%
		10			2.0%
		12	5.0%	1.0%	
Polen, et al, 1986	200	9 to 12	18.0%	0	—
Bosworth, 1987	190 athletes	9 to 12	1.1%	—	—
Buckley, 1988	3,403	12	6.6%	—	—
Johnson, 1989	1,775	11	11.0%	0.5%	5.7%
Windsor, 1989	901	9-12	5.0%	1.4%	3.0%
Ross, 1989	13,461	6	—	—	2.0%
		8	—	—	2.3%
		10	—	—	2.2%
		12	4.6%	1.4%	3.1%
Ringwalt, 1989	11,531	7	3.2%	0.7%	Male MS
		8	3.1%	0.5%	2% to 3.2%
		9	3.3%	0.6%	Female MS
		10	3.3%	0.5%	0.5% to 0.7%
		11	3.2%	0.5%	Male HS
		12	3.0 %	0.3%	1.1% to 18% Female HS 0 to 4%
Krowchuck, 1989	295 athletes	9 to 12	—	—	1.4%
Hubbell, 1990	5,252	10	12.0%	4.0%	8.0%
Terney, 1990	2,113	9	—	—	4.3%
		10	—	—	4.8%
		11	—	—	4.6%
		12	—	—	4.2%
		9 to 12	6.5%	2.5%	4.4%
Johnson, 1990	2,600	12	4.7%	1.3%	3.0%
Johnson, 1991	2,350	12	5.0%	0.5%	2.9%
Faigenbaum, 1998	965	5 to 7	2.6%	2.8%	2.7%

Adapted with permission from Rogol AD, Yesalis CE III: Anabolic-androgenic steroids and the adolescent. *Pediatr Ann* 1992;21:175–188.

Reports of steroid use by young athletes have appeared for over 20 years, with use patterns summarized in **Table 10.1**. Since these reports were first issued, the rates of use have not appreciably increased or decreased over time. Use patterns and rates are influenced by many factors, including the following: age and makeup of the study population; association with a peer group that uses steroids; knowledge of the beneficial effect of these substances; denial of the detrimental effects; association with other risk-taking behaviors; and dissatisfaction with current size and overall body image. Young athletes generally obtain information about the onset of action, duration of action, potential side effects, and options for administration from peers, coaches, strength-training specialists, or "muscle magazines," rather than from medical authorities.

Use of anabolic-androgenic steroids does not appear to be limited by socioeconomic status, nor is its use limited only to athletes. The proportion of adolescents using these substances solely for the purpose of physique enhancement may be more common.

Methods of administration

Anabolic-androgenic steroids can be taken orally or injected. Both forms have similar systemic and side effects. The principal differences between the two include onset of action, duration of action, and the length of time detection is possible. Injectable forms are considered to be more potent and longer lasting, but also of higher risk. Infection can develop at the site of injection, and needle sharing among athletes carries the risk of human immunodeficiency virus (HIV) and hepatitis B virus (HBV) transmission.

Oral anabolic-androgenic steroids, including the 17-alpha steroid derivatives and androstenediol, androstenedione, and dehydroepiandrosterone, are converted by the liver to testosterone following ingestion. Injectable forms, such as Durabolin and Boldenone, however, do not require hepatic conversion to an active form.

Adverse effects

Adverse effects from anabolic-androgenic steroid use have been reported in virtually every organ system of the body (**Figure 10.1**). Some adverse effects are reversible; others are not.

One serious and irreversible adverse effect unique to the skeletally immature individual is epiphyseal closure. A single cycle of anabolic-androgenic steroids may result in permanent epiphyseal closure and arrest of linear growth. Tendon strains have also been associated with anabolic-androgenic steroid use. These have been attributed to muscle strength gains that exceed the strength of the related tendon.

Effects on the cardiovascular system include predictable, but reversible elevations in blood pressure, increases in total cholesterol, and reduction in high-density lipoprotein levels. An increased risk of arteriosclerotic heart disease and possible cardiomyopathy are also concerns.

Negative effects on the hepatobiliary system include transient elevation in liver enzymes and bilirubin. Peliosis hepatis (blood-filled cysts in the liver) has been associated with traumatic rupture and may result in fatal hemorrhage.

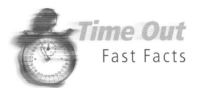

Most young athletes obtain information about steroids and other ergogenic aides from sources other than medical authorities.

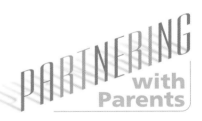

Is there any ergogenic effect of vitamin, mineral, or protein supplements?

No. In an otherwise healthy individual consuming a balanced diet, many studies have demonstrated no benefit from vitamin, mineral, or protein supplementation.

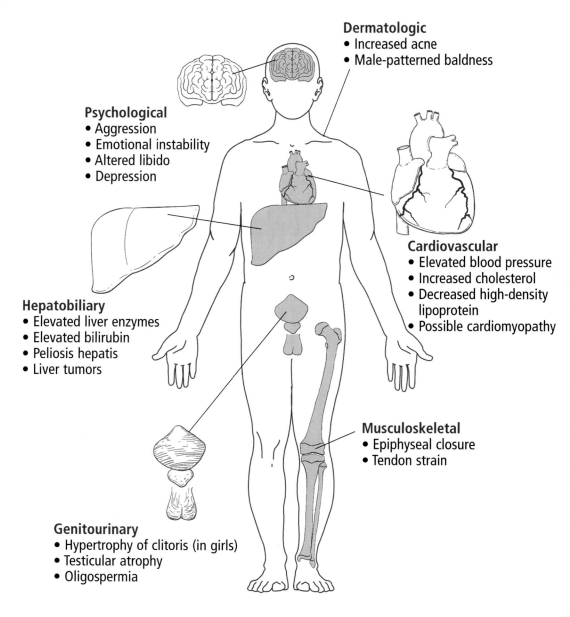

Dermatologic
- Increased acne
- Male-patterned baldness

Psychological
- Aggression
- Emotional instability
- Altered libido
- Depression

Cardiovascular
- Elevated blood pressure
- Increased cholesterol
- Decreased high-density lipoprotein
- Possible cardiomyopathy

Hepatobiliary
- Elevated liver enzymes
- Elevated bilirubin
- Peliosis hepatis
- Liver tumors

Musculoskeletal
- Epiphyseal closure
- Tendon strain

Genitourinary
- Hypertrophy of clitoris (in girls)
- Testicular atrophy
- Oligospermia

Figure 10.1
Body systems affected by anabolic steroid use.

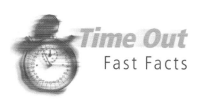

Time Out
Fast Facts

A single cycle of anabolic-androgenic steroids may result in permanent closure of growth plates.

Liver tumors, such as a benign hepatoma or potentially fatal hepatic carcinoma, have also been reported, although the true incidence in young people is not known.

Dermatologic problems, including increased acne and male-pattern baldness, are not life threatening, but may be the most obvious clinical signs.

In females, the androgenic effect of anabolic-androgenic steroids results in masculinization, including irreversible hypertrophy of the clitoris, irreversible thickening of the vocal cords, and hirsutism. In males, the genitourinary system is adversely affected in multiple ways. Testicular atrophy, oligospermia, abnormal sperm morphology, prostatic hypertrophy, and prostatic cancer have all been reported in adults. In younger individuals, the effects of these drugs on the genitourinary system, the degree to which they adversely affect fertility, and the degree to which the effects are reversible, requires additional study.

Psychological effects are a common, but not always predictable consequence of anabolic-androgenic steroid use. Aggression ("roid rage"), emotional instability, altered libido, and even a steroid-induced psychosis have been reported. Depression may occur as part of a withdrawal syndrome. The risk of drug dependency is increased in individuals who start taking anabolic-androgenic steroids before age 16 years.

Other substances with anabolic effects

Another drug that has anabolic effects but is not in the steroid family is clenbuterol, a beta-2 agonist approved for treatment of asthma in some countries. This medication can have anabolic effects in that it promotes protein synthesis and increases lean body mass. With oral and inhaled routes of administration, clenbuterol also has abuse potential for its stimulant effects. Physicians also need to be aware of certain restrictions that are placed on the use of other inhaled beta-2 agonists in elite competition. If young athletes are competing at the Olympic level and require the use of beta-2 agonists for control of reactive airway disease, their sport's appropriate governing body must be notified prior to competition.

Stimulants

Caffeine

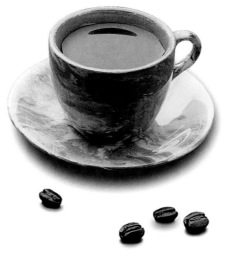

Because of the large number of consumer products containing caffeine, stimulants are perhaps the most widely available ergogenic substances. Caffeine, a xanthine derivative in the same family of alkaloids as theophylline, is found in coffee, tea, chocolate, soft drinks, and both prescription and over-the-counter drugs. The ergogenic effect of caffeine is derived from multiple actions, including central nervous system stimulation, delayed onset of fatigue, and increased metabolism of free fatty acids for energy while sparing glycogen stores. The average amount of caffeine in a cup of coffee (approximately 100 mg) has a small ergogenic effect for endurance activities. Some highly caffeinated soft drinks contain as much as 71.5 mg of caffeine per 12-oz serving. Over-the-counter drugs specifically intended to be used as stimulants contain as much as 200 mg of caffeine per tablet.

Ingesting any combination of beverages or medications that contain a total of approximately 800 mg of caffeine can result in a positive drug test in events that are subject to testing for performance enhancing substances. However, caffeine levels do not have to be illegally elevated to have adverse effects. Caffeine acts as a diuretic, which can result in dehydration. This can lead to diminished muscular strength and endurance, as well as greater risk of a heat-related injury.

Nicotine

Nicotine is another widely available stimulant that is used by many young people. Smokeless tobacco is an attractive, acceptable alternative to cigarettes to young athletes who underestimate its dangers. Any benefit from the stimulant effect is more than outweighed by health risks.

Ephedrine

Ephedrine, a chemical found in the plant genus Ephedra, is contained in many nonprescription drugs, foods, and nutritional supplements. Ephedrine has ergogenic properties similar to amphetamines. Young athletes are likely to

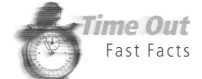

Fast Facts

The increased metabolic activity and alteration in cardiovascular cooling associated with amphetamine use may predispose athletes to heat injury.

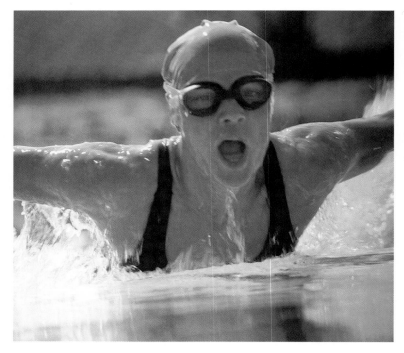

consume products containing ephedrine in herbal teas, medications (eg, Ma Huang, ginseng, gingko biloba), nonprescription cold medications, and nonprescription medications used specifically to attempt to reduce fatigue and to enhance mental alertness.

Amphetamines

Amphetamines are the most potent ergogenic drugs in the stimulant category. Illicit production of methamphetamine in home-based laboratories has increased availability to individuals in all age groups. Amphetamines increase cardiac output and metabolism of free fatty acids. Central nervous system stimulation from amphetamines can increase aggression, increase mental alertness, and decrease perception of fatigue. Heat-related injury may occur from increased metabolic activity and alterations in cardiovascular cooling. Athletes in a withdrawal phase of amphetamine abuse may experience depression and a marked reduction in athletic performance.

One area of medical and ethical controversy is the use of amphetamine derivatives and other related medications (eg, methylphenidate) in athletes with attention deficit and hyperactivity disorder (ADHD). In athletic competition where complicated play strategy and team member assignments require concentration, athletes with ADHD would presumably perform better with medical treatment. Increasing the dose of methylphenidate for athletes with ADHD during competition has also not been proven to be necessary or safe. Therefore, young athletes who regularly take methylphenidate for ADHD should be allowed to continue with their usual dose of medication on days of athletic competition. Young athletes who are competing at the Olympic level should be aware that methylphenidate and other medications used for treating ADHD are banned substances.

Beta Blockers

Beta blockers are compounds that slow the heart rate and lower blood pressure. Beta blockers have little ergogenic potential except in sports such as shooting, archery, and combination sports (eg, biathalon) where fine motor control and relief from the "jitters" are critical components of competition. Physicians who care for athletes in these sports should be aware that beta blockers are prohibited substances.

Human Growth Hormone

Human growth hormone is a polypeptide hormone produced endogenously by the anterior lobe of the pituitary gland. With the advent of recombinant DNA technology, human growth hormone has become more widely available to athletes. Both the natural compound and the synthetic drug accelerate linear growth in the skeletally immature individual and increase body weight and muscle mass, regardless of skeletal maturity status.

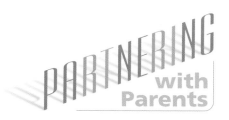

Are there any dangers inherent in vitamin, mineral, or protein supplementation?

Taken in large doses, some vitamin supplements, especially the fat-soluble vitamins, can have deleterious effects. Most are without serious side effects however, other than the substantial costs.

Detection of polypeptide hormones by conventional urine drug screening is complicated by the fact that very little of the parenterally administered product is excreted in the urine, and the synthetic product is essentially indistinguishable from the naturally occurring compound.

While increased linear growth and muscle size may enhance performance in selected sports, an insulin-like effect on glucose metabolism may negatively affect performance. Other significant side effects of exogenous human growth hormone supplementation include increased serum cholesterol and triglycerides, cardiac enlargement, hypogonadism, and changes of acromegaly of facial bones.

Blood Doping

Use of exogenous erythropoietin (EPO) and/or blood transfusions to enhance performance in endurance sports has been observed for decades. Both techniques are referred to as "blood doping." Increasing the hematocrit and hemoglobin concentration improves the availability of oxygen to the exercising muscle and consequently improves aerobic capacity and muscle endurance.

Erythropoietin is a glycoprotein produced endogenously by the kidneys. The synthetic compound is a result of recombinant DNA technology and is virtually indistinguishable from the naturally occurring substance. Production of red cells increases in direct proportion to the dose of EPO used. EPO doping can result in a hematocrit in excess of 60%, whereas transfusions rarely elevate the hematocrit above 50%.

Blood components for transfusions are obtained from donors or are harvested from the athlete well in advance of competition and then reinfused within days of competition. Detection of transfused blood is expensive and requires blood sampling. Blood doping detection techniques include analysis of red blood cell types (for homologous transfusions) and cell age (for autologous transfusions).

In athletes, dehydration during competition increases hematocrit. A hematocrit above 55% increases the risk for hyperviscosity syndrome, and possibly stroke, heart failure, and even death. Young athletes who use blood doping as an ergogenic aid are at increased risk for hyperviscosity syndrome because of their higher sweating rates and consequent increased risk of dehydration with exercise.

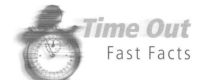

Time Out
Fast Facts

Doping with exogenous erythropoietin may result in hematocrits in excess of 60%.

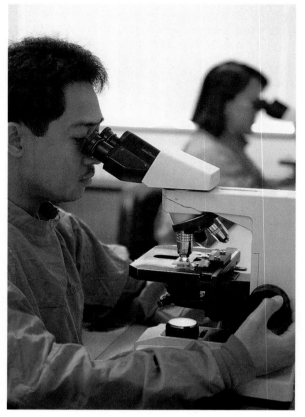

Blood doping with transfusions also carries the added risk of HIV or HBV infection. Physicians who care for young endurance athletes should be aware of the potential abuse of EPO and blood transfusions and counsel their patients regarding the dangers of this practice.

Diuretics

Diuretics may be used in sports settings to reduce body weight, reduce fluid retention from anabolic-androgenic steroid use, or serve as a masking agent for drug testing. Physicians may be asked to certify a minimum weight for athletes in sports in which competitors are matched by weight. In sports with weight categories, such as wrestling, football, and crew, young athletes may use diuretics as part of a strategy to reach the lowest possible weight. Diuretics may also be abused in sports such as bodybuilding, gymnastics, and ballet, where lower weight or a leaner appearance is rewarded.

Diuretics may be used or requested for control of fluid retention or hypertension in individuals who use anabolic-androgenic steroids. Athletes may be more open to discussing their use of diuretics rather than anabolic-androgenic steroids. However, physicians should be aware of the possibility of a more serious drug use problem. When drug testing is performed, diuretics may be used as a masking agent in an attempt to circumvent detection of other substances. Because of this abuse, diuretic agents such as furosemide are banned in competitions subject to doping control programs.

Drug Testing

Drug testing for ergogenic substances is an expensive and complex issue. Therefore, widespread testing for young athletes is not practical or feasible. However, young athletes who compete in events sanctioned by national sports federations may be selected for drug testing according to standards set by the governing body for each sport.

Some categories of drugs are restricted only in specific sports, such as beta-blockers in shooting sports. Other drug categories, such as amphetamines and anabolic steroids, are banned in all sports. Because many prescription and nonprescription drugs have effects that may enhance performance, young athletes who are subject to drug testing should be sure that anything they take is not banned.

In recent years, school systems and youth organizations have instituted voluntary drug testing for young athletes in an effort to curb abuse and provide athletes with an additional weapon to combat peer pressure to use drugs. These programs typically focus on psychoactive substances and are less likely to screen for drugs used exclusively for ergogenic purposes, such as anabolic steroids. The appendix includes policy statements from both the American Academy of Pediatrics and the American Academy of Orthopaedic Surgeons that specifically address steroid use.

Categories of ergogenic drugs and doping techniques are listed in **Table 10.2.**

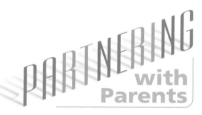

Why do studies on the effects of anabolic-androgenic steroids often fail to demonstrate improved performance, despite obvious physical changes in athletes that use them and testimonials to their effects?

For ethical reasons, doses of steroids that are administered to subjects in scientific studies are far less than those used by athletes.

Table 10.2 *Common Performance Enhancing Substances*

Anabolic-androgenic steroids	*Oral*
	17-alpha methyl testosterone (eg, Android)
	17-alpha ethyl testosterone (eg, Maxibolin)
	1-methyl testosterone (eg, Primobolan)
	Androstenediol (eg, "Andro" food supplements)
	Androstenedione
	Dihydroepiandrosterone (eg, "DHEA" food supplements)
	Injectable
	19-nortestosterone ester derivatives (eg, Durabolin)
	Testosterone ester derivatives (eg, Oreton)
	Testosterone cypionate derivatives (eg, Virilon)
	Boldenone (eg, Equipoise)
Stimulants	Amphetamines (eg, Adderall)
	Caffeine (eg, NoDoz, Vivarin, Excedrin, Midol)
	Methylphenidate (eg, Ritalin)
	Pemoline (eg, Cylert)
	Ephedrine derivatives (eg, Pseudoephedrine)
	Beta-2 agonists (eg, Albuterol)
Beta blockers	Propanolol
Polypeptide and glycoprotein hormones	Human growth hormone
	Adenocorticotropic hormone (ACTH)
	Human chorionic gonadotrophin (hCG)
Blood doping	Erythropoietin (EPO)
	Autologous blood transfusions
	Homologous blood transfusions
Diuretics	Furosemide
	Hydrochlorothiazide
	Mannitol
	Spironolactone
	Acetazolamide

FINISH LINE

The use of performance enhancing substances and other doping techniques is unethical, unhealthy, and potentially life threatening. Physicians need to be aware of the potential for abuse of these substances by all athletes, as well as nonathletes. Many substances have ergogenic effects and may be banned for competitors at national and international events. Physicians should be aware of drug control policies for their athletes and avoid prescribing or recommending a medication that may disqualify the athlete from an event. Counseling and sound medical advice are critical for athletes using or contemplating the use of performance enhancing substances.

Providing medical information should not be construed as tacit approval for the use of performance enhancing substances. Conversely, the use of scare tactics that emphasize the negative side effects of illicit ergogenic substances is ineffective as a deterrent to their use in young athletes.

Changes in the pattern of use by young athletes are more likely to be achieved by providing positive counseling regarding alternatives to illegal and dangerous techniques. Healthy alternatives include programs in strength training and conditioning, programs in sports nutrition, and camps or coaching in which emphasis is placed on sport skill acquisition and training.

For More Information

1. American Academy of Pediatrics Committee on Sports Medicine and Fitness: Adolescents and anabolic steroids: A subject review. *Pediatrics* 1997;99:904–908.

2. Brower K: Anabolic steroids: Addictive, psychiatric, and medical consequences. *Am J Addict* 1992;1:100–114.

3. Johnson MD: Anabolic steroid use in adolescent athletes. *Pediatr Clin North Am* 1990;37:1111–1123.

4. Pasquale M: Stimulants and adaptogens: Part I. *Drugs in Sports* 1992;1:26.

5. Yesalis CE (ed): *Anabolic Steroids in Sport and Exercise.* Champaign, IL, Human Kinetics, 1993.

Chapter 11

Psychological Issues

DANIEL GOULD, PHD
RUSSEL MEDBERY

Opinions vary as to whether organized sports for children are beneficial or harmful. The potential beneficial effects include character development, confidence, leadership, teamwork, and achievement orientations; however, these attributes do not simply appear as a result of participating in sports. Similarly, participation in organized sports does not necessarily foster an environment of excessive stress, lower self-esteem, or apathy. Research has shown that the psychological benefits are more likely to occur when competent, adult supervision is supplied by coaches and parents who understand children and who know how to structure programs that result in a positive learning experience. When these adults fail to understand the unique psychological makeup of the young athlete or treat children like elite adult athletes, these negative effects are likely to occur.

Physicians caring for young athletes can provide qualified youth sport leadership in the psychological domain by: 1) helping parents understand the psychology of young athletes; 2) helping to create developmentally appropriate policies, regulations, and coaching; and 3) recognizing and managing psychological issues of concern and referring young athletes to pediatric mental health experts when appropriate. Many excellent references address the diagnosis and management of specific clinical disorders, including depression, substance abuse, and anorexia/bulimia. This chapter focuses on psychological issues that can be recognized and managed by primary care physicians.

For conditions that require more specialized care, educational or clinical sport psychology experts may be consulted (see For More Information, p 113). Clinical sport psychologists are licensed to diagnose and treat individuals with emotional disorders (eg, severe depression, suicidal tendencies).

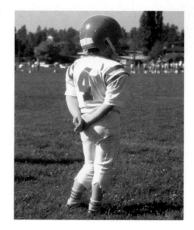

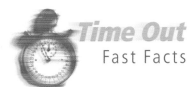

Time Out
Fast Facts

The psychological benefits of sports are more likely to occur when supervision is supplied by adults who understand children and know how to structure programs that result in a positive learning experience.

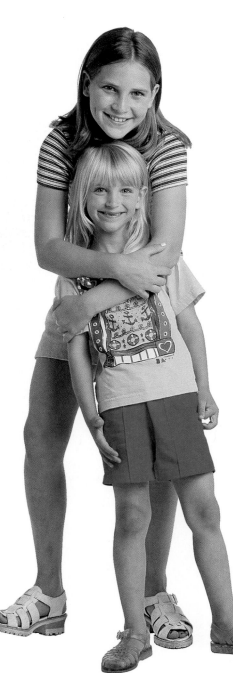

In addition to extensive training in psychology, they receive additional training in sport and exercise psychology and the sport sciences.

Educational sport psychology consultants, however, are not trained to treat individuals with emotional disorders, nor are they licensed psychologists. Rather, they have specialized training in sport and exercise science and the psychology of human movement. These specialists may have graduate training in psychology and counseling. They are "mental coaches" who, through group and individual sessions, educate athletes about psychological skills and their development, including anxiety management, confidence and self-esteem development, and improved communication.

Although there will be times when a young athlete should be referred to a sport psychology specialist, in most instances the physician should be able to serve as an educational resource for parents and coaches of young athletes. This chapter focuses on ten common issues that physicians are most frequently asked about children's sports. The information contained is based on the latest pediatric sport psychology research and the professional opinions of leading developmental sport psychologists.

Components of a Youth Sport Program

Parents should learn as much as they can about the philosophy of the overall sports program, particularly that of the coach. Signs of a desirable coach include: 1) considerable positive interaction with the athletes, 2) strong emphasis on teaching sports skills and sportsmanship, and 3) a consistent philosophy that puts the young athlete's physical, social, and psychological development before winning. Discipline has its place, but should be used infrequently and never in a demeaning way. Ineffective or undesirable coaches provide little effective teaching and commonly use negative feedback and punishment, often conveyed in a demeaning manner. They also espouse a philosophy that places winning before the child's development.

One of the best ways for parents to learn about a coach is to ask specific questions about the coach's philosophy of coaching, such as:

1. What are the coach's objectives in working with young athletes?

2. How does he or she achieve these objectives in practices and games?

3. How much does each child play and how is playing time determined?

4. Do children get individual attention?

5. What role does the coach expect from parents?

If possible, parents should be encouraged to attend several practice sessions to observe the type of interaction that occurs between the coach and the athletes. If this is not possible, parents should meet with the parents of other team members to inquire about the program and coach.

The Role of Parents in a Child's Sport Experience

Certainly parents should be involved in their child's youth sport experience; however, research has shown that too little or too much involvement can have negative psychological effects. For example, overinvolvement can lead to increased stress and burnout, which is physical or emotional withdrawal from a previously enjoyable activity as a result of long-term stress. Underinvolvement can negatively affect the child's sports participation and motivation. In addition, underinvolved parents have no way of knowing what is happening in their child's program.

Table 11.1 shows a list of potential parent roles and responsibilities that has been developed by the American Sport Education Program as part of their sport parent program. An appropriate balance between too little and too much involvement can be found by using these guidelines, as well as responding to the child's sports experience.

Table 11.1 *Sport Parent Responsibilities and Code of Conduct*

Responsibilities

1. Encourage your children to play sports, but do not exert undue pressure. Allow your child to choose to play, and to quit, if he or she wants.

2. Understand what your child wants from sports and provide a supportive atmosphere for achieving his or her goals.

3. Set limits on your child's participation in sports. You need to determine when your child is physically and emotionally ready to play and to ensure that the conditions for playing are safe.

4. Ensure that the coach is qualified to guide your child through the sports experience.

5. Keep winning in perspective, and help your child do the same.

6. Help your child set realistic performance goals.

7. Help your child understand the valuable lessons sports can teach.

8. Help your child meet the responsibilities to the team and the coach.

9. Discipline your child appropriately when necessary.

10. Allow coaches to do the coaching—do not meddle or coach from the stands.

11. Supply the coach with information about any injuries or other medical conditions your child may have. Ensure that your child takes any necessary medications to games and practices.

Code of Conduct

1. Remain in the spectator area during games.

2. Do not advise the coach on how to coach.

3. Do not make derogatory comments to coaches, officials, or parents of either team.

4. Do not try to coach your child during the contest.

5. Do not drink alcohol at contests or come to a contest after drinking too much.

6. Cheer for your child's team.

7. Show interest, enthusiasm, and support for your child.

8. Be in control of your emotions.

9. Help when asked by coaches or officials.

10. Thank coaches, officials, and other volunteers who conduct the event.

Reproduced with permission from American Sport Education Program, 1994: *SportParent*. Champaign, IL, Human Kinetics, 1994, p 29.

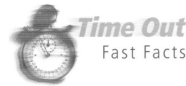

Parent as Coach

Parents are appropriate and often necessary in the role of coach to their children in entry-level sports. In fact, 60% of the estimated 2.5 million volunteer youth sport coaches in the United States coach their own children. Because most parents have no formal training as coaches, participation in a youth sport coaches certification program and a first aid program are recommended prerequisites.

As children become more intensely involved in sports, the issue of parent as coach becomes more problematic. While a number of outstanding athletes were coached by a parent, some evidence suggests that coaching one's own child can lead to increased stress and burnout. Children may confuse coaching feedback and criticism with a lack of unconditional parental love. Parent-coaches also face the dilemma of remaining impartial, trying not to show favoritism towards their own child, but also not overcompensating by being extra hard on their own child.

Given these concerns, parents should be encouraged to coach their children in sports at the entry levels of play. However, as children move to higher levels of play, it may be easier to provide unconditional support if the child plays for another coach.

Stress and Sports

Pediatric sport psychology research clearly shows that most children who participate in sports do not experience excessive stress. Therefore, children should not be discouraged from participating in sports because of competitive stress concerns. However, this research has also shown that excessive stress can be a problem for certain children in specific situations. If only 10% of children experience excessive stress, this could still translate to millions of children nationwide. To increase awareness and to help reduce stress from sports, sport psychologists have identified personal and situational factors associated with heightened stress in young athletes (**Table 11.2**). Physicians who are familiar with this profile are better able to identify children who are experiencing unhealthy levels of stress and are at risk.

To help children with stress or who are at high risk of experiencing stress, parents and coaches need to be educated about what situations create stress for young athletes and what strategies are effective for reducing stress. A positive sports environment, without negative feedback or criticism, can bolster confidence and enjoyment while reducing stress. Stress can also be alleviated by reducing social evaluation (eg, "How did you play?" not "Did you win?") and the importance placed on winning (eg, no more "fiery" pregame pep talks). Finally, sport psychologists can adapt adult anxiety reduction techniques, such as progressive muscle relaxation, breath control, and mental training strategies, for use with children. General directions like "just relax" or "you can do it" are not enough to help children manage stress.

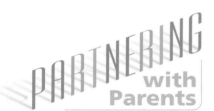

Children and Burnout

Burnout is a growing concern in competitive sports for children. It is thought to occur when early specialization in a sport and long, intense hours of training cause children to lose interest in the sport (**Table 11.3**). Children as young as age 4 years begin participating in sports such as gymnastics, swimming, or tennis and may be competing at an international level by their early teens. When careers end early or performance declines prematurely, burnout is suspected.

Recent studies have contributed to the general understanding of burnout as a special case of sport withdrawal where a young athlete discontinues or curtails sport involvement that was once considered pleasurable. However, children withdraw from sports for reasons other than burnout, but burnout should be suspected when other obvious reasons for withdrawal are not apparent.

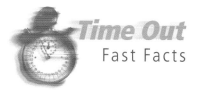

Time Out
Fast Facts

Most children who participate in sports do not experience excessive stress.

Table 11.2 *Characteristics of Children at Risk for Stress During Competitive Situations*

Personal Characteristics

1. High trait anxiety disposition (a personality disposition that predisposes a child to see competition and social evaluation as psychologically threatening)
2. Low self-esteem
3. Perfectionistic personality
4. Low performance expectancies relative to his or her team
5. Low self-performance expectancies
6. Frequent worries about failure
7. Frequent worries about adult expectations and social evaluation by others
8. Less perceived fun
9. Less satisfaction with his or her performance, regardless of winning or losing
10. Perceived importance to parents that he or she participate in sport
11. Outcome goal focus (places a great deal of focus on winning and losing, as opposed to self-improvement)

Situational Characteristics

1. Defeat or victory— children experience more stress after losing than winning.
2. Event importance— the more importance placed on a contest, the higher the state of anxiety experienced by the participants.
3. Sport type— other things being equal, individual sports are more stressful than team sports.

Reproduced with permission from Weinberg RS, Gould D: *Foundations of Sport and Exercise Psychology.* Champaign, IL, Human Kinetics, 1995, p 457.

Table 11.3 *Sample Training Schedule*

5:00 AM	Wake up
5:15 AM	Eat a light breakfast (don't forget vitamins)
5:30–7:00 AM	Practice (Monday, Wednesday, Friday weightlifting)
8:00 AM–3:00 PM	School
	• miss every other Friday to travel to meets
	• physical therapy 1:30 PM to 3:00 PM 3 days/wk
3:30–6:30 PM	Practice
7:00 PM	Dinner
8:00–10:00 PM	Study (Monday team meetings; Wednesday religious group meetings)
10:00–10:30 PM	Free time/relax
10:30 PM	Sleep

Adolescents who experience a burnout typically have a one-dimensional view of themselves as athletes rather than students, family members, musicians, or school activity leaders. In addition, these young athletes often have a limited sense of control of their own destinies, both in and out of sports. Their parents and/or coaches make the important decisions regarding their lives, with little or no input from them. Prominent factors associated with burnout are shown in **Table 11.4**. Unlike the transient stress experienced by most athletes before a contest, the child with burnout has stress that constantly builds.

Encouraging Children to Participate in Sports

American children are increasingly sedentary, and as a result, have greatly increased their health risks. In addition, children who do not participate in sports cannot derive the social and psychological benefits that come from well-run programs. Therefore, parents should encourage their children to become involved in sports.

One of the best ways to encourage children to become involved in sports and physical activities is for parents to engage in those activities with them. Parents are encouraged to engage in physical play with very young children (girls as well as boys), play ball with them, swim, dance, bike, run, and hike. Sharing in an active lifestyle sends a message to children that physical activity is fun and rewarding.

While parental involvement typically increases a child's activity level, some children may still prefer more sedentary activities, such as watching television or playing video games. Potential conflict may be the result. Studies have shown that children who are pushed into activities they do not want to do or dislike are not likely to develop the intrinsic motivation needed to sustain a lifetime of involvement. At the same time, if children are not exposed to sports, they will never fully appreciate what they are missing. Parents must then walk a fine line between encouraging and exposing children to sports without pushing them into activities in which they have no

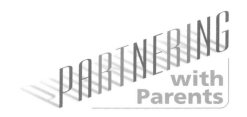

PARTNERING with Parents

How can I encourage my child to participate in sports without forcing him into a negative experience?

Never force children to participate. Offer a variety of activities and let them select one or more to try. Often children will agree to join activities with their friends. Teach by example by being an active parent. Remember that organized sports are not for everyone. Children can still be physically active by participating in other nonsports activities and free play.

Table 11.4 *Factors Associated with Burnout in Young Athletes*

1. Very high self- and external expectations
2. Win-at-all-costs attitude
3. Parental pressure
4. Long practices with little variety
5. Inconsistent coaching practices
6. Overuse injuries
7. Excessive time demands
8. High travel demands
9. Love from others determined by winning and losing
10. Perfectionism

Reproduced with permission from Weinberg RS, Gould D: *Foundations of Sport and Exercise Psychology.* Champaign, IL, Human Kinetics, 1995, p 458.

interest. One possible solution is to ask the child to select from one of several activities, with the understanding that if they do not enjoy the activity after 2 or 3 weeks, they do not have to continue. Moreover, the coach should be informed of the child's reluctance to participate so that he or she will be sure to provide a positive, encouraging environment. More often than not, children want to continue with an activity after a low-pressure trial period. However, if they still have no interest in the program after trying it for the designated time, they should be allowed to stop participating. Follow this with an opportunity to try a different sport and assure them that they can always go back to the first sport again if they wish.

While patience and persistence may pay off, parents may reach a point when they realize that despite active encouragement to participate, competitive sports may not be right for their child. Nonetheless, children should still be encouraged to engage in some regular physical activity. Free play, recreational sports, and/or individual exercise programs provide healthy options for children who are not interested in or ready for competitive sports.

Quitting Sports

Children cite many reasons for participating in sports, including fun, improving skills, being with friends, fitness, challenge, and feeling worthy/successful. A strong sense of self and competence are particularly important for children to remain interested in participating. Children usually quit when they do not feel worthy relative to the activity ("I don't play well."), when one or more of their important motives for participating are not met ("My friends quit."), or when they become interested in other activities ("Scouts and soccer meet at the same time, and I like Scouts more."). Finally, studies have shown that children often quit one sport only to continue on in another—a phenomenon that has been labeled sports transferring.

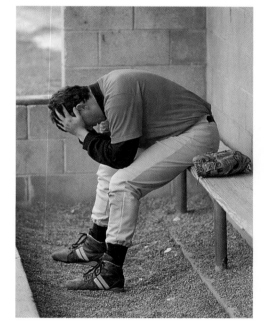

Children may discontinue a sport for many good reasons; however, if they quit because of a negative experience or if they have a low sense of self-worth, the basis for these feelings should be addressed. If the basis for these feelings cannot be reversed, the child may be best served by sitting out for the season. After the decision to discontinue is made, a search for more positive options should ensue.

Developing Self-Esteem in Sports

One of the greatest potential benefits of youth sports participation is the development of self-esteem and self-worth. Parents and coaches play a role in ensuring that this occurs, while the physician plays an important role in identifying children with low self-esteem.

Symptoms of low self-esteem include low levels of self-confidence, often expressed with phrases such as "I can't," "I am no good," and "I stink." These children may also have difficulty making friends, are often afraid to take risks or engage in activities in which their performance is critically evaluated, and are generally anxious about participating in sports. Young athletes with low self-esteem may exhibit little effort because they feel that, despite their best efforts, they will fail. If a more positive experience is not found, referral to a sport psychology specialist should be considered.

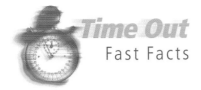

Time Out
Fast Facts

Discipline is important in a youths' sports program but should be used infrequently and never in a demeaning way.

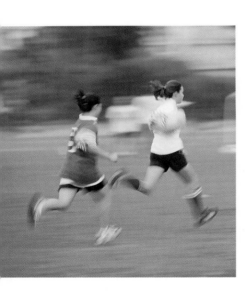

Coaches and parents are particularly important in helping build self-esteem in these children. Coaches who use the following strategies on a regular basis enhance self-esteem in young athletes:

1. Ensuring success by breaking down skills into smaller parts so that they can be more easily learned and mastered;

2. Modifying activities so that children can be more successful (eg, lower baskets in basketball);

3. Providing plenty of rewarding statements;

4. Ensuring that praise is sincere;

5. Maintaining realistic expectations;

6. Rewarding effort as much as outcome;

7. Creating an environment that reduces fear of trying new skills; and

8. Being enthusiastic.

When a Child Fails in Sports

A very difficult situation for parents is knowing what to say when their child fails in sports. Every child reacts differently to failure; some may appear unaffected, whereas others have a great deal of difficulty trying to cope.

Parents must show unconditional love and emotional support when their child fails or feels as if he or she has failed a sport. Involved parents need to be aware of the possibility of getting so caught up in their child's athletic success that they subtly, or not so subtly, convey their disappointment in the child when they lose or fail. Generally, parents should refrain from giving corrective advice because the child often misinterprets this advice as criticism. While some parents wait to give advice until after the child has had time to deal with the mistake or loss, a better solution may be to let the coach provide the advice; after all, that is his or her job.

Parents who feel compelled to give advice should follow a three-fold "psychological sandwich" approach to error correction. First, mention what the child did correctly ("Good try, you stayed right in there on that pitch."), as this will help reduce the child's frustration in making the error. Second, provide information to correct the error made ("Watch the ball all the way."). End with an encouraging remark ("Stick with it—it's tough, but you'll get it.").

Learning the Right Values Through Sports

Most parents want their child to develop character and good moral values such as honesty, integrity, and compassion through their sports participation. Although a child has the potential to develop such attributes and values, remember that these values must be taught and modeled—they do not simply appear with participation in sports.

Parents should first identify the values they would most like to instill in their child, and then assess the values of the organization and the coaches who are working with their children. Studies have shown that young athletes model the values of the people they spend time with and admire. At the organizational level, parents should become familiar with league rules and speak with other parents to find out how athletes, coaches, and parents are treated. At the team level, parents should learn what values the coach emphasizes, whether his or her actions are consistent with those values, and whether the players, parents, and coaches are treated with respect. On the field, parents should learn whether rules are reinforced and whether all players are treated in a fair, consistent manner. They should also observe the types of values the coaches and other parents display in front of the athletes, and determine if winning is given more importance than effort, improvement, and enjoyment. Finally, parents should have a role in reinforcing desirable values, identifying undesirable behaviors, and serving as appropriate role models.

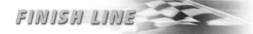
FINISH LINE

> Participation in organized sports has many potential benefits for psychological development in young athletes. However, benefits will only be derived if competent qualified adult leadership is provided throughout the youth sports experience. The physician plays an extremely important role in educating parents and coaches as to the best strategies for ensuring that the best possible psychological development is afforded young athletes.

For More Information

1. American Sport Education Program: *SportParent.* Champaign, IL, Human Kinetics, 1994.

2. Association for the Advancement of Applied Sport Psychology *(www.aaasponline.org)*

3. Gould D: Intensive sport participation and the prepubescent athlete, in Cahill BR, Pearl AJ (eds): *Intensive Participation in Children's Sports.* Champaign, IL, Human Kinetics, 1993, pp 19–38.

4. Petlichkoff LM: The drop-out dilemma in youth sports, in Bar-Or O (ed): *The Child and Adolescent Athlete.* Cambridge, MA, Blackwell Science, 1996, pp 418–430.

5. Smoll FL, Smith RE: *Children and Youth in Sport: A Biopsychological Perspective.* Madison, WI, Brown & Benchmark Publishers, 1996.

6. Sport Psychology Division of the U.S. Olympic Committee (719-578-4579) for a list of qualified sports psychologists.

7. Weiss M: Psychological effects of intensive sport participation on children and youth: Self-esteem and motivation, in Cahill BR, Pearl AJ (eds): *Intensive Participation in Children's Sports.* Champaign, IL, Human Kinetics, 1993, pp 39–70.

8. Weinberg RS, Gould D: *Foundations of Sport and Exercise Psychology.* Champaign, IL, Human Kinetics, 1999.

section three
Basic Management Concepts

Section Editor
William A. Herndon, MD

Chapter 12

Playability Issues

WILLIAM A. HERNDON, MD
FREDERICK R. REED, JR, MD

When or whether or not an athlete may return to play following an injury may be one of the most difficult decisions a physician must make. Unfortunately, in most situations, there are no standardized criteria to guide the decision-making process. Therefore, these decisions can be very subjective, depending on the type of injury or illness, age of the athlete, sport, level of play, and how far recovery and rehabilitation have progressed. This chapter focuses on *general* return to play issues, not issues regarding whether a child or adolescent should participate in sports at all. Specific recommendations for return to play, as well as participation issues are covered in other chapters of this text.

Responsibility for Return to Play Decisions

Many individuals, aside from the athlete, the parents, and the athlete's physician, may be involved or ask to be involved in the return to play decision. Coaches, athletic trainers, physical therapists, school administrators, and sometimes even the media seek to have input. However, in these situations the physician-patient relationship has been established and takes precedence over these other relationships (except the parental relationship), so that the treating physician has a legal responsibility for the ultimate medical care of the athlete and for the risks associated with return to play.

All decisions should focus on the safety of the athlete. Therefore, the risks associated with return to play must be assessed, along with the role of other factors such as protective equipment and position or technique changes that can reduce the risk and make return to play safe for the athlete. In addition, the athlete's desire to return to play must be taken into account. The level of risk depends on the nature of the injury or illness, the specific sport, and the level of recovery that has occurred. Information from coaches, athletic trainers, and physical therapists can be invaluable in estimating risk associated with return to play. However, the saying "when in doubt, keep the player out" should

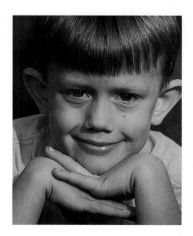

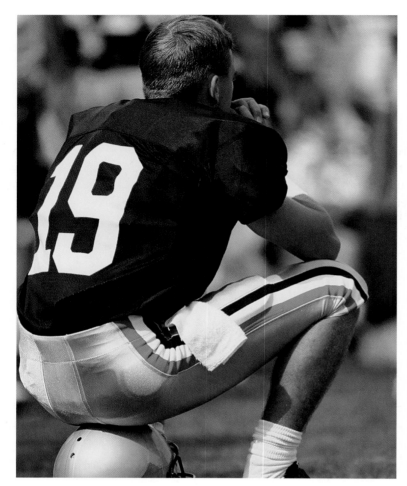

be remembered. The athlete's well-being must be the priority, even though coaches and sometimes family members may try to influence the physician's decision. A consensus among the coaching staff, the administration, and the physician should be established in writing, in the preseason, giving the physician total authority to make return to play decisions.

Essential Elements of Return to Play Decisions

Return to play decisions usually need to be made either on the sidelines during the event or later in the office or training room. On the sidelines, an acute injury or medical illness must be evaluated and a decision made about whether the athlete is fit to return to play. Making these decisions on the sidelines is usually not easy, as they are often made in the "heat of battle" while emotions are running high, adequate medical information sometimes is not available, and pressure from the coaching staff or parents is great.

Decisions made in the office or training room are typically less urgent, less emotional, and based on more complete medical data. In this setting, a discussion with parents and coaches about risks is also less emotional. A number of questions must be posed and answered before an athlete can return to play.

1. What is the diagnosis?

2. Has the injury healed completely and been adequately rehabilitated?

3. Has range of motion, flexibility, and strength been restored?

4. Is the athlete's general fitness level satisfactory?

5. If there is an increased risk in return to play or practice, do the athlete, coach, and parents understand the risks?

6. Can any measures such as changes in equipment, training, or technique be implemented to prevent further injury?

General Playability Issues

Injuries will always occur in athletic participation and can never be completely prevented. However, problems from the medical conditions that follow are often preventable. Each of the following conditions is discussed only briefly here; guidelines regarding specific injuries and medical conditions are presented in greater detail in other chapters.

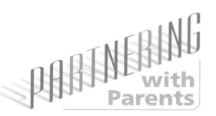

What should a physician do when an athlete seems physically ready to return to play but the athlete is reluctant or unwilling to resume participation?

Remember that the physician is an advocate for the patient. Never force an athlete to return if he or she is not ready. Be prepared to investigate the reason that the athlete does not feel prepared to return. Often there are psychological stressors involved and the athlete is looking for an "out."

Concussion

Concussions occur from head trauma and result in a temporary loss of neural function. Signs and symptoms may include any of the following: dizziness, headache, confusion, visual disturbances, amnesia, loss of consciousness, drowsiness, nausea, or vomiting. Slurred speech, disorientation, lack of coordination, inappropriate emotions, and auditory abnormalities can also be seen. Loss of consciousness and amnesia are the signs that have formed the basis for most concussion grading scales. However, these signs vary widely, depending on the athlete and the situation. Most athletes do not lose consciousness, and there is great variability in the range of amnesia. All grading scales are based on anecdotal evidence, and experts continue to disagree on how to use these grading scales in managing athletes with head injury.

An athlete who has sustained a concussion should not be allowed to return to play while symptomatic or displaying signs of a concussion. In most instances, this means that they should not return to play the same day. However, if the athlete has not been rendered unconscious, is asymptomatic, and shows no signs of change in neurologic or physical status for 15 minutes from the time of concussion, the physician should instruct the athlete to perform some physical activity that increases intracranial pressure such as sit-ups or running sprints. If symptoms recur, the athlete should not return to play that day. If there are no symptoms after this activity, the athlete can return to play if this was his or her first concussion. Return to play decisions following a more serious concussion are less well defined. There is lack of scientific evidence regarding the exact number of days needed to recover from a concussion. Therefore, decisions regarding return to play must be made on an individual basis and must include factors such as recovery of symptoms, findings from subsequent physical examinations, and the number of concussions the athlete has sustained. More detailed information on concussions is provided in Chapter 18.

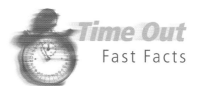

Time Out
Fast Facts

An athlete who has sustained a concussion should not be allowed to return to play while displaying any signs or symptoms of head injury.

Brachial Plexus Injuries

Brachial plexus neurapraxia, or "burners and stingers," occur with a sudden stretch to the brachial plexus in which the head and neck are laterally deviated away from the involved shoulder or forced lateral flexion toward the involved shoulder, causing nerve compression. Athletes have temporary paresis, paralysis, or dysesthesia as a result. Management consists of rest and anti-inflammatory medication, if necessary, as this condition typically resolves spontaneously. Many factors are involved in return to play decisions: the athlete must be asymptomatic; the neurologic examination must be normal; the neck and shoulder range of motion and strength must be within normal range; and there must be no tenderness in the cervical spine. Recurrent injuries warrant further evaluation.

Neck Injuries

Cervical spine injuries

Trauma to the cervical spine is extremely serious and requires thorough examination, including cervical spine radiographs, to assess the severity of the injury and implications for treatment. The most common neck injury is a cervical sprain. Athletes with a cervical sprain should not return to play until

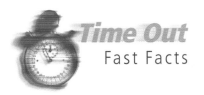

Developmental narrowing of the spinal canal should not necessarily preclude an individual from participating in contact sports.

they are asymptomatic and have full range of motion and strength in the neck. However, return to play is prohibited in athletes with acute fractures and/or dislocations of the cervical spine until complete healing and rehabilitation has occurred. If the injury requires surgical cervical fusion, in most cases the athlete probably should not return to contact sports. Consultation with a neurosurgeon or orthopaedist is advised in making return to play decisions after these types of injuries. More detailed information on spinal injuries is provided in Chapter 31.

Acute transient quadriplegia

Acute transient quadriplegia (ATQ) is a condition that results in temporary loss of motor and/or sensory function in all extremities. Careful diagnostic studies should be performed, including cervical spine radiographs and MRI to identify any pathology or anatomic variant that may have contributed to the injury. Studies have demonstrated a relationship between ATQ and developmental narrowing of the cervical spine. However, ATQ differs from a transient or complete quadriplegia that occurs secondary to an unstable fracture or dislocation of the cervical spine, or that occurs as a result of a degenerative condition of the spine. Athletes with this condition are not predisposed to complete quadriplegia, and recent studies have suggested that developmental narrowing of the spinal canal should not preclude an individual from contact sports. However, once an episode of transient quadriplegia has occurred, the physician is at great risk for liability by allowing an affected athlete to return to play, since there is no consensus among the experts.

Acute Musculoskeletal Injuries

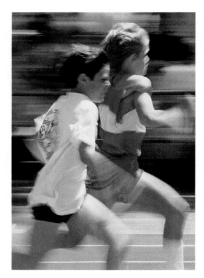

Return to play decisions following acute musculoskeletal injuries are relatively straightforward and are usually based on common sense. Athletes with minor contusions and strains usually can return to most activities with simple and adequate protection of the injury, if the athlete feels comfortable, and performance is not altered. Conversely, athletes who sustain fractures and/or dislocations should not be allowed to return to play. Instilling a local anesthetic to diminish pain so the athlete can continue to participate is not acceptable.

Return to play after an injury has healed depends on the sport, the nature of the injury, and time lost from participation. Rehabilitation of previous injuries is extremely important in preventing further injury. The focus of rehabilitation should be on return of range of motion, strength, and flexibility, followed by a systematic progression through a hierarchy of sport-specific skills designed to prepare the athlete to resume full participation. Chapter 29 provides detailed information on general rehabilitation principles.

Blunt Abdominal Trauma

Blunt trauma to the abdomen may injure the spleen, liver, kidneys, and sometimes even the large or small intestines. Athletes with possible intra-abdominal organ injuries should not be allowed to return to play until the abdomen has been medically cleared. Question these athletes about a history of infectious mononucleosis with splenomegaly, as this condition precludes contact sports for at least 4 weeks because of the risk of injury to the enlarged spleen from abdominal trauma.

Dehydration

Dehydration is a preventable condition that may lead to heat stress and even more dangerous heat-related injuries. All athletes are at risk, even adults who underestimate fluid requirements, but children are at greater risk because of increased body surface area. Coaches, parents, athletic trainers, and physicians must ensure that adequate fluids are available and that frequent breaks are given for athletes to rehydrate. Fluid intake, usually with water or an electrolyte sports drink, must be encouraged every 15 to 20 minutes during practice and play. Athletes who become dehydrated should not return to play until they have been adequately rehydrated. Hydration levels may be easily monitored and recorded by measuring the athlete's body weight before and after each practice. More than 5% loss of body weight that is not regained prior to the next practice should be cause for withholding the athlete from activity.

Heat-Related Illnesses

Heat-related illnesses range from minor muscle cramps or syncope to the very dangerous heatstroke. As described in Chapter 8, heat-related illnesses are caused by a combination of factors, including environmental temperature, humidity, dehydration, lack of acclimatization, and fatigue. No matter what the cause, these conditions are always preventable. Athletic participation is precluded until the athlete is asymptomatic.

Exercise-Induced Asthma

An acute episode of asthma can prevent participation in an athletic event. However, a history of asthma or exercise-induced asthma almost never precludes participation in virtually any sport. Many exercise-induced episodes are preventable with the use of preexercise bronchodilators and avoidance of airway cooling and drying. When acute bronchospasm subsides, return to play is acceptable when the patient is no longer short of breath, and has no subjective sensation of shortness of breath. Chapter 22 provides detailed information on this topic.

Overuse Injuries

Overuse injuries in young athletes range from stress fractures to various types of apophysitis. Almost all stress fractures require a period of rest from sports participation, whereas most apophysitis do not preclude participation unless the athlete has a limp or is favoring the injured part. Treatment usually focuses on keeping the athlete playing while protecting the injured part from further symptoms or injury by modifying training techniques or equipment, using orthotics, or changing positions on a team. During this period of time, alternative or modified activities may be undertaken and are often advisable. Unfortunately, sometimes athletes must simply stop playing for a time to allow their injuries to heal or symptoms to decrease. Generally, it is not possible to resolve a serious overuse problem if the athlete is allowed to continue to play. A period of relative rest, continued cardiovascular fitness, and a strengthening program for noninjured parts, followed by appropriate rehabilitation and graded return to play is usually very successful and is the preferred method to prevent further injury and diminished quality of play.

FINISH LINE

Return to play decisions can be difficult. While many sources are available to help, the physician has the ultimate responsibility. All decisions should be in the athlete's best interest, and conservatism should be the rule.

For More Information

1. Wojtys EM, Hovda D, Landry G, et al: Current concepts: Concussion in sports. *Am J Sports Med* 1999;27:676–687.

2. Dyment PG (ed): *Sports Medicine: Health Care for Young Athletes,* ed 2. Elk Grove Village, IL, American Academy of Pediatrics, 1991.

3. Garrick JG: Determinants of return to athletic activity. *Orthop Clin North Am* 1983;14:317–321.

4. Torg JS, Pavlov H, Genuario SE, et al: Neurapraxia of the cervical spinal cord with transient quadriplegia. *J Bone Joint Surg* 1986;68A:1354–1370.

5. Torg JS, Naranja RJ Jr, Pavlov H, Galinat BJ, Warren R, Stine RA: The relationship of developmental narrowing of the cervical spinal canal to reversible and irreversible injury of the cervical spinal cord in football players. *J Bone Joint Surg* 1996;78A:1308–1314.

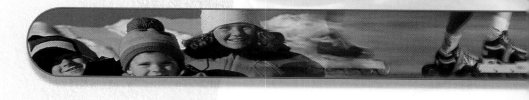

Chapter 13

Injury Prevention

WILLIAM R. BARFIELD, PHD
RICHARD H. GROSS, MD

With over 20 million American youths participating in organized community sports, and millions more involved with interscholastic sports, the number of injuries occurring in organized sports in the United States has risen to 3 million annually. Approximately 770,000 of these injuries require a visit to a physician, and between 45,000 and 90,000 require hospitalization. Children are now competing in sports at younger ages, with reports of 6-year-old children running full marathons, 8-year-old children swimming 10 miles daily, and young gymnasts and tennis players spending hours working to perfect skills in hopes of becoming an Olympic champion or a professional athlete.

As the level and intensity of children's participation in sports increases, the need for effective injury prevention strategies also increases. The rapid changes in youth sports over the past generation have resulted in incomplete information in injury patterns and prevention strategies. For example, the sudden increase in girls' participation in sports has resulted in an increased incidence of significant knee injuries, but the factors that contribute to these injuries are just beginning to come to light. Only 20 years ago, girls' interscholastic sports were almost nonexistent compared with boys' sports. Now there is almost equal participation. Until injury risk factors and risk reduction strategies have been identified, injury prevention programs cannot reach their full potential.

This chapter focuses on injury risk factors and prevention strategies as they relate to the physical and psychological characteristics of the young athlete and the physical environment, which includes fields, other playing surfaces, equipment, coaches, and officials. Examples of effective injury prevention strategies abound, including the effect of altering coaching and officiating techniques with regard to "spearing" techniques in high school football and the dramatic reductions in injury in gymnasts once the trampoline was removed from competition.

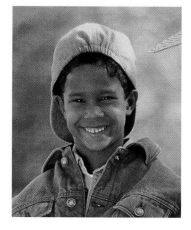

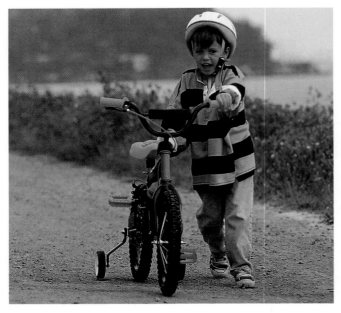

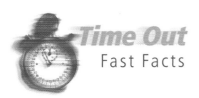

Time Out
Fast Facts

Preseason conditioning programs are essential in helping prevent injuries to athletes during an athletic season.

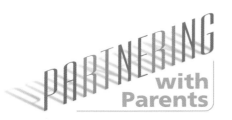

with Parents

Do stretching programs really prevent repetitive use injuries?

Although this would seem logical and is often advocated, there are no studies that show that stretching reduces the incidence of injuries. However, there is probably no harm incurred from proper stretching. Most people continue to advocate stretching as part of a regular exercise program.

Factors Contributing to Injury
The Athlete

Younger children participating in sports generally have a lower rate of injury and sustain less severe injuries than their older counterparts. In fact, bicycling is a much more hazardous activity than sport participation in this age group. The velocity of play in sports is lower, and training is generally less intense than that seen in preadolescent and adolescent athletes. At about age 12 years, some children begin to drop out of sports programs, presumably because they are less talented, lose interest, lose motivation, develop other interests, or are not selected for competitive teams. Adolescents who continue to participate in sports experience a rapid increase in the rate and severity of injury. However, this peak in sports-related injury rate does not differ from the overall injury rate among adolescents.

During early adolescence, the level of physical maturity and strength varies widely among athletes. Rapid gains in strength occur in boys during the process of maturation. Therefore, when participation is governed by age or grade level, it is very difficult to avoid physiologic mismatching, particularly when size and strength are important factors for performance. If late maturation contributes to an athlete's diminishing success, his or her self-esteem may suffer.

Some sports, such as football, use weight rather than age to determine levels of competition, which can minimize mismatching athletes at the same maturation level. A preadolescent and a fully mature adolescent may weigh the same, but one may be significantly stronger than the other. Matching by weight or maturity is less important for injury prevention in noncontact sports, such as running, swimming, or gymnastics. In fact, later maturing athletes may have a competitive advantage in these sports.

Athletes with a history of musculoskeletal injury, especially those who have not completed an adequate rehabilitation program, are at increased risk of injury. Also at risk are those athletes who begin training with a low level of fitness. Proper management of injuries is the key to a safe return to play. Much of the emphasis on injury prevention in young athletes could be better termed "reinjury prevention." For example, contusions are the most common musculoskeletal injury in young athletes. Prevention of reinjury following a contusion depends on the adults involved with the young athlete. Whether the adult responsible is the coach, the athletic trainer, or the parents does not matter. What does matter is that the contusion is allowed to heal, that passive stretching of the injured area is avoided, and that the athlete demonstrates adequate strength and motion of the part before returning to play.

Life stress is often an unrecognized factor in injury. Death of a family member, divorce, or other real or threatened losses render young athletes more susceptible to injuries. The goals of the coach or other involved adult may differ from those of the athlete; oftentimes the athlete is less committed to achievement. In these unfortunate situations, the athlete may perceive that the only way "out" is to be injured.

Another factor that contributes to injury is use of anabolic-androgenic steroids in conjunction with training. Steroids do, in fact, result in gains in strength and weight, but at an unacceptable cost. Physicians, coaches, athletic trainers, and parents must be knowledgeable about steroids and their effects so that young athletes can be warned about their deleterious long-term effects. More detailed information about steroids and other performance enhancing substances is provided in Chapter 10.

Environmental Risk Factors

The condition and design of facilities, proper equipment (including fit, design, and application), coaching, officiating, and weather conditions (especially temperature and humidity) comprise the environment of the young athlete. Some environmental factors are obvious, such as field conditions; others are more subtle, such as the coach's knowledge of injury rehabilitation. The coach can help prevent injury by using safe training regimens, careful supervision, appropriate motivation, and modifying activities according to ability.

Epidemiologic studies conducted in recent years have provided valuable information on hazardous environmental factors. These factors include inappropriate techniques, such as spearing, and unsafe equipment, such as trampolines and stationary bases. Between 1979 and 1992, a total of 15 athletes were killed because of mishaps with movable soccer goals in which the goal cage tipped over and crushed a player. However, improvements to equipment have also prevented injuries. In baseball, the introduction of helmets, soft baseballs, breakaway bases, and face masks for younger players have reduced injuries.

The Coach

The coach is a pivotal figure in a young athlete's life; it is the coach who is often responsible for the great gains or losses for the athlete. Coaches who advocate "playing with pain," restricting fluids during hot weather, or returning to play prior to proper rehabilitation after injury may actually increase their players' risk of injury. Within the past two decades, training programs for youth coaches have focused on creating programs that provide the optimum environment for young athletes. In addition to sport-specific training, topics such as injury prevention, rehabilitation, and psychological factors are now included in the curriculum. Less well studied at present is the role of officiating in injury prevention; in a study of men's soccer, 30% of injuries were the result of foul play. Since many rules are designed to protect athletes from injury, it is logical to assume that better enforcement of rules would reduce injuries.

Strategies for Prevention of Injury
The Preparticipation Physical Evaluation

The preparticipation physical evaluation (PPE) can be a useful tool in injury prevention. Its goal is to identify underlying medical problems, prior injuries, or risk factors for further injury before "clearing" a young athlete for sports participation. An assessment of general health, fitness, flexibility, strength, joint stability, and alignment can provide treatment or preconditioning recommendations. The PPE also provides a forum to explore the

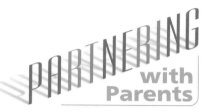

What are the most important factors in preventing heat injury?

Proper conditioning, attention to adequate fluid intake, and avoidance of exercise during times of maximal heat stress are all important in preventing heat illness.

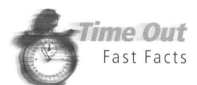

Time Out
Fast Facts

Athletes with a history of musculoskeletal injury, especially those who have not completed an adequate rehabilitation program, are at increased risk of injury.

Coaches can help prevent injuries by using safe training regimens and appropriate motivation, and by modifying activities according to ability.

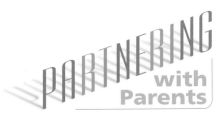

Can mouth guards and protective eyewear reduce the incidence of dental and eye injuries?

Yes. However, they must be constructed of approved materials and be properly fitted. There is some feeling that properly fitted mouth guards may also reduce the likelihood of concussion. Information on these can be obtained from the American Ophthalmologic Society and the American Dental Association.

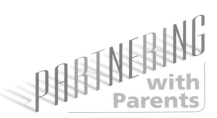

What is the best way to ensure that protective athletic equipment is safe, effective, and constructed of appropriate material?

For protective eyewear and mouth guards, look for the endorsement of the American Academy of Ophthalmology (AAO) and the American Dental Association (ADA). Bicycle helmets should display an approval by Snell or ANSI, the American National Standards Institute. These devices, as well as other sports equipment, are critically evaluated by several organizations including ANSI, ASTM (American Society for Testing Materials), and NOCSAE (National Operating Committee on Standards for Athletic Equipment).

athlete's goals and motivation and to discuss overall health issues such as nutrition, weight control, and drug use. Psychological factors are often omitted from the PPE, but with the documented effect of poor social support, inadequate social skills, and negative life events on injury rate, this is a fruitful field for investigation. The issues surrounding the PPE and its format are detailed in Chapter 6.

Coaching

The coach plays a vital role in injury prevention. Ideally, the coach will be aware of a player's injury history, health status, history of negative life events that may impact his or her performance, and optimal learning style. The coach is responsible for creating an environment that emphasizes the needs of the athlete first, particularly with regard to improving skills and techniques; therefore, he or she must be knowledgeable in sport-specific training techniques. Effective coaches will accommodate training restrictions that result from injury and will insist that injuries be properly diagnosed and treated before the athlete is allowed to return to full activity.

Developing graduated training methods that build confidence and skill is difficult, but essential for team success. Procedures for injury assessment and first aid are critical, as are climate-specific considerations such as adequate fluid replacement and training restrictions in hot climates.

Despite the clear benefits of having knowledgeable and well-trained coaches, many youth coaches are volunteers with little or no experience. Currently, there are insufficient numbers of properly trained coaches to staff the increasing number of organized sports for young athletes. Training programs for youth sport coaches are available and encouraged. These programs, such as the American Coaching Effectiveness Program, typically include information on growth and development, psychological issues, injury prevention, and first aid guidelines and training techniques for specific sports and sport skills.

Training and Equipment

When possible, the coach should inform athletes about the expected level of fitness that must be achieved before preseason practice begins to minimize the incidence of stress injury. In addition to general fitness, sport-specific training can be effective in reducing injuries common to certain sports. For example, to prevent elbow and shoulder injuries in throwing athletes, a preseason conditioning program should be initiated to help prevent injuries that are otherwise common. Such a program might include stretching and strengthening exercises for the shoulder girdle, instruction in proper throwing techniques, and the timing for cessation of throwing and gradual increase in throwing activity.

Injury prevention strategies for all sports cannot be detailed in one chapter, but those for the most popular sports are summarized in **Table 13.1**. The nature of the sport and the demands of the sport determine the types of injury most likely to occur (contact versus noncontact and strenuous versus nonstrenuous activity), and can help to identify the strategies for injury prevention. However, for all sports, the following general strategies are recommended: 1) the rules of play must be followed; 2) the athlete must have adequate preseason conditioning; 3) proper protective equipment must be used; and 4) all previous injuries must be adequately rehabilitated prior to return to play.

Table 13.1 *Sport-Specific Suggestions for Injury Prevention**

Ballet/Dance

Common Injuries	Prevention Strategies
Repetitive hyperextension of the spine	Initiate a program of strengthening and stabilization exercises for the trunk.
Sprains, tendinitis, stress fractures of the lower extremity	Initiate a stretching and strengthening program for tight hip flexors and weak abductors/external rotators; work the hip within available range of motion.
Talar impingement	Treat precursor conditions (shin splints, metatarsalgia).
Snapping hip (iliopsoas tendinitis, trochanteric bursitis)	Initiate a program of strengthening and proprioception exercises for the ankle and calf; encourage low-impact training (Pilates method, pool workouts).
	Avoid pointe work until strength and skill permit; ensure that pointe shoes are fitted professionally.
	Limit pointe work and pliés if the ankle is swollen or if there is any restricted joint motion.
	Ensure calcium intake is adequate.

Baseball/Softball

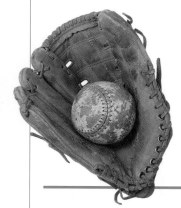

Common Injuries	Prevention Strategies
Throat injuries (to catchers)	Use proper protective equipment (helmets, throat guards for catchers, breakaway bases).
Head and eye injuries	
Rotator cuff impingement/tendinitis	Limit the number of throws and teach proper throwing technique.
Medial epicondylitis	Initiate a program of strengthening for the shoulder and a graduated preseason training program.
Ankle injuries	

Basketball

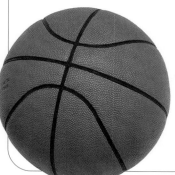

Common Injuries	Prevention Strategies
Patellar tendinitis	Initiate a program of stretching, strengthening, and overall conditioning exercises.
Ankle injuries	Use braces and taping for ankles.

*Injuries and prevention strategies are not listed in any particular sequence. Both lists provide general examples and are not intended to represent every injury or prevention strategy.

Continued

Table 13.1 *Sport-Specific Suggestions for Injury Prevention—cont'd*

Field Hockey

Common Injuries	Prevention Strategies
Ankle sprains	Use proper protective equipment (lace-up ankle braces and/or tape).
Knee sprains	
Back pain (often discogenic or vertebral end plate)	Initiate a program of strengthening exercises for the quadriceps and hamstrings.
	Initiate a program of exercises to maintain overall flexibility and neutral spine posture.

Football

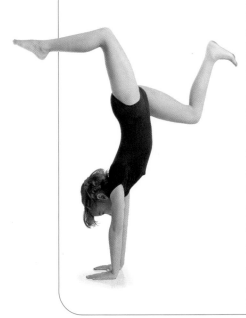

Common Injuries	Prevention Strategies
Concussions	Teach proper tackling techniques.
Neck injuries	Use proper protective equipment (helmets, face masks, mouth guards.
Stingers and burners	
Low back stress fractures	Ensure frequent water breaks are scheduled in high temperature/high humidity conditions. Remove helmet frequently.
Pelvic contusions	
Dehydration	Ensure proper hydration during practice and competition.
Heat-related illnesses	

Gymnastics

Common Injuries	Prevention Strategies
Repetitive flexion, hyperextension, and compression stresses at the thoracolumbar junction and on the lumbar vertebrae	Initiate a program of strengthening exercises for the abdomen and trunk and exercises to maintain the spine in a neutral position.
Capsulitis and dorsal impingement at the wrist	Use tape or braces to protect the wrist.
Radial epiphysitis	Limit weight bearing and impact on the upper extremities to protect the elbow and wrist.
Osteochondritis dissecans at the elbow	Limit extreme or repetitive abduction and external rotation of the shoulder.
Ulnar collateral sprains of the elbow	Initiate a program of strengthening exercises for the rotator cuff and scapular stabilizers.
Shoulder instability	
Tendinitis of the biceps and supraspinatous muscles	

Ice Hockey

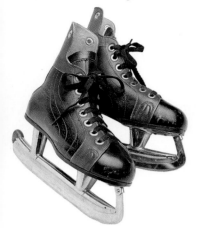

Common Injuries

Concussions

Lacerations about
the head and face

Acromioclavicular sprains

Glenohumeral subluxa-
tions/dislocations

Ligament sprains in
the knee

Contusions of the
quadriceps

Prevention Strategies

Use proper protective equipment (mouth guard,
well-padded full-cage helmet with good strap *around*
the chin) (Note: Many helmets are equipped with
only a strap that goes under the chin).

Initiate a program of strengthening exercises for the
upper body, especially the rotator cuff and scapular
stabilizers, and the quadriceps and hamstrings.

Ensure that the net can slide out of the holes
in the ice when athletes strike the pipes.

Increase padding in the thigh guard by using football
thigh pads because these are larger and thicker.

Lacrosse

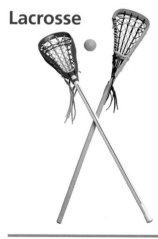

Common Injuries

Contusions/lacerations
about the face

Ankle sprains

Knee sprains

Back pain (often disco-
genic as a result of
repetitive flexion)

Prevention Strategies

Use proper protective equipment (head gear with
good face mask, mouth guard, lace-up ankle braces
and/or tape).

Initiate a program of strengthening exercises
for the quadriceps and hamstrings.

Initiate a program of exercises to maintain overall
flexibility and good posture.

Martial Arts

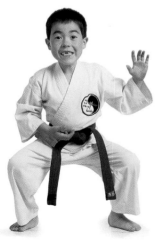

Common Injuries

Concussions

Contusions about the
head

Rib fractures

Renal contusions

Hand trauma

Anterior tibial
compartment syndrome

Prevention Strategies

Use proper protective equipment for the head
and chest (covering the ribs and kidneys).

Wear gloves, mouth guards, and shin guards.

Recognize signs and symptoms of anterior
compartment syndrome.

*Injuries and prevention strategies are not listed in any particular sequence. Both lists provide general examples and
are not intended to represent every injury or prevention strategy.

Continued

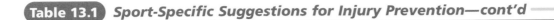

Table 13.1 *Sport-Specific Suggestions for Injury Prevention—cont'd*

Skiing

Common Injuries	Prevention Strategies
Tibial shaft fractures	Check bindings for proper adjustment.
Ulnar collateral ligament tear of the thumb	Ski within capabilities.
	Wear a helmet.

Snowboarding

Common Injuries	Prevention Strategies
Hand and wrist fracture	Use proper protective equipment (wrist splints, releasable bindings, soft-shell boots for beginners).
Shoulder dislocations	Wear a helmet.
Ankle fractures	

Soccer

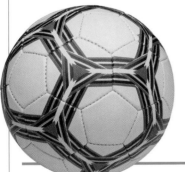

Common Injuries	Prevention Strategies
Concussion	Teach proper "heading" techniques and avoid excessive heading.
Contusions about the head	Avoid heading a water-soaked ball.
Tibial shaft fractures	Use shin guards.

Swimming

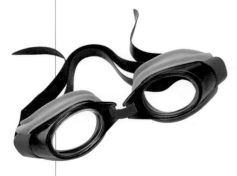

Common Injuries	Prevention Strategies
Rotator cuff impingement/tendinitis	Initiate program of strengthening, stretching, and flexibility exercises for the shoulder, rotator cuff, upper back and scapular stabilizers.
Medial patellofemoral pain (from breaststroke)	Limit use of hand paddles or devices that create added resistance in the water.
Spondylolysis	Use fins to provide greater leg drive and reduce demands on the shoulder.

Tennis

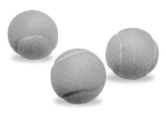

Common Injuries

Rotator cuff impingement/tendinitis

Medial epicondylitis

Lateral epicondylitis

Spondylolysis

Prevention Strategies

Initiate a program of strengthening and flexibility exercises for the back, shoulder, and abdominal muscles, especially strengthening the rotator cuff and scapular stabilizers and improving flexibility in the hamstrings and hip flexors.

Use proper mechanics and equipment to prevent elbow injuries.

Track and Field

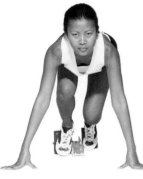

Common Injuries

Stress fractures of the lower extremity

Sesamoiditis

Shin splints

Iliotibial band syndrome

Prevention Strategies

Ensure proper diet and conditioning, gradually increasing speed and intensity.

Initiate a cross training program.

Ensure good shoe fit.

Avoid downhill running and sudden stops.

Wrestling

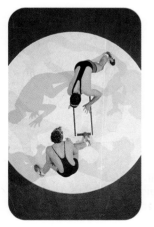

Common Injuries

Glenohumeral subluxation/dislocation

Acromioclavicular and sternoclavicular sprains

Meniscal tears

Skin infections (herpes virus, bacteria [impetigo], tinea corporis)

Auricular hematomas (with resultant cartilage deformity [cauliflower ear])

Prevention Strategies

Initiate a preseason program of strengthening exercises for the rotator cuff, scapular stabilizers, quadriceps mechanism, and hamstrings.

Avoid quick stops in dangerous positions during practice and competition.

Ensure that mats are cleaned daily with commercial antiseptic solution.

Teach athletes to seek medical attention for rapid treatment of any questionable skin lesions to prevent spread of infection.

Conduct skin checks before tournaments.

Use proper protective equipment (snug-fitting head gear with ear protectors).

Drain any blood in the auricle promptly to prevent cartilage deformity.

*Injuries and prevention strategies are not listed in any particular sequence. Both lists provide general examples and are not intended to represent every injury or prevention strategy.

FINISH LINE

The success of injury prevention for the young athlete depends on the knowledge, commitment, and motivation of key adults involved with the athlete. General strategies include identification of "at risk" athletes through the PPE, treating and rehabilitating prior injuries, and matching athletes with appropriate sports and levels of competition. Coaches who are knowledgeable in child development and healthy training practices contribute to safer sports play. A safe environment, including playing surfaces, facilities, and equipment also reduces injury. Sports injuries can also be avoided by adjusting training and competition to accommodate the athlete's tolerance.

Since each sport has specific demands in training and competition, injury prevention can also focus on sport-specific issues. When predictable stresses lead to predictable injuries, preventive intervention has its greatest potential. Through careful attention to individual and environmental factors, sports injuries in young athletes can be significantly reduced.

For More Information

1. Bijur PE, Trumble A, Harel Y, Overpeck MD, Jones D, Scheidt PC: Sports and recreation injuries in US children and adolescents. *Arch Pediatr Adolesc Med* 1995;149:1009–1116.

2. Bramwell ST, Masuda M, Wagner NN, Holmes TH: Psychosocial factors in athletic injuries: Development and application of the social and athletic readjustment rating scale (SARRS). *J Human Stress* 1975;1:6–20.

3. Hergenroeder AC: Prevention of sports injuries. *Pediatrics* 1998;101:1057–1063.

4. Jones BH, Cowan DN, Tomlinson JP, Robinson JR, Polly DW, Frykman PN: Epidemiology of injuries associated with physical training among young men in the army. *Med Sci Sports Exerc* 1993;25:197–203.

5. Kibler WB (ed): *The Sport Preparticipation Fitness Examination.* Champaign, IL, Human Kinetics, 1990.

6. Maron BJ, Poliac LC, Kaplan JA, Mueller FO: Blunt impact to the chest leading to sudden death from cardiac arrest during sports activities. *N Engl J Med* 1995;333:337–342.

7. Mueller FO, Cantu RC, Van Camp SP (eds): *Catastrophic Injuries in High School and College Sports.* Champaign, IL, Human Kinetics, 1996.

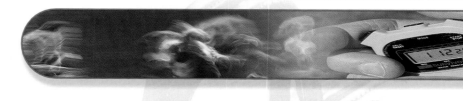

Chapter 14

Medical Management on the Sidelines

LARRY G. MCLAIN, MD

In the past, most team physicians, particularly at the high school level, have been orthopaedic surgeons. However, because of the large number of sporting events that require a medical presence, pediatricians, family physicians and others with an interest in sports medicine have also served as excellent team physicians. These physicians have received a favorable reception because of their qualifications to handle the medical and psychological issues of the young athlete and the injury issues related to physical and skeletal immaturity. With the proper dedication and commitment, these physicians can be excellent advocates for young athletes in caring for musculoskeletal injuries, injury prevention, fitness promotion, and school health.

General Attributes

Team physicians must be dedicated, available, committed to self-education about sports medicine issues, willing to develop and work with a sports medicine team (athletic trainers, coaches, administrators, physical therapists, and athletes and their parents), and possess a calm, diplomatic approach to clinical problem-solving. However, standards for training and assessing the competence of team physicians are not well defined. Many physicians who are currently team physicians were self-taught or have learned by doing. Physicians in training now have greater elective opportunities in sports medicine and the option of participating in sports medicine fellowship programs. Additional training in sports medicine is available through continuing education programs or team physician courses sponsored by national level sports medicine organizations.

Benefits

Serving as a team physician provides a valuable service to schools, teams, and athletes, and also offers many benefits. These include increased access

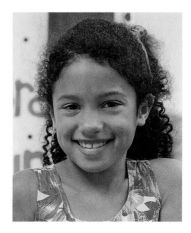

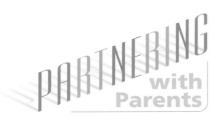

Officials, coaches, and players are often in a hurry for injured players to be removed from the playing field. When is it appropriate to do so?

Team physicians should resist pressure to remove an injured participant until he or she has completed an initial assessment and determined that the injured athlete can be moved safely and without risk of further injury.

When EMS arrives on the scene of a significant athletic injury, who should be in charge of the scene—EMS or the team physician?

Because this responsibility varies from community to community, it is not the who so much as it is that there is a plan in place that designates the who. It is advisable to meet with EMS personnel prior to the beginning of the season to establish the details of access to the site, communications, equipment, management of the scene, and evacuation.

to adolescents in a nonoffice setting, an opportunity to build and promote a practice in the community, and the personal satisfaction and enjoyment that comes from working with young athletes.

Risks

Despite the many positive aspects of being a team physician, concerns about liability and the adequacy of professional training and preparation remain. Physicians making medical diagnoses, recommending treatment, and/or determining readiness to return to play are expected to adhere to the same standards on the sidelines as they would use in their offices. On the sidelines, many diagnostic tools are obviously lacking, such as the controlled environment of the office and immediate availability of imaging modalities. In addition, the physician on the sidelines is often pressured to make an immediate return to play decision, and often, the patient is uncooperative. However, these compromises in the medical setting do not justify compromises in medical decision making. Rather, the challenges of the sideline setting demand a greater reliance on clinical acumen.

These daunting legal challenges cannot be eliminated; however, they can be mitigated by ensuring that the athlete's best interests always come first. An athlete should not be allowed to return to play until a diagnosis is known and the risk of further injury has been identified. In addition, a record of the decisions and recommendations made on the sideline should be maintained. Open communication with the athlete, parents, coach, and/or athletic trainer can help prevent or resolve any conflicts or misunderstandings that can jeopardize optimal medical care.

Good Samaritan legislation offers some protection for volunteer physicians rendering emergency care. However, these statutes vary between states and cannot be relied on to cover all of the team physician's activities. Team physicians who are paid for their work or who have formal contracts to provide sports medicine services tend not to be covered under Good Samaritan laws. Because malpractice coverage varies by policy and state, team physicians are encouraged to review their policies before committing to a team.

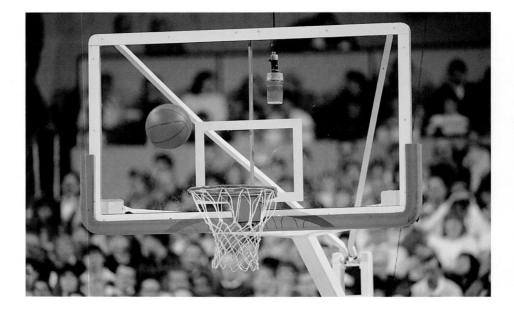

Table 14.1	*Common Medical, Neurologic, and Orthopaedic Emergencies*

Medical	Neurologic
Sudden cardiac death, cardiac arrest	Head injuries (concussion)
Exercise-induced asthma (EIA)	Cervical spine injuries
Acute episode of asthma	**Orthopaedic**
Diabetes mellitus (hypoglycemia)	
Syncope	Unstable extremity fractures
Seizures	Difficult joint dislocations (neurovascular compromise)
Heat illness and dehydration	
Bee sting allergy and other anaphylactic reactions	
Blunt abdominal trauma	

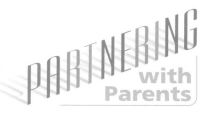

Duties and Responsibilities

Team physicians are responsible for the events they cover medically and may be responsible for determining an athlete's ability to safely participate. These responsibilities should be specified in advance to ensure that athletes, coaches, parents, athletic trainers, and administrative staff all understand and agree.

After clarifying duties and responsibilities, the team physician can begin the planning process. Planning issues involve personnel, equipment, procedures, and documentation. Sideline settings will vary according to what is needed and what is available. Some of the more common emergency situations are listed in **Table 14.1**. Knowing what to expect and having an emergency plan in place can significantly decrease the anxiety associated with potentially catastrophic injuries.

Sideline Organization

All aspects of field supervision must be well organized before the start of competition. Although the incidence of catastrophic injury is low, the potential for serious injury exists, and plans to handle the worst-case scenario must be in place. Led by the team physician, precompetition planning sessions with school administrators, coaches, athletic trainers, and the emergency medical system (EMS) in the area must occur to clarify roles. It is advisable to stage a mock emergency on the practice field to prepare for the possibility of such an event. This could include stabilization, movement, and even cardiopulmonary resuscitation (CPR) for an athlete with serious head and/or neck injuries. Other clinical situations to be considered include caring for an athlete with asthma, heatstroke, a severe traumatic musculoskeletal injury, or a cardiac arrhythmia.

Team physicians must coordinate a group of competent, well-qualified health care professionals to care for athletes on an emergency basis. Sideline organization also includes coordination with the EMS team to ensure that the proper equipment is on-site, that the hospital has been notified and is on alert during the competition, that the EMS response time is acceptable, and that EMS is available on an on-call basis or at the site of the competition. Finally, the team physician must check the availability and function of the equipment that must be present on the sideline (**Table 14.2**).

PARTNERING with Parents

Where should an injured athlete be assessed?

Many times the initial evaluation must take place on the field or sideline. Often it is difficult to adequately diagnose and assess the extent of injury or determine readiness to return to play in that setting. Occasionally, it is necessary to further evaluate the athlete in a locker room or other private location away from the excitement of the competition and without the distraction of coaches, teammates, and parents. Injured athletes can be more thoroughly examined by removing equipment and clothing without compromising the privacy of the athlete.

Table 14.2   *Suggested Sideline Equipment*

Stretcher	Elastic bandages - 12
Backboard	Ice, plastic bags
Cervical spine immobilizer (C-collar)	Compression dressings - 8
Blankets - 2	Blood contamination kit
Crutches - adjustable	Knife or clippers for face mask removal
Slings - 2	Bag for disposal of contaminated waste
Splints - 2 (upper and lower extremity)	

Table 14.3   *Suggested Contents for the Sideline Medical Bag*

Equipment

Stethoscope
Otoscope/ophthalmoscope
Penlight
Tongue blades - 2
Tape
Needles - 4
Syringes - 4
Thermometer
Blood pressure cuff
Reflex hammer
Finger splints - 3
Latex gloves - 4 pairs
Steri-strips - 1 box
Scalpel
Forceps
Nylon suture
Bandage scissors
Cotton swabs - 1 box
Betadine
Eye shield
Saline irrigation solution

CPR Equipment

Airway/endotracheal tube*
Laryngoscope*
Bulb syringe
Ambu bag
Medications*
    Atropine (1-mg prefilled syringe)
    Epinephrine (1:10,000 solution)
    Lidocaine (100-mg prefilled syringe)

General Medications

Analgesics
Acetaminophen (325-mg tablets)
Ibuprofen (600-mg tablets)

Antibiotics
Erythromycin (500-mg tablets)*
Penicillin (500-mg tablets)*

Skin Preparations
Antibiotic ointment
Steroid cream
Silver sulfadiazine cream
Insect repellent
Antifungal cream
Skin glue

GI Medications
Antacids
Loperamide
Lomotil

Eyes, Ears, Nose, Throat
Antibiotic eye drops
Proparacaine eye drops

Miscellaneous
Albuterol inhaler
Diphenhydramine
Dexamethasone
Epi-pen
Insulin, regular*
Glucagon*
Diazepam*

*These medications are optional, given the sideline setting and the proximity to resources that have or can supply these medications.

The Sideline Medical Bag

In addition to the equipment on the sideline, the team physician must have a personal medical bag. Experience has shown that the "old black bag" is both too small and highly susceptible to the elements. The medical bag that is favored by many experienced team physicians is a fishing tackle-type box that can be found in sporting goods or hardware stores. Advantages of this type of "bag" are size, ability to be locked, and the capacity of withstanding the elements.

Table 14.3 lists suggested equipment and drugs for the medical bag. Because this list represents the minimum requirements and is not intended to be all-inclusive, each physician may alter the contents of the bag to his or her own preferences. Contents may also vary depending on the sport, level of competition, and availability of EMS. While most clinical situations on the sideline usually do not require the team physician to render lifesaving care or referral to a medical facility, the medical bag should contain only essential supplies for dealing with an emergency until help arrives.

Before a Competition

The team physician should arrive at least 30 minutes before the start of competition and perform the following duties:

- Survey the playing field for any dangerous conditions;

- Check all medical supplies and equipment;

- Check the availability of telephones to ensure that EMS is available;

- Conduct introductions with the visiting coaches because the visiting team may not have their own team physician;

- Conduct introductions with the officials and referees and inform them of where he or she will be on the sidelines during the game; and

- Develop and agree upon "stopping play" guidelines with officials to allow the medical team access to the field.

During a Competition

Once the competition begins, the team physician should be stationed on the sidelines with an unobstructed view of the playing field and should have easy, rapid access to the field. Anticipation of possible injuries is a valuable habit to acquire, and the physician must concentrate only on the action on the field. If the team physician is examining an athlete on the sidelines, someone else should be designated to watch the field.

A significant responsibility of the team physician is to determine the extent of any injury or illness occurring during the game and to determine the diagnostic and therapeutic intervention the situation requires. The team physician must also decide if the injured athlete is able to return to play. The circumstances dictate that the physician must have total authority to make this decision. While the game setting is highly charged and emotional, the team physician should not be unduly influenced by nonmedical issues. Calm, rational, and objective decisions are necessary to safeguard both the athlete and the physician.

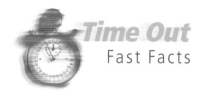

Time Out
Fast Facts

Team physician courses are available through the American College of Sports Medicine for individuals who are interested in acquiring more training in this area.

Team physicians who are paid to provide sports medicine services are often not covered under Good Samaritan laws.

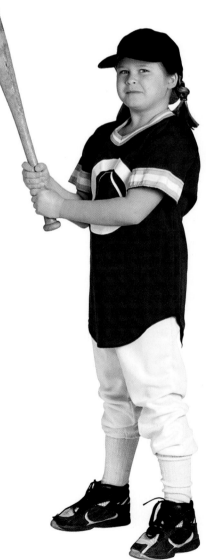

FINISH LINE

The requirements for a team physician include dedication, availability, and commitment to providing high-quality medical care to young athletes. The responsibility is great, but the benefits of being a team physician are many. Any physician who is considering accepting this great responsibility should review his or her malpractice insurance before accepting.

Efficient, effective sideline management is an essential component of providing proper care to the injured athlete. Developing a well-organized, team approach that includes appropriately trained personnel who are available to cover games is a key responsibility of the team physician. Physicians should be involved with coaches and school administrators in preseason planning. Proper protective equipment must be available on the sideline, as should appropriate means for transporting an injured athlete to the hospital. Communication among all members of the sideline team is critical, particularly with the transport team and the hospital receiving the injured athlete.

For More Information

1. Herbert DL: Practice guidelines take center court: How to limit liability. *Phys Sportsmed* 1996;24:81–83.

2. McKeag DB, Hough DO, Zemper ED (eds): *Primary Care Sports Medicine.* Dubuque, IA, Brown & Benchmark, 1993, pp 191–200.

3. Mellion MB, Walsh W: The team physician, in Mellion MB (ed): *Sports Medicine Secrets.* Philadelphia, PA, Hanley & Belfus, 1994, pp 1–4.

4. Puffer JC: Organizational aspects, in Cantu RC, Micheli LJ (eds): *ACSM's Guidelines for the Team Physician.* Philadelphia, PA, Lea & Febiger, 1991, pp 95–100.

5. Rubin A: Emergency equipment: What to keep on the sidelines. *Phys Sportsmed* 1993;21:47–54.

Chapter 15

Female Athletes

LETHA YURKO-GRIFFIN, MD, PhD
SALLY S. HARRIS, MD, MPH

The number of young girls participating in sports and exercise has dramatically increased since 1972, as a result of Title IX of the Educational Amendment Act. Title IX mandated colleges and universities who wished to keep their government funding to provide students of all races and genders with equal opportunity in all areas of college life, including sports participation. The requirements to field competitive athletic teams at the collegiate and university level fueled the development of high school and recreational sports for young women. It also required investigators to more clearly define the physiologic limits for young women and their response to the stresses of anaerobic and aerobic exercise.

At about the same time, society became enamored with fitness, and the concept of the female physique transitioned from a soft, full-figured form into a well-proportioned, muscularly toned body. Athletic adolescent girls became emulated and admired by their peers, rather than being scorned or chided for being unfeminine. According to a poll conducted by the Women's Sport Foundation, 99% of all parents believe that sports and fitness activities provide important benefits to girls. According to US government statistics, women's sport participation increased by 700% during the 1980s, with the number of girls' high school teams increasing from 15,000 to 70,000.

Psychological Concerns

The psychological benefits of sports for young women are many, including contributing to a group effort and learning to be "team players." They learn to be competitive and aggressive in a positive sense, to be confident leaders, and to experience the thrill of winning. They also learn to win graciously and to accept defeat with dignity, gaining from each defeat lessons for future improvement. These traits will later help young women succeed in the competitive business world.

Both parents can now serve as sport mentors for their daughters, improving the relationship between girls and their parents. Moreover, young women can

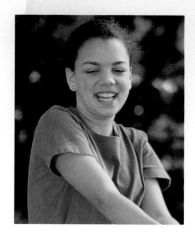

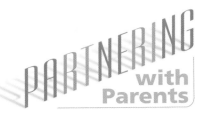

Can boys and girls compete equally in the same sports?

There are no significant differences in height, weight, strength, endurance, motor skill development, or injury risk between prepubertal boys and girls. Therefore, girls can compete equally with boys on a coeducational basis until approximately age 10 to 12 years.

now increase their overall fitness just as their male counterparts have done for years. A young girl's heart, lungs, and muscles adapt to the rigors of training by becoming more efficient, and her bones and muscles become stronger. Not only do these adaptations improve a young girl's sport participation, but they also improve her overall quality of life.

However, sport participation is not without risk of harm to the female athlete's psychological being, as well as her physical being. With puberty, boys grow bigger and stronger, rapidly increasing in body size and muscle development. Girls, however, experience increases in height and weight, but frequently these changes are not accompanied with a comparable increase in muscle mass. Therefore, while boys "grow into their sport" and become bigger and stronger to enhance their performance, girls may "grow out of their sport." They develop breasts and hips, a disadvantage when the lean prepubertal look is desired in sports such as skating, dance, and gymnastics. With puberty, a girl's increase in muscle growth is not proportional to her increase in height, and she may become frustrated and discouraged as she attempts to change sport techniques to accommodate her new body. Moreover, while overall attitudes are changing regarding the acceptance of athleticism in girls, many teenage girls feel time-stressed by sports and wish to spend less time in their sport and more time socializing in nonathletic pursuits.

When caring for girls during this developmental age, the physician should be suspicious of the athlete who presents with symptoms far greater than physical findings or has multiple minor injuries in a short period of time. In these situations, the athlete may be looking for an excuse or "an acceptable escape" from sports. Talking with the athlete in the absence of the coach, athletic trainer, and parents may provide an environment in which she can express her frustration and fears and allow the physician and athlete to work together to find an acceptable solution.

Impact of Gender Differences

Prior to puberty, there are no significant differences between boys and girls in height, weight, strength, endurance, motor skill development, or injury risk. Therefore, until approximately ages 10 to 12 years, girls can compete equally with boys on a coeducational basis. After puberty, girls' higher body fat and lower muscle mass per total body weight puts them at a significant physical disadvantage compared with boys, and coeducational sports participation is no longer equitable. Other gender differences limiting sports performance in girls after puberty include lower upper body strength and lower maximal aerobic capacity, the latter caused by lower blood volume, fewer red blood cells, lower hemoglobin content, smaller hearts, and lower stroke volume (**Table 15.1**).

The performance gap between boys and girls is wider than that explained by these physiologic differences alone and is thought to be caused in part by limited opportunity and less adequate training programs for female athletes. Training programs have the ability to produce similar and relative improvements (percent change) in strength and endurance in boys and girls, although the absolute magnitude of change will be greater in boys after puberty because of greater baseline muscle mass and aerobic capacity.

Medical Concerns

Medical concerns unique to the female athlete include menstrual irregularities such as delayed menarche and secondary amenorrhea, the relationship between phases of the menstrual cycle and sports performance, iron deficiency anemia, nutritional deficiencies, breast problems, and the triad of disordered eating, amenorrhea, and osteoporosis.

Menstrual Cycle and Sports Performance

Scientific research has been unable to prove any significant impact of different phases of the menstrual cycle on sports performance, although subtle effects on some measures of fitness have been shown. World records have been set by athletes in all phases of menstruation. Similarly, oral contraceptives have not been found to have any significant effects on sports performance, and, in fact, have been associated with a decreased risk of stress fractures. Regular exercise appears to have some beneficial effects on menstruation, such as lighter flow and reduced symptoms of premenstrual syndrome and dysmenorrhea. Current research is addressing whether hormone levels may affect the risk of soft-tissue injury, particularly ligament tears of the knee.

Menstrual Irregularities

Menstrual irregularities such as delayed menarche (no menarche by age 16 years), oligomenorrhea (3 to 9 menses per year), and secondary amenorrhea (0 to 2 menses per year in women who have already established menstrual cycles) are more prevalent in female athletes. Prevalence of secondary amenorrhea is estimated at 2% to 5% in the general population, 10% to 20% in female athletes, and up to 66% in some groups of elite athletes such as long-distance runners. In the past, these menstrual irregularities were thought to occur as a direct consequence of intensive training because of the failure of these girls to attain and maintain a critical level of body fat thought to be needed to initiate and maintain menses. However, research has disproved the critical fat hypothesis. The etiology of the menstrual disorders is thought to be caused by many factors, including an overall "energy drain" in which energy intake is inadequate to meet energy demands, resulting in a hypothalamic amenorrhea that appears to be an adaptive response of the body to conserve energy. Other contributing factors include low body fat, high training intensity, suboptimal nutrition, physical and emotional stress, history of previous menstrual irregularities, and eating disorders.

Mild delays of 1 to 2 years in the onset of menarche are common among adolescent athletes and may often occur because of a selection process whereby girls who are naturally late in maturing maintain a prepubertal body type (longer legs, narrower hips, smaller breasts, less body fat) longer. This gives them a physical advantage over girls who mature early, and enables them to experience greater success and therefore longer involvement in sports. More extreme delays in menarche, out of context with family history of age at menarche, are likely to involve a component of nutritional deprivation.

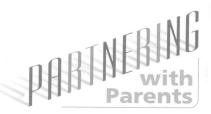

What are common sports problems for girls?

Medical concerns unique to female athletes include menstrual irregularities; the triad of disordered eating, amenorrhea and osteoporosis; iron deficiency anemia; nutritional deficiencies, and breast problems.

Table 15.1   Anatomic and Physiologic Gender Differences

Parameter	Postpubertal Girls	Postpubertal Boys	Impact
Oxygen pulse (efficiency of cardiorespiratory system)	Lower	Higher	Higher oxygen pulse provides boys an advantage in aerobic activity.
Vo₂max (reflects level of aerobic fitness)	Lower	Higher	Boys have greater aerobic capacity.
Metabolism (BMR)	6% to 10% lower (when related to body surface area)	6% to 10% higher (when related to body surface area)	Girls need fewer calories to sustain same activity level as boys.
Thermoregulation	Equals boys	Equals girls	Equal ability to adequately sweat in a hot environment to decrease core body temperature.
Endocrine system Testosterone	Lower	Higher	Boys have increased muscle size, strength, aggressiveness.
Estrogen	Higher	Lower	Unknown if related to increase in ligamentous laxity or in rate of ACL injuries.
Height	64.5"	68.5"	Increased height and weight in boys give them structural advantages.
Weight	56.8 kg	70.0 kg	
Limb length		Longer	Boys can achieve a greater force for hitting and kicking.
Articular surface	Smaller	Larger	May provide boys with greater joint stability; boys have greater surface area to dissipate impact force.

The primary medical concern regarding delayed menarche and secondary amenorrhea is the potential adverse effects on bone density associated with these hypoestrogenic states. There are no long-term effects on fertility once menses have resumed. However, amenorrheic athletes should be counseled about contraception since ovulation can precede onset of menses, making pregnancy possible. Girls with delayed menarche have decreased bone density for their age and are at increased risk for stress fractures and scoliosis. It is unclear whether normal bone density accretion is merely postponed until menses begin, or whether an irreplaceable period of time is lost during which

Table 15.1 *Anatomic and Physiologic Gender Differences—cont'd*

Parameter	Postpubertal Girls	Postpubertal Boys	Impact
Body shape	Narrower shoulders Wider hips Legs 51.2% of height More fat in lower body	Wider shoulders Narrower hips Legs 52% of height More fat in upper body	Girls have lower center of gravity and therefore greater balance ability; girls have increased valgus angle at the knee that increases knee injuries; boys and girls have different running gaits.
% Muscle/Total body weight*	~36%	~44.8%	Boys have greater strength and greater speed.
% Fat/Total body weight	~22% to 26%	~13% to 16%	Girls are more buoyant and better insulated; they may be able to convert fatty acid to metabolism more rapidly.
Age at skeletal maturation	17 to 19 years	21 to 22 years	Girls develop adult body shape/form sooner than boys.
Cardiovascular system Heart size Heart volume Systolic blood pressure	 Smaller Smaller Lower	 Larger Larger Higher	Stroke volume in girls is less, necessitating an increased heart rate for a given submaximal cardiac output; cardiac output in girls is 30% less than in boys; the risk of hypertension may be less in girls.
Hemoglobin		10% to 15% > per 100 mL blood	The oxygen carrying capacity of blood is greater in boys.
Pulmonary system Chest size Lung size Vital capacity Residual volume	 Smaller Smaller Smaller Smaller	 Larger Larger Larger Larger	Total lung capacity in boys is greater than in girls.

*There are no appreciable differences in these parameters prior to puberty; therefore, prepubertal boys and girls can compete on a fairly equal basis.

bone density would normally be increasing. In the case of secondary amenorrhea, it is well known that significant loss of bone density can occur, between 4% and 20% per year in some girls. Therefore, it is possible for a young athlete with several years of amenorrhea to have the bone density equivalent to an elderly postmenopausal woman. Oligomenorrhea has been associated with milder loss of bone density.

The loss of bone density associated with amenorrhea and oligomenorrhea is irreversible and places oligomenorrheic girls at increased risk of stress fractures in the short term, and at increased risk of premature osteoporosis

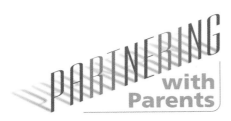

Which amenorrheic female athletes should receive medical care?

Girls whose menarche is delayed beyond age 16 years or those who have secondary amenorrhea for more than 6 months should be monitored for potential loss of bone density and considered for estrogen supplementation.

What is the best way to manage amenorrhea?

The first steps in treatment consist of a combination of increased caloric intake, decreased training intensity, and increased body fat. The goal is to stimulate menses to occur or resume naturally.

in the long term. Failure to achieve normal bone density for age because of amenorrhea is of particular concern for teenage girls because adolescence is a critical period of time during which 48% of bone density is accrued. Although exercise normally improves bone density because of the mechanical forces on bones associated with the impact loading or muscular tension of exercise, this beneficial effect does not occur in the absence of adequate levels of estrogen. Therefore, amenorrheic runners generally have a lower bone density than their sedentary peers (**Figure 15.1**).

Initial treatment of delayed menarche or secondary amenorrhea consists of a combination of increased caloric intake, decreased training intensity, and increased body fat and calcium supplementation, with the goal of triggering menses to occur or resume naturally. Athletes are often resistant to these interventions. A small change, such as 10% to 20%, in these parameters can be effective. A recent study showed success in reversing amenorrhea in endurance athletes by reducing training by 1 day per week and increasing caloric intake by 360 kcal/day in the form of a sports drink over a 15-week period of time. However, other medical causes of primary or secondary amenorrhea, such as pregnancy, reproductive dysfunction, pituitary tumor, hypothyroidism, and other hormone imbalances, should be ruled out before making the diagnosis of "athletic amenorrhea." The following laboratory studies should be ordered for these athletes: Pregnancy test, thyroid stimulating hormone (TSH), prolactin, follicle stimulating hormone (FSH), and dehydroepiandrosterone sulfate (DHEAS), if there are signs of excessive androgen.

Athletes with delayed menarche beyond age 16 years, or secondary amenorrhea lasting longer than 6 months, should be monitored for potential loss of bone density and considered for estrogen supplementation, usually done in

Figure 15.1
Lumbar Spine Bone Mineral Density—Amenorrheic Athletes.

Adapted with permission from Marcus R, Cann C, Madvig P, et al: Menstrual function and bone mass in elite women distance runners: Endocrine and metabolic features. *Ann Intern Med* 1985;102:158–163.

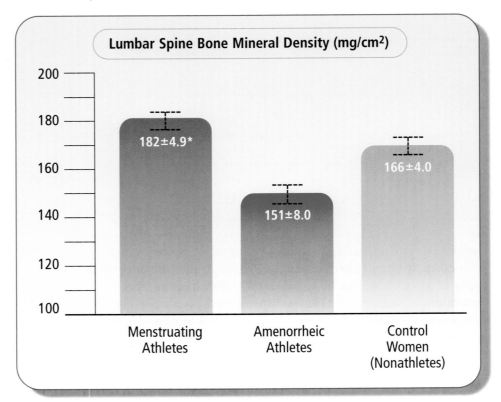

*mean ± standard error

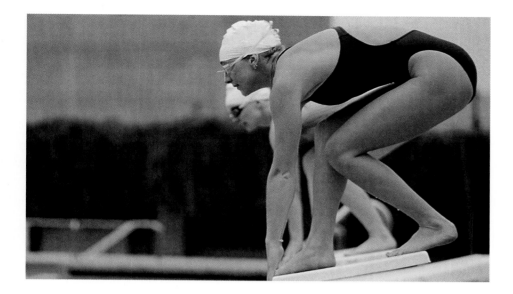

the form of oral contraceptive pills, to protect bone density. The appropriate time to initiate estrogen therapy remains controversial as research addressing long-term follow-up of bone density in adolescents is lacking. Currently, the American Academy of Pediatrics does not recommend hormone therapy for girls within 3 years of menarche, especially if the girl is younger than age 16 years. It is recommended that estrogen supplementation be delayed until after age 16 years unless there is a history of stress fracture or if 2 or more years of amenorrhea have occurred after menarche. Dual emission X-ray absorptiometry (DEXA) is useful for establishing a baseline measurement of bone density and for monitoring bone density to determine when estrogen supplementation is indicated. An increased calcium intake of 1,500 mg/day is recommended, ideally through dietary sources, or in the form of a 500-mg calcium supplement if dietary intake is inadequate.

The Female Athlete Triad: Disordered Eating, Amenorrhea, and Osteoporosis

Female athletes may be at greater risk for disordered eating because of influences unique to the athletic environment, in addition to the societal emphasis on thinness that all girls experience in the United States. While some athletes with eating disorders meet the diagnostic criteria for anorexia nervosa or bulimia nervosa, many do not, but still engage in a variety of unhealthy weight control techniques that are referred to as disordered eating. The prevalence of disordered eating is difficult to obtain and is often underreported. It is estimated that 15% of adolescent female competitive swimmers and 32% of female collegiate athletes have disordered eating, characterized by use of one method of disordered eating (such as vomiting, diet pills, fasting, diuretics, or laxatives) twice weekly for at least 3 months. However, eating disorders affect athletes in a wide variety of sports.

Risk factors that make athletes more vulnerable to disordered eating include the desire to optimize performance, a "win-at-all-costs" mentality, pressure to meet weight or body fat goals, heightened awareness of physique and body image, personality traits of perfectionism and compulsiveness, the drive for

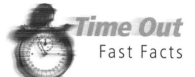

Time Out
Fast Facts

Athletes at highest risk for disordered eating

1. Sports emphasizing a lean appearance (gymnastics, diving, figure skating, dance, synchronized swimming)

2. Sports emphasizing body leanness for optimal performance (long-distance running, swimming, cross-country skiing)

3. Sports utilizing weight classifications (rowing, weight lifting, judo, tae kwon do)

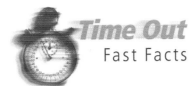

**Common Harmful
Health Consequences
of Disordered Eating**

Reproductive dysfunction

Irreversible bone loss

Psychological problems

Cardiovascular problems

Gastrointestinal problems

Thermoregulatory dysfunction

Death (10% to 15%
for anorexia)

**Adverse Effects of
Disordered Eating on
Athletic Performance**

Decreased strength, endurance,
speed, and coordination

Slower reaction time

Inability to concentrate

Electrolyte imbalances
and dehydration

Increased susceptibility to injury

Amenorrhea, loss of bone density,
and stress fractures

excellence, and the ability to block out distraction and pain. In female athletes with eating disorders, up to 70% believe these practices are harmless and will improve performance. However, the harmful effects of eating disorders are well known. In addition to the well-recognized morbidity of eating disorders for a variety of organ systems and the 10% to 15% death rate in individuals with anorexia, there are numerous adverse effects on performance.

Preventive measures include increased awareness of disordered eating by athletes, parents, coaches, and athletic trainers. It is important to create a supportive environment in which concerns about weight can be discussed. The emphasis should not be that weight loss improves performance, but rather the role of good nutrition and fitness in optimizing athletic performance, setting realistic goals and methods for weight management, and discouraging purging behaviors. A good health history addressing exercise habits, diet, and weight can identify problems. There are many warning signs of disordered eating (**Table 15.2**).

Treatment requires early identification and a multidisciplinary approach, including medical evaluation, and nutritional and psychological counseling. Most athletes can continue in their sport if cooperative with treatment and in the absence of conditions for which exercise could be harmful, such as severe weight loss, cardiac compromise, electrolyte abnormalities, hypotension, dehydration, or stress fracture.

Breast Problems

Nipple irritation and abrasions that result from excess friction can be alleviated by adhesive bandages or tape applied over the nipples, lubricants, and a good sports bra. Sports bras can also prevent breast and shoulder discomfort that can result from inadequate breast support during exercise. A good sports bra is made of soft, nonabrasive, mostly nonelastic, breathable material with good supportive features and few seams and fasteners. Breast injuries caused by direct trauma are uncommon, but can result in formation of a hematoma. These injuries are managed with analgesics, support, and protection from reinjury.

Table 15.2 *Warning Signs of Disordered Eating*	
Compulsive exercising above or beyond the requirements of the sport	Frequent bathroom trips after meals (for purposes of purging)
An increasingly restrictive diet	Binge eating and fasting
A preoccupation with food, calories, and body weight	Eating secretly or avoiding eating with others
Dissatisfaction with one's own body	Wearing baggy or layered clothing
Fear of becoming fat even when one's weight is average or below average	

Anemia

Iron deficiency anemia is one of the most common medical conditions seen in female athletes. Prevalence of iron deficiency anemia ranges up to 20% in studies of adolescent female athletes and is particularly high in cross-country runners. An additional 20% to 60% of female athletes are deficient in iron, but not yet anemic (low ferritin, normal hemoglobin). It is important to realize that iron stores are depleted before clinically recognized anemia occurs.

The most common cause of iron deficiency in women is inadequate dietary intake of iron to compensate for menstrual losses. Vegetarian diets are common among female athletes and place them at higher risk. Therefore, female athletes should be questioned about dietary intake of iron and screened for anemia as appropriate. Even mild anemia has been shown to have adverse effects on performance, particularly endurance events. Monitoring ferritin levels, in addition to a hemoglobin or hematocrit, can help detect mild forms of anemia in which hemoglobin and hematocrit are in the lower range of the normal spectrum, but actually represent a mild anemia relative to the individual's normal baseline. It is unclear whether nonanemic iron deficiency impairs performance, although it is likely to represent a preanemic state. Iron deficiency anemia should be treated with supplementation of 50 to 100 mg of elemental iron three times per day (eg, 325 mg of ferrous sulfate three times per day) for 2 months to correct the anemia. Treatment at the same dose for 6 to 8 months is necessary to replenish iron stores and restore normal ferritin levels.

Nutritional Requirements

With the exception of iron and calcium, nutritional requirements for female athletes do not differ significantly from those of male athletes. Adolescent females in general underestimate caloric needs and ingest inadequate amounts of iron and calcium. The average 15- to 17-year-old girl ingests only about 750 mg of elemental calcium per day, far below the recommended daily allowance (RDA) of 1,300 mg. A balanced diet of 3,000 kcal/day is required to obtain the RDA of 15 mg of iron, and female athletes often ingest less than

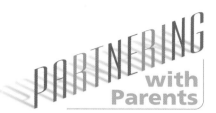

What is the best way to evaluate my daughter for anemia?

Monitoring ferritin levels, in addition to a hemoglobin or hematocrit, can help detect mild forms of anemia. Sometimes, the hemoglobin and hematocrit are in the lower range of the normal, but these levels actually represent a mild anemia relative to the individual's normal baseline.

Table 15.3 *Iron Content of Foods*

Food	Milligrams of Iron
Liver (3 oz)	7
Turkey, pork, beef (3 oz)	4 to 5
Shrimp (3 oz)	3
Chicken breast (3 oz)	1
Fish (3 oz)	1
Egg (1)	1
Dried fruit (4 oz)	3 to 4
Kidney beans (½ cup)	3
Cream of Wheat (½ cup)	9
Fortified cereal (½ to ¾ cup)	18

Table 15.4 *Calcium Content of Foods*

Food	Milligrams of calcium
Whole milk (1 cup)	300
Cottage cheese (1 cup)	200
Cheese (1 oz)	200
Yogurt (1 cup)	350 to 400
Canned salmon or sardines (3 oz)	275
Tofu (4 oz)	150
Broccoli (1 cup)	200
Eggs (2)	50
Calcium-fortified orange juice (1 cup)	200 to 250

2,000 kcal/day. In addition, many female athletes eat few meat or dairy products, the primary sources of iron and calcium respectively, in an attempt to "eat healthy" and reduce fat intake.

Preventive efforts should emphasize adequate dietary intake of iron and calcium over supplements because of the greater bioavailability in food sources. Vegetarians can be advised of a number of nonmeat sources of dietary iron (**Table 15.3**), and encouraged to eat iron-fortified cereals. A daily multivitamin containing the RDA of 15 mg of iron is recommended if dietary sources appear inadequate. Calcium can be obtained from low-fat dairy sources, a variety of nondairy foods, and calcium-fortified orange juice (**Table 15.4**). If dietary sources are inadequate, a 500-mg daily calcium supplement is recommended to achieve the RDA of 1,300 mg for eumenorrheic adolescents, and 1,500 mg for amenorrheic adolescents.

Common Musculoskeletal Injuries

The anatomic and physiologic uniqueness of each sex as an athlete, combined with the nature of the sport, has an impact on injury patterns. Increased laxity in girls may be a factor in the increased incidence of ankle sprains, glenohumeral and patella subluxations or dislocations, and patella overuse problems. A wider pelvis, increased valgus of the knee, and foot pronation also contribute to the increased incidence of patellofemoral tracking abnormalities. A lack of upper body strength has been reported to be a predisposing factor in shoulder overuse problems. Unique neuromuscular reflex patterns and less strength per total body weight may be related to the increased incidence of noncontact anterior cruciate ligament injuries in girls.

The role, if any, of estrogen and the relative lack of testosterone in injury patterns is not yet clearly understood. It is known that there are estrogen receptor sites on ligaments. The impact of the lack of testosterone available to stimulate muscle strength and bulk has long been studied, yet much is still to be learned regarding risk factors in gender-specific injury patterns. **Table 15.5** lists some of the more common musculoskeletal injuries in adolescent female athletes. Specific musculoskeletal problems and their appropriate management are detailed in Section 5 of this text.

Table 15.5 *Common Musculoskeletal Injuries in Adolescent Female Athletes*

Shoulder	Laxity:
	Impingement
	Subluxation
Spine	Scoliosis
	Apophysitis
	Spondylolysis
Foot	Forefoot overuse problems
	(corns, calluses, bunions, metatarsalgia)
Knee	Patellofemoral stress syndrome
	Patella subluxation and dislocation
	Anterior cruciate ligament injuries

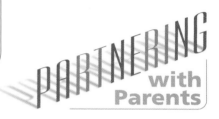

Conditioning and Rehabilitation

Prevention of musculoskeletal injury through proper conditioning, including a well-designed weight training program, is essential for adolescents when competition in sports is increasing and young bodies are changing rapidly under the influence of puberty. At one time, weight training was not advised for young athletes, especially young girls. It was thought that young girls lacked adequate testosterone to benefit from such programs and that they were at significant risk of sustaining injuries to their growth centers and developing musculoskeletal systems. However, research has proved that these beliefs are unfounded and has shown that weight training improves fitness by increasing muscle strength and endurance, enhances the cardiovascular system, and indirectly increases bone strength and self-esteem.

In general, weight training will not result in muscles that appear to be over-proportioned. It is true that a muscle working at its maximum capacity will generally increase in size as a result of increasing its metabolic processes to handle the greater workload. However, the degree to which a muscle hypertrophies depends not only on the applied load, but also on diet, and on the amount of anabolic hormone (primarily testosterone) available. Females genetically have less testosterone; therefore, the degree of muscle bulk they will develop with properly applied resistance and good nutrition is less than that of males.

A unique weight training method practiced by many girls, especially those in dance, is the Pilates method. This conditioning technique, named for the physical trainer who developed it about 75 years ago, emphasizes proper body alignment, flexibility, and strength through lengthening. Many exercises can be done on mats, but some use specialized pieces of equipment consisting of movable carriages containing pulleys, cables, and springs that are easily adaptable to young developing bodies.

If young girls use weights as a part of their conditioning program, they must be properly instructed in their use, ensure that they are well hydrated when lifting, and remember to stretch after warming up and before lifting.

Why do girls so often complain of pain on the anterior aspect of the knee?

A wider pelvis, increased valgus of the knee, and foot pronation contribute to the increased incidence of patellofemoral tracking abnormalities.

FINISH LINE

Young girls should be encouraged to participate in sports and exercise regularly. With proper injury prevention and with prompt recognition and treatment of a medical or orthopaedic problem when it arises, the psychological and physiological benefits of sports and exercise far outweigh the risks of injury.

For More Information

1. Agostini R (ed): *Medical and Orthopaedic Issues of Active and Athletic Women.* Philadelphia, PA, Hanley & Belfus, 1994.

2. Arendt EA: Orthopaedic issues for active and athletic women. *Clin Sports Med* 1994;13:483–503.

3. Drinkwater BL (ed): *The Female Endurance Athletes.* Champaign, IL, Human Kinetics, 1986.

4. Hunter-Griffin LY (ed): *Athletic Training and Sports Medicine,* ed 2. Park Ridge, IL, American Academy of Orthopaedic Surgeons, 1991, pp 921–932.

5. Griffin LY: The female athlete, in DeLee JC, Drez D Jr (eds): *Orthopaedic Sports Medicine: Principles and Practice.* Philadelphia, PA, WB Saunders, 1994, pp 356–373.

6. Ireland ML: Special concerns of the female athlete, in Fu FH, Stone DA (eds): *Sports Injuries: Mechanisms, Prevention, and Treatment.* Baltimore, MD, Williams & Wilkins, 1994, pp 153–187.

7. Nattiv A, Arendt EA, Riehl R: The female athlete, in Zachazewski JE, Magee DJ, Quillen WS (eds): *Athletic Injuries and Rehabilitation.* Philadelphia, PA, WB Saunders, 1996, pp 841–851.

8. Pearl AJ (ed): *The Athletic Female.* Champaign, IL, Human Kinetics, 1993.

9. Puhl JL, Brown CH (eds): *The Menstrual Cycle and Physical Activity.* Champaign, IL, Human Kinetics, 1986.

10. Wells CL (ed): *Women, Sport & Performance: A Physiological Perspective.* Champaign, IL, Human Kinetics, 1985.

Chapter 16

Physically Challenged Athletes

FRANK M. CHANG, MD

Children with disabilities currently have the best opportunity ever to participate in sports and athletic activities. Strong voices advocating for the disabled, increased awareness of the lay community, and legislation such as the Americans with Disabilities Act have resulted in significant changes in attitude among children, parents, and school boards. These children are being mainstreamed into the classroom and given the opportunity to participate in academic and athletic opportunities with their able-bodied peers.

The term "physically challenged" refers to individuals with chronic musculoskeletal or neurologic disabilities that can be classified as congenital or acquired. **Tables 16.1** and **16.2** describe many common disabilities and the appropriateness for participation in specific sports. Physically challenged children who are encouraged to participate in sports will most likely improve their health, endurance, and flexibility, as well as their self-esteem.

Guidelines Based on Specific Ability/Disability

Amputations

Amputations are congenital or acquired. Acquired amputations can be traumatic, or therapeutic, in which part of a limb may be removed by necessity because of a malignancy or vascular insufficiency. Amputations are further classified by the functional level remaining: 1) in the lower extremity, ankle, below-knee, above-knee, and hip disarticulation; 2) in the upper extremity, wrist, below-elbow, above-elbow, and shoulder disarticulation. Determining the proper functional level is important as it helps ensure that athletes will compete against others with similar abilities.

Children with congenital deficiencies of the lower extremities usually lack the corresponding muscles and associated soft tissues, and they may also be missing other less obvious soft-tissue structures. Children with congenital short femurs or proximal focal femoral deficiencies usually also have an

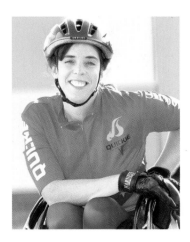

Table 16.1 Participation Possibility Chart: Individual Sports

	Archery	Bicycling	Tricycling	Bowling	Canoeing/kayaking	Diving	Fencing	Field events*	Fishing	Golf	Horseback riding	Rifle shooting
Amputations												
Upper Extremity	RA	R	R	R	RA	R	R	R	R	RA	R	RA
Lower Extremity (above knee)	R	R	R	R	R	R	—	R	R	R	R	R
Lower Extremity (below knee)	R	R	R	R	R	R	R	R	R	R	R	R
Cerebral palsy												
Ambulatory	R	R	R	R	R	R	—	R	R	R	R	R
Wheelchair	R	—	—	R	R	—	—	—	R	—	—	R
Spinal cord disruption												
Cervical	RA	R	R	R	RA			—	R	RA	X	RA
High thoracic: T1-T5	R	R	R	R	R		RA	R	R	RA	—	R
Low thoracolumbar: T6-L3	R	R	R	R	R	R	RA	R	R	R	R	R
Lumbosacral: L4-Sacral	R	R	R	R	R	R	R	R	R	R	R	R
Neuromuscular disorders												
Muscular dystrophy	RA	R	R	R	IA	—		—	R	R	X	RA
Spinal muscular atrophy	RA	—	R	R	—	—		R	R	R	—	RA
Charcot-Marie-Tooth	R	R	R	R	R	R	R	R	R	R	R	R
Ataxias	R	—	R	R	—	—		R	R	—	—	R
Others												
Osteogenesis imperfecta	R	—	R	R	R	—	R	R	R	—	—	R
Arthrogryposis	R	—	—	R	R	—	—	R	R	—	R	R
Juvenile rheumatoid arthritis	RA	—	—	RA	R	—	—	—	R	—	—	R
Hemophilia	RA	R	R	R	R	R	R	R	R	R	R	R
Skeletal dysplasias	R	R	R	R	R	R	R	R	R	R	R	R

R = Recommended; A = Adapted; X = Not recommended; I = Individual

* Clubthrow, discus, javelin, shot

Continued.

Table 16.1 *Participation Possibility Chart: Individual Sports—cont'd.*

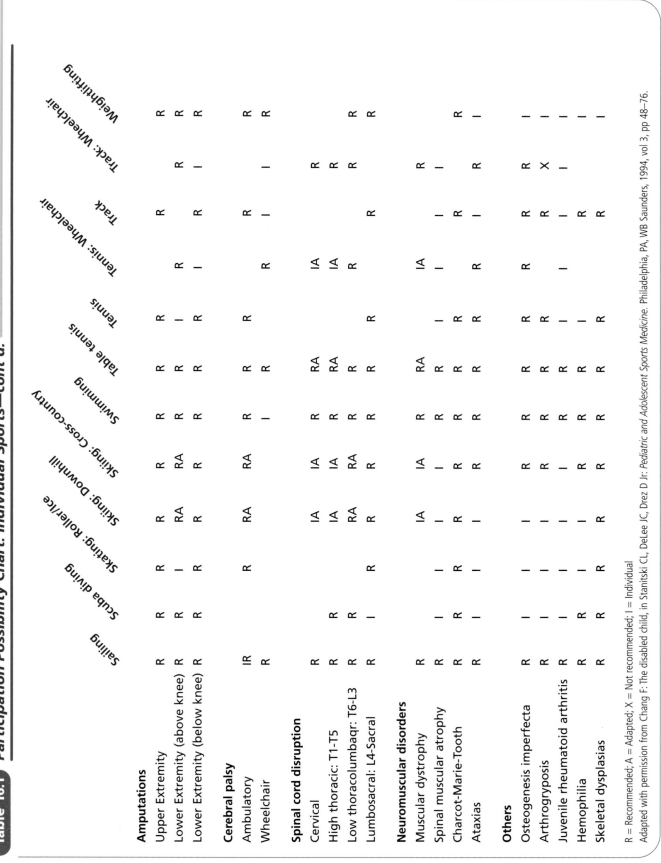

	Sailing	Scuba diving	Skating: Roller/Ice	Skiing: Downhill	Skiing: Cross-country	Swimming	Table tennis	Tennis	Tennis: Wheelchair	Track	Track: Wheelchair	Weightlifting
Amputations												
Upper Extremity	R	R	R	R	R	R	R	R		R		R
Lower Extremity (above knee)	R	R	I	RA	R	R	R	R	R	R	R	R
Lower Extremity (below knee)	R	R	R	R	R	R	R	R		R		R
Cerebral palsy												
Ambulatory	IR		R	RA	R	R	R	R	R	R	R	R
Wheelchair	R				—	R	R		R	—	—	R
Spinal cord disruption												
Cervical	R			IA	IA	R	RA		IA		R	
High thoracic: T1-T5	R	R		IA	IA	R	RA		IA		R	
Low thoracolumbar: T6-L3	R	R		RA	RA	R	R		R	R	R	R
Lumbosacral: L4-Sacral	R	—	R	R	R	R	R	R	R	R	R	R
Neuromuscular disorders												
Muscular dystrophy	R		IA	IA	R	RA			IA		R	R
Spinal muscular atrophy	R	—	—	—	R	R	R	—	—	—	—	
Charcot-Marie-Tooth	R	R	R	R	R	R	R	R	R	R	R	R
Ataxias	R	—	—	R	R	R	R	R	R	—	R	—
Others												
Osteogenesis imperfecta	R	—	—	R	R	R	R	R	R	R	R	—
Arthrogryposis	R	—	—	R	R	R	R	R	R	R	X	—
Juvenile rheumatoid arthritis	R	—	—	—	R	R	R	—	—	—	—	—
Hemophilia	R	R	—	R	R	R	R	R	R	R		—
Skeletal dysplasias	R	R	R	R	R	R	R	R	R	R		—

R = Recommended; A = Adapted; X = Not recommended; I = Individual

Adapted with permission from Chang F: The disabled child, in Stanitski CL, DeLee JC, Drez D Jr: *Pediatric and Adolescent Sports Medicine.* Philadelphia, PA, WB Saunders, 1994, vol 3, pp 48–76.

Table 16.2   *Participation Possibility Chart: Team Sports*

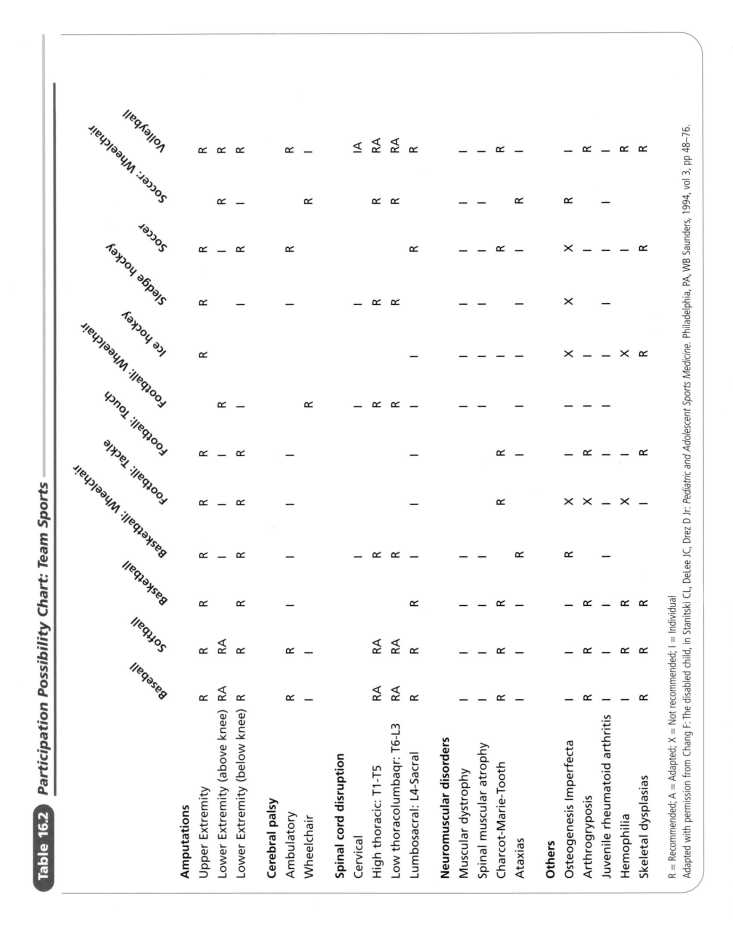

	Baseball	Softball	Basketball	Basketball: Wheelchair	Football: Tackle	Football: Touch	Football: Wheelchair	Ice hockey	Sledge hockey	Soccer	Soccer: Wheelchair	Volleyball
Amputations												
Upper Extremity	R	R	R	R	R	R	R	R	R	R	R	R
Lower Extremity (above knee)	RA	RA	RA	—	—	—	—	R	—	—	R	R
Lower Extremity (below knee)	R	R	R	R	R	R	—	R	—	R	—	R
Cerebral palsy												
Ambulatory	R	R	—	—	—	—	R	R	—	R	R	R
Wheelchair	—	—	—	R	—	R	R		—	—	—	—
Spinal cord disruption												
Cervical	RA	RA	—	—	—	—	—		—	—	R	IA
High thoracic: T1-T5	RA	RA	R	—	—	R	R		R	R	R	RA
Low thoracolumbaqr: T6-L3	RA	RA	R	—	—	R	R		R	R	R	RA
Lumbosacral: L4-Sacral	R	R	—	—	—	—	—	—	—	R	—	R
Neuromuscular disorders												
Muscular dystrophy	—	—	—	—	—	—	—	—	—	—	—	—
Spinal muscular atrophy	—	—	—	—	—	—	—	—	—	—	—	—
Charcot-Marie-Tooth	R	R	R	R	R	—	R	R	—	R	R	R
Ataxias	—	—	R	—	—	—	—	R	—	—	R	—
Others												
Osteogenesis Imperfecta	—	—	R	X	—	—	—	X	X	X	R	—
Arthrogryposis	R	R	R	R	R	R	—	R	—	—	—	R
Juvenile rheumatoid arthritis	I	—	—	—	—	—	—	—	—	—	—	—
Hemophilia	—	R	R	X	X	—	—	X	X	—		R
Skeletal dysplasias	R	R	R	R	R	R	R	R	R	R	R	R

R = Recommended; A = Adapted; X = Not recommended; I = Individual

Adapted with permission from Chang F: The disabled child, in Stanitski CL, DeLee JC, Drez D Jr: *Pediatric and Adolescent Sports Medicine*. Philadelphia, PA, WB Saunders, 1994, vol 3, pp 48–76.

associated anterior cruciate deficient knee manifested by positive drawer and Lachman signs. It is
important to understand this condition so that it
will not be mistaken as an acute rupture of the
anterior cruciate ligament. Many of these patients
are fitted in a below-knee prosthesis. The rigid
prosthesis has less flexibility and elasticity than a
normal lower leg and will also increase the risk of
an injury to the remaining knee ligaments. When
participating in sports with significant potential
for knee injuries, a second prosthesis with medial
and lateral hinges and a thigh lacer for additional
support and suspension should be prescribed to
protect the knee.

Children wearing prosthetic limbs are at
increased risk for skin problems. With prosthetic
lower limbs, the weightbearing forces must be
transferred to the skeleton through the skin and
underlying soft tissues. Some amputee levels pose
more difficulty for the prosthetist to transfer these
forces successfully. For any lower extremity ampu-
tation above the level of the ankle, the skin and
soft tissues transferring the weightbearing forces
are more susceptible to breakdown and pressure
necrosis.

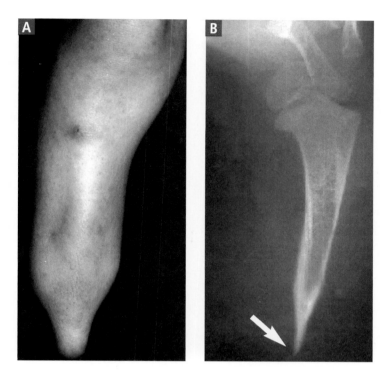

Figure 16.1 Stump overgrowth. **A** Clinical photograph of bony
overgrowth of the tibia in a below-knee amputee. **B** Radiograph
shows bony spike that impales the skin and interferes with
prosthetic wear.

Stump overgrowth is also a constant problem in children with amputations (**Figure 16.1**). This occurs most frequently in the fibula, followed by
the tibia, humerus, radius, ulna, and femur. During this process, the bone
grows through whatever soft tissues the surgeon left to cushion the end of the
stump. As the child runs and jumps, the skin is at high risk for breakdown. To
prevent skin breakdown from occurring, the child, parents, coaches, and physical education teachers should be made aware of the potential problem. If the
end of the stump begins to feel bonier, or erythema and skin irritation begins,
the child should be evaluated for stump overgrowth. The overgrown stump
should be revised surgically to prevent the potential complications. In a young
child, several stump revisions may be necessary at 2- to 3-year intervals prior
to skeletal maturity.

Cerebral Palsy

Cerebral palsy is a nonprogressive central nervous system deficiency that
is present around the time of birth and can be loosely extended to present
during early childhood. In children with cerebral palsy, inadequate motor
control and lack of coordination are considered more significant problems
for sports than susceptibility to injuries. Impaired hand-to-eye coordination
results in difficulty in controlling racquets, bats, golf clubs, and other sports
equipment. Difficulty catching and throwing and perceptual problems,
such as judging the speed of a ball, are considered challenges, but not insur-
mountable obstacles. Running with speed is more difficult. However, these
deficiencies in coordination can be improved and overcome to some extent
with practice.

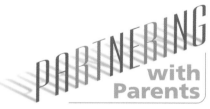

*My child has cerebral palsy
but is active. What type of
injuries can I expect?*

Overuse symptoms are common,
as are muscle strains because of
muscle tightness. Patellar overload and anterior knee pain are
also common. Proximal migration
of the patella may occur as a
result of flexed knee gait.

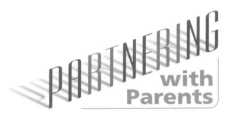

Why does my teenager with cerebral palsy have activity-related back pain?

A hip flexion contracture leads to secondary increase in lumbar lordosis. This results in symptomatic spondylolysis and back pain.

Children with cerebral palsy are susceptible to overuse symptoms and are at increased risk of muscle strains because of muscle tightness. These children are frequently less active, so the muscles do not have the opportunity to stretch on a regular or frequent basis. Muscle imbalance magnifies the problem, resulting in tightness and contractures of major muscle groups. The spastic muscles are usually an agonistic group of muscles. For example, the triceps surae group of muscles attached to the Achilles tendon is frequently spastic, overactive, and tight compared with the antagonistic ankle dorsiflexors.

The tightly contracted muscles result in joint stress. Patellar overload is common and will frequently evolve into true chondromalacia. Both growth and spasticity result in progressive tightening of the hamstrings and quadriceps muscles, causing a shortened stride length and increased pressure across the patellofemoral joint. In more severe cases, the tight hamstrings produce a crouched or flexed knee gait. When allowed to persist, proximal migration of the patella occurs. The increased pressure gradually results in increased wear and damage to the articular surface of the patella. The symptoms are the same as in able-bodied children with patellar overload symptoms, but the problem is accentuated and more resistant to treatment. In addition, the tension on the quadriceps mechanism can produce a syndrome similar to "jumper's knee" in adolescents. The constant pull of the patellar tendon results in fragmentation of the lower pole of the patella radiographically, with pain and tenderness clinically.

Muscle tightness and imbalance across the hip joint will gradually affect the normal development of the hip joint, and in more severe cases, the hip joint will subluxate and eventually dislocate. Coxa valga and acetabular dysplasia may develop in children who are less severely affected, and acetabular dysplasia may become symptomatic as the joint undergoes degenerative arthritic changes. As these changes occur, increased activity such as running and jumping will result in hip pain.

Head Injuries

Children with head injuries are functionally very similar to children with cerebral palsy; however, neurologic function may improve in these children as the injured tissue recovers. Visual field defects, present in some children with head injuries, increase the potential for injuries and can cause problems if an object such as a ball passes through the child's "blind spot."

Meningomyelocele

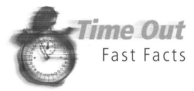

In children with meningomyelocele, judgment may be impaired due to intellectual compromise.

In children with meningomyelocele, development of an abnormal spinal canal results in a damaged spinal cord that is inadequately protected; therefore, the patient has altered motor function and sensation below the involved level. The sensory level usually corresponds to the motor level, and the involvement may be asymmetrical. In addition to motor and sensory deficits, bowel and bladder functions are impaired. Hydrocephalus is frequently associated with this condition and increases the risk for impaired cerebral function and mentation and damage to the motor cerebral cortex.

A child with meningomyelocele is typically able to participate in sports in a manner similar to a child with a spinal cord injury. However, the varying degrees of intellectual compromise associated with this condition may cause the child difficulty in understanding the rules of the sport or may result in perceptual problems that may affect performance. Children with severe hydrocephalus should wear adequate head protection to prevent head injury and shunt damage.

Sports participation for these children depends on several factors, the two most important being the child's neurologic functional level and the severity of hydrocephalus. The functional level of the spinal cord will determine the motor function of the lower extremities, and the severity of hydrocephalus will determine the degree of mental retardation and spasticity. Classification of children with meningomyelocele is based on their functional level (ie, the lowest nerve root level that is functioning). For example, if the child can actively dorsiflex the ankle, but has no active plantar flexion, he or she is functioning at the L5 level, or the fifth lumbar nerve root is functioning, but there is no function below that level.

Children with low lumbar and sacral level involvement can function almost normally; however, patients with low lumbar involvement may require orthoses to stabilize the foot and ankle. Children with involvement at the midlumbar level also may require braces to stabilize the knee. Those with higher level involvement function best in a seated position, and those with midlumbar level involvement may perform physical athletic activities better in a wheelchair compared with ambulation in braces.

Children who wear braces and participate in sports may develop pressure sores and skin breakdown; therefore, lack of sensation is a concern. Children sitting in wheelchairs for prolonged periods of time are also susceptible to pressure sores and skin breakdown from the seat of the wheelchair. Individuals with normal sensation who experience discomfort will automatically shift positions as the pressure increases or as the tissues become ischemic, but children with inadequate sensation do not have these same protective mechanisms. To avoid these problems, the child, parents, and coaches must be educated to inspect the skin frequently until the skin pressure tolerances can be determined. Children must be taught to shift their weight frequently and to use their upper extremities to lift themselves off their seats. To decrease excessive pressure while sitting in the wheelchair, specially designed cushioned seats to evenly distribute the weight and dissipate pressure are available. In addition, children with meningomyelocele have problems with thermoregulation.

Because weightbearing stimulates skeletal development, children with meningomyelocele are more susceptible to fractures secondary to osteopenia. When the muscles are not functioning and are not stressed by weightbearing, the bones receive less stimulation and the skeletal elements become osteopenic.

Fractures in these children are more difficult to diagnose. Individuals with altered or absent sensation often report no associated pain. The injured area may appear locally inflamed, so a fracture can easily be mistaken for an infection with swelling, erythema, increased local temperature, and a low-grade fever. Immobilization of a fractured extremity results in the bone becoming

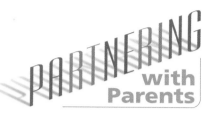

What are good sports options for children with meningomyelocele?

Typically, a child with meningomyelocele and motor deficit can participate in sports in a manner similar to a child with a spinal cord injury. Examples of common activities include competitive wheelchair racing, basketball, and decathlon events.

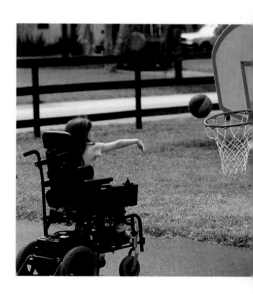

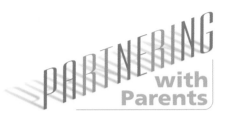

What are other sports problems in kids with meningomyelocele?

Fractures are more difficult to diagnose and can be mistaken for infection.

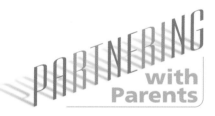

Are heat- and cold-related illnesses a problem in children with a spinal cord injury?

Thermoregulation is a problem in children with spinal cord injuries above T8. They have dysautonomia, a condition in which they cannot maintain normal body temperatures. Therefore, precautions must be taken to avoid heat- and cold-related illness.

even more osteoporotic and susceptible to refracture when immobilization is completed. Gradual, progressive weightbearing after a fracture or recent operation and the use of functional braces can help to prevent a refracture. Limiting the time of immobilization and nonweightbearing will decrease the incidence of refracture.

Children with meningomyelocele are also susceptible to muscle strains. The lowest spinal level of functioning muscles is usually less than 100% normal strength. Since children with spinal defects are less active, the overall motor power is not as well developed. Some muscles are also tighter than normal and prone to strains because of muscle imbalance and decreased flexibility.

Spinal Cord Injuries

Although spinal cord injuries in children are uncommon, they account for 13% to 15% of all spinal cord injuries, with boys affected twice as often as girls. Spinal cord injuries are typically traumatic and associated with spinal fractures. Children younger than age 10 years may have spinal cord injuries with no associated fractures because of their generalized ligamentous laxity.

The problems experienced in association with spinal cord injury are similar to meningomyelocele. Spinal cord injuries, except in special circumstances such as Brown-Sequard lesions, are typically transverse lesions with symmetric involvement. Spinal cord injuries can involve the cervical spinal levels and compromise upper extremity function. Intellectual function is usually intact unless the child has had an associated head injury.

In children with insensate skin, shoes, orthotics, and wheelchairs can cause excessive localized pressure that leads to skin irritation, blisters, skin breakdown, soft-tissue infections, and osteomyelitis. In addition to educating the children to be aware of their skin and the interface with their braces, wheelchairs, and foot wear, coaches, physical education instructors, and parents also should be aware of the potential problems and check the skin periodically for redness, calluses, and blisters. Even if the child has no history of skin problems associated with a brace, the added stress of competitive sports can cause excessive skin pressure. In addition, children are constantly growing. With growth, brace fit will change and will eventually lead to altered pressure sites.

In children with higher level lesions, thermoregulation is a problem. Children with spinal cord injuries above T8 cannot maintain normal body temperatures. Maintenance of body temperature is dependent on heat dissipation and heat production. Heat production mechanisms, such as shivering, and heat dissipation mechanisms, such as perspiration, are absent below the level of the spinal cord injury. The higher the neurologic level, the more difficult it is for the patient to compensate for changes in ambient temperature. Children with meningomyelocele have similar problems with thermoregulation. Precautions must be taken when participating in winter sports, and the children must be closely observed in very warm environments. In a survey of the competitors at the 1990 US Junior National Wheelchair Games, almost half of the athletes participating in track and field events listed hyperthermia as a problem and 9% of those competing in swimming listed hypothermia.

Down Syndrome

The abnormal collagen produced in association with Down syndrome results in generalized ligamentous laxity and decreased muscle tone. The ligamentous laxity causes hyperflexibility of joints and related problems, such as flexible flatfeet and joint instability with associated subluxations and dislocations. Judgment may also be impaired because of intellectual compromise and compounded by the fact that children with Down syndrome frequently do not report discomfort or pain and may continue to participate despite the presence of symptoms.

Atlantoaxial subluxation

Atlantoaxial instability and occipitocervical instability have been reported intermittently since 1965. Atlantoaxial subluxation affects approximately 15% of children with Down syndrome and is potentially the most devastating problem associated with this condition. The subluxation is caused by laxity of the annular ligament of C1 and is magnified by the generalized hypotonia. The space available for the spinal cord consequently diminishes (**Figure 16.2**). As C1 displaces on C2, the spinal cord can impinge on the odontoid or the posterior ring can impinge on the spinal cord. Excessive motion at this level can result in permanent damage to the spinal cord. If the motor tracks are injured, the patient is left a quadriplegic or quadriparetic with respiratory compromise.

Beginning in 1983, the Special Olympics required screening for atlantoaxial instability in athletes with Down syndrome prior to participation in any sport that places excessive stress on the head or neck, including gymnastics, diving,

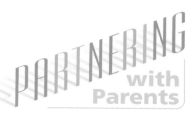

What are the preparticipation physical evaluation (PPE) recommendations for clearance of children with Down syndrome regarding the cervical spine?

Clearance that rules out atlantoaxial instability includes a negative neurologic history/exam and normal flexion/extension lateral radiographics. These exams should be repeated every two to three years.

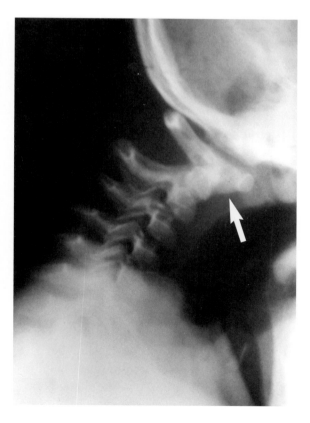

Figure 16.2 Flexion radiograph shows forward displacement of C1 on C2.

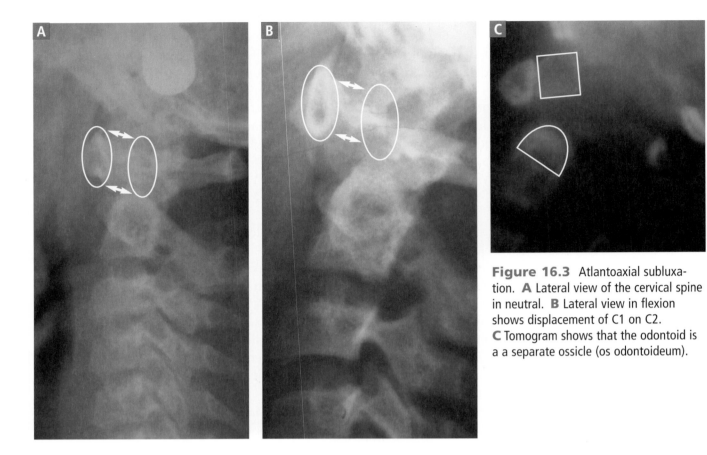

Figure 16.3 Atlantoaxial subluxation. **A** Lateral view of the cervical spine in neutral. **B** Lateral view in flexion shows displacement of C1 on C2. **C** Tomogram shows that the odontoid is a a separate ossicle (os odontoideum).

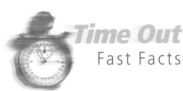

Time Out
Fast Facts

The Special Olympics has instituted screening for atlantoaxial instability for the following sports:

  gymnastics

  diving

  pentathlon

  butterfly stroke and breast stroke in swimming

  diving start in swimming

  high jump

  warm-up exercises.

pentathlon, butterfly and breast stroke in swimming, diving starts in swimming, high jump, and warm-up exercises that place undue stress on the head and neck muscles. This requirement has raised awareness of the problem, and many school districts also now require screening prior to participation in physical education.

Atlantoaxial subluxation is best detected with lateral views of the cervical spine in maximum flexion and extension. Flexion-extension views are then compared to assess the atlanto-dens interval (ADI) (**Figure 16.3**). Statistically, the development of neurologic symptoms is greatest between ages 5 to 10 years. Neurologic symptoms include neck pain, stiff neck, torticollis, progressive weakness or change in sensation in any extremity, decreasing endurance, loss of bowel or bladder control or a change in bowel habits, increased clumsiness, or a change in gait pattern.

The ADI is normally less than 2.5 mm, but the highest acceptable value is 4.5 mm in a child with Down syndrome. In an asymptomatic child with an ADI of greater than 4.5 mm, activities that increase risk to the cervical spine should be restricted. This includes sports such as tumbling, gymnastics, diving, soccer, high jump, football, butterfly and breast stokes in swimming, and skiing. If the ADI is excessive (greater than 6.0 mm) or the child has neurologic symptoms, the child is a candidate for a cervical surgical stabilization. Screening is recommended by some organizations and should be done prior to enrolling the child in any high-risk activities, at the onset of school, or in the presence of neurologic symptoms. Although some physicians still recommend follow-up screening at 3- to 5-year intervals until skeletal maturity, this is controversial. The American Academy of Pediatrics agrees with the recommendation to evaluate atlantoaxial instability in patients with Down syndrome who have neurologic symptoms. However, lateral radiographs of the cervical spine as a screening procedure for otherwise asymptomatic patients has potential but unproven value in preventing spinal cord injury in young athletes with Down syndrome.

Knee and hip problems

Two other joints may cause problems in children with Down syndrome. The patellofemoral joint may be unstable and chronically subluxate or dislocate, and occasionally the hip joint may become unstable. Patellofemoral joint laxity can intensify any anatomic abnormalities, such as genu valgus, patella alta, or a hypoplastic medial femoral condyle, and can result in instability. Recurrent subluxations and acute dislocations may not produce reports of pain in a child with Down syndrome. Treatment is more difficult because, in addition to ligamentous laxity, the children are also relatively hypotonic and nonoperative management frequently fails. Surgical realignment of the extensor mechanism may be necessary on rare occasions.

Hip instability is an even more difficult problem to treat. Excessive joint laxity can result in a distended hip capsule that allows the hip to dislocate. Parents will describe audible clunking or popping sounds, with usually very little evidence of symptoms. Some children with Down syndrome will even actively dislocate their hip for attention or self-stimulation. Nonoperative

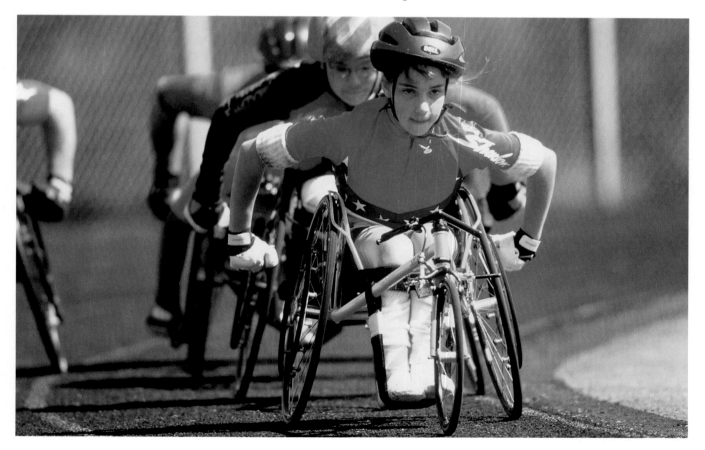

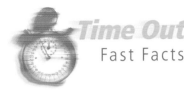

Physically challenged children who are encouraged to participate in sports will most likely improve their health, endurance, flexibility, and most important, their self-esteem.

measures, such as temporary casting or prolonged abduction bracing, produce inconsistent results. Even surgical correction with femoral or pelvic osteotomies, combined with capsulorrhaphy and prolonged postoperative casting, do not always ensure permanent hip stability. Although hip damage and eventual degenerative changes do occur, the natural history of this problem is not well documented. The instability does appear to diminish somewhat with progressive growth and development.

Foot problems

Children with Down syndrome normally have flexible flatfeet; however, most are asymptomatic. If planovalgus deformities are symptomatic, orthotics may help to minimize symptoms and excessive shoe wear.

Hearing Impairment

Hearing-impaired children are not predisposed to any specific injuries and can participate in all sports, but they are at a disadvantage because communication with other participants is compromised. Not only can they not hear someone giving instruction, but often their speech is also impaired. They also lack the ability to receive auditory cues. Because they do not have any visible physical disabilities, these children tend to play with other able-bodied children, leaving them at some disadvantage. Since the inner ear is connected to the vestibular apparatus, balance may be affected.

Hearing aids are useful for some children. Lip reading and signing will facilitate communications, but have obvious disadvantages during the heat of competition, especially in sports involving other team members or other competitors. For hearing-impaired children to experience maximum success in sports, they may elect to participate in individual activities like tennis, skiing, and running where the need for communication is minimal.

Visual Impairment

Participation without eyesight in sports is, at best, a difficult situation. Occasionally, auditory cues can be substituted during some sports such as skiing, and special programs have been developed at a few ski resorts. As the proficiency and skills of the skier increase, the individual can ski faster and on more difficult terrain.

Other sports have been successfully adapted in recent years. Rock climbing, speed skating, tandem bicycling, and competitive swimming are all gaining popularity with visually impaired athletes.

Children with head injuries may also have limitations in their field of vision depending on the anatomic location of the lesion. Awareness of the location of the visual field defect is important for safety and in choosing a sport that will not be significantly affected by the child's "blind spot."

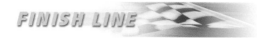

FINISH LINE

> Participation in sports is as important for physically challenged children as it is for their able-bodied counterparts. Prior to participation, physically challenged children should be evaluated by a physician to identify sports commensurate with their abilities.

For More Information

1. American Academy of Orthopaedic Surgeons: Sports and recreational program for the child and young adult with physical disability. Proceedings of the Winter Park Seminar, Winter Park, CO. Chicago, IL, American Academy of Orthopaedic Surgeons, 1983.

2. Chang FM: Sports programs for the child with a limb deficiency, in Herring JA, Birch JG (eds): *The Child With a Limb Deficiency.* Rosemont, IL, American Academy of Orthopaedic Surgeons, 1998, pp 361–377.

3. Chang FM: The disabled athlete, in Stanitski CL, DeLee JC, Drez D Jr (eds): *Pediatric and Adolescent Sports Medicine.* Philadelphia, PA, WB Saunders, 1994, vol 3, pp 48–76.

4. Sussman MD (ed): *The Diplegic Child.* Rosemont IL, American Academy of Orthopaedic Surgeons, 1992.

section four
Medical Conditions

4

SOCCER
ALL STAR
WORLD CUP KICK-OFF ACTION
MATCH

Section Editors
Steven J. Anderson, MD
Gregory L. Landry, MD

Cardiac Conditions

R E G I N A L D   L .   W A S H I N G T O N ,   M D

Cardiac conditions such as dysrhythmias, hypertension, and heart disease can affect a child's ability to safely participate in sports. Signs and symptoms such as murmurs, syncope, and chest pain may also affect a child's ability to be physically active. It is important to establish the safety of physical activity for these children and to encourage them to participate at levels that are appropriate for their specific condition. Most of these children can participate in physical activities without limitations, but there are exceptions. All children with cardiac conditions should be evaluated individually to determine their physical limitations before they increase their physical activity. Prior to any increase in physical activity, children should undergo a preparticipation physical evaluation (PPE). This chapter highlights the cardiovascular components of the PPE and reviews the most common cardiovascular disorders in children. Those with known congenital defects require specialty evaluation that is beyond the scope of this chapter.

Murmurs

Heart murmurs are commonly heard in children and by some estimates, up to 85% of young athletes have audible heart murmurs detected on screening examinations. Most heart murmurs are considered functional or "innocent." Often, heart murmurs are first identified during the PPE. Once detected, further evaluation should seek to answer these questions:

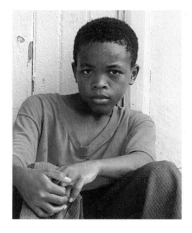

1. Is the murmur functional or organic?

2. If the murmur is organic, should participation in physical activity be limited?

3. What type of evaluation should be completed before participation in physical activity is allowed?

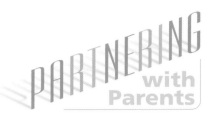

Are heart murmurs commonly found on the preparticipation physical evaluation (PPE)?

Heart murmurs are common and found in up to 85% of youngsters undergoing the PPE.

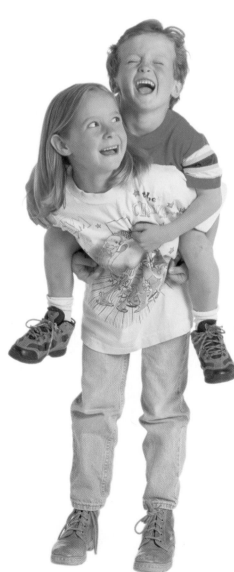

Functional Murmurs

Still's murmur

The most common type of murmur in children is Still's murmur, which is characterized by a medium- to high-pitched, slightly vibratory or moaning murmur heard only during systole. It is easiest to hear along the lower left side of the sternum, although it radiates widely from the apex of the heart to the upper left side of the sternum. The child should lie in a supine position during auscultation because the sound decreases dramatically when the child is sitting or standing. The murmur occurs only during systole and is never heard during diastole. These murmurs are usually intermittent and become louder when cardiac output increases, for example with anxiety, fever, or exercise.

Venous hum

Another common functional murmur is the venous hum. This continuous blowing or "humming" murmur is best heard above or below the clavicles on either side when the child is sitting. However, it is generally inaudible when the child is supine or when the return of venous blood from the neck to the heart is obstructed by gently compressing the jugular vein. If the murmur persists despite performing these maneuvers and continues to be heard when the child is supine, the differential diagnosis must include a patent ductus arteriosus (PDA). A child with a suspected PDA should be examined by a cardiologist before increasing physical activity.

Organic Murmurs

Organic murmurs are generally characterized by their harshness rather than by their intensity. Organic murmurs are not vibratory in nature, but they are audible with the child in any position. Organic murmurs may be caused by minor defects in the atrial or ventricular septa or by more complex cardiovascular problems such as narrowing of the aortic or pulmonary valves or cyanotic heart disease. If there is any suspicion of such problems, the child should be referred to a cardiologist.

Evaluation of Heart Murmurs

A complete evaluation consists of a thorough history and physical examination, an electrocardiogram, a radiograph of the chest, and often, an echocardiogram. An assessment for heart murmurs should begin with a thorough history of the child and the immediate family members. The history should also document any adverse responses to exercise or activity and relevant symptoms, such as near syncope, syncope, chest pain, palpitations, and/or decreased exercise tolerance. The physical examination should include a thorough evaluation of the cardiovascular system, including peripheral pulses, auscultation, and blood pressure. An electrocardiogram, a chest radiograph, an echocardiogram, or an exercise stress test may provide additional information. However, these tests should be selected and interpreted by someone experienced in diagnosing and treating congenital heart disease.

The presence of an organic murmur alone does not preclude physical activity or sports participation. Many children with organic murmurs have good cardiovascular function and are capable of full, active involvement in

Table 17.1 *Elements of Patient History When Assessing for Dysrhythmias*

Questions about the patient's history	Questions about the family history
1. Number, frequency, and duration of the episodes	1. Sudden death
2. Time of day when the episodes occur	2. Syncope
3. Relationship of these episodes to meals or exercise	3. Near syncope or dizziness
4. Severity of the symptoms	4. Seizures
5. Recent use of medications, caffeine, or illicit substances	5. Supraventricular tachycardia
6. Associated symptoms, including headache, nausea, vomiting, incontinence, tingling of the extremities, loss of vision, or syncope	6. Prolonged QT syndrome
	7. Hypertrophic cardiomyopathy
	8. Congestive cardiomyopathy
	9. Arrhythmogenic right ventricular dysplasia

all physical activities. Guidelines for advising these children about participating in sports are contained in the proceedings from the 26th Bethesda Conference on Cardiovascular Abnormalities in the Athlete.

Dysrhythmias

A variety of tests can be used to diagnose and characterize dysrhythmias. Particularly important, however, is obtaining a thorough patient and family history (**Table 17.1**). An electrocardiogram and occasionally long-term recording devices (24-hour Holter monitor or activity monitors) also provide useful information.

Not all children with dysrhythmias require medical treatment or restrictions from physical activities. For instance, dysrhythmias originating from wandering atrial pacemakers or the sinus node are usually benign and do not require treatment. A child with these conditions may participate in athletic activities without any restrictions.

Children with premature ventricular contractions (PVCs) may report that their heart is "skipping beats." An electrocardiogram will reveal an irregular rate originating from the ventricle. The rhythm is irregular, and the extra beat is followed by a compensatory pause. The next beat following the compensatory pause is more forceful and is perceived by the patient as a skipped beat. No treatment is required if the PVCs are uniform, appear singly (not in couplets), and disappear when the heart rate exceeds 140 beats/min. However, if the above criteria are not met, further evaluation by a cardiologist is warranted before athletic participation can be allowed.

Supraventricular tachycardia (SVT) is also known as paroxysmal atrial tachycardia (PAT). In this dysrhythmia, abnormally rapid conduction of an atrial impulse into the ventricle causes episodic increases in heart rate. A child with SVT or PAT requires further evaluation and perhaps medical treatment before participation is approved.

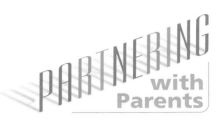

What elements of the history on the PPE should raise suspicion from the cardiac point of view for possible unexpected sudden death?

A history of syncope during exercise raises concern; a family history of premature myocardial infarction (MI) in first and second degree relatives or the observation of stature and body habitus indicating Marfan syndrome is a concern.

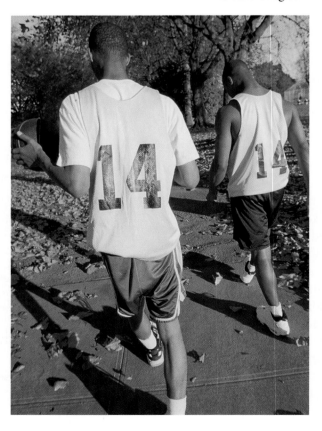

Children who have complete heart blocks or complex dysrhythmias (atrial flutter, atrial fibrillation, junctional tachycardia, and ventricular tachycardia) should be evaluated and treated by a cardiologist before participating in athletic activities.

Near Syncope and Syncope

Children who experience episodes of near syncope report dizziness and lightheadedness, either with exercise or without. They often feel cold, clammy, and sweaty and have thready peripheral pulses and low blood pressure. With syncope, however, these symptoms are followed by loss of muscle tone and loss of consciousness. Syncope and near syncope may be associated with underlying cardiac conditions, including vasodepressor syncope (fainting), primary and secondary cardiovascular syncope, vascular syncope, and noncardiovascular syncope.

Vasodepressor syncope is caused by a sudden fall in blood pressure with subsequent loss of consciousness. Associated signs and symptoms may include dizziness, lightheadedness, pallor, diaphoresis, nausea, hyperventilation, and tachycardia. This type of syncope can be triggered by anxiety or fear in response to the sight of blood, loud noises, or other environmental stimuli. Typically, the syncopal episode lasts less than 1 minute and is preceded by prodromal symptoms. If the environmental stimulus is identified and eliminated, participation in sports may continue. If the episodes persist, continued participation in sports is not recommended until the athlete is evaluated by a cardiologist.

Primary and secondary cardiovascular syncope may result from congenital heart problems that cause low cardiac output or dysrhythmia. As such, patients with syncope should be evaluated for underlying congenital heart problems before participating in sports.

Vascular syncope (also known as orthostatic or neurocardiogenic syncope) occurs when blood pools in the lower parts of the body and reduces the amount of blood returning to fill the left ventricle. During a tilt test examination, children with this type of syncope will demonstrate a normal increase in heart rate, followed by a precipitous fall in heart rate and/or blood pressure. Often, severe problems, such as seizures, develop. These children often require medication before being allowed to participate in athletic activities and should be examined by a cardiologist.

Noncardiovascular syncope is caused by hypoxia, hypoglycemia, hyperventilation, seizures, vertigo, hysteria, and severe migraines. The history and physical examination will help determine which tests or specialty consultations should be obtained prior to sports participation. Activity restrictions should be determined individually and depend on the cause of the syncope. Syncope must be properly diagnosed and treated, if necessary, before the child participates in athletic activities.

Chest Pain

Young athletes rarely complain of chest pain. However, when they do, cardiovascular causes must be ruled out first. To make this determination, an evaluation of the characteristics of chest pain will help determine its cause:

1. Duration

2. Quality

3. Factors that provoke the pain

4. Factors that relieve the pain

5. Location and radiation of the pain

Chest pain can be caused by injury to the musculoskeletal system or can originate from conditions affecting the lungs, pleura, mediastinum, myocardium, or pericardium. Musculoskeletal pain usually can be related to a specific episode of trauma and is characterized by localized pain and tenderness that occurs with specific movements and/or activities. Some common causes of chest wall pain include contusions or fractures of the ribs or sternum, strains of the pectoralis or intercostal muscles, costochondritis, and/or costosternitis.

Nonmusculoskeletal pain or pain from abnormalities of the heart or lungs occurs without antecedent trauma, is less well localized, and is less clearly related to specific movements and/or activities. Inflammation or infection of the pleura or pericardium may be associated with chest pain. Chest pain is also frequently reported as a component of asthma.

Cardiac causes of chest pain tend to produce symptoms that are worse with stress on the cardiovascular system. Pain from myocardial ischemia can occur with hypertrophic cardiomyopathy or aortic stenosis. A history of syncope, palpitations, or exercise intolerance raises concern for these conditions. Echocardiography is recommended for patients with features of Marfan's or Turner's syndrome and chest pain because of the possibility of dissection of the aorta.

Fortunately, chest pain in children is rare. However, because of the potential for serious underlying conditions, each case of chest pain needs to be explained satisfactorily before the child is cleared to participate in athletic activities.

Systemic Hypertension

Evaluation of blood pressure requires the use of appropriately sized cuffs. Larger athletes often require a thigh cuff for use on the arm. If blood pressure is elevated initially, repeat measurements should be taken after a few minutes and, if necessary, after the athlete lies down for several minutes. If the blood pressure is still elevated, the athlete should be questioned about the use of stimulants (caffeine, nicotine, cold or cough medications) and anabolic or corticosteroids, which can increase blood pressure. If signs and symptoms of systemic hypertension persist, the athlete should be evaluated for target-organ damage, such as retinal changes (by ophthalmoscope examination), left ventricular mass (by echocardiography), and renal damage (analysis of blood and urine, and perhaps imaging studies). Children with target-organ damage may need to be restricted from isometric exercises or some high-contact dynamic sports.

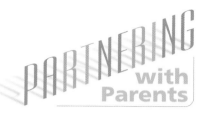

What is the greatest cardiac risk for a young athlete?

Sudden death while participating in sports is the greatest cardiac risk. Therefore, the screening PPE is critical to identify athletes who are at risk.

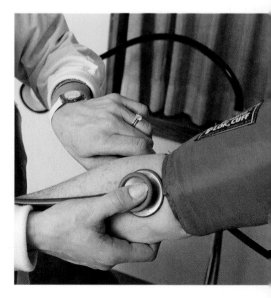

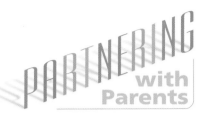

How should my child with hypertension be evaluated prior to participation?

Hypertensive children with target-organ damage should be referred to a cardiologist to undergo graded exercise tests. These tests measure peak blood pressures during exercise.

Children with severe, untreated, or unresponsive hypertension should avoid sports that involve prolonged periods of isometric exercises or stress and high-contact sports that might directly damage organs. If a child has interest in a sport that involves a high isometric component, prolonged hand grip stress testing should be performed before sports participation is approved.

Acquired Heart Disease

Some children may have acquired heart disease. For instance, rheumatic fever can damage the aortic and mitral valves. Therefore, children who have had rheumatic fever should be evaluated by a cardiologist before beginning an athletic activity.

Individuals who have had a Kawasaki syndrome without cardiovascular complications may participate in all activities. However, if the child has arteritis or coronary artery aneurysms, approval by a cardiologist should be obtained before participation is allowed.

Mitral valve prolapse is present in approximately 8% of children, but most of them can participate in physical activities. Children with mitral valve prolapse and a history of syncope, chest pain that is intensified by exercise, dysrhythmias, significant mitral insufficiency, or a family history of sudden death should be examined by a cardiologist before participating in vigorous physical activities.

Congenital Heart Disease

Congenital heart diseases include a number of specific conditions and occur at a rate of 8 per 1,000 live births. It is impractical to define the same limits for all children with congenital heart disease because some may have only minor defects, while others may have complex, inoperable defects. Furthermore, children who have undergone corrective or palliative surgery may not have achieved successful results. Because of these factors, children with congenital heart conditions need to be evaluated individually according to the guidelines established by the Bethesda Conference.

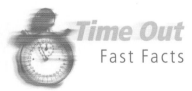

There are between 10 and 25 cases of sudden cardiac death reported each year.

Sudden Cardiac Death

The incidence of sudden cardiac death in children is estimated to be 7.5 per million per year of participation in males and 1.5 per million per year of participation in females. This accounts for between 10 and 25 cases of sudden death reported each year. Most of these studies, however, do not include a death that may occur during physical education classes, intramural sports, or casual recreational sports.

The most common cardiac causes of sudden death include hypertrophic cardiomyopathy, congenital coronary artery anomalies, aortic stenosis, myocarditis, dilated cardiomyopathy, mitral valve prolapse, and dysrhythmias.

Screening echocardiograms have been suggested to identify some of the causes of sudden death. Most experts believe that in most settings, screening echocardiograms are not indicated because of the high cost of the procedure and the low frequency of disorders that are detected.

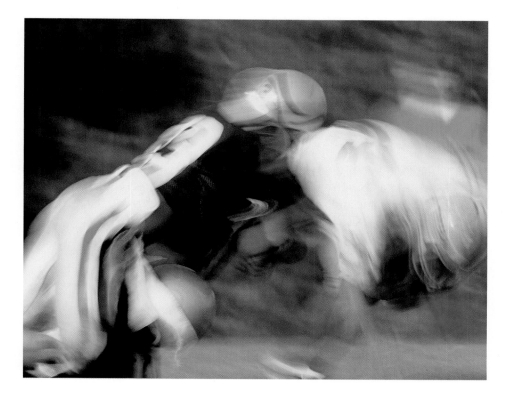

Hypertrophic Cardiomyopathy

Most patients who die suddenly have hypertrophic cardiomyopathy and have had prodromal symptoms, although it is believed they may have kept these symptoms to themselves. These athletes frequently will have had presyncope or syncope with or without exercise prior to the fatal event. Chest pain and palpitations may also have been experienced during exercise. It is important to emphasize, however, that some of these athletes may have been asymptomatic for years. A systolic murmur will often be appreciated, but only when the athlete is standing or with a Valsalva maneuver, and these murmurs are often very soft. Therefore, it is important during a PPE to examine the athlete in several positions and to do so in a quiet room. If this diagnosis is suspected, a referral to a cardiologist should be done before participation is allowed.

Anomalies of the left coronary artery are also frequently mentioned as a cause of sudden cardiac death. These athletes may or may not have had symptoms of syncope associated with activity and/or chest pain. This is a difficult diagnosis to make when the athlete has a negative family history, a normal physical examination, and a normal electrocardiogram. However, if symptoms lead to the suspicion of this diagnosis, activity should be restricted and the athlete should undergo evaluation of the coronary arteries immediately.

Athletes with aortic stenosis and mitral valve prolapse will have heart murmurs or abnormal auscultatory findings that should lead to the suspected diagnosis. Athletes who have the physical appearance of Marfan's syndrome should be screened to exclude the possibility of a dilated aorta. Athletes who have an acute febrile illness followed by prolonged fatigue may have acute myocarditis that also may lead to an acute cardiac death.

Although the incidence of sudden cardiac death is rare in this age group, a high index of suspicion should prevent some cases from occurring.

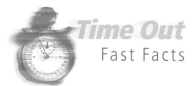
Time Out
Fast Facts

The most common cardiac causes of sudden death include hypertrophic cardiomyopathy, congenital coronary artery anomalies, aortic stenosis, myocarditis, dilated cardiomyopathy, mitral valve prolapse, and dysrhythmias.

FINISH LINE

Before participating in any sports, children should undergo a complete physical examination that includes a thorough personal and family history of any cardiac conditions. Most individuals who experience cardiac symptoms during physical activity will not appear to have cardiac disease on initial assessment, so specific laboratory tests may be necessary to evaluate the athlete further.

Most children with cardiovascular conditions can participate in most, if not all, physical activities. Decisions regarding sports participation in children who have cardiovascular disease must be made individually. It is the primary responsibility of their health care providers to evaluate their individual cardiovascular problems and set individual limits of physical activity, with appropriate consultation with a cardiologist.

For More Information

1. 26th Bethesda Conference: Recommendations for determining eligibility for competition in athletes with cardiovascular abnormalities: January 6–7, 1994. *J Am Coll Cardiol* 1994;24:845–899.

2. American Academy of Pediatrics, Committee on Sports Medicine and Fitness: Athletic participation by children and adolescents who have systemic hypertension. *Pediatrics* 1997;99:637–638.

3. American Academy of Pediatrics, Committee on Sports Medicine and Fitness: Cardiac dysrhythmias and sports. *Pediatrics* 1995;95:786–788.

4. Kanter R: Syncope and sudden death, in Garson A, Bricker JT, Fisher D, Neish S (eds) *The Science and Practice of Pediatric Cardiology*, ed 2. Baltimore, MD, Williams & Wilkins, 1998, vol 2, pp 2169–2199.

Chapter 18

Head Injuries

B R Y A N   W .   S M I T H ,   M D ,   P H D

Head injuries, though they range from uncomplicated to catastrophic, are never simple. Annually, hundreds of thousands of head injuries occur in organized athletic activity. While collision sports such as boxing, football, and ice hockey are associated with a high risk of head injury, sports such as basketball, soccer, baseball, and wrestling also pose significant risk. Recreational activities such as biking, in-line skating, skiing, and skateboarding result in numerous emergency department visits for head injuries.

Controversy exists within the medical community regarding treatment of concussion, the most common head injury in sports. Numerous guidelines for the management of concussions have been developed; however, scientific support and consensus from medical specialists is still lacking. This chapter reviews the differential diagnoses and pathophysiology of the athletic head injury, outlines the signs and symptoms of concussion, and describes the evaluation of the athlete with a head injury. Management and return to play decisions also will be presented.

Differential Diagnosis/Pathophysiology

Epidural Hematoma

Epidural hematomas typically occur as the result of damage to the middle meningeal artery via a temporal skull fracture (**Figure 18.1**). Most often, the mechanism of injury involves a high-impact event, such as being struck by a baseball. Typically, the injured athlete will experience a lucid period, followed by a severe headache and progressive obtundation. Prompt recognition and subsequent treatment in an emergency department with neurosurgical expertise can prevent significant brain injury and save the athlete's life.

Subdural Hematoma

High-impact trauma to the skull can injure venous structures beneath the dura mater, resulting in a subdural hematoma (**Figure 18.2**). Falls or high-speed collisions are the usual mechanism of injury. With a concomitant skull fracture, signs and symptoms can evolve in minutes. However, without

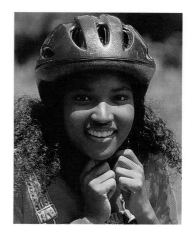

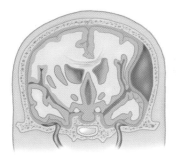

Figure 18.1 Epidural hematoma.

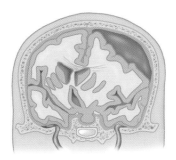

Figure 18.2 Subdural hematoma

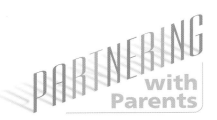

My child has had more than one concussion. Should this be evaluated?

Young athletes with multiple concussions or persistent symptoms may require neuropsychological testing or neurologic referral to assist the team physician in making a return to play decision.

a fracture, signs and symptoms may take days to develop. Usually, the athlete is unconscious for some period of time. Even in the best of circumstances, significant morbidity can occur because of resultant brain damage.

Second-Impact Syndrome

Second-impact syndrome is a rare condition believed to be caused by a loss of autoregulation of the vascular components of the brain. Second-impact syndrome may occur when an athlete sustains a second head trauma before recovering from an initial head injury. Resultant massive cerebral edema occurs over seconds to minutes, frequently progressing to death. This condition is most often reported in boxers and football players, with a majority of cases reported in young athletes. Despite several unanswered questions regarding the etiology and prevention of this syndrome, second-impact syndrome has been a driving factor in the development of most concussion management and return to play guidelines.

Malignant Brain Edema Syndrome

Malignant brain edema syndrome is a poorly understood and rare condition that can occur in young children following a single head trauma. The pathophysiology resembles second-impact syndrome, with the loss of vascular autoregulation and resultant diffuse cerebral hyperemia. Neurologic decline to coma and death may take minutes to hours. Therefore, prompt recognition and management at an appropriate medical facility is vital.

Cerebral Concussion

A cerebral concussion is defined as a transient traumatic disruption of cognitive function. Because this neuronal insult causes an increased demand for glucose intracellularly, a transient mismatch in glucose delivery and use occurs. This mismatch is believed to alter regulation of cerebral blood flow. These changes are believed to result in a heightened vulnerability for further injury until normal function has been restored.

Several signs and symptoms have been reported in athletes who have sustained a concussion (**Table 18.1**). *An athlete who has sustained a concussion*

Table 18.1	*Signs and Symptoms of Concussion*	
Headache	Amnesia	
Sleep disturbance	Posttraumatic	
	Retrograde	
Dizziness	Hyperexcitability	
Confusion	Vomiting	
Nausea	Visual disturbances	
Unsteadiness	Tinnitus (ringing in the ears)	
Difficulty concentrating	Lightheadedness	
Disorientation	Fatigue	
Loss of consciousness		
Irritability		

should not be allowed to return to practice or competition while symptomatic or displaying any signs of a concussion. To date, there is no precise correlation between symptoms and the length of time the brain is injured intracellularly. Loss of consciousness and amnesia are the signs that have formed the basis for most concussion grading scales. However, signs are quite variable in their occurrence and resolution. Most individuals who sustain concussions do not lose consciousness. Those who sustain a concussion may experience varying degrees of amnesia or no amnesia at all.

The scientific literature contains more than 15 concussion grading schemes that assess the severity of injury. The variability of symptoms complicates the "grading" of the injury. All of the grading scales are based on clinical observations. As such, the grades tend to be variable, and experts continue to disagree on how to use these grading scales in managing athletes with concussions.

Post-Concussive Syndrome

Post-concussive syndrome is characterized by varying degrees of headache, irritability, concentration and memory impairment, dizziness, sleep disturbance, and fatigue. Although the incidence is unknown, this syndrome may be more common than recognized. Symptoms may last weeks to months and are probably the result of alterations in neurotransmitter function. In most patients, symptoms that persist for more than 1 week should be evaluated either with CT or MRI to rule out structural pathology. If cognitive dysfunction is suspected, neuropsychological testing may be useful to document the degree of dysfunction. Neurologic referral should be considered in protracted cases. Return to play should be dictated by the full resolution of symptoms and normal diagnostic study results.

Clinical Evaluation and Management

Initial evaluation and management depend on the athlete's level of consciousness. If the athlete is unconscious, the cervical spine must be immobilized prior to transport to prevent possible catastrophic damage to the spine. An open airway must be established next and adequate ventilation ensured. During this period, circulation needs to be monitored and supported, as necessary. If the patient has signs of neurologic deterioration, such as posturing or pupillary abnormalities, intubation with moderate hyperventilation should be initiated.

Initially, an athlete who is conscious or rapidly awakening should be managed in the same way as an unconscious athlete, beginning with an evaluation for cervical spine injury. If a cervical spine injury is suspected or cannot be ruled out, the spine should be immobilized before the athlete is moved off the field. If the athlete is ambulatory, escort the athlete to the sideline, noting any abnormality in gait, balance, and orientation. It is best to move the athlete to a less congested location to avoid unnecessary outside stimulation and interference with medical evaluation and treatment. In the unconscious athlete, prompt transport to a trauma center or comparable medical facility with neuroimaging and appropriate specialists should be considered.

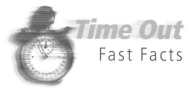
Time Out
Fast Facts

Head and spinal cord injury is uncommon in children under 15 years of age but increases markedly in those 15 to 18 years of age.

Proper equipment—such as bicycle helmets and helmets for in-line skaters—significantly reduces the risk of serious head injury.

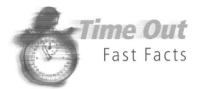

Time Out
Fast Facts

An athlete with a concussion should not be allowed to return to practice or competition while symptomatic or displaying signs of a concussion.

History

The athlete should be questioned about the mechanism of injury and any symptoms that he or she is experiencing. Pay close attention to the patient's affect. It is not uncommon for the athlete to be hyperexcitable, irritable, sullen, or moody following a concussion. If the athlete avoids answering the questions, it is possible that he or she cannot answer the questions because of the injury. It is important to recognize that athletes usually want to play and may attempt to deceive the examiner by hiding their injuries so that they may be allowed to return to play.

Orientation needs to be evaluated by questioning the athlete concerning person, place, and time. For example, ask the athlete to identify his or her school, opponent, position played, and the current score (remember to block the scoreboard from the athlete's view). Assess memory by asking the athlete to recall the mechanism of injury and the events prior to the injury (eg, menu for pregame meal, the score at half time, etc). Both short- and long-term memory can be evaluated by asking the athlete three to five words to recall immediately and at the end of the examination.

Physical Examination

The next part of the evaluation consists of a complete neurologic examination, including a cranial nerve assessment, gross visual field examination, pupillary and funduscopic examination, otoscopic examination of each tympanic membrane for blood in the middle ear, a generalized examination for

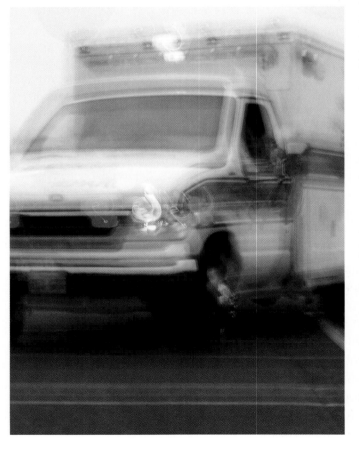

strength and sensation, and a check of deep tendon reflexes. Positive findings on these tests are rare in the athlete with a concussion. However, when present, prompt transport to the hospital is often warranted. The absence of these signs does not exclude a potentially serious brain injury.

The last phase of the evaluation involves testing concentration and coordination. An athlete with a concussion usually shows abnormalities of concentration and/or coordination. To assess concentration, ask the athlete to recite the months of the year backwards. It is important to note the speed as well as the accuracy. For the second test, the serial sevens test, instruct the athlete to start at 100 and subtract seven repeatedly, ending at zero. While accuracy is important, also note whether the athlete becomes frustrated, confused, or takes an inordinate amount of time to complete the task. Some individuals may be unable to complete either test, particularly the serial sevens test, even under normal conditions. Preseason baseline testing for comparison may be useful. Coordination is assessed by observing the athlete's gait and by having the athlete perform a Romberg test.

When the athlete is on the sidelines, reevaluation should be performed after 15 minutes to determine

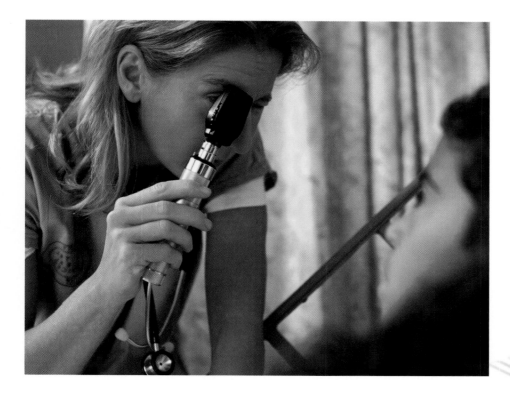

whether signs and symptoms have resolved. During this time, someone should stay on the bench with the athlete. With a football player, take the helmet to keep the athlete from returning to the field without medical clearance. If signs and symptoms of a concussion clear within 15 minutes, repeat the assessment after a brief period of exercise (eg, 40-yd dash, jumping jacks, five push-ups or sit-ups). If signs or symptoms return with exercise, the athlete should not return to play.

Diagnostic Tests

Standardized Assessment of Concussion

The standardized assessment of concussion (SAC) is a diagnostic tool that is designed to assess orientation, immediate memory, concentration, and delayed recall in an objective manner. It takes approximately 5 minutes to administer and has been designed for use on the field by physicians, athletic trainers, and coaches. There are three versions available to minimize practice effects when the athlete repeats the test. Ideally, the athlete should be tested before preseason practice to provide a baseline value. Research using the SAC on both high school and collegiate football players has been promising; however, additional research is necessary to validate this tool and better understand its applicability to athletes from all sports.

Imaging

Imaging studies may provide useful diagnostic information if concussion symptoms worsen or fail to resolve within a reasonable time frame. Usually, CT is more readily available, less expensive than MRI, and is considered quite adequate to evaluate for both gross blood in the cranium and evidence of skull fracture. However, whether all athletes with brief (seconds) loss of

PARTNERING with Parents

My child had a head injury and was not allowed to return to play that day. Was that a good idea?

It depends. If the athlete loses consciousness or has symptoms and signs that last for more than 15 minutes after the injury, he or she should not return to play that day. However, if he or she does not lose consciousness, has no symptoms, and shows no signs of change in neurologic or physical status for 15 minutes after the injury, the physician should instruct the athlete to perform some physical activity, such sit-ups, push-ups, Valsalva maneuver, that increases intracranial pressure. If symptoms recur after the activity, the athlete should not return to play or practice for the remainder of that day. If the athlete remains asymptomatic after the activity, he or she can return to activity if this was the first concussion.

consciousness require imaging is debatable. The length of time the athlete was unconscious, the duration and progression of symptoms, and the physician's experience in evaluating head injuries must be considered when ordering an imaging study. More subtle pathology, such as vascular malformations and minor bleeding, can be identified on an MRI scan. Therefore, MRI is preferred in more protracted cases, typically, if symptoms have not resolved in 1 week.

Neuropsychological testing

Cognitive skills can be evaluated with one of many neuropsychological tests. These tests are typically performed by neuropsychologists and require 3 or more hours to complete. While these tests have been shown to be sensitive in the assessment of concussion, their utility, availability, and cost make them impractical for routine evaluation of concussion. In patients with multiple concussions or persistent symptoms, neuropsychological tests may provide objective information to assist the physician in making return to play decisions.

Treatment

Standard treatment for most concussions is rest and observation for as long as the athlete is symptomatic. Most concussions resolve without sequelae. Analgesics play no defined role in the acute treatment of concussion. Most athletes can be managed at home by a responsible caregiver (eg, parent) who has been given thorough instructions on the signs of neurologic deterioration.

All athletes rendered unconscious should be observed closely for at least 24 hours and perhaps hospitalized. In these cases, the athlete is allowed to eat and

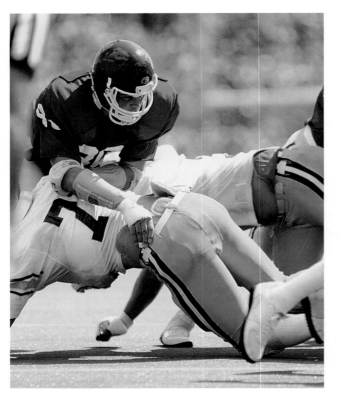

to sleep, but should be awakened every 2 to 3 hours if he or she has any symptoms prior to going to sleep. Worsening symptoms, new symptoms, and/or deteriorating neurologic signs warrant urgent reexamination by a physician, and transport to the hospital for imaging studies and possible consultation with a neurosurgeon. As the athlete recovers, daily follow-up by the physician is the preferred method of management while the patient is symptomatic.

Return to Play

Many factors influence the decision to return the athlete to play following a concussion. Current recommendations in the literature are based on clinical experience rather than on scientific research. Adherence to even the most conservative guidelines is no guarantee against an undesirable outcome.

The athlete who shows signs and symptoms of concussion should never be allowed to return to any physical activity that may result in additional head trauma. In many situations, this decision requires trusting the athlete to honestly answer questions about the resolution of symptoms. Therefore, it is important to establish rapport with the athlete, if possible, and to inform the athlete of the magnitude of the situation. In the middle of a competition, athletes, their coaches, and even their parents may not be objective about the risks of concussions.

If the athlete has not been rendered unconscious, is asymptomatic, and shows no signs of change in neurologic or physical status for 15 minutes from the time of concussion, the physician should instruct the athlete to perform some physical activity, (eg, sit-ups, push-ups, knee bends, Valsalva maneuver) that increases intracranial pressure. These activities may cause symptoms to recur, and if they do, the athlete should not return to play or practice for the remainder of that day. If the athlete remains asymptomatic after physical activity, he or she can return to activity if this was the first concussion. Any documented loss of consciousness or symptoms and signs that last for more than 15 minutes should result in the athlete being restricted from play for that day.

Return to play decisions following a concussion that is more involved than that described in the previous paragraph represent a clinical judgment for which there is no consensus among experts. There is a lack of scientific evidence when it comes to the exact number of days needed to recover from a concussion. The severity of the concussion, the number of previous concussions, the risk for further injury, and the family's understanding and acceptance of the potential for risk and complications must be considered in making these decisions. Each concussion sustained places the athlete at greater risk for subsequent injury. Established return to play guidelines suggest restrictions ranging from 1 week to the rest of the season depending on the degree of injury and the number of previous concussions sustained during the season. Since second-impact syndrome has been reported primarily in adolescent athletes, it could be postulated that the autoregulatory control in a developing brain is not as mature in this age group as in adults. Therefore, a greater degree of conservatism should be considered when returning young athletes back to activity after concussions.

Current guidelines should not be viewed as fixed standards of care, but as starting points in the decision tree. Inaccuracies in grading scales put some athletes at increased risk for harm when they are allowed to return to play prematurely or subject others to unnecessary restrictions when it is safe to return to play. A potential benefit of standard concussion guidelines is increased consistency in concussion management and decreased "doctor shopping" by athletes seeking more lenient return to play standards. In clinical practice, return to play decisions should be made on an individual basis. This takes into account the recovery of symptoms, as well as how the athlete performs on subsequent physical examinations at rest and following a physical activity challenge.

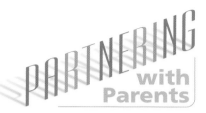

How soon should my child return to sports after a head injury?

No one should be allowed to return to physical activity while symptomatic. Younger athletes are the most prone to second-impact syndrome. Therefore, a greater degree of conservatism should be considered when returning young athletes back to activity.

FINISH LINE

Head injuries frequently occur in sports, and because of the potential for a catastrophic outcome, all head injuries should be considered serious. Established grading scales and return to play guidelines may assist in the clinical decision-making process, but should not substitute for the clinical judgment of the examining physician. All individuals involved in sports, including athletes, coaches, parents, teachers, athletic trainers, and team physicians should recognize the symptoms of a head injury and understand the need to seek prompt medical attention in the event of such injury. All medical personnel should be reminded that any unconscious athlete should be considered to have a cervical spine injury unless proven otherwise.

Even with disagreement between sports medicine experts pertaining to returning the athlete to play following a concussion, there is consensus in the literature on one point: *An athlete who has sustained a concussion should not be allowed to return to practice or competition while symptomatic or displaying signs of a concussion.*

For More Information

1. Cantu RC: Return to play guidelines after a head injury. *Clin Sports Med* 1998;17:45–60.

2. McCrea M, Kelly JP, Kluge J, Ackley B, Randolph C: Standardized assessment of concussion in football players. *Neurology* 1997;48:586–588.

3. National Collegiate Athletic Association: Concussion and second-impact syndrome, in Halpin T, Dick RW (eds): *1999–2000 NCAA Sports Medicine Handbook,* ed 12. Indianapolis, IN, NCAA Publications, 1999, pp 47–49.

4. Report of the Quality Standards Subcommittee: Practice parameter: The management of concussion in sports (summary statement). *Neurology* 1997;48:581–585.

5. Wojtys EM, Hovda D, Landry G, et al: Current concepts: Concussion in sports. *Am J Sports Med* 1999;27:676–687.

Chapter 19

Eye Injuries

JOHN B. JEFFERS, DVM, MD

Most coaches tell their young athletes to "keep your eye on the ball." Many sports require athletes to wear protective equipment for every part of the body except the eyes. The American Academy of Pediatrics and the American Academy of Ophthalmology strongly recommend the use of protective eyewear for all athletes for all sports and recreational activities. During childhood and adolescence, muscle coordination and reaction time are still developing, making young athletes particularly vulnerable to eye injuries. If young athletes become comfortable with wearing eye protectors early on, they will develop the habit of wearing them throughout their athletic careers and significantly decrease the overall incidence of severe eye injuries later. In fact, when properly fitted, sport-appropriate eye protectors have been found to reduce the risk of significant eye injury by at least 90%.

Preparticipation Physical Evaluation

Ideally, the preparticipation physical evaluation (PPE) should include a complete eye examination. However, most athletic programs use only a table-top visual screening device to measure acuity, muscle balance, and stereoacuity. Whether a complete examination or screening is performed, it is important to obtain pertinent past ocular history by asking the following questions:

1. *Is the athlete wearing glasses or contact lenses (rigid or nonrigid)?*
   Severe myopia, or nearsightedness carries a potential for retinal detachment.

2. *Has the athlete had refractive surgery?*
   Trauma to the eye may cause a rupture of the globe.

3. *Has the athlete had previous eye trauma or intraocular surgery?*
   Scarred or weakened tissue can predispose the athlete to eye injuries.

4. *Does the athlete have amblyopia, or lazy eye?*
   This would make the athlete functionally one-eyed.

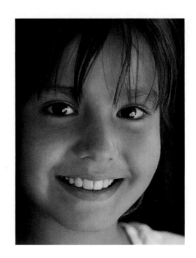

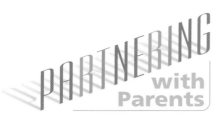

What should young athletes know about preventing eye injuries?

The American Academy of Pediatrics and the American Academy of Ophthalmology strongly recommend the use of protective eyewear for all sports and recreational activities.

Common Sports-Related Eye Injuries

In 1997, an estimated 32,789 sports- and recreation-related eye injuries were treated in hospital emergency departments in the United States. Basketball was associated with the most injuries with 7,673 (23%), followed by baseball and softball together with 3,560 (11%). In the age group from 5 to 14 years, baseball and softball had the highest incidence of eye injuries with 1,803 cases. In the past, the baseball and softball injuries occurred while batting, but recent experience indicates that being hit by misjudged balls—fly balls, "bad hop" grounders, and line drives—is now the most common cause of eye injury. For the age group from 15 to 24 years, basketball was associated with the most eye injuries with 3,361. **Table 19.1** lists specifications for eye protectors.

For most types of bodily injury, risk of injury is related to the nature of the sport. Contact or collision sports have a greater potential for causing injury compared with noncontact or noncollision sports. However, even noncontact sports can cause eye injuries. For example, although racquetball is classified as a noncontact sport, balls or racquets travel at high speeds, and impact with an eye can cause potentially devastating injuries. A general rule of thumb is that the more intraocular damage there is, the less orbital damage and vice versa. The force of the impact has to be dissipated somewhere in the tissues. Signs and symptoms of serious eye injury are listed in **Table 19.2**. For many common sports, the risk of eye injury is as follows:

1. **Low-risk sports:** Track and field, cross-country running, bicycling, tennis (singles).

2. **High-risk sports (protection is available):** Hockey (ice, roller, street, or field), football, baseball, softball, basketball, tennis (doubles), racquet sports (racquetball, squash, handball, badminton), lacrosse, swimming.

Table 19.1 *Specifications for Eye Protectors*

1. Regular glasses and contact lenses do not protect the eyes from injury.

2. For most sports, polycarbonate lenses that are 3 mm thick at the center offer the best protection. For sports that pose low risks of eye injury, polycarbonate lenses that are 2 mm thick at the center are acceptable.

3. All eye protectors should be made with sturdy polycarbonate frames with molded temples. Glasses that are hinged at the temple tend to bend when struck. Some sports eye protectors have neon-colored cushions at the nose and temple that young athletes like and are more likely to wear.

4. Lenses of eye protectors should be treated to resist fog.

5. Eye protectors should be fitted by an experienced ophthalmologist, optometrist, or optician. Most complaints about wearing eye protectors concern poor fit.

6. Face protectors (shields or cages) attached to helmets may be made of polycarbonate or wire. Most collision sports, such as hockey, lacrosse, and football, require the use of face protectors. The helmet must fit properly and be secured with a chin strap for maximum protection.

7. Standard goggles may not fit athletes with very narrow facial features. In these athletes, a sturdy metal frame with polycarbonate lenses will usually suffice.

Table 19.2 *Signs and Symptoms of Serious Eye Injury*

1. Sudden complete or partial loss of vision	7. Flashing lights or perception of large floaters
2. Complete or partial loss of visual field	8. Irregularly shaped pupil
3. Pain, with or without eye movement	9. Foreign body sensation
4. Photophobia, or light sensitivity	10. Red eye
5. Diplopia, or double vision	11. Blood in the anterior chamber
6. Protrusion of one eye	12. Halos around lights

3. **Very high-risk sports (protection is not available or permitted):** Boxing, full-contact martial arts. (Wrestling is also considered a high-risk sport; however, the NCAA now allows the use of previously prohibited eye protectors.)

Sharp Injury

Eye injuries may be caused by contact with blunt or sharp objects. For example, sharp objects include fingers that can poke an eye or fingernails that can lacerate the eyelid, cornea, or sclera. In addition, nonprotective eyewear can shatter and lacerate the eye and eyelid.

Blunt Injury

More often, eye injuries are caused by blunt objects that strike the eye. Common injuries of this type include edema and ecchymosis of the lids, orbital fracture, corneal abrasion, traumatic iritis, traumatic hyphema, traumatic cataract, and edema of the retina. When a blunt force strikes the eye, the anteroposterior diameter suddenly decreases and the equatorial diameter suddenly increases (imagine a round balloon pressed between the palms) (**Figure 19.1**). This distortion of the globe often causes the intraocular or intraorbital tissues to tear and hemorrhage.

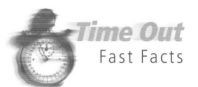

Time Out
Fast Facts

High-risk sports for eye injuries

Hockey

Football

Baseball

Softball

Basketball

Tennis (doubles)

Racquet sports (racquetball, squash, handball, badminton).

Lacrosse

Wrestling

Paintball

Figure 19.1
A blow to the globe may occur if the ball is small enough to fit inside the bony orbit. Forces are transmitted to suddenly decrease the anteroposterior diameter of the eye and increase equatorial diameter.

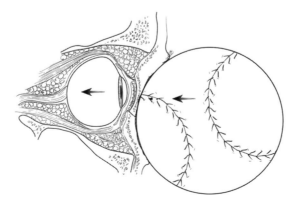

Figure 19.2 If sufficient force is transmitted to the globe, it may increase intraorbital pressure sufficient to fracture the thin floor or medial wall of the orbit, causing a "blowout" fracture.

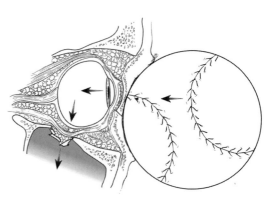

Fractures

Fractures can also occur as a result of sports injuries. As intraocular and intraorbital pressures increase, the thinner walls of the floor and medial aspect of the orbit often fracture, causing a "blowout fracture" (**Figure 19.2**). Another mechanism for a floor fracture is a severe impact on the inferior rim of the orbit that causes the bone to buckle. Extraocular tissues may become entrapped in the fracture sites and limit movement of the eye, resulting in double vision. In large floor fractures, when the orbital edema and hemorrhage subside, periocular tissue sinks into the sinus cavity and causes enophthalmus, or sunken eye. Because the roof of the orbit is also the floor of the brain, a forceful blow to the superior orbital rim can fracture the roof and introduce an infection. If such an injury is suspected, athletes should be instructed not to blow their noses to decrease risk of sinus organisms gaining access to the orbit and causing secondary infection.

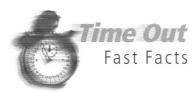

Time Out
Fast Facts

Before evaluating an eye injury, wash your hands.

Clinical Evaluation

Before an athlete is examined, it is critical that the physician or examiner wash his or her hands. If water is not available, alcohol wipes may be used instead. A list of equipment for conducting emergency eye examinations is provided in **Table 19.3**. First, identify the mechanism of injury and determine the direction and magnitude of the injuring force. For example, was the athlete struck

| Table 19.3 | *Emergency Kit for Sport-Related Eye Injuries* |

1. Card to test near vision
2. Penlight with blue filter
3. Fluorescein strips
4. Sterile eyewash in a plastic squeeze bottle (saline)
5. Plastic or metal eyeshields
6. Topical anesthesia, such as proparacaine hydrochloride 0.5%
7. Cotton applicator sticks (for removal of foreign bodies)
8. Plastic sandwich bags to make ice packs or moist chambers
9. Tape
10. Topical ophthalmic antibacterial solution, such as polymyxin B and trimethoprim or sulfacetamide 10%
11. Topical ophthalmic antibacterial ointment, such as erythromycin or bacitracin
12. Topical cycloplegic solution, such as tropicamide 1%

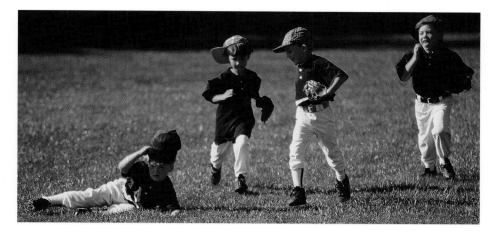

by a slow ground ball or a 90 mph pitch? This information may suggest the extent of potential injuries. Second, apply a topical anesthetic to control pain because a comfortable athlete will be more cooperative. However, never use topical anesthesia to mask pain so that the athlete can continue playing. Third, measure baseline visual acuity before manipulating or examining the eyes with your hands or penlight. Later, any improvement or worsening can be measured against this baseline. Hold a card designed to measure near vision (or any printed material) approximately 14″ from the eye and measure the size of the smallest print (in cm) that the athlete can read. If the card is held closer than 14″, measure its distance from the athlete's face. If the athlete is unable to read any print, hold up a few fingers at a distance and ask the athlete to count them. Document the distance and acuity. Athletes with poorer vision may be tested using hand movements. Light perception is a test for minimal vision. With no light perception, all vision is lost.

In the case of chemical or particle exposure (eg, exposure to field markings or dust from artificial turf), forego the initial test for visual acuity. Instead, immediately flush the affected eye with large amounts of clean water or any potable solution for 15 to 30 minutes, depending on the amount and concentration of chemical or particles involved. Physiologic saline or eyewashes in plastic squeeze bottles also work well. Contact lenses are best left in place during the initial irrigation. They may be removed later.

Next, check eye movements in all directions and note any limitations. Check pupillary response to light. Dilation of the pupil in an injured eye indicates an afferent defect. After this, administer appropriate first aid. After the initial examination and treatment, protect the injured eye with an eye shield. Depending on the severity of the injury, the athlete may require a repeat evaluation before returning to play. If there is any doubt about the diagnosis or the severity of the injury, refer the athlete to an ophthalmologist.

Treatment

Edema and Ecchymosis of the Eyelids

Place a small amount of crushed ice, about the size of a golf ball, in a plastic sandwich bag, wrap the bag in gauze, and apply it to the injured area. Be careful to place very little weight on the injured eye. The bag may be taped to the forehead to help keep it in place and to avoid manual pressure against the eye. This is best done with the athlete sitting.

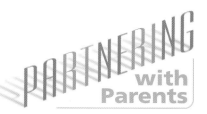

Are eye injuries common in baseball?

Baseball and softball had the highest incidence of eye injuries in children between ages 5 and 14 years. Eye protection for baseball includes face guards attached to the helmet and sports goggles that can include a corrective lens for kids who wear glasses.

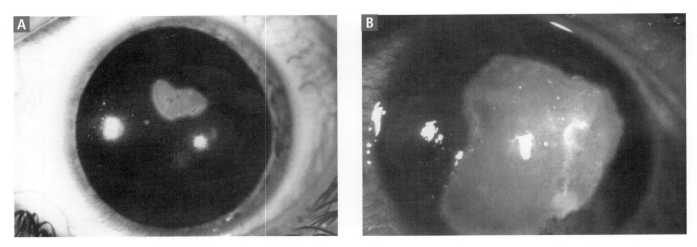

Figure 19.3 **A** A small corneal abrasion. **B** A large corneal abrasion.

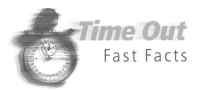

Protruding Edematous Conjunctiva

When left exposed, a protruding edematous conjunctiva tends to become dry and infected. Instead of applying an antibiotic ointment (which makes reexamination difficult), create a moist chamber to prevent the tissues from drying by taping a piece of plastic wrap or one side of a plastic sandwich bag tightly around the orbit and nose.

Lacerations of the Eyelid or Eyeball

In the case of lacerated eyelids or eyeballs, measure visual acuity and cover the injured eye with an eye shield. Refer the athlete to an ophthalmologist. Save any avulsed tissue in saline and send this with the athlete.

Corneal Abrasions

Apply topical antibiotic drops or ointment and cycloplegic drops. But remember, ointment and dilation blur vision, so the athlete may not be able to return to play immediately (**Figure 19.3**). Small abrasions can be treated without patching the eye. If a patch is used, it should be applied with just enough pressure to keep the eyelid closed. Do not patch patients who wear contact lenses.

Traumatic Iritis

When the iris is contused, an acute, painful iritis with photophobia results. Vision is blurred, and the pupil is small on the affected side. Apply topical steroid drops and cycloplegic drops. Do not use topical steroid drops for corneal abrasions. An athlete with this injury should be examined by an ophthalmologist.

Traumatic Cataract

This condition is most commonly characterized by a foreign body that penetrates the lens, which causes immediate blurred vision, an opaque lens, and sometimes intraocular hemorrhage. A severe, forceful blow to the eye often results in a cataract. Using an eye shield, protect the eye with a traumatic cataract, with or without subluxation or luxation of the lens, and refer the athlete to an ophthalmologist.

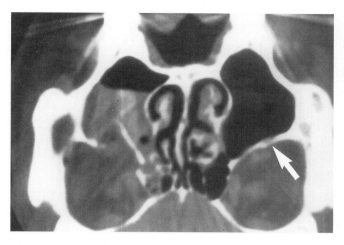

Figure 19.4 This CT scan shows blood in the maxillary sinus secondary to an orbit fracture.

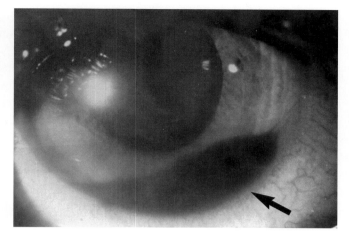

Figure 19.5 A layer of blood is appreciated over the lower iris when viewed with a penlight with magnifying loupes, if necessary.

Orbital Fracture

In the case of a suspected orbital fracture, advise the athlete against blowing his or her nose and prescribe oral antibiotics and a decongestant nasal drop or spray (**Figure 19.4**). This injury also requires immediate examination by an ophthalmologist.

Traumatic Hyphema

A hyphema is a contusion to the iris that causes bleeding in the anterior chamber of the eye (**Figure 19.5**). The signs and symptoms may be identical to that of traumatic iritis, but with the penlight with magnifying loupes, the layer of blood can be appreciated over the lower iris. Immediate management consists of measuring visual acuity, covering the injured eye with an eye shield, and keeping the athlete's head elevated. This injury also requires immediate examination by an ophthalmologist.

Return to Play Guidelines

Depending on the injury and on the physician's evaluation, an injured athlete may return to play immediately. A recovering athlete may return to play when an ophthalmologist has determined that the ocular tissue has had sufficient time to heal. Especially in the case of a traumatic hyphema, remember that the athlete may sustain another blow that could trigger a Valsalva maneuver that increases the pressure inside the eye and causes bleeding. In addition, the injured eye must be free of pain and discomfort and have adequate recovery of vision. For all athletes, the use of sport-appropriate, well-fitting protective eyewear is strongly recommended.

Functionally One-Eyed Athletes

Functionally one-eyed athletes must be identified during the PPE. By definition, the athlete's weaker eye has visual acuity worse than 20/40 (best corrected), while the stronger eye has visual acuity of 20/40 or better (best corrected). The most common cause of this condition is amblyopia,

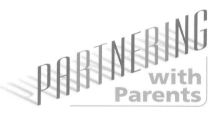

My child has limited vision in one eye. Are there some sports he should avoid?

These young athletes should not participate in boxing or full-contact martial arts.

or lazy eye. However, prior trauma, serious eye disease, or intraocular surgery may cause severe scarring and greatly decrease the vision in the eye.

This athlete must take extra precautions to protect the better eye from sports-related injuries that could have serious consequences in the athlete's lifestyle. The functionally one-eyed athlete may participate in most sports as long as appropriate, well-fitted protective eyewear is worn. When a helmet is required, both an eye protector and the face shield or cage should be worn. The athlete should not be allowed to participate in sports that pose very high risks of eye injury, such as boxing and full-contact martial arts. The athlete should always wear eye protectors during sporting events, but it is also strongly recommended that he or she wear glasses with polycarbonate lenses during all waking hours. These individuals will be unable to obtain an unrestricted driver's license in 40 states.

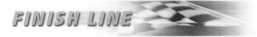

Injuries to the eye that result in significant pain or a change in visual acuity require evaluation by an ophthalmologist. Ideally, all young athletes should wear protective eyewear appropriate for the sport, especially in higher risk sports such as basketball, wrestling, hockey, paintball, football, baseball, softball, doubles tennis, and other racquet sports.

For More Information

1. Jeffers JB: An on-going tragedy: Pediatric sports-related eye injuries. *Semin Ophthalmol* 1990;5:216–223.

2. Larrison WI, Hersh PS, Kunzweiler T, Shingleton BJ: Sports-related ocular trauma. *Ophthalmology* 1990;97:1265–1269.

3. Turriff T: *Product Summary Report—Eye Injuries Only—Calendar Year 1997*. Chicago, IL, Prevent Blindness America, 1998.

4. Vinger PF: Athletic eye injuries and appropriate protection, in *Focal Points: Clinical Modules for Ophthalmologists*. San Francisco, CA, American Academy of Ophthalmology, 1997, vol 15, pp 1–14.

5. Vinger PF: The eye and sports medicine, in Duane TD, Tasman W, Jaeger EA (eds): *Duane's Clinical Ophthalmology*. Philadelphia, PA, JB Lippincott, 1994, vol 5, pp 1–103.

Chapter 20

Maxillofacial Injuries

S T E V E N   M .   S U L L I V A N ,   D D S

Many sports-related injuries involve the maxillofacial, or face and jaw, region. Fortunately, the use of face masks and mouth guards have reduced the number of injuries in many sports, but significant injuries still occur and are even more prevalent in contact sports without mandatory protection.

Most maxillofacial injuries occur in children between the ages of 8 and 15 years. Boys sustain two to three times as many injuries as girls as the result of the larger number of male participants and sport selection. Changes in the craniofacial skeleton during development may predispose children to certain types of maxillofacial injuries. With dental injuries, the anterior teeth, especially the maxillary central incisors, are most frequently injured. Children are also predisposed to contact injuries of the lower jaw because the emerging permanent teeth are proportionately large compared with the other facial structures. While crown fractures are the most common injuries to the permanent teeth, the primary teeth tend to be displaced.

Time from injury is one of the most critical concerns with injuries such as root fracture, displacement, and tooth avulsion. Treatment delays can markedly affect outcome and contribute to root resorption, posttraumatic infection, or delayed tooth loss. Almost any athlete who sustains a dental injury should be evaluated by a dentist.

Common Dental Injuries

The clinical evaluation should include inspection of both the hard tissues, which include teeth and supporting bone, and the soft tissues of the oral cavity (**Figure 20.1**). Any lacerations to the soft tissues should be examined carefully, especially if tooth fractures are evident. Tooth fragments that have become embedded in the soft tissues may not be apparent. All teeth and tooth fragments should be located, and if there is any suspicion of ingestion or aspiration, radiographs of the chest and abdomen may help find the missing teeth (**Figure 20.2**). Any trauma that causes a fracture of a tooth or alveolus can also cause a fracture of basal bone; therefore, the occlusion and temporomandibular joints should be evaluated as well. The temporomandibular joints can be evaluated quite simply by assessing the range of motion and identifying

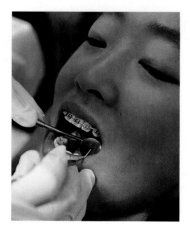

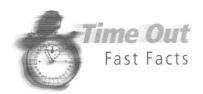

Fractures into the dentine or of the crown that involve the pulp chamber (exposed pink or bleeding pulp) require immediate attention.

whether the mouth opens in a normal, straight manner. Deviations to one side could indicate a fracture of the condylar process. Another possible sign of an injury is a malocclusion, which may be caused by a fracture of the mandible or maxilla (**Figure 20.3**).

If the initial clinical evaluation performed on the playing field reveals injuries beyond simple superficial chips of the crown, the patient should be referred immediately to an oral and maxillofacial surgeon or emergency department for a more thorough evaluation and appropriate treatment.

Fractures of the Tooth Crown

When a crown fracture occurs, the first and most important task is to protect the neurovascular components, or the pulp, within the central portion of the tooth (**Figure 20.4**). Esthetics, at this point, are a secondary consideration and can be dealt with at a later time. If exposed, the pulp can become contaminated and possibly destroy the tooth. These injuries could require further invasive treatment, such as endodontic therapy, in addition to restoration of the fractured crown. Crown fractures typically will involve fractures of the enamel structure, which are usually only superficial chips. Fractures into the dentin, however, are more serious. Not only do they produce discomfort and disfigurement, but they can compromise the pulp as well. On clinical inspection, these fractures expose the outer enamel component and the cream- to yellow-colored dentin underneath. Fractures of the crown that involve the pulp chamber are identified by exposed pink or bleeding pulp. This type of fracture requires immediate attention.

Emergency treatment of fractured teeth by the dentist includes placing a calcium hydroxide base

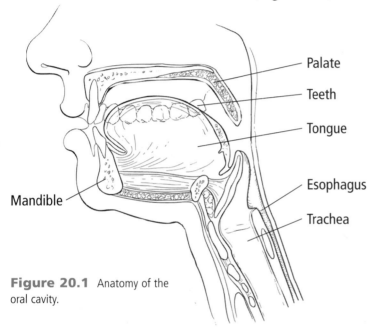

Figure 20.1 Anatomy of the oral cavity.

- Palate
- Teeth
- Tongue
- Esophagus
- Trachea

Mandible

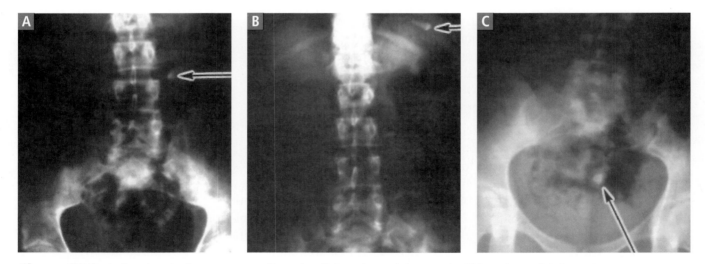

Figure 20.2 Aspirated teeth often appear on radiographs. **A** Premolar tooth in stomach. **B** Premolar tooth in lower thorax. **C** Premolar tooth in the abdomen.

Reproduced with permission from The Academy of General Dentistry: Prevention and management of ingested foreign bodies. *General Dentistry* 1993;41:422–444.

and restoring the tooth using an acid-etched composite restorative material. Ideally, the team physician should have these materials on hand to treat the fracture temporarily until definitive treatment can be rendered. Immediate follow-up with the athlete's dentist or specialist is imperative.

Tooth Displacement Injuries

Injuries caused by high-velocity impact and injuries sustained at the alveolar level may displace or completely avulse the teeth and fracture the supporting alveolar bone. The upper and lower front teeth are most often displaced. With all displacement injuries, it is important to determine whether the tooth or the entire alveolar process has been displaced. This is accomplished by cleaning the oral cavity and then palpating the alveolar process to identify which components move. If the teeth alone move, they may be repositioned into the socket quite readily. If the teeth and alveolar process both move, there is a more serious fracture. Though uncomfortable, this is one of the most important steps in initial management of this injury. Teeth that show minor mobility (less than 1 mm) typically will not require any further stabilization, though further injury must be avoided. Teeth that move more than 1 mm require splinting for 7 to 10 days. Splints should be applied by a dentist in a controlled environment where the teeth and jaws can be positioned properly and the splinting material can be applied in a dry field.

Early treatment of a more severe displacement injury (more than 1 to 2 mm) involves repositioning and

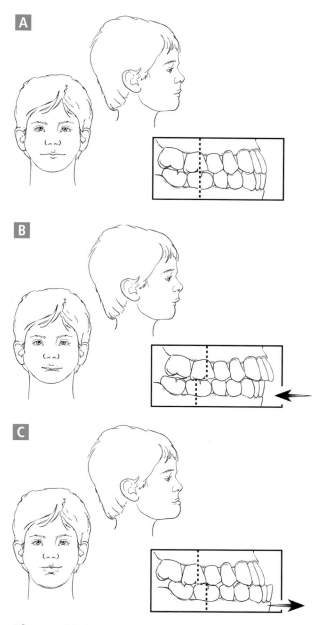

Figure 20.3 Evaluation of the temporomandibular joint should include assessment of possible malocclusion. **A** Normal bite. **B** Overbite. **C** Underbite.

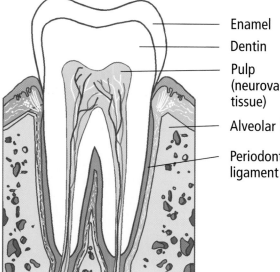

Enamel

Dentin

Pulp (neurovascular tissue)

Alveolar bone

Periodontal ligament

Figure 20.4 Anatomy of a tooth.

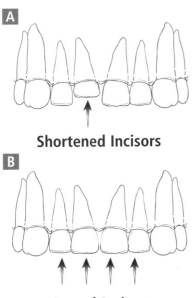

Shortened Incisors

Normal Incisors

Figure 20.5 With severe displacement injuries, the normal crown can appear shorter **A** than those of the normal adjacent teeth **B**.

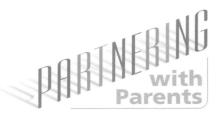

After a child loses a tooth as a result of a sports injury, how long should it be splinted?

Typically, teeth that move more than 1 mm require splinting for 7 to 10 days.

stabilizing the tooth, followed by further evaluation and management. With all displacement injuries, time is extremely important. Studies show that if the displaced teeth are repo-sitioned within 90 minutes of injury, fewer sequelae ensue, including loss of the tooth or root resorption. In nearly 50% of patients, displacement injuries may proceed to necrosis of he pulp; therefore, close observation and follow-up by a dentist or endodontist is necessary.

Some of the more severe displacement injuries are intrusive displacement injuries in which the normal crown appears shorter than those of adjacent teeth, or appears in infraocclusion, as if it failed to erupt (**Figure 20.5**). These injuries occur most often with teeth that have fully formed roots. In children ages 6 to 8 years, teeth that intrude minimally will often re-erupt passively because the roots of their teeth have not yet formed completely. Intruded permanent teeth require either orthodontic or surgical repositioning and endodontic therapy. In any case, immediate treatment by a dentist should be arranged.

Avulsion Injuries

Avulsions of the maxillary central incisors are some of the most common dental injuries in children because these teeth have recently or are in the process of erupting and have loosely structured periodontal ligaments. The ideal treatment of an avulsed tooth is early replantation and stabilization. Once again, time is critical. If immediate replantation is not possible, the tooth should be stored in an appropriate medium that will nourish the cellular components of the root surface. Physiologic saline is an ideal storage medium, and tooth preserving mediums are also available commercially. If neither of these is available, milk or the athlete's saliva can suffice. The root surface should not be cleaned or touched (ie, pick up the tooth by the crown only), except to gently remove any superficial contaminants. Often, the storage medium passively washes away the debris. Any attempts to clean the root surface can harm periodontal membrane cells and prevent successful replantation.

Prevention of Dental Injuries

One of the most important preventive measures for dental injuries is the use of mouth guards and face masks. The National Collegiate Athletic Association (NCAA) estimates that 200,000 dental injuries per year can be prevented by this simple measure alone. Since the introduction of mandatory mouth guards and padded helmets with face masks, the incidence of dental injuries in football has been reduced from 10% to 0.35 to 0.45%. Mouth guards should cover all tooth surfaces and include occlusal coverage as well to prevent vertical crown fractures.

Mouth guards offer a substantial degree of protection to the teeth and oral soft tissue, as well as protect athletes from concussion. An ideal mouth guard has the following characteristics:

• Soft and comfortable, but firm enough to withstand trauma

• Fabricated easily at a low cost

• Adaptable over a dental appliance in the mouth

- Does not interfere with speech or breathing

- Does not deteriorate after prolonged use

- Does not have an offensive odor or taste and is not toxic

The three types of mouth guards commercially available are the stock mouth guard, mouth-formed, and custom-made protectors. Stock mouth guards are preformed, over-the-counter, and worn as manufactured. They are inexpensive, but are bulky and must be held in place by clenching the teeth, which tends to interfere with breathing and speech. Mouth-formed protectors are usually thermoplastic and reasonably priced. They are placed in boiling water to soften, dipped in cold water for an instant, and then placed over the maxillary arch and under the upper lip using a constant pressure upward and backward for about 30 seconds. Custom-formed (vacuum) mouth guards are fabricated over a dental cast using a vacuum-formed material. They are the most comfortable and interfere least with breathing and speech. However, they are also the most expensive because they require at least two visits to the dentist for proper fitting. Mouth-formed protectors offer the best compromise between fit and cost for most young athletes. Athletes must be cautioned to avoid trimming the mouth guard excessively because this will reduce its protective effect. Nervous chewing of the mouth guard also reduces fit and protection. Damaged mouth guards should be replaced.

Mandibular Fractures

The most common mandibular fracture involves the condylar process, followed by fractures of the mandibular angle (**Figure 20.6**). As tooth follicles develop near the mandibular angle and ramus, the bone quantity in that area diminishes and predisposes the posterior mandible to fractures. Approximately 50% of all mandibular fractures occur in areas posterior to the teeth, while the remaining 50% are distributed among the mandibular body, anterior mandible, and dentoalveolar components (less than 4%).

An athlete who is believed to have a mandibular fracture should be evaluated to ensure that the airway is open. The oral cavity should be inspected to identify whether there are loose or missing teeth, to find these teeth, and to ensure that the airway is patent. With mandibular fractures, the most common finding is malocclusion, which is easily assessed by asking the patient if his or her teeth meet differently now than they did before the incident. Gross malocclusions indicate mandibular fractures, whereas minor malocclusions suggest greenstick fractures or effusions into the temporomandibular joints. Additional signs and symptoms of mandibular fractures include bruising in the mouth, mucosal tears, crepitus at the fracture sites, palpable irregularities along the bone surfaces if bones are significantly displaced, and numbness of the lower lip and chin on the side of the fracture if it crosses the mandibular canal. Significant edema can develop and, on occasion, profuse bleeding can develop as well if the inferior alveolar artery is cut by severely displaced bones.

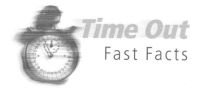

Time Out
Fast Facts

Use of a mouth guard and face mask is one of the most important preventive measures for avoiding dental injuries.

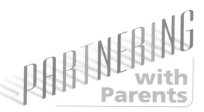

PARTNERING with **Parents**

After a child has a tooth knocked out during sports participation, how should the tooth be cared for?

The coach, athletic trainer, or team physician may have physiologic saline on hand to store the tooth until the child reaches the emergency department. The root surface should not be cleaned or touched. Transport of the tooth in a clean, dry gauze in a bag is the next alternative.

Figure 20.6 Bony anatomy of the mandible.

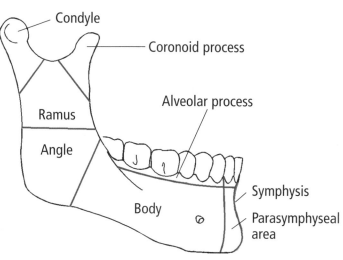

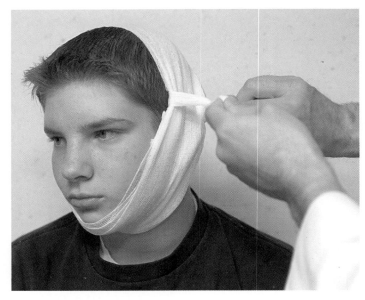

Figure 20.7 The mandible may be stabilized temporarily by wrapping elastic bandages under the chin and over the head.

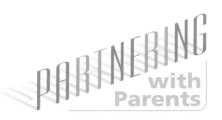

Which dental injuries should be referred for professional evaluation?

If the athlete has an on-field injury that is more serious than a simple crown chip, he or she should be referred immediately to an oral and maxillofacial surgeon or to the emergency department for a more thorough evaluation.

Any athlete who sustains a mandibular fracture should be fully immobilized, including the head and neck, and evaluated for injury to the cervical spine. Open mandibular fractures require immediate care by an oral and maxillofacial surgeon. The mandible may be stabilized temporarily by wrapping elastic bandages around the head, beginning under the chin and going over the top of the head to hold the mouth closed (**Figure 20.7**). The mandible can also be stabilized with wires, but this procedure should be performed only by individuals who have been trained to do so. Inappropriately placed wires can dislodge teeth and cause their eventual loss.

Patients with mandibular fractures should receive definitive treatment as quickly as possible, certainly no later than 7 to 10 days following the injury. Treatment includes simple closed reduction by wiring the jaws together and open reduction with rigid internal fixation. Typically, in 6 to 8 weeks, the mandible will regain 75% of its pre-injury strength.

Midfacial Fractures

The most common midfacial fracture in young athletes is a nasal fracture. A prominent structure on the face, the nose is vulnerable to injury, especially when helmets and face masks are not worn. Nasal fractures should be evaluated, and epistaxis, if present, should be controlled with constant direct pressure to the nose with the athlete in a sitting position. If a bag of crushed ice is available, pressure can be applied with it to facilitate vasoconstriction and reduce bleeding.

Nasal fractures involving the nasal septum are easily diagnosed by exerting an upward pressure on the columella. Typically, the nasal septum will be extremely tender when moved slightly, which suggests possible separation of the septum from the maxillary crest. Deviations of the nose or saddle-nose deformities suggest displacement of the nasal bones on either side (**Figure 20.8**). Septal hematomas must be identified and aspirated promptly to avoid septal necrosis.

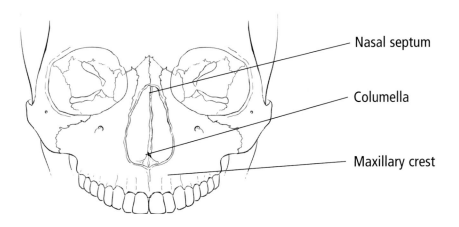

Nasal septum

Columella

Maxillary crest

Figure 20.8 Principal structures of the midface.

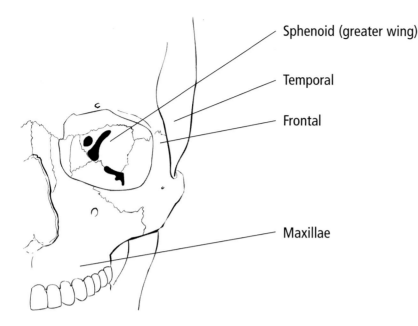

Figure 20.9 Bony anatomy of the zygomatic complex.

Usually, nasal fractures can be managed on an outpatient basis. Nasal reduction should be managed by a specialist, and is ideally performed immediately before swelling develops or within 4 days for children and 10 to 12 days for adolescents. Treatment, administered under local or IV sedation, includes manipulating and elevating the nose, packing it for internal support, and splinting it for external support. In general, the internal packing should remain in place for approximately 24 to 48 hours to prevent septal hematomas from forming, as well as to provide outward support for the nasal bones. External nasal splints are generally worn for 7 to 10 days. Recommendations about returning to play will depend on the extent of the injury, the stability of the fracture, the options for protective head gear, and the risk of further injury or potential injury. The patient should not participate in athletic activity without protective facial equipment for 4 to 6 weeks to allow the injury to heal completely and also to avoid re-injury.

Fractures of the zygomatic complex often occur in contact sports where protective head gear is not worn. Fortunately, because children have not yet developed air cells in their bones, fractures of the zygomatic complex are not common in children younger than age 10 or 12 years. The zygoma articulates with four other bones: the temporal, the frontal, the maxillae, and the greater wing of the sphenoid (**Figure 20.9**). Therefore, a fracture of the zygomatic complex can be evaluated by palpating several areas: at the temples near the brow bone, along the rim below the eye, and inside the mouth along the roof under the cheekbones (**Figure 20.10**). Typically, step defects will be noted, and the zygoma may move. However, it is not uncommon for the zygoma to become impacted, posteriorly and medially, into the maxillary sinus, and therefore seem rather stable, even though it is displaced. Epistaxis is also a fairly common finding. Blood from the maxillary sinus will ultimately drain through the nose. The patient may also have periorbital ecchymosis, diplopia, and numbness over the cheek.

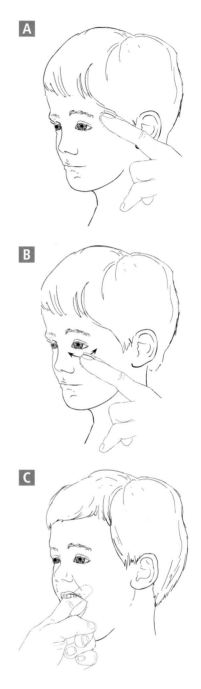

Figure 20.10 Evaluation for a fracture of the zygomatic complex. **A** Palpate at the temples near the brow bone. **B** Palpate along the orbital rim below the eye. **C** Palpate inside the mouth along the roof under the cheek bones.

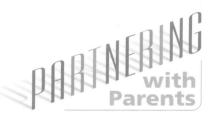

Following a fracture of the nose, how quickly should evaluation and treatment be done?

Reduction of the fracture under ideal conditions is performed immediately, before swelling develops. However, within 4 days for children and 10 to 12 days for older adolescents is acceptable.

All fractures of the zygomatic complex should immediately raise concern about eye injuries, which are true emergencies. It is important to examine baseline visual acuity (eg, the ability to read a newspaper at arm's length) to evaluate the pupil, to assess whether structures passing through the superior orbital fissure have been compromised, and to evaluate the extraocular movements. A consultation with an ophthalmologist is mandatory to reassess visual acuity and to check for occult eye injury. Following a clinical evaluation for any eye injuries, the patient should be instructed to avoid blowing the nose and to follow up immediately with a maxillofacial surgeon so that axial and coronal CT scans can be performed to ascertain the degree of displacement. Displaced fractures require surgery, including open reduction and stabilization with rigid fixation. These fractures typically heal in approximately 6 weeks, and athletes may be allowed to return to play afterwards.

Maxillary fractures in children are rare and account for a very small percentage of all facial fractures, for several reasons. First, the bones of the maxilla are fairly elastic. Second, the maxilla is buttressed by adjacent facial bones, as well as deciduous teeth. Third, the maxillary sinuses have not yet developed air cavities. All of these factors result in a structure that is difficult to fracture under normal conditions.

Athletes with suspected maxillary fractures require careful examination for dental injuries as well, and any loose or missing teeth should be found. The most obvious clinical finding in a maxillary fracture is a malocclusion. Often, patients will notice that the teeth do not come together as they did prior to the injury. Sometimes, an open bite malocclusion, seen when the upper teeth do not overlap or touch the lower teeth, will be evident. Along with the malocclusion, step defects at the zygomatic buttress, bruising, periorbital swelling, diplopia, facial lengthening, and/or epistaxis may also suggest a maxillary fracture. These athletes require examination at the emergency department and consultation with the appropriate specialist.

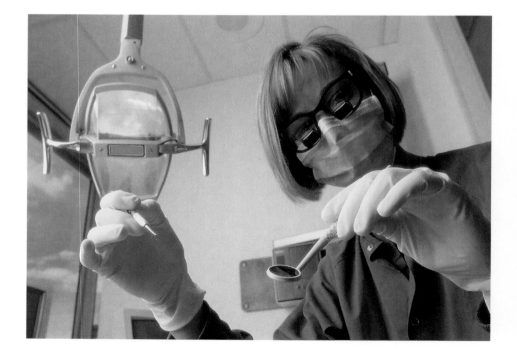

Typically, maxillary fractures in children can be treated surgically with closed techniques. In the operating room, the occlusion will be reestablished and a functional reduction accomplished. Maxillary fractures are usually stabilized in 4 to 6 weeks, with or without the use of maxillomandibular wiring. In general, open reduction with internal fixation is contraindicated in patients with multiple unerupted permanent teeth. For these patients, closed reductions can achieve good results as well. The use of protective head gear, such as face masks, reduces the incidence of maxillary fractures.

Maxillofacial Lacerations

Most lacerations of the maxillofacial region are associated with or are a direct result of injuries to the teeth. Lacerations of the lips and mouth are fairly common. Inside the mouth, lacerations of the mucosa that are less than 5 mm in length do not require suturing. However, lacerations longer than 5 mm that penetrate through the lip, for example, require layered closure to prevent unsightly scarring.

Lacerations that require surgical repair should first be debrided and cleansed, and then covered with pressure dressings to control hemorrhaging until the patient can be transported for definitive treatment. Fortunately, the vessels of the facial structures are fairly elastic, and direct pressure will stop the bleeding adequately. Extremely large or unstable lacerations may need to be tacked temporarily using a 3.0 or 4.0 silk suture after infiltration with a local anesthetic into the vestibules of the corner of the mouth. With tongue lacerations, untrained clinicians may find it more difficult to effect local anesthesia. However, in urgent situations when temporary tacking sutures are required, injection of the anesthetic agent into the tongue itself, though uncomfortable, will often suffice. Small resorbable sutures are preferred for tongue lacerations. Typically, a 4.0 or 5.0 suture applied in a layered fashion achieves excellent results.

Lacerations outside the mouth, like any cutaneous injury, require immediate care beginning with control of bleeding, primary cleansing of the wound, inspection for foreign bodies, and application of gauze pressure bandages. Any patient with a laceration that has been contaminated by soil may require a tetanus booster.

After lacerations are repaired, guidelines for returning to play should be established based on the extent of the injury, its location, and the likelihood of re-injury. Whenever possible, protection of the injured area is advisable.

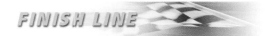

Most injuries to the teeth will require consultation of a dentist. Simple contusions and lacerations to the face can be managed in the office, but when a more complex laceration occurs with or without a suspected fracture, an appropriate specialist must be consulted to assist with management.

For More Information

1. Ranalli DN: Sports dentistry. *Dent Clin North Am* 1991;35:609–858.

2. Andreasen JO (ed): *Traumatic Injuries of the Teeth.* St Louis, MO, CV Mosby, 1972.

3. Fonseca RJ, Walker RV (eds): *Oral and Maxillofacial Trauma.* Philadelphia, PA, WB Saunders, 1991.

Chapter 21

Chest and Abdominal Injuries

P. Cameron Mantor, MD
David Tuggle, MD

Although uncommon, serious injuries to the lungs, liver, spleen, and other organs can occur in young athletes, particularly in those who participate in contact sports. Coaches, athletic trainers, and physicians alike should be aware of the potential thoracic and abdominal injuries that can occur in the young athlete.

The most common bony injuries to the chest are rib fractures, costochondral separations, clavicle fractures, and sternoclavicular dislocations. Fractures of the scapula or sternum are rare. These injuries are usually associated with collisions between athletes or between an athlete and a fixed object. Stress fractures of the bones of the thorax are not uncommon, especially from repetitive throwing or in athletes who participate in contact sports.

Abdominal injuries also occur when children participate in contact sports. The extent of injury is related directly to the amount of force involved. Injuries to abdominal organs can lead to significant morbidity and even permanent impairment. The organs most vulnerable to injury are the spleen and liver, followed by the kidney, pancreas, and gastrointestinal tract. Children with known liver or spleen enlargement are at higher risk of injury.

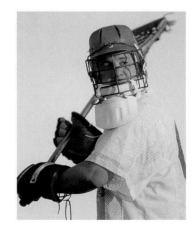

Anatomy/Biomechanics

The thorax is a flexible cage. Each rib articulates posteriorly with the vertebral column, and the first seven ribs articulate with the sternum (**Figure 21.1**). Ribs eight, nine, and ten articulate with the cartilage superior to them, and the 11th

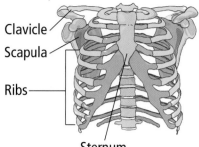

Clavicle

Scapula

Ribs

Sternum

Figure 21.1 Bony anatomy of thoracic cage.

and 12th cartilages are free. The tip of the 12th rib is at the level of the second lumbar vertebra, and the 10th rib is the lowest anterior rib seen. The clavicle lies anterior to the first rib, making the first rib difficult to feel. The second rib is easy to locate because the costal cartilage articulates at the junction of the manubrium of the body of the sternum. The sternal angle is opposite the second costal cartilage and is a key landmark in the chest that is used when counting the ribs. The scapula protects the posterior ribs and vertebral column and is encased in muscle and fascia.

The bony thorax is very flexible in young children. However, as children get older, the bones of the thorax become more rigid and are more prone to fracture. Children assume adult bone physiology at about age 8 years. The flexibility of the bony thorax is important to the young athlete. Most sports injuries to the thorax impair the athlete's performance because of the pain associated with the injury.

Clinical Evaluation

History

Identifying the mechanism of injury is crucial in diagnosing the injury. It is also important to know whether the force came from another player or from a fixed structure. Blows of great force can be delivered over a very small surface area, resulting in significant damage.

The most common symptom of all thoracic injuries is pain, which may be difficult to localize and may be associated with shortness of breath.

Physical Examination

The examination should start with observation of the athlete's respirations. Viewing the quality and rate of respirations provides valuable clues about the severity of injury. Gentle palpation of the chest wall may localize the area of injury. Pain and swelling can be a sign of muscle injury or fracture. Rib fracture is the most common injury, and significant displacement of a fractured edge of a rib could cause a pneumothorax. Palpation of the neck and supraclavicular area may reveal crepitus consistent with a pneumothorax caused by rib fractures. With multiple rib fractures, flail chest and subsequent respiratory distress are possible. An athlete who cannot move or use his or her arm may have a fracture of the clavicle on that side. Gentle palpation of the bone generally identifies the fracture. Sternal fractures are less common, although sternoclavicular dislocations can be seen. Auscultation of the chest may reveal decreased breath sounds on the injured side, which may be the result of splinting from pain and decreased ventilation or pneumothorax. Tympany to percussion also suggests pneumothorax.

Abdominal injuries typically affect soft tissues and viscera. Palpation may reveal tenderness, guarding, or rigidity. Bowel sounds should be present; their absence may indicate a possible bowel injury or peritonitis.

Diagnostic Tests

Radiographs of the chest are the single most useful test in identifying specific thoracic injuries. A rib series may be more useful in identifying obscure nondisplaced fractures. Anteroposterior views will best demonstrate clavicle fractures. Lateral views are most useful in evaluating the presence of a sternal fracture.

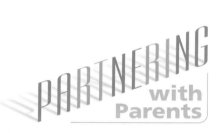

What evaluation will the doctor recommend for a suspected rib fracture?

Chest radiographs are the single most useful test in identifying rib fractures and underlying cardiopulmonary injuries.

What should coaches know about rib fractures?

These fractures may be associated with an undetected pneumothorax and possibly delayed distress. Pain management includes prescription analgesics. Rib binders may also be helpful.

Radiographs of the abdomen are less helpful in detecting significant abdominal injuries. More frequently, ultrasound and CT scan will be necessary.

Treatment

Definitive diagnosis and treatment of most chest injuries require transport to a hospital where appropriate studies can be performed.

Immobilization of rib fractures is impossible; however, taping or elastic bindings may alleviate some pain. Surgical treatment is rarely indicated for sternal or scapula fractures. Most athletes simply require limited activity until the pain subsides.

Nonsteroidal anti-inflammatory drugs are typically recommended for pain management. Narcotics may be used in certain circumstances; however, they promote respiratory depression in some patients and thus are of less benefit.

Intrathoracic Injuries

Life-threatening chest injuries include pneumothorax, tension pneumothorax, hemothorax, cardiac contusion, pericardial tamponade, and pulmonary contusion.

Simple Pneumothorax

A pneumothorax develops when air enters the pleural space, but cannot escape (**Figure 21.2**). A rib fracture usually causes direct injury to the lung parenchyma. This injury can occur when a football player sustains a particularly forceful tackle or a bicyclist falls during a high-speed race. Air accumulates and compresses the lung on the affected side, causing a ventilation-perfusion mismatch. Characteristic signs and symptoms include chest pain and difficulty breathing. Auscultation of the chest reveals decreased breath sounds, and percussion reveals hyperresonance. Radiographs confirm the diagnosis.

Athletes should be taken to the emergency department for examination and probable chest tube placement. Simple pneumothorax does not require needle decompression. If rib fractures are present, complete return to unrestricted activity may take up to 6 weeks.

Tension Pneumothorax

The etiology of a tension pneumothorax is similar to that of a simple pneumothorax, but it differs clinically in that air continues to accumulate within the pleural space. The entrapped air causes progressive collapse of the lung on the affected side (**Figure 21.3**). Shifting of the mediastinum may decrease cardiac output and compromise lung function on the opposite side. A tension pneumothorax is a medical emergency that must be recognized and treated promptly. Patients have severe dyspnea and tachypnea. If left untreated, this injury will lead to respiratory arrest. In addition to decreased breath sounds

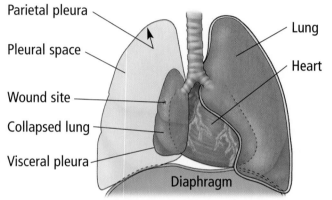

Figure 21.2 Pneumothorax occurs when air leaks into the pleural space from an opening in the chest wall or surface of the lung. The lung collapses as air fills the pleural space, and the two pleural surfaces are no longer in contact.

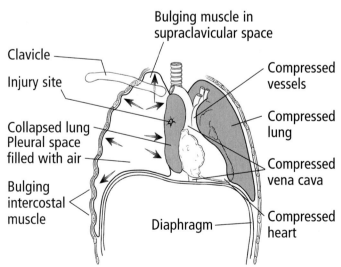
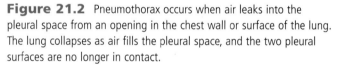

Figure 21.3 Tension pneumothorax can develop if a penetrating chest wound is bandaged too tightly and air from a damaged lung cannot escape.

and hyperresonance, signs of tension pneumothorax include tracheal deviation away from the side of injury and distention of the jugular vein. Immediate intervention includes needle decompression with a large angiocatheter placed anteriorly in the second intercostal space. This procedure relieves the tension pneumothorax, but the athlete must be transported to the emergency department for placement of a chest tube.

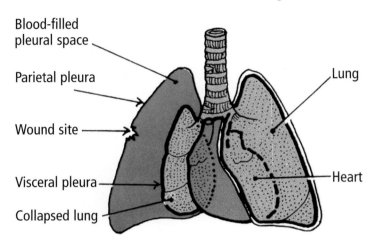

Blood-filled pleural space

Parietal pleura

Wound site

Visceral pleura

Collapsed lung

Lung

Heart

Figure 21.4 Hemothorax is a collection of blood in the pleural space produced by lacerated blood vessels in the chest.

Hemothorax

A hemothorax occurs when blood accumulates within the pleural space following either blunt or penetrating trauma, with resulting injury to the lung parenchyma or an intercostal vessel (**Figure 21.4**). Bleeding is usually self-limited and rarely requires surgical intervention; however, the blood must be removed from the chest cavity to prevent complications, such as infection, empyema, or chronic atelectasis of the lung.

The clinical significance of this injury depends on the amount of blood lost and the extent to which the fluid itself impairs respiratory function. Symptoms such as dyspnea and tachypnea are related to the amount of ventilatory compromise. Auscultation of the chest reveals decreased breath sounds, and percussion reveals dullness on the affected side. Radiographs confirm the diagnosis. The athlete needs immediate transport to the emergency department for placement of a chest tube.

Cardiac Contusion

A cardiac contusion is caused by direct trauma to the anterior chest wall or sternum, which may occur in any contact sports. Athletes typically report chest discomfort related to trauma, but may be otherwise asymptomatic. The clinically important consequences of this condition are arrhythmias, which, if severe, can lead to an abrupt cardiac collapse. Definitive diagnosis outside of the emergency department is very difficult. The focus of management is to identify arrhythmias and initiate prompt pharmacologic therapy. Once resolved, further risk of sudden dysrhythmia is low. Long-term medical therapy is rarely necessary, and prompt return to full physical activity can be expected.

Pericardial Tamponade

Pericardial tamponade is an accumulation of fluid within the pericardial sac. Although most frequently associated with penetrating injuries, blunt injuries, such as an unprotected blow to the sternum, can also cause this injury. The pericardial sac is firm and fibrous, so the accumulation of fluid can lead to significant hemodynamic compromise. This is caused by the inability of the heart to fill, which severely reduces cardiac output and leads to shock. The hallmark signs and symptoms of cardiac tamponade, called Beck's triad, include jugular vein distention, hypotension, and muffled heart tones. Differentiating cardiac tamponade from a tension pneumothorax can be difficult. If this injury is suspected, the athlete should be transported to the emergency department immediately. Cardiac ultrasonography is an

Radiographs of the abdomen are less helpful in detecting significant abdominal injuries. More frequently, ultrasound and CT scan will be necessary.

Treatment

Definitive diagnosis and treatment of most chest injuries require transport to a hospital where appropriate studies can be performed.

Immobilization of rib fractures is impossible; however, taping or elastic bindings may alleviate some pain. Surgical treatment is rarely indicated for sternal or scapula fractures. Most athletes simply require limited activity until the pain subsides.

Nonsteroidal anti-inflammatory drugs are typically recommended for pain management. Narcotics may be used in certain circumstances; however, they promote respiratory depression in some patients and thus are of less benefit.

Intrathoracic Injuries

Life-threatening chest injuries include pneumothorax, tension pneumothorax, hemothorax, cardiac contusion, pericardial tamponade, and pulmonary contusion.

Simple Pneumothorax

A pneumothorax develops when air enters the pleural space, but cannot escape (**Figure 21.2**). A rib fracture usually causes direct injury to the lung parenchyma. This injury can occur when a football player sustains a particularly forceful tackle or a bicyclist falls during a high-speed race. Air accumulates and compresses the lung on the affected side, causing a ventilation-perfusion mismatch. Characteristic signs and symptoms include chest pain and difficulty breathing. Auscultation of the chest reveals decreased breath sounds, and percussion reveals hyperresonance. Radiographs confirm the diagnosis.

Athletes should be taken to the emergency department for examination and probable chest tube placement. Simple pneumothorax does not require needle decompression. If rib fractures are present, complete return to unrestricted activity may take up to 6 weeks.

Tension Pneumothorax

The etiology of a tension pneumothorax is similar to that of a simple pneumothorax, but it differs clinically in that air continues to accumulate within the pleural space. The entrapped air causes progressive collapse of the lung on the affected side (**Figure 21.3**). Shifting of the mediastinum may decrease cardiac output and compromise lung function on the opposite side. A tension pneumothorax is a medical emergency that must be recognized and treated promptly. Patients have severe dyspnea and tachypnea. If left untreated, this injury will lead to respiratory arrest. In addition to decreased breath sounds

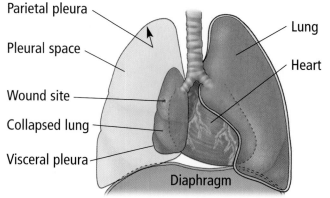

Figure 21.2 Pneumothorax occurs when air leaks into the pleural space from an opening in the chest wall or surface of the lung. The lung collapses as air fills the pleural space, and the two pleural surfaces are no longer in contact.

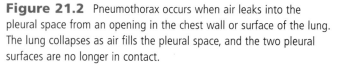
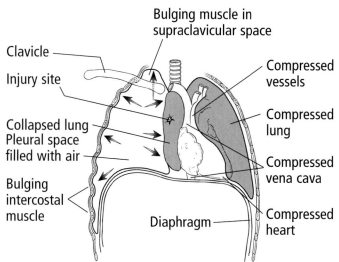

Figure 21.3 Tension pneumothorax can develop if a penetrating chest wound is bandaged too tightly and air from a damaged lung cannot escape.

and hyperresonance, signs of tension pneumothorax include tracheal deviation away from the side of injury and distention of the jugular vein. Immediate intervention includes needle decompression with a large angiocatheter placed anteriorly in the second intercostal space. This procedure relieves the tension pneumothorax, but the athlete must be transported to the emergency department for placement of a chest tube.

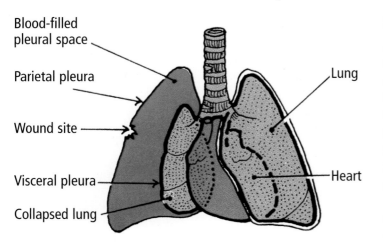

Blood-filled pleural space

Parietal pleura

Wound site

Visceral pleura

Collapsed lung

Lung

Heart

Figure 21.4 Hemothorax is a collection of blood in the pleural space produced by lacerated blood vessels in the chest.

Hemothorax

A hemothorax occurs when blood accumulates within the pleural space following either blunt or penetrating trauma, with resulting injury to the lung parenchyma or an intercostal vessel (**Figure 21.4**). Bleeding is usually self-limited and rarely requires surgical intervention; however, the blood must be removed from the chest cavity to prevent complications, such as infection, empyema, or chronic atelectasis of the lung.

The clinical significance of this injury depends on the amount of blood lost and the extent to which the fluid itself impairs respiratory function. Symptoms such as dyspnea and tachypnea are related to the amount of ventilatory compromise. Auscultation of the chest reveals decreased breath sounds, and percussion reveals dullness on the affected side. Radiographs confirm the diagnosis. The athlete needs immediate transport to the emergency department for placement of a chest tube.

Cardiac Contusion

A cardiac contusion is caused by direct trauma to the anterior chest wall or sternum, which may occur in any contact sports. Athletes typically report chest discomfort related to trauma, but may be otherwise asymptomatic. The clinically important consequences of this condition are arrhythmias, which, if severe, can lead to an abrupt cardiac collapse. Definitive diagnosis outside of the emergency department is very difficult. The focus of management is to identify arrhythmias and initiate prompt pharmacologic therapy. Once resolved, further risk of sudden dysrhythmia is low. Long-term medical therapy is rarely necessary, and prompt return to full physical activity can be expected.

Pericardial Tamponade

Pericardial tamponade is an accumulation of fluid within the pericardial sac. Although most frequently associated with penetrating injuries, blunt injuries, such as an unprotected blow to the sternum, can also cause this injury. The pericardial sac is firm and fibrous, so the accumulation of fluid can lead to significant hemodynamic compromise. This is caused by the inability of the heart to fill, which severely reduces cardiac output and leads to shock. The hallmark signs and symptoms of cardiac tamponade, called Beck's triad, include jugular vein distention, hypotension, and muffled heart tones. Differentiating cardiac tamponade from a tension pneumothorax can be difficult. If this injury is suspected, the athlete should be transported to the emergency department immediately. Cardiac ultrasonography is an excellent tool to use in diagnosing this injury. Once diagnosed, therapy includes volume resuscitation, needle decompression of the pericardial sac, and possibly surgical intervention.

Pulmonary Contusion

A pulmonary contusion is a common and potentially life-threatening injury associated with significant external chest trauma. This type of contusion can occur after a significant blow to the chest wall, with or without associated rib injuries. The significance of the underlying pulmonary injury is related to the amount of force imparted to the chest wall and the amount of fluid and blood accumulated within the pulmonary parenchyma. The degree of ventilation-perfusion mismatch is also related to the severity of illness. Symptoms range from mild tachypnea requiring minimal therapy to complete respiratory failure, which may require mechanical ventilation. Diagnosis is based on radiographic evidence of pulmonary injury.

Treatment includes supplemental oxygen and judicious use of analgesics. If hypoxemia persists, intubation and mechanical ventilation may be necessary. All patients with pulmonary contusions must be observed for signs and symptoms of pneumonia, including a cough, fever, elevated white blood cell count, and the presence of infiltrate on chest radiograph. Prompt treatment with pulmonary physiotherapy and antibiotics is necessary on confirmation of pneumonia. If the patient's respiratory status continues to deteriorate, acute respiratory distress syndrome may develop. Referral to a critical care facility is usually necessary at this point, as mortality can reach 50%.

Return to Play

Most thoracic injuries are bony in nature. Typically, with thoracic injuries such as rib fractures, return to play may take 6 weeks or longer, depending on the number of ribs fractured. Some authorities recommend 3 months of recovery before organized contact sports are resumed. Chest protectors are available to protect previously injured ribs. Return to play for other diagnoses vary and should be deferred to the athlete's treating physician.

Abdominal Injuries

Contusion to the Abdominal Wall

Contusions to the abdominal wall can occur from a forceful hit in any athletic event. Findings that include bruising and pain over the affected area associated with muscular contraction aid in establishing a diagnosis. Treatment usually requires little more than icing the affected area for 12 to 24 hours. The athlete can return to play as soon as the pain has resolved or no longer limits activity. Occasionally, enough force is imparted to the abdominal muscles to cause bleeding and formation of a hematoma. Treatment is the same as for contusion, but recovery may take weeks.

Muscle Strain

Muscle strains can also occur in sporting events. Fast, vigorous stretching of the muscle fibers during contraction leads to acute discomfort and muscle spasm. The discomfort is aggravated by the continued use of the strained muscle. Return to play is delayed with this injury. Muscle strain may also result from overuse of the muscles, such as that which occurs with weight

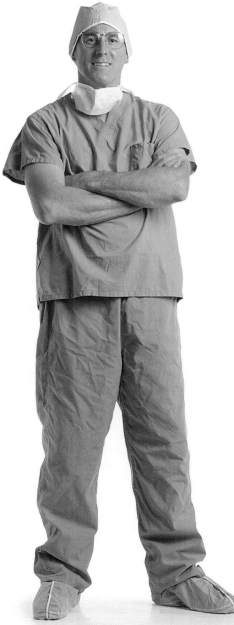

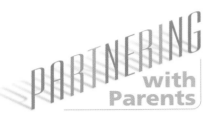

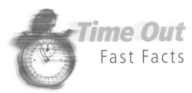

lifting. In these instances, the discomfort is mild at first and becomes more severe with continued injury to the muscles. Patients with abdominal muscle strain should discontinue the activity that caused the injury and follow gradual rehabilitation until recovery is complete.

Injuries to the Spleen

Blunt trauma to the upper left quadrant of the abdomen or the lower rib cage often results in injury to the spleen. The amount of abdominal discomfort may be minimal, despite the presence of a significant injury. On occasion, irritation of the diaphragm from bleeding, inflammation, or enlargement may cause referred pain to the left shoulder. If the injury causes significant intra-abdominal bleeding, systemic signs such as tachypnea, tachycardia, and hypotension may develop. Immediate treatment with intravenous fluid resuscitation is necessary as patients with significant bleeding may progress to shock. Therefore, athletes with a suspected spleen injury require immediate transport to the emergency department. The most useful diagnostic test is an abdominal CT scan, although occasionally ultrasound is more readily available. These modalities are also useful for following the patient's recovery.

Nonoperative management is appropriate for patients whose vital signs are stable and who have no other significant intra-abdominal injury that would require laparotomy; however, this course of management will then require close, continual monitoring by the surgical staff. If blood transfusion requirements reach 40 mL/kg, then surgery is required.

For patients who remain stable, observation in an intensive care unit for up to 24 hours is adequate. Continued observation and bed rest for 3 days, with evaluation of hemoglobin levels, is necessary prior to discharge. Once discharged, these patients should remain under "house arrest" for 3 weeks. If evaluation at this point reveals good recovery, and repeat ultrasound or CT scans document complete healing, patients may be released from the house, but should be restricted from physical activity for another 3 months. Once evaluation reveals a completely healed spleen, athletes may return to full physical activity; however, they should be cautioned about the possibility of re-injury if they return before the spleen is completely healed. Although uncommon, delayed rupture of the spleen, usually as a consequence of a recurrent forceful blow to the same area, has been reported.

Surgical options, if necessary, include splenorrhaphy, or suturing the spleen, and splenectomy. If a splenectomy is indicated, immunizations and antibiotic prophylaxis should be considered as well. The management of splenic injuries has improved in recent years because of an increased awareness of postoperative sepsis. After surgery, patients will need 6 to 8 weeks to recover before resuming physical activity.

Injuries to the Liver

The causes of hepatic injuries are similar to those of splenic injuries. The liver, although larger than the spleen, is fairly well protected by the rib cage and abdominal wall musculature. The hepatic capsule is also significantly stronger than that of the spleen. However, if the liver is enlarged secondary to viral or other etiologies, then it would be more susceptible to injury than normal.

Common injuries include contusions, lacerations, and fractures. The most common symptom is pain over the area of injury. Injuries that cause intra-abdominal bleeding will produce signs and symptoms of shock. Athletes should be transported to the emergency department to undergo a CT scan. Plain radiographs are of little help unless associated musculoskeletal injuries are suspected.

Most athletes with hepatic injuries can be treated nonoperatively. Indications for surgery include hemodynamic instability and the need for blood transfusions of 40 mL/kg or more. Hepatic resection is rare. Follow-up care is similar to that for splenic injuries. Return to full physical activity will take 6 to 8 weeks.

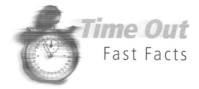

Prevention of abdominal and rib injuries includes the use of rib protectors for use in hockey and football.

Injuries to the Pancreas

The pancreas is a relatively protected organ located in a retroperitoneal position in the middle of the epigastrium. A direct blow, as with a fist, a ski pole, or a bicycle handlebar, to the body of the pancreas as it overlies the vertebral column is the usual mechanism of injury. Signs and symptoms include diffuse, nondescript abdominal pain with occasional vomiting. Most cases of pancreatic contusion resolve spontaneously unless there is a significant injury to the parenchyma or the main pancreatic duct. Diagnosis of pancreatic injury includes testing for serum amylase and lipase, as well as radiologic evaluation with either an ultrasound or CT scan.

Nonoperative treatment is most often indicated; however, significant injuries to the parenchyma or main duct may require surgical intervention.

Injury to the Kidneys

The kidneys are located deep in the retroperitoneal space where they are protected to some extent by the lumbar musculature as well as the lower rib cage. Significant blows to this area can cause injuries that vary from simple contusions to fractures through the capsule that carry the potential for significant hemorrhage into the retroperitoneal space. Signs and symptoms include mild to moderate discomfort in the region of the kidney, along with microscopic or macroscopic hematuria. Diagnostic imaging should include an abdominal CT scan with contrast.

Nearly all renal injuries can be managed nonoperatively. Complete healing, as evidenced by CT scan, should occur within 3 months. Once healed, athletes should be able to return to full activity.

Injuries to the Gastrointestinal Tract

Intestinal injuries are caused by direct blows to the abdomen that force the bowel against the spine or the firm retroperitoneum. Signs and symptoms of bowel injury may be absent if the bowel sustains only simple contusions. Athletes typically seek medical care only if a transmural injury has occurred. In the absence of a perforation, the patient may have diffuse pain from the physical injury and nausea caused by an ileus. Diagnosis is very difficult, and therapy is supportive with cessation of oral intake and IV fluid therapy. If a significant injury results in perforation, then fever, diffuse pain, and peritonitis will be present, and surgical resection is indicated. This injury can occur anywhere from the duodenum to the colon, with the injuries to the latter less common. Once physically recovered from the laparotomy, usually within 6 weeks, athletes can return to physical activity.

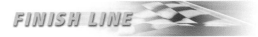

Significant abdominal and thoracic injuries remain uncommon in young athletes. However, if injuries occur and are missed, significant morbidity and mortality are possible.

For More Information

1. Billups D, Martin D, Swain RA: Training room evaluation of chest pain in the adolescent athlete. *South Med J* 1995;88:667–672.

2. Barrett GR, Shelton WR, Miles JW: First rib fractures in football players: A case report and literature review. *Am J Sports Med* 1988;16:674–676.

3. Galan G, Penalver JC, Paris F, et al: Blunt chest injuries in 1,696 patients. *Eur J Cardiothorac Surg* 1992;6:284–287.

Chapter 22

Exercise, Asthma, and Anaphylaxis

DAVID M. ORENSTEIN, MD
GREGORY L. LANDRY, MD

Asthma is one of the most common chronic medical conditions of childhood, affecting up to 15% of all children. Nearly all people with asthma have symptoms triggered by and/or exacerbated by exercise. Asthma induced by exercise, or exercise-induced asthma (EIA), affects patients with asthma, as well as a number of individuals without previously recognized asthma. As many as 10% of high school and college athletes have been diagnosed with EIA. Still, asthma and EIA are underdiagnosed in part because symptoms of EIA often manifest after, not during, exercise and may resolve spontaneously. Further, athletes with EIA might not wheeze, the classic sign of asthma, but rather cough or report chest tightness, shortness of breath, or even chest pain.

Exercise can also produce urticaria, angioedema, and anaphylaxis, all of which may occur together in the same syndrome or individually. Urticaria is characterized by localized nonpitting edema of the superficial dermis. Usually there are well-circumscribed wheals that often coalesce to form larger wheals. Angioedema is well-demarcated localized edema that involves deeper layers of skin and subcutaneous tissue. Anaphylaxis is a life-threatening illness that usually involves upper airway distress and/or hypotension in previously sensitized individuals. Signs and symptoms of asthma can occur with these entities, but are rare.

Because asthma and anaphylaxis are two distinct clinical entities, they will be discussed separately.

Pathophysiology of Exercise-Induced Asthma

The pathophysiology of EIA is related to the function of the airways to humidify and warm inspired air to body temperature before it reaches the intrathoracic airways. These functions are handled efficiently when ambient

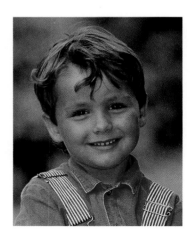

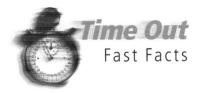

EIA is underdiagnosed because usually it is a self-limited condition, and symptoms often occur after, not during, exercise.

air is already warm and humidified or minute ventilation is low. However, when ambient air is very cold or dry and/or when minute ventilation is increased with exercise, warming and humidifying is incomplete. The cool, dry air that reaches the bronchi is a major stimulus for EIA. The resultant bronchospasm and airway inflammation cause airway constriction and produce coughing, chest tightness, and/or shortness of breath. If inflammation already exists, EIA is even more likely to occur. Particles and other toxic components of polluted air almost certainly make signs and symptoms worse.

The exact sequence of cellular events leading to airway narrowing is not fully known, but mediators of inflammation derived from mast cells may be partly to blame. Support for this theory comes from an observed refractory period in almost half of patients with EIA. In these individuals, the asthma response to successive exercise challenges will diminish. This observation is consistent with a depletion of inflammatory mediators from mast cells where replenishment is incomplete if the interval between exercise challenges is 1 hour or less.

Clinical Evaluation

History

EIA is most likely to occur with, or especially after, a period of relatively intense exercise of at least 6 to 8 minutes. If the ambient air is cold and dry, the likelihood of an episode is increased. Exercise bouts that are less than or greater than 6 to 8 minutes are less likely to prompt EIA, with the possible exception of extremely intense brief bursts, as these may also provoke bronchoconstriction. For reasons that are not yet clear, swimming is less likely than other sports to stimulate EIA, although it is thought to be related to the high humidity in most swimming pools. Signs and symptoms can include any one or combination of coughing, wheezing, chest tightness, difficulty breathing, or chest pain. Symptoms typically last from 10 to 60 minutes and resolve spontaneously. Inhalation of a ß-agonist bronchodilator, such as albuterol, can hasten resolution of symptoms. Outdoor sporting events, especially those held in cold weather, are more likely to produce symptoms of asthma than are indoor events.

Physical Examination

The athlete with EIA will often have a normal physical examination between episodes. Careful attention to the nose and sinuses may reveal abnormalities because of the association between asthma and allergic rhinitis (and sinusitis). Auscultation of the lungs may reveal unilateral adventitious sounds, which suggest a foreign body, a pneumonia, or a mass.

Children with asthma may not take good breaths because these cause coughing. However, athletes must be encouraged to take good breaths. Forced expiration may produce coughing, wheezing, or rhonchi, which suggest asthma, but are not specific findings for this diagnosis.

A careful examination of the heart is also necessary because cardiac disease may produce exercise-induced cough and exercise-induced intolerance, such as EIA.

Diagnostic Testing

Diagnosing EIA is usually relatively straightforward. An athlete who coughs, wheezes, reports chest tightness, difficulty breathing, or chest pain during or after exercise is likely to have EIA. If the athlete is known to have asthma, he or she can expect increased symptoms of asthma with exercise, and formal testing is seldom needed. In athletes not previously known to have asthma, diagnosis of EIA can be established by a therapeutic trial of ß-agonist inhalation (eg, two puffs of albuterol) 15 minutes before exercise. If this approach is not successful, pulmonary function testing can help identify individuals with large and small airways obstruction. However, athletes with exercise-related airway obstruction may have normal baseline pulmonary function. In these individuals, a bronchial provocation test can be performed using exercise, cold air, methacholine, or histamine.

With an exercise challenge, pulmonary function testing is performed prior to exercise and every 3 to 5 minutes after exercise for 15 or 20 minutes. The exercise challenge should last 6 to 8 minutes and should raise the athlete's heart rate to 180 beats/minute. Typically, in an athlete with EIA, forced expired volume in 1 second (FEV_1, a measure of large airway function) and/or midexpiratory flow (sometimes called FEF_{25-75}, a measure of small airway function) will decrease. Decreases of 15% to 20% are required to confirm the diagnosis. False-negative tests may occur if the exercise challenge fails to recreate the airway obstruction.

Athletes occasionally have signs and symptoms of EIA, but do not meet the diagnostic criteria for EIA when given a bronchial provocation test. This may occur because the athlete exercises in cold, dry air, so the test does not recreate the environment that provokes the symptoms. In these instances, empiric treatment may still be prudent.

Differential Diagnosis

Few conditions are confused with EIA. The condition that is most difficult to distinguish from EIA is vocal cord dysfunction (VCD). This unusual and probably psychogenically mediated adduction of the vocal cords is seen primarily in elite athletes. VCD produces symptoms that are very similar to EIA, but is not responsive to bronchodilators. Diagnosis is made with either formal pulmonary function tests before and after exercise (in which the inspiratory loop of the flow-volume curve is flattened, while FEV_{25-75} and FEV_1 are preserved), or with direct visualization of the adducted vocal cords by flexible fiberoptic laryngoscopy after exercise. Flow-volume loops must be specifically requested because they are not routinely performed as part of an exercise provocation study.

Other conditions that mimic EIA include viral or bacterial lung infections that can produce coughing or shortness of breath that worsens with exercise, and trauma to the larynx or chest that causes pain or difficulty breathing that is more pronounced with the deep breathing associated with exercise. Gastroesophageal reflux should also be considered as a potential trigger for EIA. Cardiac causes of chest pain and cough should be considered in the differential diagnosis.

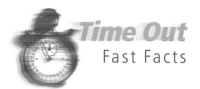

Time Out
Fast Facts

A child with well-controlled asthma or exercise induced bronchospasm should be able to participate in virtually any sport.

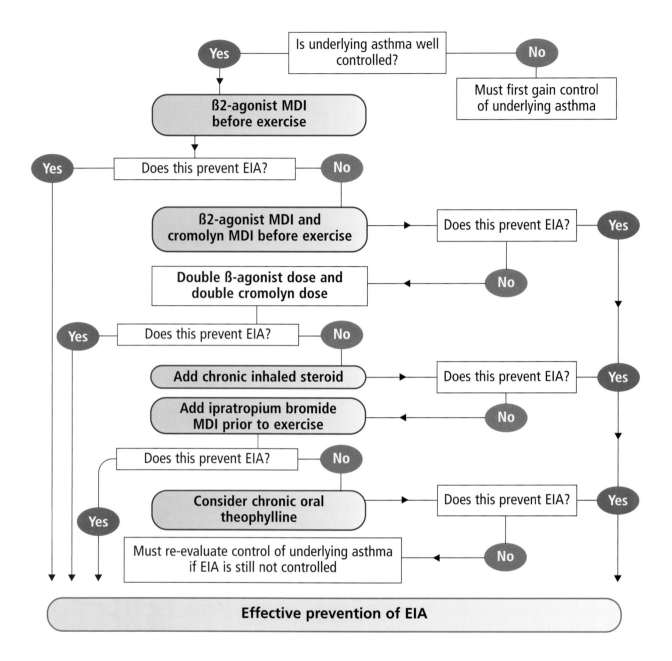

Figure 22.1 Flow chart for selecting drugs to prevent EIA.

Adapted with permission from Bar-Or (ed): *The Child and Adolescent Athlete.* Oxford, England, Blackwell Science Ltd, 1996, pp 448–450.

Treatment and Prevention

Usually, EIA is easily treated and prevented (**Figure 22.1**). If EIA occurs, two puffs of a ß-agonist bronchodilator such as albuterol will almost always reverse the airway obstruction and relieve the symptoms. Prevention is also possible and should be the preferred method of treatment, instead of relying on rescue treatment once symptoms appear. The first step in prevention is taking two puffs of a ß-agonist bronchodilator 15 minutes prior to exercise. If a ß-agonist is not tolerated, then cromolyn sodium or nedrocromil can be used in the same way. If these medications used independently do not prevent EIA, advise the athlete to use both agents before exercise. If necessary, the athlete may double the number of puffs of both agents. Some of the oral leukotriene inhibitors, such as montelukast, also help prevent EIA, but are not typically used for treatment of simple EIA.

Table 22.1 *Drugs Commonly Used for Exercise-induced Asthma (EIA)*

Medication	Route of Administration	Effectiveness in EIA	Legal or Banned	Prophylaxis (P); Therapeutic (T)
Cromolyn sodium	Aerosol	Good	Legal	P
Nedrocromil sodium	Aerosol	Good	Legal	P
ß₂-agonists				
Salbutamol	Aerosol	Excellent	Legal	P, T
Salbutamol	Oral	Good	Banned	P, T
Terbutaline	Aerosol	Excellent	Legal	P, T
Terbutaline	Oral	Good	Banned	P, T
Occiprenaline	Aerosol	Excellent	Legal	P, T
Salmeterol	Aerosol	Excellent	Legal	P, T
Clenbuterol	Aerosol	Excellent	Legal	P, T
Theophylline	Oral	Good	Banned	P, T
Iprathropium bromide	Aerosol	Fair	Legal	T
Steroids				
Beclomethasone	Aerosol	Unknown	Legal	P, T
Budesonide	Aerosol	Fair	Legal	P, T
Prednisone	Oral	Unknown	Banned	T
Prednisolone	Oral	Unknown	Banned	T

Adapted with permission from Bar-Or (ed): *The Child and Adolescent Athlete*. Oxford, England, Blackwell Science Ltd, 1996, pp 448–450.

If treatment with these agents does not prevent EIA, the athlete should be asked to demonstrate the proper technique for using the inhaler. Other considerations include the possibility that the inhaler canister is empty or the medication has expired. If these causes have been explored, the diagnosis should be questioned and referral to an asthma specialist is indicated. In most patients, the diagnosis of EIA is correct, but the athlete has underlying asthma, with chronic, inadequately controlled airway inflammation. Pulmonary function testing will show baseline airway obstruction with incomplete response to an inhaled bronchodilator. This inflammation must be controlled. Long-term treatment with an inhaled anti-inflammatory agent, such as cromolyn sodium, nedrocromil, or inhaled corticosteroids, will usually reduce inflammation.

Most of the drugs now in use for treating and preventing asthma are legal for use in scholastic, collegiate, and international competition (**Table 22.1**). In addition, the United States Olympic Committee Drug Control Program operates a hotline (1-800-233-0393) to keep physicians, coaches, and athletes aware of changes in regulations regarding accepted and banned drugs.

Nonpharmacologic treatment may help some athletes with EIA. For example, a scarf may be tied around the nose and mouth to help warm and humidify inspired air. Sometimes, warm-up exercises before practice or competition can induce a refractory period (in about half of patients with asthma), and thus make the competition less asthmagenic. To induce a refractory period, the athlete must exercise long enough and with enough intensity to actually induce some bronchospasm. There are

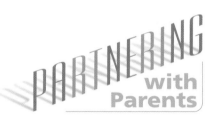

How can my children prevent symptoms of EIA from occuring?

Most patients with EIA can prevent symptoms by modifying the intensity of their activity, avoiding cold, dry air, or allergens, or by pretreating with ß₂-agonists or inhaled anti-inflammatories.

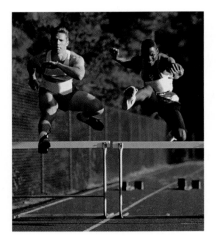

no universal warm-up exercises, and routines will likely vary among athletes; however, 10 to 15 minutes of exercise is usually sufficient to induce sweating. If the athlete has a refractory period, subsequent exercise bouts will be less likely to induce symptoms for about 2 hours. For high school and college athletes, the suggestion of changing sports may not be practical, but parents of younger children may be advised to help their children select lower risk sports. However, because pharmacologic treatment is so effective, few athletes will have to abandon their sport of choice, and no young person with EIA should be excluded from sports or physical activity.

Most athletes with asthma respond well to exercise training. Many professional and Olympic athletes have managed to attain high levels of sports performance, despite having asthma. Youngsters with asthma should be encouraged to exercise and participate in sports.

Pathophysiology of Exercise-Induced Anaphylaxis

Exercise can produce urticaria, angioedema, and anaphylaxis separately or together in the same syndrome. Classic exercise-induced anaphylaxis (EIAna) was first described 20 years ago. Since then, hundreds of patients have described a similar pattern of initial signs and symptoms of EIAna.

In more than half of patients with classic EIAna, food or drugs are a coprecipitant with exercise. In one study, the most common food was celery, followed by the more common food allergens such as shellfish and wheat. EIAna has also been reported after ingestion of a variety of medications. Jogging is the most common precipitating type of exercise, but EIAna has been associated with other types of exercise as well.

Clinical Evaluation

History

Athletes often report the same pattern of initial signs and symptoms, including fatigue, generalized warmth, pruritus, and erythema. Information about an athlete's last meal and/or medication regimen in relationship to beginning exercise is important. Some athletes may report that symptoms develop if they exercise too soon after eating any meal.

A serious episode is characterized by a variety of airway problems, including choking, stridor, and dysphagia, and abdominal pain and vomiting. Symptoms typically last between 30 minutes and 4 hours. About one third of patients experience syncope in association with EIAna, but only one death has been reported in the medical literature.

Physical Examination

Soon after the initial signs and symptoms develop, large urticaria (between 1 and 2.5 cm) develop with angioedema. However, in some athletes, only small punctate (2 to 4 mm) urticaria develop. This is usually called cholinergic urticaria because it is thought to be triggered by cholinergic response in the skin as the result of temperature changes. This form of urticaria, called variant EIAna, is rarely associated with angioedema, bronchospasm, or hypotension.

Treatment and Prevention

Epinephrine is the treatment of choice. However, as with any anaphylactic reaction, IV fluids, antihistamines, and oxygen are helpful if epinephrine does not resolve the symptoms. Some athletes will improve spontaneously if they stop exercising.

For most athletes, the key to treatment is prevention. All athletes with EIAna should be referred to an allergy specialist because of the high association of this condition with food allergies. Athletes who are food sensitive should undergo skin testing and be encouraged to keep a food diary to help better identify offending foods. Some athletes may be able to safely exercise only in the morning after an overnight fast.

Prophylactic antihistamines are helpful for some athletes. Diphenhydramine and hydroxyzine were regarded as most effective, but their strong sedative effects may limit their use in some individuals. Any of the nonsedating antihistamines may be beneficial. Athletes should be counseled to use antihistamines liberally until more is known about the precipitating factors in his or her case. Some athletes will always require pretreatment to be able to exercise symptom free. These athletes should not exercise alone and should carry an emergency epinephrine kit with them at all times.

Coaches and physicians should also keep an emergency epinephrine kit in the first aid kit or medical bag. The kit must be kept out of heat and light, and its expiration date checked frequently.

Venom Allergies

Another cause of anaphylaxis is an allergic reaction following a sting from a venomous insect, most commonly yellow jackets, honey bees, wasps, hornets, and ants. Reactions to these bites are responsible for about 50 deaths in the United States each year. Most systemic reactions are immediate and produce the symptoms of anaphylaxis described above.

Epinephrine must be given to these individuals immediately, followed by transport to the emergency department. Large local reactions to stings produce induration and erythema within 24 to 72 hours. In these instances, a severe systemic reaction is not likely. However, athletes who experience this type of large reaction may be at risk for a systemic reaction in the future. Therefore, they should carry an emergency epinephrine kit with them at all times. Most allergy specialists would not recommend immunotherapy for these individuals.

Athletes who have experienced an anaphylactic reaction to a sting should be referred to an allergy specialist to identify the specific venom allergy and to discuss immunotherapy. This type of therapy has been shown to significantly reduce reactions to subsequent stings in most patients. These athletes must carry an emergency epinephrine kit at all times.

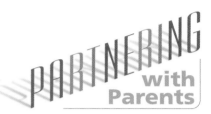

My child develops severe reactions to bee stings without systemic signs and symptoms. Should she carry an Epi-pen?

She should carry an Epi-pen. Severe local reactions do not have the same serious complications as anaphylaxis and do not require treatment with epinephrine. However, these patients may be at greater risk for anaphylaxis with future stings.

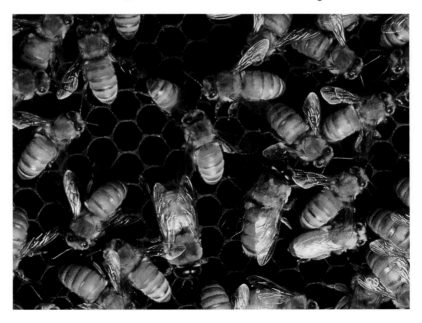

FINISH LINE

Exercise-induced asthma (EIA) is very common but often undiagnosed. Signs and symptoms include coughing, chest tightness, chest pain, difficulty breathing, and/or wheezing during, or more commonly, after 6 to 8 minutes of vigorous exercise. EIA is most likely to occur with endurance exercise in cool, dry air. In most athletes, it is readily prevented by taking two puffs of inhaled albuterol, cromolyn sodium, or nedrocromil prior to exercise. Once it is recognized and treated, EIA should not prevent athletes from enjoying a full athletic career.

Exercise-induced anaphylaxis (EIAna) can produce urticaria, angioedema, and anaphylaxis either separately or together. Most athletes with this condition have a related food or medication allergy. Injection of epinephrine usually resolves symptoms, but treatment is largely preventive. Referral to an allergy specialist and liberal use of prophylactic antihistamines are recommended. For athletes who are allergic to venomous insect stings, an emergency epinephrine kit should be carried at all times.

For More Information

1. DuBaske LM, Horan RF, et al: Exercise-induced allergy syndromes, in Weiler JM (ed): *Allergic and Respiratory Disease in Sports Medicine.* New York, NY, Marcel Dekker, 1997, pp 253–278.

2. Graft DF, Valentine MD: Insect sting allergy, in Kaplan AP, Kersey R (eds): *Allergy,* ed 2. Philadelphia, PA, WB Saunders, 1997, pp 652–663.

3. Lemanske RF Jr, Busse WW: Asthma. *JAMA* 1997;278:1855–1873.

4. McFadden ER Jr, Gilbert IA: Exercise-induced asthma. *N Engl J Med* 1994;330:1362–1367.

5. Volcheck GW, Li JT: Exercise-induced urticaria and anaphylaxis. *Mayo Clin Proc* 1997;72:140–147.

Chapter 23

Acute Illnesses

PAUL R. STRICKER, MD

Whether children join an organized sport, play during school recesses, or run around in the backyard, physical activity is important to their overall health and well-being. Like other youngsters, young athletes can become ill from a variety of infections. Team sports, in particular, which place children in close contact with each other for extended lengths of time, may increase a child's risk of contracting an infection.

Physicians should be aware of the potential implications of a sick young athlete. Important considerations include the relationship between exercise and the immune system, the severity of the illness and its impact on the ability of the athlete to either continue participation or require a period of rest, the type of illness and the risks for serious sequelae, the danger of contagion to other individuals or team members, and treatment options and their effects on performance.

Exercise, Immunity, and Infection

The effects of exercise on the immune system have been and continue to be an area of active research. Investigators are currently working to understand how exercise induces changes in the immune system. Studies are investigating both the short- and long-term effects of exercise upon quantitative and functional measures of the immune system, including neutrophils, lymphocytes, and immunoglobulins. Short-term exercise is defined as physical effort that is performed on a treadmill, stationary bicycle, or hand cycle for short bursts of activity lasting from seconds to minutes. Long-term exercise includes consistent aerobic activity several times a week at levels around or above 75% maximum oxygen uptake ($Vo_{2\ max}$), as well as high-intensity or endurance sports such as long-distance running, cross-country skiing, swimming, and competitive bicycling.

During physical activity, many physiologic changes occur, and changes in one body system (eg, hormonal changes) can affect other systems as well. For example, with exercise, levels of epinephrine and cortisol rise. Epinephrine peaks during exercise and then diminishes during recovery, while cortisol rises more steadily and remains elevated for a longer period

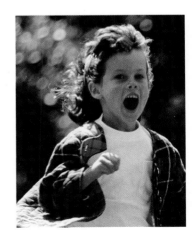

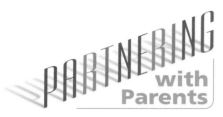

When should an athlete be released to return to practice or games following an acute febrile illness?

Athletes should not compete or practice with a fever because of the increased risk of myocarditis and dehydration. Once the fever has resolved, be sure that exercise tolerance is normal so that an athlete is not at increased risk of injury or suboptimal performance.

of time. Quantitative changes in immune components include increases in neutrophils and lymphocytes with epinephrine, as well as delayed increases in neutrophils and decreases in lymphocytes corresponding to the rise in cortisol, with a return to baseline in a few hours. This decrease in lymphocytes includes a change in lymphocyte subsets such as the decreased ratio of CD4 (T-helper) cells to CD8 (suppressor T) cells. In long-term exercisers, cortisol levels often remain elevated even at rest, and significant increases in cortisol appear in many athletes who overtrain. The catabolic nature of prolonged elevation of cortisol and its effects on lymphocytes may contribute to susceptibility to infection.

Functional assessment of immune components also reveals changes with exercise. Neutrophil chemotaxis and phagocytosis are diminished with endurance training. Salivary IgA concentration is decreased with short-term exercise and even suppressed below baseline with long-term, high-intensity training. Natural killer cell activity actually increases, but decreases during recovery back to baseline. These changes cause concern about the athlete's ability to ward off pathogens during periods of recovery from intense exercise. These effects of exercise on the immune system can be found in **Table 23.1**.

Although exercise can affect the quantity and activity of immune system components, it remains unclear whether athletes are actually more susceptible to infections. Researchers tend to agree that, in general, individuals who exercise at a moderate level ($< 60\%$ $Vo_{2\,max}$) enhance immune function and may experience shorter duration of illness compared with those who do not exercise. However, an increasing body of evidence supports the idea that elite athletes may be at greater risk for infections than individuals who exercise at a more moderate level. Increasing training volume and intensity ($> 80\%$ $Vo_{2\,max}$) can increase the risk of upper respiratory infections, and continuing to exercise with an infection such as

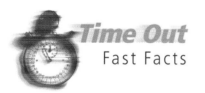

Regular exercise of moderate intensity seems to enhance immune function.

Table 23.1 *Effects of Exercise on the Immune System*

Quantitative Changes	Activity	
	Short-term	Long-term
Total white blood cells	↑↑	↑*
Neutrophils	↑↑	↑
Lymphocytes	↑	↓
Ratio of CD4 (T-helper cells) to CD8 (suppressor T cells)	↓	↓
Salivary IgA concentration	↓	↓↓
Functional Changes		
Neutrophil activity	↑	↓
Natural killer cell activity	↑	↑

*Although long-term exercise induces increased white blood cell (WBC) count with each bout, this increase is less severe in athletes compared with those who have not participated in a long-term exercise program. In addition, the actual resting WBC count in long-term exercisers is often decreased.

Adapted with permission from Stricker PR, Green GA: Infections in athletes, in Mellion MD (ed): *Sports Medicine Secrets,* ed 2. Philadelphia, PA, Hanley & Belfus, 1999, p 165.

mononucleosis or viral meningitis actually prolongs the duration of the illness. Based on animal data, an individual who exercises during the incubation period of Coxsackie B virus infection may be at increased risk for myocarditis.

Upper Respiratory Infections

Although viral upper respiratory infections (URI) can affect any individual at any time of the year, rates of infection in the general public usually peak in the fall and winter when many viruses are predominant. During these times, youngsters are in school, attend classes, play together, and participate in team training in close proximity with many other children, hence sharing of infectious agents is more common. All athletes should be reminded to maintain good personal hygiene by washing their hands frequently and by not sharing water bottles.

Such techniques may help reduce the spread of infection, yet an athlete engaged in high-intensity exercise may have an increased risk for URI. Studies show that the risk of URI is higher in long-distance runners when they increase their training mileage and also during the 2 weeks after a race. Other data demonstrate that the risk of URI increases with longer periods of training and a higher intensity of effort. In fact, many athletes report that they contract more infections during various times in the competitive season when they train intensely and during and after major competitions. Elevated cortisol levels and temporary exercise-induced suppression of immune function may negatively impact the immune system, but other variables, such as fatigue, psychological stress, and inadequate recovery time, are also involved.

As previously mentioned, evidence also suggests that moderate levels of exercise can enhance immune function and lower the risk of URI. The effects of exercise on the risk of URI remain a complicated issue because it is difficult

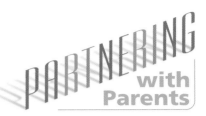

Can my child exercise while taking an antihistamine-decongestant for a cold?

In general, yes. However, these agents tax the cardiovascular system and decrease the body's ability to regulate temperature. Make sure the child is well hydrated and used good judgment when exercising in the heat.

What vitamins, minerals, or other dietary supplements can reduce the likelihood of illness during an athletic season?

To date, there is no evidence that any of the above reduce the risk of illness during training. Children require a well-balanced diet, plenty of fluids, adequate rest, and should avoid over training.

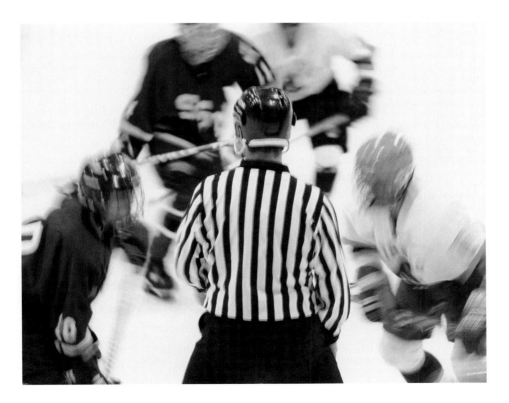

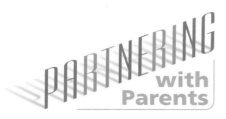

How can I decide whether to let my child practice when he is ill? Should I always take him to the doctor?

If symptoms are "above the neck" and there is no fever, it is generally believed to be safe to continue exercising as symptoms allow. If there is any question about his ability to tolerate exercise, it is best to check with the physician.

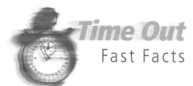

Time Out
Fast Facts

Splenic rupture associated with mononucleosis is infrequent, but it does present a real risk during the first 3 weeks after onset of symptoms.

to isolate the effects of exercise from those of the psychological stress associated with training and competition, environmental and weather conditions, exposure to individuals who are ill, inadequate nutrition, and other potentially significant but unknown stressors.

Effects of Infections on Exercise Capacity

Unfortunately, there are few well-designed studies that examine the effects of illness on the body's response to exercise. One prospective study found that subclinical viral infections did not decrease performance. However, active infections and illnesses that cause fever can be detrimental to athletes. Fevers affect the body's ability to regulate body temperature, increasing the risk of heat exhaustion and heatstroke. Fever may also worsen dehydration, especially if the athlete also has diarrhea. Acute viral infections that cause fever have been shown to decrease muscle strength and endurance from a combination of decreased exercise tolerance, dehydration, fatigue, direct viral effects on muscle tissue as evidenced by myalgias, and elevated cardiac output because of fever. For example, moderate to severe cases of infectious mononucleosis often render an athlete unable to train, probably because of decreased muscle strength and endurance.

Athletes often want to continue to train and compete despite an illness, and the physician is regularly faced with decisions regarding return to play. In general, if symptoms are confined above the neck, such as a runny nose or nasal congestion, athletes may continue at whatever level they can tolerate. However, athletes with systemic symptoms such as fever, myalgias, and elevated resting heart rate should refrain from intense exercise with high cardiac demand. Risks of serious sequelae, including dehydration, heat exhaustion, prolonged illness, and myocarditis, may preclude a rapid return to physical activity and competition. Return to play depends on absence of fever, decreased symptoms, and a return to a normal resting heart rate, which may require 7 to 14 days of rest.

Specific illnesses require special considerations. In particular, mononucleosis carries with it the well-known risk of splenic rupture associated with splenomegaly. Although the risk of splenic rupture is small (less than 0.5% of patients), it can occur during the first 4 to 21 days after symptoms appear. An athlete may return to activities 4 weeks after the onset of the illness if other symptoms are significantly diminished, and he or she feels well enough to begin some moderate exercise. However, if there is any clinical concern or question about the status of the spleen, diagnostic imaging with ultrasound or CT scan can confirm the presence of splenomegaly because palpation by physical examination is unreliable.

Varicella infection precludes sports participation because it is highly contagious. Athletes may return to play when afebrile and all lesions are scabbed over.

The Role of Antibiotics

Athletes intent on training through an illness may ask for an antibiotic at the first sign of a runny nose. If this is the case, the physician should reassure the athlete and take the opportunity to explain the course of viral infections and their unresponsiveness to antibiotics. If a medication can be taken to reduce symptoms without interfering with potential drug testing or causing excessive

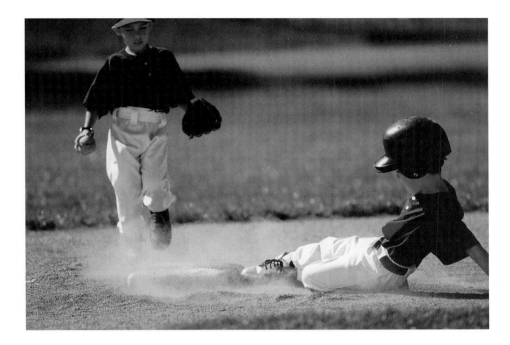

drowsiness, its use would be appropriate. Conversely, athletes who resist taking an antibiotic for a bacterial infection should also be reassured that the antibiotic is indicated. Although limited, studies show that various antibiotics, such as ampicillin, amoxicillin, tetracycline, and trimethoprim/sulfamethoxazole, have no adverse effects on aerobic capacity or strength. However, an antibiotic should be selected carefully to avoid side effects such as nausea, diarrhea, photosensitivity, and allergic reaction.

FINISH LINE

Significant research investigating the response of various immune factors to exercise is ongoing. Moderate exercise tends to enhance immune function, while prolonged, intense exercise may compromise immunity and increase the risk of URI.

Exercise during certain viral illnesses, such as Coxsackie B virus and mononucleosis, is not without potential serious complications. Fortunately, even though the potential sequelae are dangerous, these illnesses are less frequent than the common cold. In these cases, examination of the athlete is key to assess whether the illness is confined locally or is manifesting systemic symptoms, and to plan treatment and return to activity. Treatment should focus on relieving symptoms without producing other undesirable effects and shortening the course of the illness, if possible.

For More Information

1. American Academy of Pediatrics, Committee on Sports Medicine and Fitness: Medical conditions affecting sports participation. *Pediatrics* 1994;94:757–760.

2. Brenner IK, Shek PN, Shephard RJ: Infection in athletes. *Sports Med* 1994;17:86–107.

3. McDonald W: Upper respiratory tract infections, in Fields KB, Fricker PA, Delaney MJ, Fallon KE (eds): *Medical Problems in Athletes.* Malden, MA, Blackwell Science, 1997, pp 6–10.

4. Nieman DC: Immunity in athletes: Current issues. *Gatorade Sports Science Institute Sports Science Exchange* 1998;11:1–6.

5. Stricker PR, Green GA: Infections in athletes, in Mellion MB (ed): *Sports Medicine Secrets,* ed 2. Philadelphia, PA, Hanley & Belfus, 1999, pp 165–169.

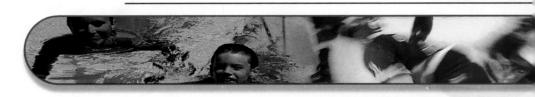

Chapter 24

Chronic Conditions

HELGE HEBESTREIT, MD
ODED BAR-OR, MD

Patients with chronic medical conditions face additional risks when they participate in sports. These risks depend not only on the specific condition, but also on the severity of the condition and on the sport, environment, coaching, supervision, training regimen, and level of competition. Despite the risks, a child or adolescent with a chronic condition may also benefit from increased physical activity and/or sports participation. Some of these benefits are disease-specific and, in fact, physical activity is part of the treatment regimen for some diseases. In addition, most children and adolescents with chronic medical conditions can experience many of the same benefits from physical activity as other children, including improved fitness and motor coordination as well as psychological benefits, such as improved self-esteem, body image, social development, and concentration. Last, but not least, an active child may be more likely than an inactive child to adopt a habit of lifetime physical activity. In adults, a high level of physical activity is linked to reduced cardiovascular morbidity and mortality.

The extent to which children with chronic health conditions can engage in physical activity should be based on the demands of the sport, the impact of the condition on performance, and the potential risks of an acute or chronic worsening of the patient's condition as the result of participation (**Table 24.1**). Each patient must be considered individually and reevaluated on a regular basis.

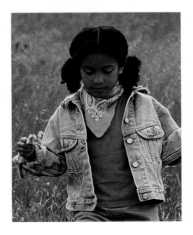

Insulin-Dependent Diabetes Mellitus

Insulin-dependent diabetes mellitus (IDDM) is an autoimmune process that destroys pancreatic ß-cells. The prevalence of IDDM in children and adolescents is about 1 in 1,000. Currently, the only effective treatment for the long-term management of insulin deficiency is subcutaneous injections of insulin. However, with this therapy, insulin levels are not controlled by blood glucose concentrations. Instead, the rate of insulin release from the injection site is

Table 24.1   Risks and Benefits of Exercise in Children with Chronic Health Conditions

Condition	Risks of Exercise	Benefits of Exercise
Insulin-dependent diabetes mellitus	• Hypoglycemia • Ketoacidosis	• Increased physical fitness • Improved overall health • Increased sensitivity to insulin • Possibly, fewer long-term complications
Bronchial asthma	• Asthma attack	• Increased physical fitness • Improved self-esteem, body image, and social development • Fewer hospital visits and days absent from school
Cystic fibrosis	• Dehydration • Arterial oxygen desaturation • Hypoglycemia (children with CF-related diabetes mellitus) • Ketoacidosis (children with CF-related diabetes mellitus) • Possibly, worsening of cor pulmonale	• Increased physical fitness • Improved self-esteem • Improved overall health • Possibly, decreased morbidity and mortality
Juvenile rheumatoid arthritis	• Flare-up of arthritis • Injuries • Possibly, increased mortality (children with cardiac involvement)	• Increased physical fitness • Increased strength in muscles and ligaments • Improved joint protection • Increased bone mineral content
Epilepsy	• Seizures	• Increased physical fitness • Improved self-esteem • Improved overall health
Hemophilia	• Bleeding (into joints, muscles, and other organs)	• Increased physical fitness • Increased levels of clotting factors • Increased strength in muscles and ligaments • Improved joint protection

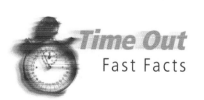

Time Out
Fast Facts

Children with diabetes who exercise consistently may decrease their risk of developing complications such as neuropathy and/or microangiopathy.

dependent on the composition of the injected insulin solution, the site of injection, and local factors such as perfusion at the injection site that may vary with the type, intensity, and duration of exercise. Most adolescents and adults with properly controlled IDDM can participate safely in most sports.

Risks of Exercise

Even patients with well-controlled IDDM may experience hypoglycemia during or up to 24 hours following exercise. The extent to which blood glucose drops depends mostly on the duration and the intensity of the activity. Endurance activities such as distance running, swimming, canoeing, or bicycling may precipitate larger drops in blood glucose. In fact, parents of children with IDDM

Table 24.2 *Recommendations to Children with IDDM Who Want to Engage in Sports*

1. Always bring a glucometer, food, and fast-acting carbohydrates to the sporting venue.

2. Inject insulin subcutaneously at a site away from an exercising muscle (eg, the abdomen). Decrease the dose of insulin by up to 30% to 50%. The magnitude of reduction depends on the type, intensity, and duration of exercise and should be based on individual guidelines provided by the physician.

3. Check blood glucose level before exercising and only exercise if it is between 100 and 200 mg/dL. If the exercise is continued for more than 15 to 30 minutes, check blood glucose again during and after exercising. Check blood glucose level again at bedtime and, if it is low, eat slow-release carbohydrates (for example, bread with cheese or sausage or yogurt) and test blood glucose level once or twice during the night.

4. Exercise only if metabolic control is good (ie, blood glucose levels between 100 to 250 mg/dL without ketonuria). If higher than 250 mg/dL, delay exercise to prevent diabetic ketoacidosis; if blood glucose level is below 100 mg/dL, eat a snack and recheck blood glucose levels before exercise.

5. Eat more carbohydrates 1 to 3 hours before exercise, especially if the exercise session is unplanned. Drink carbohydrate solutions (for example, juice or commercially available sport drinks) every 30 minutes during prolonged exercise. Replenish carbohydrate stores after exercising.

6. Remember that blood glucose levels may be low for more than 24 hours after prolonged exercise.

7. Try not to exercise during peak times of insulin activity or within 1 hour of insulin injection.

report that sports activity is the most common cause of severe hypoglycemia in their children. Severe hypoglycemia may cause loss of coordination and judgment, unconsciousness, seizures, and death. Longer-lasting effects of hypoglycemia include a reduction in the ability to concentrate. Some children with poorly controlled IDDM and very low levels of circulating insulin may experience ketoacidosis with exercise. If untreated, ketonemia and acidemia may cause extreme fatigue, coma, and eventually, death.

Benefits of Exercise

Many studies have shown that sports participation improves the physical fitness of patients with IDDM. Also, exercise may positively affect the disease process itself. For example, serum lipid profiles improve with physical training. Furthermore, evidence suggests that high levels of physical activity may reduce the risk of long-term complications of diabetes, such as neuropathy and microangiopathy. However, the effects of training programs on the long-term control of blood glucose in patients with IDDM are still controversial.

Recommendations

Children with IDDM and their parents should be thoroughly educated about the potential benefits and risks of participating in sports. Although there are general guidelines for young patients with IDDM who want to engage in sports, every child must be advised individually (**Table 24.2**). For example, since physical activity increases the body's sensitivity to insulin, the dose should be decreased during endurance exercises and additional carbohydrates should be ingested. The levels of blood glucose may need to be monitored more closely to avoid severe side effects. Sometimes, a simulation of a sports event in the exercise laboratory, with continuous monitoring of blood glu-

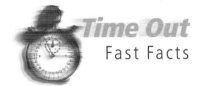
Time Out
Fast Facts

To avoid exercise-induced episodes of hypoglycemia, children with diabetes need to reduce pre-exercise doses of insulin and increase their intake of carbohydrates 1 to 3 hours before exercise.

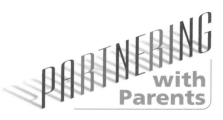

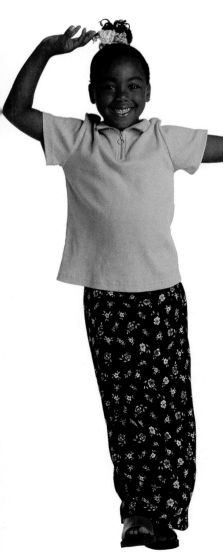

What activity restrictions are placed on children with cystic fibrosis?

Precautions vary widely. Pulmonary function and exercise stress tests can be helpful in establishing limitations in aerobic exercise.

cose, may help the child learn how to prevent exercise-induced complications. Teammates and coaches should be informed of the child's diabetes and taught how to recognize the signs and symptoms of hypoglycemia. Ready sources of glucose or carbohydrates should be available on the sideline.

Cystic Fibrosis

Cystic fibrosis (CF) occurs in 1 in 2,000 to 2,500 live births and is caused by an inherited defect of the cystic fibrosis transmembrane regulator protein (CFTR). In healthy individuals, the CFTR serves as a chloride channel in epithelial cells. Patients with cystic fibrosis have high concentrations of sodium chloride in their sweat and abnormally viscous mucus that often plugs the airways and ducts in exocrine glands, such as the pancreas. Over time, patients with CF may suffer from deterioration of lung function, loss of salt via the sweat, and exocrine and endocrine insufficiency of the pancreas, resulting in diabetes mellitus and malnutrition. Despite these problems, many patients with CF can participate in competitive sports and strenuous endurance events, such as marathons and triathlons.

Risks of Exercise

Patients with CF lose large amounts of sodium chloride through their sweat. Consequently, sweating does not increase serum osmolality. Therefore, thirst perception is impaired in patients with CF. As a result, patients with CF have an increased risk of dehydration and severe morbidity, particularly when they exercise in hot weather. In patients with advanced lung disease, desaturation of arterial oxygen occurs with exercise. This desaturation might indicate intrapulmonary right-to-left shunts or increased pressure in the pulmonary artery with right-to-left atrial shunting. In these patients, exercise may or may not add to the strain on the right heart and worsen cor pulmonale. Lastly, a type of diabetes mellitus (CF-related diabetes mellitus) will develop in about 10% of patients with CF.

Benefits of Exercise

For patients with CF, participation in physical activity increases fitness and improves their self-esteem and well-being. Specific benefits include enhanced clearance of mucus from the airways and increased strength and endurance of the muscles used in respiration. Some evidence suggests that a high level of physical activity and aerobic fitness may decrease morbidity and mortality in patients with CF.

Recommendations

Patients with CF should be encouraged to exercise as much as medically feasible. However, because of possible pulmonary decompensation caused by air trapping and a pneumothorax, scuba diving and mountain climbing should be discouraged. Before starting an exercise program, patients with advanced disease should undergo exercise testing, including oximetry, to determine an appropriate level of exercise. To prevent dehydration, patients should be encouraged to drink beverages containing salt every 15 to 20 minutes and to ingest salty foods during and after exercise, especially if they sweat a lot and ambient temperature is high. So far, the optimal concentration of sodium chloride in beverages for patients with CF has not been determined, but it should exceed 30 mmol/L. Commercially available drinks contain a lower concentration of sodium chloride, but offer better hydration than plain water.

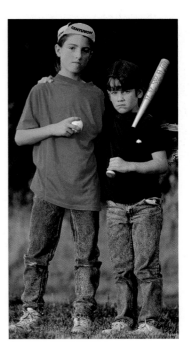

Juvenile Rheumatoid Arthritis

Juvenile rheumatoid arthritis is not a single entity, but denotes a variety of conditions that are characterized by prolonged and sometimes recurrent joint inflammation. However, most of these diseases also affect other organ systems, such as the heart, eyes, or hematopoietic system. Arthritis decreases the range of motion of affected joints and muscle wasting occurs. Also, bones adjacent to the joint weaken because of loss of mineral content.

Risks of Exercise

Exercise may induce flare-ups of arthritis that cause discomfort and limit physical activity. The affected joints may be prone to injuries because of cartilage attrition, subchondral cysts, and capsular laxity. Furthermore, the protection of surrounding muscles and ligaments deteriorates with progressive, inactivity-related atrophy. Also, the risk of fractures near the affected joints increases with increasing osteoporosis. Mortality related to exercise might increase for patients with cardiac involvement.

Benefits of Exercise

In addition to the general benefits of exercise, children with arthritis who participate in regular physical activity may achieve a better range of motion in affected joints, increase the strength of ligaments and muscles, and prevent the loss of bone mineral content.

Recommendations

Children should not be permitted to participate in sports that stress affected joints during times of acute joint inflammation. Contact sports and sports that place excessive stress on the joints, such as jogging, high-impact aerobics, and gymnastics, are higher risk, while walking, swimming, and bicycling at recreational levels may be better tolerated. All patients with systemic lupus erythematosus or HLA B27-associated arthritis should undergo electrocardiograms and echocardiograms to rule out cardiac involvement. These tests should be repeated subsequently if any signs of cardiac involvement appear. If exercise exacerbates the arthritis, cooling the joint may help to limit pain and swelling.

Epilepsy

Epilepsy is a chronic medical condition that causes randomly recurring seizures. In some patients, the seizures are provoked by flickering light, hyperventilation, missing sleep, alcohol, drugs, or sudden discontinuation of antiepileptic medication. Only in very rare cases, does exercise trigger a seizure. The overall prevalence of epilepsy in children below age 9 years is about 0.5%.

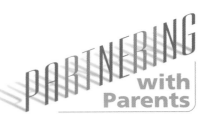

Our son has well-controlled epilepsy. Should he avoid any particular sports?

He should be able to participate in most sports. Sports such as scuba diving and mountain climbing should be avoided where the consequences of a seizure could be catastrophic. He should never swim alone.

Risks of Exercise

Commonly, a loss of consciousness occurs with epileptic seizures. Therefore, when seizures are not adequately controlled, some activities are potentially dangerous to the patient (eg, mountain climbing, diving, and swimming) or to others (eg, archery). The potential increase in physical and emotional stress from participation in sports may increase the risk of seizure activity.

Benefits of Exercise

Some evidence suggests that physical activity and a high level of fitness may have a protective effect against seizures. For a child with epilepsy, remaining active can be helpful to maintain self-esteem and general well-being.

Recommendations

Every athlete with epilepsy should be seen regularly by a physician who has experience treating seizure disorders. The decision to allow participation in sports should be based on the frequency of seizures, a possible relationship between seizures and exercise, the sport, and the athlete's adherence to anticonvulsant therapy. For high-risk sports, such as swimming, the athlete should have excellent control (ie, no seizures for 1 year or more) before participating. A few sports are considered absolute contraindications for patients with excellent epileptic control, including scuba diving, ski jumping, auto racing, motorcycling, and rodeo. For other sports, it may be helpful to consult a neurologist to assist with the risk assessment for the athlete and sport in question.

Hemophilia

Hemophilia is a disorder of inadequate blood clotting that presents with excessive bleeding. The most common types, A and B, are inherited as sex-linked recessive disorders. With hemophilia A, the level of factor VIII in the blood is decreased, and with hemophilia B, the concentration of factor IX is decreased. Because blood products occasionally contain infectious agents, patients with hemophilia were at high risk of acquiring blood-borne diseases such as HIV infection or hepatitis B or C during the 1980s, when blood was not tested and factor VIII concentrates were prepared insufficiently to eliminate such viruses. However, factor concentrates are now considered safe for these patients.

Risks of Exercise

If concentration of the factor in the plasma falls below 2% to 5% of normal, bleeding may occur with minimal trauma and may, in turn, affect the muscles and joints. Recurrent bleeding into the joints can cause hemophilic arthropathy. Children with hemophilia who have factor levels of 5% to 40% of normal have only a small risk of hemorrhage with everyday activities. However, they do have an increased risk of bleeding during surgery or after significant trauma.

Benefits of Exercise

Exercise may double the level of clotting factor in the blood, even in individuals with hemophilia. However, this benefit is clinically relevant only in the child who has a baseline level of clotting factor above 5% of normal. Exercise improves muscle strength and coordination and thereby, may improve joint stability and reduce the risk of injury.

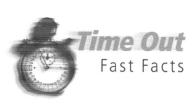

Time Out
Fast Facts

Athletes with hemophilia with factor levels of 5% to 40% have only a small risk of hemorrhaging with everyday activities. Trauma from sports may increase the risk of significant bleeds.

Recommendations

As a general rule, children with hemophilia should be encouraged to be active, even if physical activity occasionally induces bleeding. The choice of sport should be based on the level of clotting factor, interest of the child and parents in a specific type of sport, the stresses that the sport places on symptomatic joints, and the cooperation of the coach. In general, any child or adolescent with hemophilia should be advised not to engage in any sport that involves impact or collisions. However, swimming and other sports, at a recreational level, may be better tolerated. Children with a level of factor VIII or factor IX below 5% should not engage in any contact sports. They need to be restricted to archery, badminton, bicycling, dancing, fishing, golf, hiking, swimming, table tennis, and walking. Children with hemophilia and blood-borne infections (such as HIV infection) have only minor additional limitations on sports participation. Because contact sports and high-intensity exercise are discouraged anyway, sports participation is only impossible with end-stage disease.

If a child with hemophilia engages in sports, an emergency plan to treat bleeding is required. Whenever possible, the child should wear protective clothing and equipment. When bleeding occurs, cool the affected muscle or joint with cold compresses or ice packs and replenish the deficient clotting factor as soon as possible.

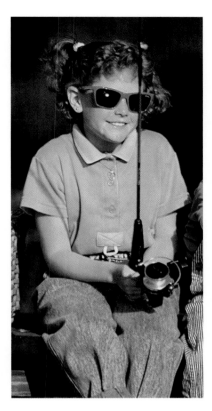

Cancer

Increasing numbers of young cancer patients are cured by chemotherapy and other therapies without major sequelae. The ability of these patients to engage in strenuous exercise is determined by the type, grade, and stage of the neoplasm itself, and also by the location of the tumor and the treatment regimen. In general, competitive sports should be avoided while cancer treatment is in progress. However, some physical activity should be encouraged during maintenance therapy. A patient who is cancer-free should be encouraged to participate in sports. However, drugs used in chemotherapy, such as anthracycline, can cause life-long effects on heart function. Currently, anthracycline is used in more than half of all young cancer patients. A cardiologist should evaluate these patients thoroughly before they engage in competitive sports.

FINISH LINE

Despite risks associated with chronic medical conditions, affected children should be encouraged to be physically active whenever possible. In many instances, the benefits of exercise will outweigh the risks and will increase the child's physical and emotional well-being.

For More Information

1. American Academy of Pediatrics, Committee on Sports Medicine and Fitness: Medical conditions affecting sports participation. *Pediatrics* 1994; 94:757–760.

2. Boas SR: Exercise recommendations for individuals with cystic fibrosis. *Sports Med* 1997;24:17–37.

3. Bar-Or O: Pathophysiological factors which limit the exercise capacity of the sick child. *Med Sci Sports Exerc* 1986;18:276–282.

4. Goldberg B (ed): *Sports and Exercise for Children with Chronic Health Conditions.* Champaign, IL, Human Kinetics, 1995.

5. Nixon PA, Orenstein DM, Kelsey SF, Doershuk CF: The prognostic value of exercise testing in patients with cystic fibrosis. *N Engl J Med* 1992;327:1785–1788.

Chapter 25

Blood-borne Pathogens

WILLIAM L. RISSER, MD, PhD

The risk of human immunodeficiency virus (HIV) infection, as well as infection through other blood-borne pathogens such as hepatitis B virus (HBV) and hepatitis C virus (HCV), is a major concern for many athletes, parents, and athletic programs. Immunization against hepatitis B virus is an important protective measure for everyone involved with athletic programs, including the laundry and janitorial staff. This chapter discusses issues related to infection and transmission of blood-borne pathogens in young athletes. The precautions outlined in this chapter for the prevention of exposure to blood and other body fluids visibly contaminated with blood should help to minimize the chance of transmission of infection among athletes, staff, and others.

Risk of Transmission and Sports Participation by Infected Athletes

During athletic activity, children and adolescents may be exposed to blood that is contaminated with HIV, HBV, or HCV. Exposure is most likely to occur in sports such as wrestling, football, or rugby, in which close physical contact occurs and bleeding wounds are common. Exposure can also occur from contact with blood on equipment, clothing, playing surfaces, or locker room floors. A list of recommended supplies and equipment for sideline wound care is provided in **Table 25.1**.

No cases of HIV transmission have been documented in the athletic setting, although an unsubstantiated report alleges that a professional Italian soccer player infected another player during a collision. Recent findings from studies of HIV transmission in health care settings are summarized in **Table 25.2**.

The risk of HIV transmission between athletes is almost certainly much lower than the risk posed to health care workers who are stuck with contaminated needles. Infection through mucous membranes or damaged skin appears to require prolonged exposure to large quantities of blood.

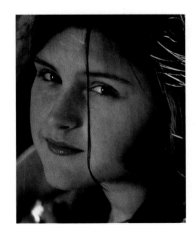

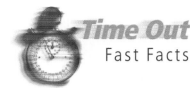
Fast Facts

Athletes are more likely to acquire HBV, HCV, and HIV through sexual activity or needle sharing than during athletic activity.

Table 25.1	Recommended Supplies and Equipment for Sideline Wound Care

- Gloves, disposable vinyl or latex
- Soap and water or alcohol-based antiseptic handwash
- Occlusive dressings
- Towels, disposable and nondisposable
- Bags for disposable blood-contaminated material
- Bags for nondisposable blood-contaminated material
- Basin for mixing bleach solution
- ¼ cup and 1 quart containers
- Clean uniforms
- Equipment for assisted ventilations
- Oral airways

Table 25.2	Routes of HIV Transmission in Health Care Settings

Type of Exposure	Infection Rate (95% confidence interval)
Needlesticks	0.2% to 0.3% (0.1% to 0.5%)
Exposure of mucous membranes or damaged skin	0.1% (0.01% to 0.5%)
Exposure of intact skin	0% (0.0% to 0.1%)

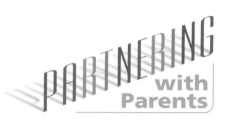
with Parents

How can I reduce my child's risk of acquiring infection with a blood-borne pathogen during sports?

Cover all wounds or skin lesions with a durable occlusive dressing. If the child is exposed, immediately cleanse the area with soap and water. Have the child vaccinated against HBV.

Findings like those above have led several sports medicine organizations to publish policy statements permitting sports participation for HIV-positive athletes, if their health allows. The risk of transmission of infection from HIV-positive athletes is felt to be extremely small, but cannot be assumed to be zero. The greatest risk of transmission continues to be through sexual activity. Thus, it is important to advise athletes to practice safe sex.

Athletes with HIV may be informed of the very small risk that they pose to others, so that these athletes can consider if they want to participate in sports that pose the greatest risk of contact with blood, such as wrestling or football. Health care providers are not authorized to notify the athletic staff or other athletes that a specific athlete is HIV-positive without the athlete's and his or her parents' informed consent. In addition to possible legal consequences, unauthorized disclosure of HIV status would probably cause the athlete to be excluded from participation. Furthermore, there are potential legal challenges to test athletes for blood-borne pathogens solely as a condition or consequence of their sports participation.

Coaches and staff should inform athletes and their families that the athletic program has a policy of nondisclosure of the infection status of athletes, and that a very small risk of transmission of HIV infection may exist in sports such as football and wrestling in which bleeding wounds and damaged skin are common. These guidelines also apply to athletes infected with HCV, although this condition is somewhat more easily transmitted than HIV.

The hepatitis B virus presents a greater transmission risk than either HCV or HIV. In Japan, a chronically infected sumo wrestler infected several of his high school team members, apparently by skin-to-skin contact. In Sweden,

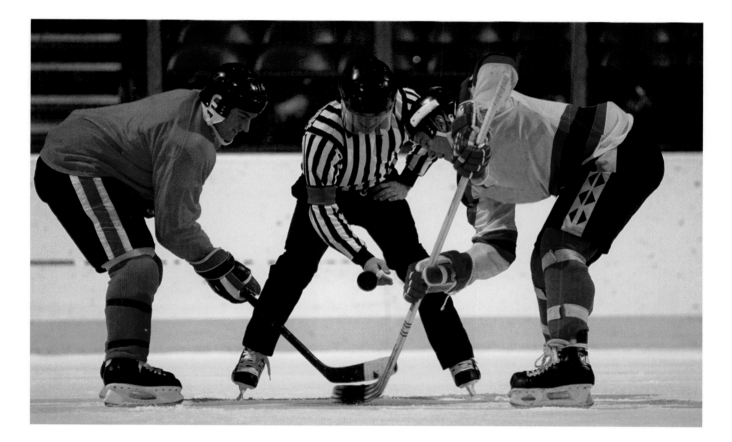

an epidemic of infection was documented among orienteers. Though the mode of transmission was not clear, the source of infection may have been basins of water that were contaminated with blood when used to wash open wounds. In health care workers, the risk of infection from percutaneous exposure to HBV may be as great as 45% if the blood is HBV e-antigen-positive.

Whether an athlete with chronic HBV should be allowed to play contact sports such as football, wrestling, or rugby is controversial. The National Collegiate Athletic Association (NCAA) recommends that athletes chronically infected with HBV "probably" should be excluded from collision sports, particularly if they are e-antigen-positive. The American Medical Society for Sports Medicine, the American Academy of Sports Medicine, and the American Academy of Pediatrics recognize the very small risk of transmission of HBV, but believe that the exclusion of chronically infected athletes from participation in sports is not warranted.

Prevention of Infection

A series of three vaccinations for HBV will protect almost all athletes from the very small risk of acquiring infection during sports participation and the greater risk of acquiring infection during sexual activity. Health care providers and coaches should urge young athletes, both children and adolescents, to be immunized if they were not immunized when they were younger. In many areas of the country, free HBV vaccinations are available to indigent youths. Because immunization in infancy has recently become standard practice, in the next few years most athletes will already have been vaccinated and probably have lifelong immunity.

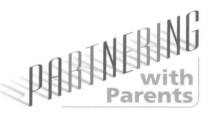

My 7-year-old child was vaccinated against HBV as an infant. Does he need a booster now or in the future?

Boosters are not currently recommended, but the longevity of protection is not known.

My daughter received the first two vaccinations 2 years ago, but never received the third. Do we have to start all over again?

No, there is no need to start over. Despite the time lapse, high seroconversion rates occur when the remaining doses are given at appropriate intervals.

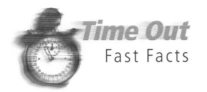

Time Out
Fast Facts

Exposure to blood-borne pathogens is most likely to occur in wrestling, football, and rugby.

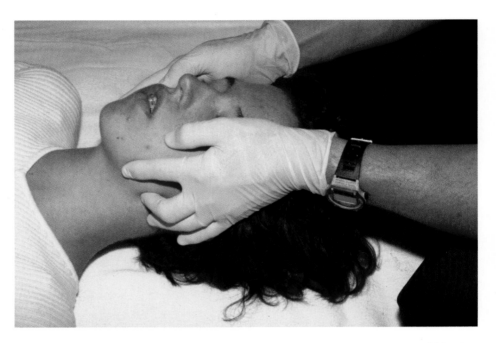

Figure 25.1 Latex gloves should always be worn when there is any chance of blood or body fluid contamination.

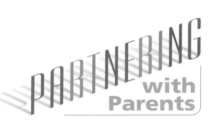

with Parents

Our daughter is HIV positive. Is it safe for her to participate in sports?

It is probably not detrimental for her to participate in sports. There may be a very small risk of infecting others in sports that are likely to result in exposure to blood or open wounds.

Administrators and coaches should initiate measures to prevent athletes from being exposed to blood and to protect those who have been exposed. It is particularly important to protect athletes and staff who may be exposed repeatedly, such as adults who give first aid, laundry workers, and cleaners who may handle bloody clothing or equipment (**Figure 25.1**). Several organizations have published guidelines for athletic settings that are based on recommendations by the Centers for Disease Control and Prevention (CDC) for health care providers and public safety workers.

A summary of the American Academy of Pediatrics' recommendations for handling blood-borne pathogens in the pediatric office are listed in **Table 25.3.** These recommendations are consistent with those written by the American Medical Society for Sports Medicine, the American Academy of Sports Medicine, and the CDC.

Implementation of these recommendations may require additional time and effort from the staff and administrators of athletic programs. However, the recommendations are not complex or demanding, and they may help protect staff and athletes from the small risk of contracting an infection with a blood-borne pathogen.

Effects of Infection on Performance

Strenuous exercise does not appear to increase the risk that athletes with asymptomatic HIV infection will become symptomatic, or adversely affect asymptomatic athletes who have HBV or HCV infections. Young athletes are rarely ill enough from symptomatic HIV infection that they will need to limit their participation in sports. Athletes who are acutely ill with a hepatitis virus should not participate until the fever is gone and they are feeling well enough. This may take several weeks.

Table 25.3 *Recommendations for Handling Blood-borne Pathogens*

1. Before and during participation, athletes and caregivers should cover damaged skin with an occlusive dressing that will remain intact during vigorous activity.

2. Athletes should be instructed to report bleeding wounds immediately. Athletes who are bleeding should be removed from play, and their wounds should be cleaned with soap and water or another skin antiseptic and covered with a durable, occlusive dressing.

3. Minor skin damage that is not bleeding may be cleaned and covered during scheduled breaks. During breaks, if an athlete's equipment or uniform is wet with blood, the equipment should be cleaned and disinfected (as described in #5) and the uniform replaced.

4. Those who treat injuries should wear disposable latex or vinyl gloves to avoid contact with blood or other body fluids visibly contaminated with blood and contaminated equipment or uniforms. After removing their gloves, medical personnel should wash their hands with soap and water or some other disinfectant.

5. Equipment and playing surfaces contaminated with blood must be cleaned until all visible blood is gone, and then disinfected with a freshly made bleach solution containing 1 part bleach in 10 parts water. The decontaminated equipment or area should be in contact with the bleach solution for at least 30 seconds. The area may be wiped with a disposable cloth after the minimum contact time or be allowed to air dry.

6. Bags used to assist with ventilation and oral airways should be available for use during resuscitation. Mouth-to-mouth resuscitation should only be performed if such equipment is not available.

7. Equipment handlers and laundry and janitorial staff should be trained in proper procedures for cleaning bloody surfaces and equipment and for handling washable or disposable materials that are contaminated with blood.

8. Depending on state regulations, school athletic programs may be required to comply with Occupational Safety and Health Administration (OSHA) or other guidelines for preventing infection. Even if it is not required, compliance with OSHA guidelines is a good way of protecting the staff.

9. Coaches and health care workers should educate athletes about the risks of transmission of blood-borne pathogens through sexual activity and needle-sharing during the use of illegal drugs, including anabolic steroids. Athletes should be taught not to share personal items such as razors, nail clippers, and toothbrushes that might be contaminated with blood.

Adapted with permission from Committee on Sports Medicine, American Academy of Pediatrics: Human Immunodeficiency virus and other blood-borne viral pathogens in the athletic setting. *Pediatrics* 1999;104:1400–1403.

FINISH LINE

Athletes and athletic program staff may have a very small risk of acquiring an infection with HIV, HBV, or HCV. Experts state that athletes infected with HIV or HCV may be allowed to play all sports. However, there is some disagreement about the participation of athletes chronically infected with HBV, especially if they are e-antigen-positive.

For More Information

1. Committee on Sports Medicine and Fitness, American Academy of Pediatrics: Human immunodeficiency virus and other blood-borne viral pathogens in the athletic setting. *Pediatrics* 1999;104:1400–1403.

2. American Academy of Pediatrics: *OSHA Materials to Assist the Pediatric Office in Implementing the Bloodborne Pathogen, Hazard Communication, and Other OSHA Standards,* ed 2. Elk Grove Village, IL, 1994.

3. The American Medical Society for Sports Medicine (AMSSM) and the American Academy of Sports Medicine: Human immunodeficiency virus and other blood-borne pathogens in sports. *Clin J Sport Med* 1995;5:199–204.

4. Guidelines for prevention of transmission of human immunodeficiency virus and hepatitis B virus to health-care and public-safety workers. *Morb Mortal Wkly Rep* 1989;38(suppl 6):1–37.

5. Mast EE, Goodman RA, Bond WW, Favero MS, Drotman DP: Transmission of blood-borne pathogens during sports: Risk and prevention. *Ann Intern Med* 1995;122:283–285.

Chapter 26

Skin Conditions

R O D N E Y   S . W .   B A S L E R ,   M D

While certain systems of the body, most notably the cardio-vascular, pulmonary, and musculoskeletal systems, benefit directly from physical activity, the integumentary (skin) system, by outward appearances, does not. Because the skin has direct contact with the environment, it often bears the burden of sports-related injuries and infections. With ever-increasing numbers of young children participating in sports activities, sports-related skin conditions will become more common. In addition, some skin diseases occur specifically or manifest differently in children and adolescents.

Injuries

Calluses and Corns

Common calluses are areas in which the stratum corneum, the outermost horny layer of the skin, becomes thickened with excess keratin (**Figure 26.1**). A corn is produced when the stratum corneum forms a conical mass that points down into the dermis, causing inflammation and pain. Most commonly seen on the feet, calluses and corns can develop anywhere the skin is subjected to friction or direct pressure. Golfers, gymnasts, and competitors in racquet sports, for example, can develop prominent calluses on their hands.

Calluses lack the tender spots seen in corns; therefore, calluses, unlike corns, are not painful or irritating. Treatment is often directed toward the prevention of blisters, which can form beneath calluses. After the affected area is soaked, the callus or corn can be pared using a pumice stone, file, or scalpel blade. Because this represents an area of friction, care should be taken to avoid removing too much excess stratum corneum. This could make the area even more tender. To reduce friction in the area, use of thin padding, or an orthotic, or a change in shoe wear should be considered.

Competitive athletes are prone to develop calluses, but simple measures such as wearing gloves and properly fitting shoes can often help prevent them.

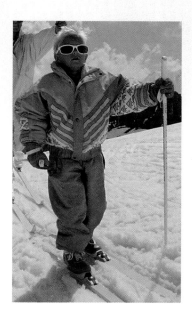

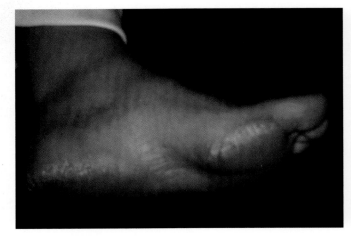

Figure 26.1 Callus

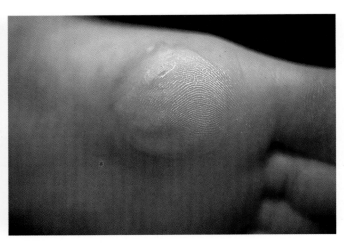

Figure 26.2 Blister

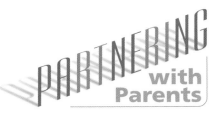

What is best way to prevent calluses?

Simple measures such as wearing gloves and taking care to have properly fitting shoes often helps prevent calluses.

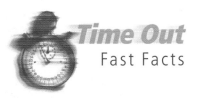

Chafing and bleeding of nipples is common in male endurance runners. Applying petroleum jelly before running and wearing a loose shirt helps.

Blisters

Blisters are tender vesicles that form at a site that is exposed to repetitive frictional or shearing forces (**Figure 26.2**). Nearly all sports expose the skin to these forces, so blisters are very common. Any moist environment softens the skin and promotes their formation.

Blisters may be filled with clear fluid or blood, depending on their severity and the site where they occur. They are best treated by draining the fluid up to three times in the first 24 hours following their appearance. The epidermal "roof" of the blister should remain intact to protect the newly forming epidermis. However, if by accident the covering skin is removed, a nonadhesive, permeable sterile membrane (DuoDerm) may be used to cover the blister for 5 to 7 days. This dressing will protect the site and promote healing.

Blisters may be prevented in a number of ways, including use of properly fitting shoes and maintaining sports equipment such as racquet grips. Also, athletic socks made of fabrics that "wick" moisture from the skin and the use of petroleum jelly to lubricate pressure points, or those parts of the foot that are in contact with the shoe, may both help prevent blister formation.

Chafing

Chafing, or irritation of the skin, occurs when opposing areas of the body, especially the inner thighs or the armpits when moist from sweat, rub together. Chafing may also occur from fabric-to-skin or equipment-to-skin contact. Tennis players and athletes who compete in endurance sports such as bicycling and cross-country running are particularly prone to this injury because of sustained, repetitive motion involved with these sports. While the inner thighs are more commonly involved, chafing may be seen also on the skin of the armpits and on the lateral aspect of the neck. In male endurance runners, chafing and bleeding of nipples is common. Application of petroleum jelly to the nipples before running and wearing a loose shirt can help.

Acute chafing is treated by applying cool compresses to the irritated area 15 to 20 minutes three times a day. When exudate is no longer weeping from the area, soothing ointments such as triple antibiotic ointment or petroleum jelly can be applied to lubricate the skin.

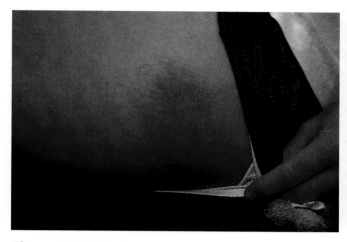

Figure 26.3 Abrasion

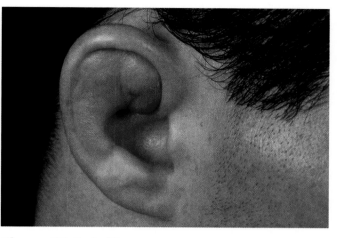

Figure 26.4 Cauliflower ear

Often, this problem can be prevented by wearing longer shorts made of fabrics, such as nylon, that minimize friction. "Bun hugger" athletic briefs, which are tight fitting briefs that extend to the midthigh, can be worn, and ointments can be used to lubricate vulnerable areas. Body powders may also reduce friction. Finally, weight loss can eliminate excess subcutaneous fat that makes upper thighs larger, resulting in a larger area of skin contact between this part of the legs.

Abrasions

Abrasions, also known as "turf burn," "mat burn," "road rash," or "strawberries," occur when the epidermis is scraped away by friction, causing punctate bleeding and exudate (**Figure 26.3**). Abrasions are localized to the area of skin that made contact with the friction-producing surface, such as artificial turf, the wooden floor of a basketball court, or a road surface.

Initial treatment should include cleansing the area with warm water and antibacterial soap or with hydrogen peroxide. Gravel or any other particulate matter should be debrided from the wound. A sterile nonadhesive membrane may then be applied to the wound and changed daily for several days. For deeper wounds, antibiotic cream or spray should be applied and then covered with a sterile nonadhesive membrane, which should be changed daily. Heavier ointments should be avoided, as they "hold in" infectious bacteria. Careful debridement, cleansing, topical antibiotic prophylaxis, and use of sterile nonadhesive membranes minimize the risk of secondary infection. Elbows, knees, and other vulnerable areas should be protected with additional clothing and pads to prevent abrasions.

Cauliflower Ear

Cauliflower ear is the thickening and distortion of the normal auricular cartilage caused by bleeding into the soft tissue of the ear (**Figure 26.4**). The inflammatory response to the blood causes destruction and scarring of the cartilage. Direct trauma or friction of the ear causes this injury, most commonly occurring in wrestlers, rugby players, and boxers who fail to use protective headgear or who use headgear that does not fit properly. A hematoma of the ear should be drained within the first several days following the injury.

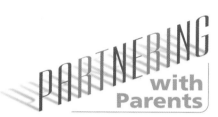

What is the first step in caring for an abrasion?

Cleanse the area with warm water and antibacterial soap or hydrogen peroxide, and then apply a sterile nonadhesive dressing.

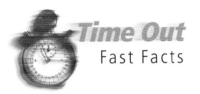

Time Out
Fast Facts

Cauliflower ear is thickening and distortion of the normal cartilage of the ear caused by bleeding in to the soft tissue between the cartilage and skin of the ear.

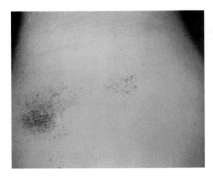

Figure 26.5 Talon noir (black heel)
Reproduced with permission from Basker RSW, Garcia MA: Acing common skin problems in tennis players. *Physician Sportsmed* 1998;26:38.

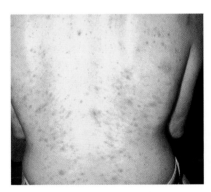

Figure 26.6 Acne mechanica
Reproduced with permission from Basker RSW, Garcia MA: Acing common skin problems in tennis players. *Physician Sportsmed* 1998;26:43.

Under sterile conditions, the blood can be aspirated with a syringe and small needle (23 or 21 gauge). The ear should be dressed with a compression dressing to prevent rebleeding. For the compression dressing, a variety of materials have been used successfully, including sterile saline-soaked cotton, flexible collodion, silicone putty, or plaster of Paris. Anything that molds to the contour of the ear will work. Gauze or elastic wrap needs to be wrapped around the head to provide gentle compression to the ear and dressing for at least 24 hours. Athletes should be advised to seek medical attention at the first sign of infection. The longer the wrestler can "stay off the mat," the less likely the ear will rebleed and the better the cosmetic result. Plastic surgeons generally do not consider any reconstructive surgery of a deformed ear until a wrestler has completed his career. Use of proper fitting headgear will usually prevent the injury.

Black Heel and Black Palm

Black heel, also called talon noir, is characterized by blue-black spots on the back or side of the heel (**Figure 26.5**). For reasons not totally understood, black heel primarily affects teenagers and young adults, especially basketball players. It is completely asymptomatic, and its palmar equivalent, black palm, affects weightlifters, golfers, and tennis players. This cutaneous curiosity requires no special diagnostic procedures or treatment, and as a rule, it resolves spontaneously at the end of the athletic season or when the athletic activity is stopped.

Acne Mechanica

The combined effects of heat, occlusion, pressure, and friction-caused especially by football and hockey equipment-lead to the appearance of inflammatory papules and pustules on the skin (**Figure 26.6**). Known as acne mechanica, this condition may be a flare-up of preexisting acne in teenagers or a new condition in prepubertal boys. As expected, acne mechanica tends to be localized under those areas that support the weight of athletic equipment, such as the shoulders, forehead, and chin in football and hockey players; the shoulders and lateral back of golfers who carry their bags; and the center of the back in weightlifters where they come into contact with the weight bench. If left untreated, cystic lesions may develop.

Systemic antibiotics do not work as well for acne mechanica as they do in treating standard acne vulgaris. Therefore, the affected area should be cleansed thoroughly after each workout with a mildly abrasive cleanser and brush. Topical astringents or 10% benzoyl peroxide often helps. The acne lesions tend to improve significantly or resolve completely at the end of the athletic season when the athletes no longer wear their equipment.

Football and hockey players should be advised to wear clean, absorbent tee shirts under their pads to prevent acne mechanica. During the off-season, the underlying acne vulgaris can be controlled with aggressive systemic and topical therapy.

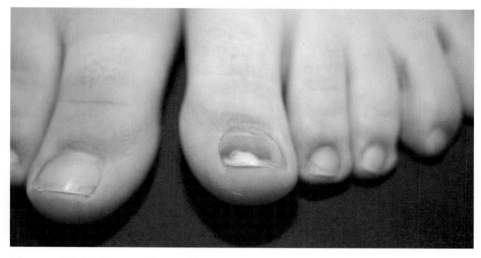

Figure 26.7 "Tennis toe" caused by hemorrhage under the nail.

Hemorrhage Under the Toenails and Fingernails

Sometimes displayed proudly by athletes as a type of "badge of courage," hemorrhage under the nails occurs in many sports, most notably running, skiing, bicycling, and tennis. In this last group, it is referred to as "tennis toe." In this type of injury, the body of the nail separates from the nail plate when the toes, for example, are repeatedly jammed into the front of the shoe (**Figure 26.7**). Although the pressure of the blood collecting under the nail plate can cause severe pain and disfigurement, serious medical consequences are rare.

In disabling cases when the patient reports such severe pain that he or she cannot walk, the blood can be drained from under the nail using a cauterizing instrument or a sterilized paper clip. In most instances, however, these hemorrhages can be treated nonsurgically with warm water soaks. Prevention includes trimming the great toe nails across in a straight line to a comfortable length. Athletic shoes must be fitted carefully for length and, more importantly, the height of the toe box.

Perniosis (Chilblains)

Perniosis, or chilblains, is an unusual injury to the skin caused by vasoconstriction in response to acute hypothermia. This condition is seen predominantly in teenage and young adult women for reasons that are not well understood, particularly in ice skaters and skiers. The distal segments of the toes, and occasionally the fingers, become blue or violet and are painful and exquisitely tender.

The simplest way to treat this condition is to advise the patient to wear heavy socks at all times, even while sleeping. Low-potency corticosteroid creams will help to eliminate inflammation without causing further vasoconstriction. To prevent perniosis, the use of any tightly fitting clothing or equipment such as gloves or ski boots should be avoided. When outdoors in cold weather, athletes should be reminded to rewarm the extremities whenever possible.

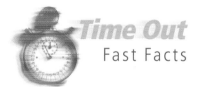
Time Out
Fast Facts

Chilblains occur when the ends of the toes, and occasionally the fingers, become blue or violet and are painful and exquisitely tender.

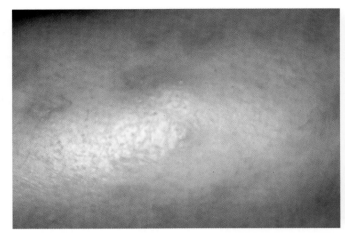

Figure 26.8 Occlusive folliculitis

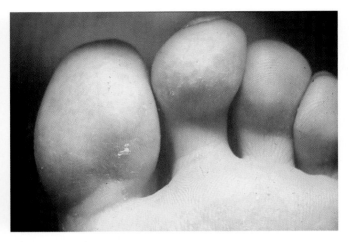

Figure 26.9 Pitted keratolysis

Infections

Occlusive Folliculitis

Occlusive folliculitis is a deep infection that is usually seen in the area under protective padding or swimsuits. Similar in appearance to acne mechanica, occlusive folliculitis produces more inflamed pustules (**Figure 26.8**). One of the more common examples of this condition is the "bikini bottom" that occurs in swimmers who wear their swimwear for long periods of time. The tender pustules may become cystic and appear in areas that coincide with the overlying clothing or equipment.

Although topical antibiotics such as clindamycin or erythromycin solutions may considerably improve mild cases, systemic antibiotics are often required. Prevention includes changing out of the swimwear as soon as possible after workouts or during long days at the beach. Also, absorbent powder applied to the involved areas after showering may also be beneficial.

Pitted Keratolysis

Malodorous footwear and athletic socks are a near universal finding among young athletes, especially young male athletes. With pitted keratolysis, however, a species of bacteria invades the epidermis and causes a particularly pungent foot odor. Besides the odor, the skin is marked by areas of white, macerated skin with distinct pits and surrounding areas of faint erythema (**Figure 26.9**). Excessive sweating is almost always present.

Affected areas should be cleansed with an antibacterial soap and treated with an over-the-counter acne preparation such as 10% benzoyl peroxide gel. Topical prescription products such as clindamycin and erythromycin solutions are also effective. Prevention includes washing the feet with an antibacterial soap, drying them with a towel, and then allowing the feet to air dry. Applying absorbent powder under socks is also quite helpful.

Plantar Warts

Plantar warts, the most common sports-related skin infection, are the painful and tender hyperkeratotic papules that can erupt anywhere on the soles of the feet. The combination of the macerating effect of perspiration,

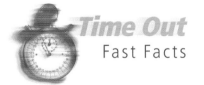

Time Out
Fast Facts

Plantar warts are painful, tender papules that can erupt anywhere on the soles of the feet. Apply a topical 40% salicylic acid plaster patch on the wart for 3 days and then remove the wart with a pumice stone.

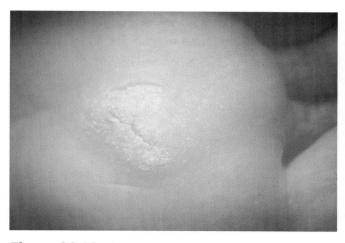

Figure 26.10 Plantar wart

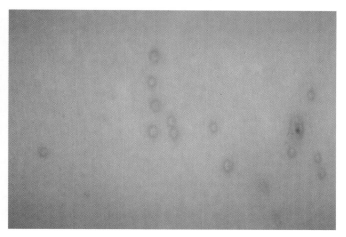

Figure 26.11 Molluscum contagiosum

exposure to the human papillomavirus, and the warm, moist environment of the locker room contribute to the development of plantar warts. In severe cases, symptoms can be nearly disabling, especially when the lesions occur over the weightbearing areas of the foot. Small black dots, which are the tips of capillaries in the skin, help differentiate these lesions from corns and calluses (**Figure 26.10**). Confluence of individual papules over a large area of the foot may result in "mosaic" plantar warts.

Aggressive therapies to excise and desiccate the wart with electric currents or lasers carry significant risks of short- and long-term disability, including the inability to walk, and can leave permanent scarring. More conservative approaches generally permit the athlete to continue competition during treatment. These include topical application of 40% salicylic acid plasters, which are left on the wart for 3 days and then vigorously pared. With mosaic warts, daily application of a solution of 5% salicylic acid and 30% formalin in ethanol is especially safe and effective. The use of shower thongs in the locker room and foot powders or a topical 10% aluminum chloride solution can diminish maceration of the skin.

Molluscum Contagiosum

Molluscum contagiosum is an infection caused by a virus of the pox group that is common among children and adolescents, particularly among young wrestlers who refer to them as "wrestler's warts" (**Figure 26.11**). Also seen with some frequency in swimmers, this infection is identified by its groups of small waxy, fleshy papules that often have central depressions or pits.

A small number of mollusca can be removed easily by curettage, although this procedure causes superficial epidermal abrasions. Freezing the papules with liquid nitrogen and then stripping them with a high-quality adhesive tape is one simple technique to treat the infection. Prevention consists primarily of avoiding infected competitors and aggressively removing lesions as soon as they appear to prevent self-inoculation. Infected wrestlers should not participate in practice or competition.

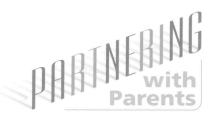

My son has wrestler's warts. Can he play if they are covered with occlusive dressings?

Infected wrestlers should not participate in practice or competition.

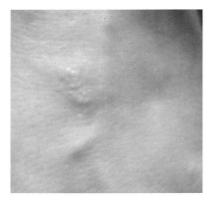

Figure 26.12 Herpes gladiatorum

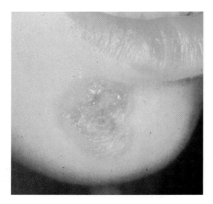

Figure 26.13 Impetigo

Herpes Gladiatorum

Herpes gladiatorum, or "wrestler's herpes," is a herpes simplex viral infection that most commonly affects the head, neck, and upper extremities. Its characteristic groups of vesicles appear on red, swollen edematous skin (**Figure 26.12**).

Systemic antiviral medications similar to those used against other types of herpes infection, including acyclovir, valcyclovir, and famcyclovir, are indicated. To promote healing, the epidermal "roof" of individual vesicles can be removed, followed by application of benzoin to the base of the lesion and injection of dilute triamcinolone intradermally under the infected areas. As with all of the skin infections in athletes, infected competitors should not wrestle until all the lesions are scabbed over, but noncontact conditioning is permissible. Contact with others must be avoided until the vesicles dry. In an athlete with a history of herpes infection, prophylaxis includes long-term, low-dose suppression therapy with one to two capsules of 400 mg acyclovir daily throughout the course of the season when the athlete may be exposed to infected individuals. Any wrestler with more than one outbreak in a season should be considered for suppression therapy.

Impetigo

Superficial bacterial infections, referred to as impetigo or pyoderma, can develop in association with nearly all contact sports and may reach epidemic proportions in wrestlers. Virulent bacterial strains, especially staphylococcal and streptococcal species, may be spread by direct contact or fomites such as equipment and improperly sterilized mats. Gymnasts are at risk for infection from abrasions received from gymnastic equipment, especially the pommel horse.

Impetigo presents as pustules or small purulent bullae on exposed areas of skin with predilection from those areas bordering mucous membranes, such as around the mouth and nose (**Figure 26.13**). These lesions rapidly progress to shallow erosions with a heavy yellow or honey-colored crust. Infected athletes cannot come into direct contact with other athletes or equipment until evidence of infection, specifically purulent drainage, has resolved. Careful attention to sterilization of mats and equipment on a regular schedule is mandatory. Athletes should be strongly encouraged to shower immediately after competition with an antibacterial soap.

Treatment of small areas of impetigo can be carried out by gently scrubbing the involved area, followed by the application of triple antibiotic or mupirocin cream three times daily. However, in most instances appropriate systemic antibiotic therapy is advised to reduce contagion and so that the athlete can return to competition as soon as possible.

Scabies

Although more correctly listed under the category of infestation rather than infection, scabies is another skin disease that can produce a "mini-epidemic" among members of an athletic team. Intense itching is the hallmark of this disease, sometimes spread by towels, uniforms, or equipment. Affected individuals usually have excoriated papules or small vesicles appearing in lines, and almost always on the webs of the fingers. Intensely pruritic papules on the skin of the penile shaft are characteristic signs of scabies.

Treatment of scabies must be aggressive and persistent. The drug of choice is 5% permethrin. Lindane and 10% crotamiton may also be used; however, 1% lotion, an effective scabicide, is still the gold standard of treatment. Permethrin should be removed by bathing after 8 to 14 hours, lindane after 8 to 12 hours, and crotamiton after 48 hours. Individuals with scabetic eczema can use corticosteroid cream to treat pruritis. As with the other skin infections, any athlete who has a suspicious rash—especially one with pruritic papules on the back of the hand, wrist, or webs of the fingers—should not compete or practice. The athlete may return to competition after appropriate treatment.

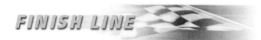

FINISH LINE

Skin conditions cause significant morbidity in athletes and may affect their ability to compete. Early recognition and treatment of many of these conditions will prevent or minimize time away from participation.

For More Information

1. Basler RS, Basler DL, Basler GC, Garcia MA: Cutaneous injuries in women athletes. *Dermatol Nurs* 1998;10:9–18.

2. Basler RSW: Managing skin problems in athletes, in Mellion MB, Walsh WM, Shelton GL (eds): *The Team Physician's Handbook*, ed 2. Philadelphia, PA, Hanley and Belfus, 1997, pp 35, 341–359.

3. Pharis DB, Teller C, Wolf JE Jr: Cutaneous manifestations of sports participation. *J Am Acad Dermatol* 1997;36(3 pt l):448–459.

4. Levine N: Dermatologic aspects of sports medicine. *Dermatol Nurs* 1994;6:179–186.

5. Bergfeld WF: Dermatologic problems in athletes. *Clin Sports Med* 1982;1:419–430.

5

Musculoskeletal Conditions

Section Editor
J. Andy Sullivan, MD

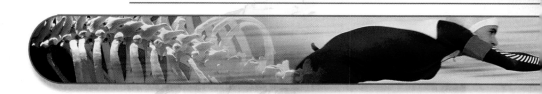

Chapter 27

Introduction to the Musculoskeletal System

J. ANDY SULLIVAN, MD

A child's skeleton differs from an adult's in many ways. These differences alter both the injury and the healing patterns that occur in children. A child's skeletal configuration becomes similar to that of an adult's around the age of 7 years. The bones continue to grow in length and width, reaching skeletal maturity at approximately age 14 years in girls and age 16 years in boys. This chapter introduces some of the most common terms and anatomic features of the musculoskeletal system. A glossary is also included in the appendices.

Anatomy

Bone Development and Structure

The most important anatomic difference between the skeleton of a child and that of an adult is the presence of the growth plate complex, consisting of the epiphysis, physis, and diaphysis (**Figure 27.1**). The primary ossification center is known as the epiphysis, which consists of the articular cartilage and the end of the long bone. The epiphysis grows circumferentially, producing the end of the bone. The physis is the cartilaginous plate, commonly referred to as the growth plate, located between the epiphysis and metaphysis. Cell division occurs here, resulting in enchondral growth and increased bone length. The physis is the weakest link in the bone-ligament complex. In an adult, if the knee is stressed to failure, the ligaments of the knee will rupture. In a child, the ligaments are stronger than the ability of the physis to remain intact, so failure usually occurs at the junction of the physis and metaphysis. This is very common about the knee and ankle.

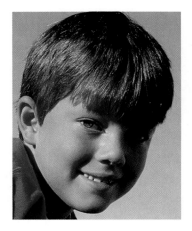

As a child nears skeletal maturity, the physis narrows and is gradually replaced by bone until it closes. The injuries produced at this time differ from those seen in immature children or in adults. This difference is most apparent in ankle injuries. In young athletes, fractures will most often occur parallel to the physis, while in adolescent athletes they will occur through the physis and into the articular surface.

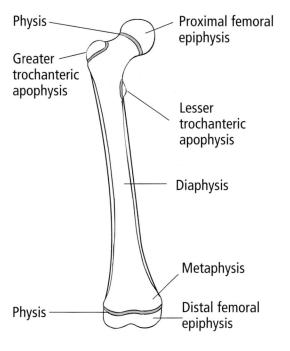

Physis — Proximal femoral epiphysis

Greater trochanteric apophysis

Lesser trochanteric apophysis

Diaphysis

Metaphysis

Physis — Distal femoral epiphysis

Figure 27.1
Components of a long bone.

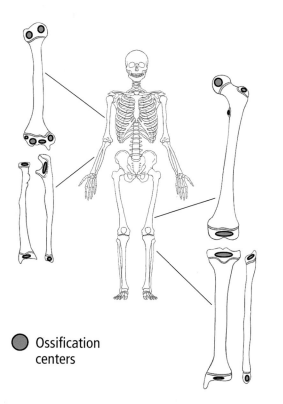

⬤ Ossification centers

Figure 27.2
Ossification centers of the upper and lower extremities.

The metaphysis is the area of the bone immediately adjacent to the physis. Enchondral ossification occurs here, producing bony trabeculae. The cortex is thin in the metaphysis and is the location of torus fractures. The bone then narrows down to the midshaft, an area called the diaphysis. In addition to this anatomic part of the bone, there is a fibrocartilaginous ring around the epiphysis called the perichondral ring. Here, bone grows radially, increasing the width of the epiphysis. This area is important in some injuries and conditions such as slipped capital femoral epiphysis.

Ossification centers appear at various ages from birth through full skeletal maturity (**Figure 27.2**). Both ossification centers and apophyses are often confused with fractures. An apophysis is an outgrowth, or prominence, of a bone that is responsible for the growth of a particular portion of the bone and provides a point of attachment for muscle groups. An example of an apophysis is the greater trochanter of the femur. With sufficient force, the muscles attached to apophyses can cause avulsion fractures. Though avulsion fractures occur most frequently about the pelvis, they can also occur through the base of the fifth metatarsal with an inversion injury of the foot, the medial epicondyle of the humerus with valgus strain at the elbow, and the transverse process of the lumbar spine.

A child's bones are more porous than an adult's, as they contain more collagen and cartilage. In fact, all long bones are first formed as cartilage models and gradually ossify, or convert into bone, until the skeleton fully matures. A child's bones are also more vascular, which contributes to their increased porosity and to their healing potential. The healing potential of a child's bones is much greater than that of an adult's. The periosteum has greater osteogenic, or bone-forming, potential and is also thicker and less likely to tear completely.

Figure 27.3 shows the principal bones in the body. In addition, a glossary of common orthopaedic terms is provided at the end of the chapter.

Anterior view

Posterior view

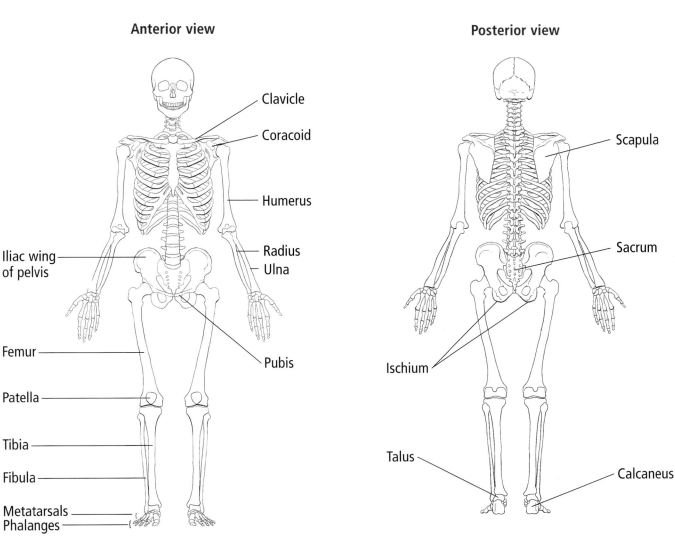

- Clavicle
- Coracoid
- Humerus
- Radius
- Ulna
- Pubis
- Iliac wing of pelvis
- Femur
- Patella
- Tibia
- Fibula
- Metatarsals
- Phalanges
- Scapula
- Sacrum
- Ischium
- Talus
- Calcaneus

Figure 27-3 Principal bones of the body.

Musculoskeletal Injuries

Fractures

A fracture is a break in the continuity of a bone. **Figure 27.4** summarizes the characteristics of different types of fractures. An open fracture is one in which the integrity of the skin is disrupted, allowing the fracture site to communicate with the outside environment. These fractures have been called compound fractures, but this term is confusing and should not be used. A closed fracture is one in which the integrity of the skin is maintained. A comminuted fracture is one in which there are more than three bone fragments. The presence of a butterfly fragment is an example of a comminuted fracture. In general, comminuted fractures are less common in children because of the porosity and elasticity of their immature bones.

When stressed, bone passes through several stages before the cortex breaks. With elastic deformation, the bone is deformed temporarily but returns to its original shape when the force is removed. With plastic deformation, the elastic limit is exceeded and the bone is deformed in shape, but the cortex is not broken.

Open fracture

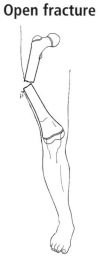

A fracture in which the skin is broken, exposing the fracture site to the environment

Closed fracture

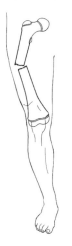

A fracture in which the skin is not broken

Comminuted fracture

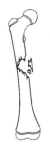

A fracture that results in three or more bone fragments

Spiral fracture

Force

A fracture caused by a twisting force that results in a spiral-shaped fracture line about the bone

Oblique fracture

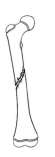

A fracture in which the fracture line is angled with respect to the long axis of the bone

Transverse fracture

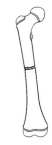

A fracture in which the fracture line is at a right angle to the long axis of the bone

Torus (buckle) fracture

A fracture that disrupts, but does not completely break the cortex (appears wrinkled or buckled)

Greenstick fracture

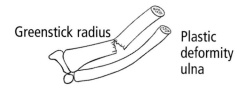

Greenstick radius

Plastic deformity ulna

A fracture that breaks one side of the cortex and causes plastic deformation of the other side

Figure 27.4 Characteristics of different types of fractures.

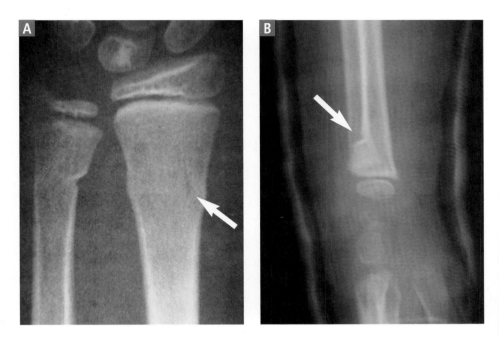

Figure 27.5
Torus fractures of the radius and ulna. **A** AP view showing the transverse line on the radius. **B** Lateral view showing buckle of the radial cortex.

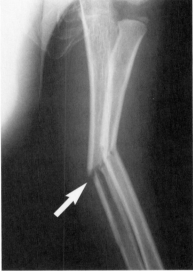

Figure 27.6 Greenstick fracture of the radius and ulna. Note one cortex is intact or in contact.

The second stage is characterized by torus, or buckle, fractures that disrupt but do not completely break the cortex. These fractures cause the cortex, usually in the metaphysis, to buckle or wrinkle (similar to wet cardboard in appearance) and may cause a transverse line to appear across the remainder of the bone, as seen on radiographs (**Figure 27.5**).

The next stage is characterized by greenstick fractures that break the cortex on one side of a bone and cause plastic deformation of the cortex on the opposite side of the bone, leaving the bone cracked and bent (**Figure 27.6**). Reduction of greenstick fractures often requires completing the fracture.

The last stage is characterized by three types of complete fractures: spiral, oblique, and transverse. Spiral fractures are caused by torsional or rotational forces, so the fracture line propagates in a spiral around the bone. With oblique fractures, the line of fracture is angled with respect to the long axis of a bone, whereas transverse fractures occur at a right angle to the long axis of a bone. Transverse fractures are usually the result of three-point bending of a long bone.

Dislocations

Dislocation is a term that is used to describe the complete dissociation of a joint. Less common in children than in adolescents, dislocations occur in the shoulder, the elbow, the hip, and more commonly, the interphalangeal joints of the fingers. A fracture-dislocation is the combination of a dislocation and a fracture near or within a joint. In children, fracture-dislocations are most common about the elbow, particularly with the Monteggia fracture in which the ulna fractures and the radial head dislocates (**Figure 27.7**). Elbow dislocations are often associated with fractures of the radial head and medial epicondyle.

With subluxation, a joint is displaced partially, but not dislocated completely. The most common examples of subluxation occur at the shoulder and/or the patella.

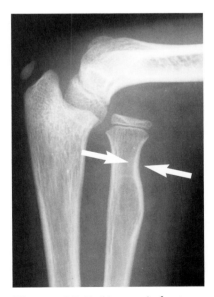

Figure 27.7 Monteggia fracture-dislocation in which the ulna is fractured and the radius is dislocated (not shown).

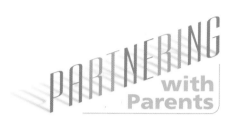

Sprains and Strains

A sprain is any injury to a ligament that ranges from a mild stretch to complete disruption of the ligament. Strain is a term used to describe an injury caused by stretching or exerting a portion of a muscle or a muscle-ligament complex beyond its limits.

Deformity, Deforming Forces, and Motion

A complete listing of the terms defined in this section is also provided in the glossary that appears at the end of the chapter.

Deformity and Deforming Forces

The terms varus and valgus can be confusing. Valgus is abduction (movement away from the midline) of a distal bone in relation to its proximal partner. Valgus of the knee or genu valgus, a knock-knee deformity, is abduction of the tibia in relation to the femur. Varus is adduction (movement toward the midline) of a distal bone in relation to its proximal partner (genu varus or bowlegs). This is more difficult to appreciate in the hip where the reference point is the greater trochanter. Coxa valga is an increase in the neck shaft angle, and coxa vara is a decreased angle.

Fracture deformity and forces can also be described by varus and valgus. A fracture with valgus deformity has the distal fragment displaced away from the midline. A valgus strain to the knee is one in which the tibia is forced away from the midline with the femur held stable. A varus force at the elbow forces the forearm toward the midline putting the lateral ligaments of the elbow under tension.

Motion

Several terms are commonly used to describe the motion of body parts relative to other body parts (**Figure 27.8**). Abduction describes any motion that carries a part of the body away from the midline, and adduction describes motion toward the midline. Flexion describes forward motion in the anatomic plane and extension describes backward motion. For example, in the anatomic position, the arm is rotated so that the palms face forward. Flexion of the elbow moves the forearm and hand forward, and extension moves them backward.

Pronation and supination describe motions of the hands and feet. With pronation, the palms of the hands turn down or backward, and with supination they turn up or forward. For example, in the upper extremity, the hands are pronated to use a keyboard, but supinated to accept change. In the feet, pronation is a combination of motions that lowers the arch or inside edge (flatfoot), and supination raises the inside edge of the foot (high arch foot). In runners who tend to pronate their feet, the inner edges of shoes wear out faster, while in those who supinate their feet, the outer edges wear out sooner. In fact, a pronated foot is very common and is often normal.

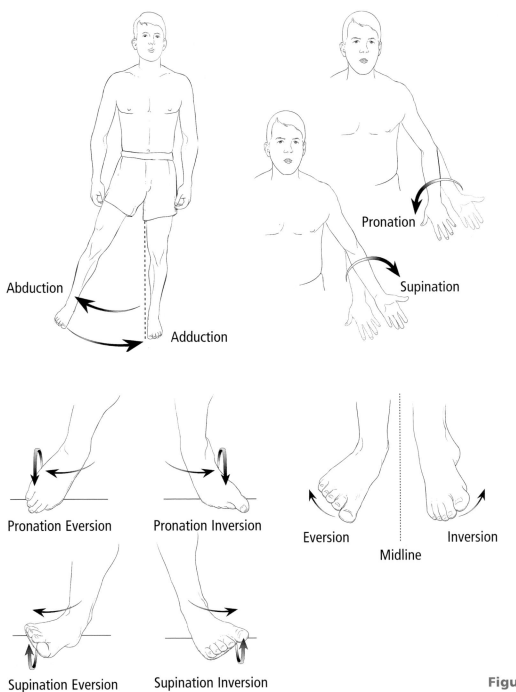

Figure 27.8 Types of motion

   Eversion and inversion are terms used to describe motions of the foot. Eversion of the foot turns the sole outward, away from the midline, and inversion turns the sole of the foot inward, toward the midline.

   Eversion, inversion, pronation, and supination are also used to describe motions about the ankle. Hence, a pronation-eversion injury would be one in which the inner edge of the foot rolls downward and inward, turning the sole upward and outward.

Table 27.1   *Basic Wound Care, Slings and Splinting Materials, and Equipment for the Office*

Wound Care Items

Topical antiseptic spray or swabs (Betadine, iodine)

Topical antibiotic ointment (Neosporin, Polysporin, etc.)

Tape - ½", 1" and 1½", both cloth and paper

Syringes (1, 5, 10, 20, 60 mL)

Suture removal kits, staple removal kits

Steri-Strips (¼", ½")

Sharps containers

Saline irrigation bottles (250, 500, 1000 mL)

Rubber gloves (sterile and nonsterile)

Needles (sizes: 18, 21, 23, 25, 27 gauge)

Medicated dressings (Xeroform, etc.)

Kerlix or Kling gauze wraps (2", 4", 6")

Hydrogen peroxide

Gauze pads (2" × 2", 4" × 4")

Elastic bandage wraps (2", 4", 6") (pick wraps with Velcro on the ends instead of metal clips)

Disposable scalpels (10, 11 and 15 blade)

Cotton applicators, cotton balls

Benzoin or Mastisol sticky spray or swabs/bullets, Collodium

Adhesive bandages (all sizes)

ABD pads

Casting and Splinting Materials

Stockinet (2", 3", 4", 6")

Webril or soft roll (2", 3", 4", 6")

Fiber glass rolls (2", 3", 4", 5")

Plaster rolls (2", 3", 4", 6") (optional)

Prefabricated fiberglass splint rolls (2", 3", 4", 5")

Moleskin (for padding the edges of the cast)

Cast shoes (S, M, L, XL)

Instruments and Tools

Tape or bandage scissors

Hemostat clamps

Heavy cast cutting shears

Electric cast saw with or without vacuum attachment

Protective ear phones (especially for when removing casts in children)

Water bucket (for dipping cast material)

Sink with plaster drain trap (to avoid clogging)

Suture kit - needle driver, hemostat, suture scissors, forceps, dissecting scissors, 4 × 4's, scalpel, sterile towels or drapes, Xylocaine, syringes, needles, suture (3-0, 4-0, 5-0 nonabsorbable), and sterile gloves

Instrument sterilization machine or fluid (or outside instrumentation sterilization service)

Otoscope/ophthalmoscope

Blood pressure cuff, stethoscope.

Woods lamp for foreign bodies in the eye, corneal abrasions, etc.

Medications*

Local anesthetics - 1% and 2% plain Xylocaine, 0.25% and 0.5% Marcaine with or without epinephrine

Injectable steroids

Acetaminophen (children's and adult, individual packets)

Ibuprofen (children's and adult, individual packets)

Benadryl (12.5 mg/25 mg, chewable)

Antacids (chewable)

Proventil/steroid MDI (inhalers)

IVF tubing, IVF bags, angiocaths (optional)

Soft Goods

Cast shoes (S, M, L, XL)

Hard and soft cervical collars (S, M, L)

Arm slings

Lateral epicondylitis straps ("tennis elbow")

Wrist splints

Foam/metal finger splints

Knee immobilizers or range-of-motion braces

Knee MCL braces, ACL braces

Simple Neoprene sleeves, Palumbo patella support braces

Velcro walking boots

Ankle braces (soft lace up and hard air cast)

Crutches (adult and child sizes)

Sport-specific items (football cervical collars, shoulder external rotation straps, etc.)

*Ensure medications are current.

Evaluating and Caring for Musculoskeletal Injuries

In evaluating a fracture or dislocation in a child, obtain a thorough history, including information about the mechanism of injury and previous injuries. The differential diagnosis of a fracture or dislocation includes sprains, strains, and contusions. Fractures about a joint may be difficult to differentiate from dislocations. Generally, dislocations are obvious unless obscured by swelling. During the physical examination, compare the injured joint or extremity with the uninjured one and note any abnormalities, including ligamentous laxity and tenderness. Early on, swelling and ecchymosis localize the injury, but later, hematomas dissect along fascial planes. Check range of motion in the joints and compare it with that of the uninjured extremity.

Splinting

After the physical examination, the extremity should be immobilized until the diagnosis is confirmed, usually by radiography. If there is any doubt about the type of injury, immobilize the injured part. Note that most office visits are for a strain or a sprain, neither of which usually requires any special supplies. Nonetheless, the office should be equipped with basic wound care items and casting/splinting materials for acute fractures or dislocations (**Table 27.1**). Keeping a small inventory of soft goods in the office can be very convenient for the patient, but a headache for the physician. Each physician should weigh the advantages and disadvantages of stocking such items before spending the time and money on the inventory. If a physician finds that it is not cost-effective or convenient to sell soft goods, athletes can be referred to local vendors or sporting goods shops when such items are needed. The medical brace bag on the sidelines should also have basic supplies (**Table 27.2**). Specific methods and devices for immobilizing injuries are outlined in individual chapters, but a few general principles apply.

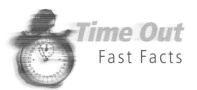

Time Out
Fast Facts

Common splinting materials for the office and sideline include wrist splints, ankle stirrups, back boards, sand bags, and plaster molds/splints.

Table 27.2 *Equipment for On-Field Brace Bag**
Large duffel bag
Hard cervical collars (S, M, L)
Arm slings (S, M, L, XL)
Long arm metal splint (posterior splint)
Elbow pads
Wrist splints
Foam/metal finger splints
Knee immobilizers
Knee pads
Short leg metal splint (posterior splint)
Ankle braces (soft lace up and hard air cast)
Crutches (adult and child sizes)
Sport-specific items (football cervical collars, shoulder external rotation straps, etc.)
*Label reusable equipment with your name and phone number.

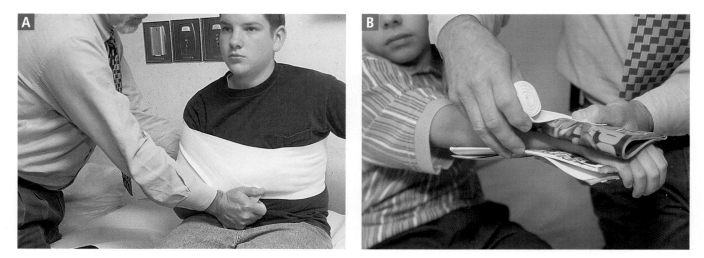

Figure 27.9 Splinting the upper extremity. **A** Use of an elastic bandage to splint the upper extremity to the body. **B** Use of a magazine and elastic bandage splint.

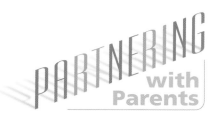

Are dislocations common in children?

Dislocations are less common in children than in adolescents and even less common than in adults.

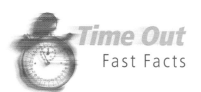

Bleeding is best controlled by direct pressure, or compression, over the bleeding area.

In an emergency, slings can be devised from a variety of articles of clothing or the arm can be wrapped to the body (**Figure 27.9**). Magazines or newspapers wrapped with an elastic bandage can be used to splint a forearm. Pillows can be used to splint the tibia or femur to the other leg. A rolled towel can be wrapped around the neck and secured with a safety pin to serve as a collar.

Gently realigning a fractured extremity while applying a splint may improve the circulation to the injured limb. However, dislocations should be splinted in the position in which they are found, without any attempt at on-field relocation until radiographs confirm the specific injury. For example, what appears to be a dislocated elbow may be a supracondylar fracture of the humerus. In addition, pulse and nerve function distal to an injury should be monitored frequently. Absence of a pulse or of nerve function necessitates urgent evaluation at the emergency department.

Controlling Bleeding

Any open injury should be covered in as sterile a manner as possible, with the coach, athletic trainer, or physician ensuring that universal precautions are followed. Almost all bleeding can be controlled by applying direct manual pressure, followed by a compression bandage. If the first bandage does not control bleeding, add another bandage on top of the first one, apply additional manual pressure, and arrange for transport to the emergency department. Tourniquets are dangerous and should not be used.

Any open injury in which a fracture or dislocation is suspected should be evaluated and treated as an emergency. All open fractures or dislocations require surgical debridement and irrigation. Therefore, if a fracture or dislocation is suspected, it is wise to refrain from giving the athlete anything to eat or drink until he or she is evaluated at the hospital. This precaution will prevent any delay in treatment if sedation or anesthesia is required.

Fractures and Healing

Fractures heal in three phases: an inflammatory phase, a reparative phase, and finally, a remodeling phase (**Figure 27.10**).

When a bone absorbs a force, except a pure compression force, one side of the cortex experiences compression while the opposite side experiences tension. In children, the periosteum is thick and strong and often remains intact on the compressed side and tears on, or is dissected off, the tensed side.

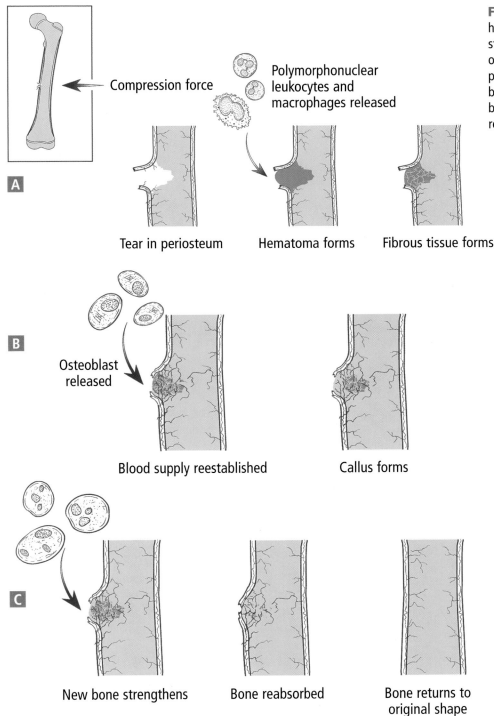

Figure 27.10 Phases of fracture healing. **A** Early inflammatory stages of healing. **B** Enchondral ossification occurs in the second phase. **C** In the third phase, new bone formation strengthens the bone, and the bone absorption remodels to restore its normal shape.

Compression force

Polymorphonuclear leukocytes and macrophages released

A

Tear in periosteum   Hematoma forms   Fibrous tissue forms

B

Osteoblast released

Blood supply reestablished   Callus forms

C

New bone strengthens   Bone reabsorbed   Bone returns to original shape

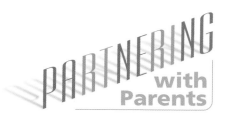

Is a fracture the same as a break?

A fracture is a break in the continuity of any bone.

How do a child's bones differ from an adult's?

Children have a growth plate complex or physis in their bones, whereas adults do not. The biomechanical properties of children's bones are different as well.

Is the growth plate susceptible to injury?

Yes. Ligaments are stronger than the growth plate, so failure during injury occurs, not at the ligaments as in adults, but at the junction of the growth plate and metaphysis bone. The growth plate can also fracture.

During the inflammatory phase, the ruptured blood vessels and medullary canal bleed, causing hematomas to form around the ends of the fractured bone. Polymorphonuclear leukocytes and macrophages are also released. The periosteum is a prime source of new bone and contains the hematoma that organizes during this phase and gradually changes to fibrous tissue. Enchondral ossification will occur in the organizing hematoma. The child may be febrile during this phase, especially if the hematoma is large.

During the reparative phase, enchondral ossification will form bone in the fractured hematoma. This is the same process that occurs at the ends of long bones in the embryo. The blood supply is reestablished to the area, and the callus gradually joins the two ends of the bone. This repair occurs more rapidly in children than in adults.

During the remodeling phase, bone formation continues to increase the strength of the newly formed bone. Osteoclastic activity causes bone reabsorption and returns the bone to its original shape.

There are many reasons that children generally heal more quickly and easily than adults. First, children have a much greater potential for bone healing than do adults, and younger children have an even better potential for remodeling. Second, the periosteum in children has a greater osteoblastic potential and increased vascularity. Third, children rarely experience the same complications from fractures as do adults. For example, delayed union, or healing that occurs much later than expected, is very unusual in children. Nonunion (failure of the bone to heal) and stiffness in adjacent joints also rarely occur in children because they have better peripheral circulation than do adults.

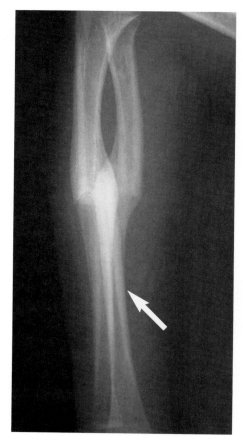

Finally, fractures may actually stimulate bones to grow in children. For example, in younger children, femur fractures that are reduced end to end may cause the bone to grow in length so that the healed leg becomes longer than the uninjured extremity. In some of these fractures, Bayonet apposition (side to side) is acceptable and, at times, desired (**Figure 27.11**).

Figure 27.11 Despite the appearance of the radius and ulna on this radiograph, function was nearly normal.

Tips on Fracture Healing in Children

1. Remodeling occurs more rapidly in fractures that occur near the physis. In general, physeal fractures heal about twice as quickly as fractures of the long bones to which they are attached. For example, radial physeal fractures will often heal in 4 weeks compared with radial shaft fractures that heal in 6 to 8 weeks.

2. Remodeling potential is greatest at the ends of bones that have the potential for growth. In the upper extremity, most growth occurs at the proximal humerus and distal radius, whereas in the lower extremity, most growth occurs at the distal femur and proximal tibia.

3. Angular deformity is more likely to remodel if it is in the same plane as the adjacent joint. Dorsal angulation at the wrist is more likely to resolve than radial or ulnar deformity.

4. Remodeling will not correct rotational deformity or intra-articular displacement.

5. Since a fracture callus will become rubbery in the inflammatory phase, the fracture will be difficult to manipulate after 10 to 14 days. In fact, a physeal fracture should not be manipulated after 5 to 7 days, except under unusual circumstances. After 5 to 7 days, the risk of damage to the physis and harm to growth are more likely to exceed the benefit of any change in position.

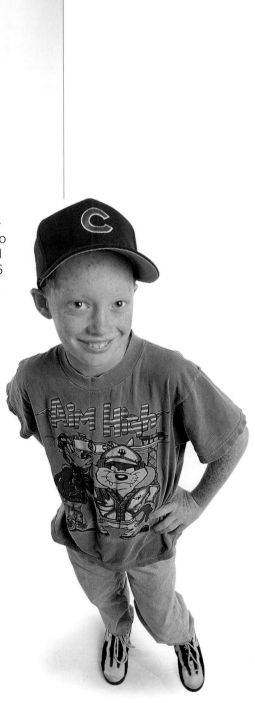

Glossary of Common Orthopaedic Terms

Arthrodesis: The surgical process of promoting bone growth across a joint to eliminate the joint and stop motion. The usual purpose is relief of pain or stabilization of a severely damaged or destroyed joint.

Capsule: A complex ligamentous structure surrounding a joint like a sleeve. It is a composite of ligaments, tendon expansions, and tendon attachments. The capsule allows motion of joints while stabilizing them, especially in rotation.

Cartilage: A cellular tissue that, in the adult, is specific to joints, but in children forms a template for bone formation and growth. Hyaline cartilage is a low-friction cellular tissue that coats joint surfaces. Fibrocartilage is tough with high collagen content, such as found in the meniscus of the knee, or the annulus fibrosus portion of the intervertebral disk.

Closed fracture: A fracture in which the integrity of the surrounding skin is intact.

Closed reduction: A procedure in which normal relationships are restored to a fractured bone or dislocated joint; no incision is needed.

Condyle: The knobby portion of the end of a long bone that articulates with another bone through a joint and serves as a point of attachment for tendons and ligaments.

Cox-, Coxa hip: Coxa vara is a varus, or adduction, deformity of the hip.

Cubitus (Elbow): Cubitus varus is a bow or adduction deformity of the elbow.

Delayed union: A delay in normal fracture healing; not necessarily a pathologic process.

Diaphysis: The shaft of a bone; the portion between the metaphyses at either end.

Dislocation: A disruption in the relationship of two bones forming a joint in which the bones have (at least momentarily) completely moved out of their normal positions. Usually, bones lie alongside one another, locked in that position until replaced by a closed or open reduction.

Epiphysis: The end of a bone; the portion that articulates with an adjacent bone to form a joint.

Extensor: Relating to the extensor side of a limb, usually the posterior surface, but is anterior on the leg from embryonic limb rotation.

External fixation: Surgical insertion of pins through the skin that are then attached to an external frame to stabilize a fracture or joint.

Flexor: Relating to the flexor side of a limb, usually the anterior surface, but is posterior on the leg from embryonic limb rotation.

Fracture: A disruption in the integrity of a bone.

Fracture-dislocation: A fracture of bone associated with a dislocation of its adjacent joint.

Fusion (Arthrodesis): A biologic "welding" process in which adjacent joint surfaces are excised to facilitate bony growth from one side of the joint to the other and stop painful joint motion. In the spine, bone graft material "welds" two vertebral bodies to create a single bone and stop motion of the adjacent vertebrae.

Genu (Knee): Genu valgum is a knock-knee deformity; genu varum is a bowleg deformity.

Internal fixation: Surgical insertion of a device that stops motion across a fracture or joint to encourage bony healing or fusion.

Kyphosis: A deformity of the spine in which the spine bends forward.

Ligament: A collagenous tissue that either binds together two bones to form a joint, or acts to suspend a structure in a certain position.

Lordosis: A deformity of the spine in which the spine sways, or extends backwards.

Malunion: Healing of a fracture in an unacceptable position. Malunions are worst when they angulate the bone away from the plane of motion of the adjacent joints.

Meniscus: A fibrocartilage structure in the knee, interposed between the femur and tibia on the medial and lateral sides.

Metaphysis: The broad portion of the bone adjacent to a joint.

Myelopathy: An abnormal condition of the spinal cord, whether through disease or compression. The usual consequences are spasticity, impairment of sensation, and impairment of bowel and bladder function.

Neuropathy: An abnormal condition involving a peripheral nerve.

Nonunion: Failure of a fracture to heal. With continued motion through a nonunion, a pseudarthrosis will form.

Open fracture: A fracture that communicates with air through a disruption of the skin.

Open reduction: An open surgical procedure in which normal or near-normal relationships are restored to a fractured bone or dislocated joint.

Osteomyelitis: Infection of bone, either bacterial or mycotic. These infections may be lifelong and are difficult to treat.

Osteonecrosis: Literally, death of bone. This term is also known as aseptic necrosis, or death of bone in the absence of infection. In children, it occurs in Legg-Calvé-Perthes disease, and in adults may occur in the femoral head (in association with alcoholism) or in the medial tibial plateau. Removing dead bone and laying down new bone is an incredibly slow process; the surrounding bony architecture usually collapses before the process occurs, leaving irreversible bony deformity and arthritis.

Osteosynthesis: The process of bony union, as in fracture healing. It is a biologic welding process that is sometimes facilitated with grafts of bone from the iliac crest and insertion of fixation devices.

Palmar: The anterior surface of the forearm, wrist, and hand.

Percutaneous pinning: Insertion of pins into bone through small puncture wounds in the skin for stabilization of a fracture or a dislocated joint that was realigned by closed reduction.

Physis: The growth plate. It is interposed between the metaphysis and epiphysis and is cartilaginous in structure.

Plantar: The sole, or flexor surface of the foot.

Pseudarthrosis: A false joint produced when a fracture fails to heal. It develops a pseudocapsule and synovial-like fluid.

Scoliosis: A deformity of the spine in which the spine bends to the right or left. With double curves, one may be to the right and the other to the left. Curves to the left in the thoracic region may be from an intraspinal tumor.

Septic arthritis: Infection of a joint, either bacterial or mycotic.

Spondylolisthesis: A slippage or subluxation of one vertebral body on the one below; the slippage can be anterior, posterior, or to either the right or left side. The common causes are degenerative changes in the disk and facet structures in adults, and a specific defect in the lamina called spondylolysis, which appears at or before early adolescence and creates a deformity that persists throughout life.

Subluxation: An incomplete disruption in the relationship of two bones forming a joint. The joint surfaces are still related to one another, but are not perfectly aligned.

Synovium: The lining of a joint that produces synovial fluid for joint lubrication.

Tendon: A highly collagenous tissue attached to muscle at one end and to a bone at the other. It transmits forces of muscular contraction to cause motion across a joint.

Tenosynovium: The sheath within which a tendon glides as it transmits muscle forces across joints.

Trochlea: A groove in a bone that articulates with another bone, or serves as a channel for a tendon to track in.

Valgus: Abduction of a distal bone in relation to its proximal partner. Valgus of the knee is a knock-knee deformity, with abduction of the tibia in relation to the femur.

Varus: Adduction of a distal bone in relation to its proximal partner. Varus of the knee is a bowleg deformity, with adduction of the tibia in relation to the femur.

Volar: The anterior surface of the forearm, wrist, and hand.

FINISH LINE

The fact that the young athlete's skeleton is still growing offers bene-fits and risks over their adult counterparts. In the child, alignment does not have to be perfect if there is sufficient growth left for remodeling to occur. The disadvantage is that the growth plate is a weak link and, if injured, can cease to grow fully or partially or can cause angular deformity or limb-length inequality.

Fractures heal more rapidly in children. Most fractures can be man-aged with closed techniques and casting and typically heal in 4 to 8 weeks. Surgical treatment is rarely needed. Nonunion is rare.

Physeal fractures, open fractures, and angular deformity about the joint are considered urgent conditions and require specialized care.

For More Information

1. Green NE, Swiontkowski MF (eds): *Skeletal Trauma in Children*, ed 2. Philadelphia, PA, WB Saunders, 1998.

2. Letts RM, Baxter MP (eds): *Management of Pediatric Fractures.* New York, NY, Churchill Livingstone, 1994.

3. Stanitski CL, DeLee JC, Drez D Jr (eds): *Pediatric and Adolescent Sports Medicine.* Philadelphia, PA, WB Saunders, 1994, vol 3.

Diagnostic Imaging

W E Y T O N   T A M ,   M D

C hanges in computer technology over the past decade have produced a number of highly sophisticated imaging modalities, such as computed tomography (CT), magnetic resonance imaging (MRI), ultrasonography, and scintigraphy (bone scans). Given the wide variety of high-quality images available today, physicians must understand the indications for and the appropriate time to order specific images.

Guidelines for Ordering Imaging Studies

Lack of communication is the enemy of patient care, whether it is between physician and patient or between physicians. Therefore, in the initial communication with the radiologist, physicians must specify the exact areas to be evaluated, the views desired, and the diagnoses under consideration. Inadequate communication may result in an order for an inadequate or inappropriate study. Providing a clinical history for the radiologist can help in the selection and interpretation of an appropriate imaging study. This is especially true with the more sophisticated imaging modalities. In clinically confusing cases, consultation with the radiologist helps to direct the approach to the study and often improves the final interpretation.

Obtaining previous imaging studies, when available, may better focus the diagnostic possibilities by showing how the patient's condition has changed over time. Often, prior related imaging studies or their reports are available. Therefore, whenever possible, all imaging studies should be interpreted in conjunction with a review of all other previously related images. If these previous reports or images originate from another facility, they should be made available to the consulting radiologist.

Comparison views of the contralateral extremity are helpful because children have multiple ossification centers at various stages of maturity. However, in the absence of a comparison view, refer to standard imaging texts, such as Keats' *Atlas of Normal Roentgen Variants*. By consulting this type of reference, the additional expense of imaging and the resulting irradiation of the contralateral normal extremity can be avoided.

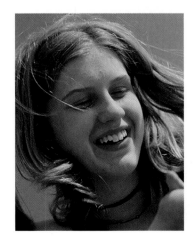

Figure 28.1
Imaging of the young athlete.

RADIOGRAPH
• acute trauma to bone or soft tissue
• bone or joint pain
• myositis ossificans

CONSIDER CONSULTING RADIOLOGIST
• if unsure of imaging modality of choice
• if complex case
• if unsure of necessity of intravenous contrast

FURTHER RADIOGRAPHIC IMAGING

COMPUTED TOMOGRAPHY
• detailed evaluation of complex or intra-articular fracture
• acute head or visceral trauma
• further evaluation of potential myositis ossificans

MAGNETIC RESONANCE
• soft-tissue trauma (joint, muscle, bone marrow) or infection to extremities
• combination of soft-tissue and bone trauma
• problem solver

BONE SCAN
• excellent sensitivity, poor specificity
• confirm infection or occult fracture
• reflex sympathetic dystrophy

ARTHOGRAPHY
• aging technique, used for evaluation of rotator cuff or TFCC tear
• increasingly used in combination with MRI for glenoid and acetabular labral tears

ANGIOGRAPHY
• detailed evaluation of vessels, especially with altered distal pulses
• especially with extremity dislocation
• especially with displaced extremity fracture

FOLLOW-UP RADIOGRAPH (10–14 DAYS)
• confirms occult fracture

STRESS VIEWS
• ligamentous injury
• physeal plate injury
• further evaluation of potential myositis ossificans

COMPARISON VIEW OF CONTRALATERAL EXTREMITY
• ligamentous injury
• physeal plate injury
• consider use of standard reference text

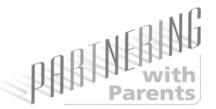

A bone scan to check a stress fracture is a useful radiographic technique. What is it?

Bone scans are used to evaluate occult or stress fractures, osteomyelitis, and occasionally, reflex sympathetic dystrophy. It is a radiographic procedure involving an injection and a low dose radioisotope. The patient is scanned several hours later and the isotope is "picked up" on the scan in the injured areas.

Common Imaging Techniques

Figure 28.1 shows the suggested hierarchy for ordering imaging studies for the young athlete.

Radiography

Conventional radiography (X ray) is the mainstay of imaging. With few exceptions, almost all imaging should begin with radiographs, especially for those patients with a history of trauma. Radiographs are almost universally available, inexpensive, and require the least amount of imaging time. Indications include acute bone trauma; soft-tissue, bone or joint pain; screening for radiopaque foreign bodies; and evaluation of bone infection.

Follow-up radiographs in 7 to 14 days provide an inexpensive means of confirming a diagnosis of radiographically occult fractures (**Figure 28.2**). At times, however, in circumstances that require a rapid diagnosis (eg, an athlete with an upcoming competition), the more sophisticated and costly imaging techniques such as a CT scan, MRI, or bone scan should be considered.

Anteroposterior and lateral views

Anteroposterior (AP) and lateral views should be obtained in patients with traumatic injuries, whenever clinically possible. Radiographs of the extremities, especially those involving the forearm or leg, should include the joint above and below the involved bone. At the very least, two views obtained at 90° from one another should be obtained.

Stress views

Stress views allow for indirect evaluation of ligamentous injuries. These views include, but are not limited to, flexion-extension views of the cervical spine, weightbearing views, and varus-valgus stress views. The joint of interest can either be stressed by the physician, the radiology technician, the patient (weightbearing), or by the use of weights. Note that if the patient has acute trauma, the presence of a physician is often required when obtaining stress views.

Flexion-extension views of the cervical spine obtained following acute trauma can evaluate spinal stability. However, obtaining these views requires that the patient be conscious and able to communicate the presence of neurologic change, such as pain or dysesthesia. These views should be actively performed by the patient, with a physician supporting the head (**Figure 28.3**).

Figure 28.2 Follow-up radiographs are useful for identifying some suspected fractures. **A** Normal AP view. **B** Normal lateral view. **C,D** Repeat radiograph 3 weeks later show periosteal new bone consistent with an undisplaced fracture.

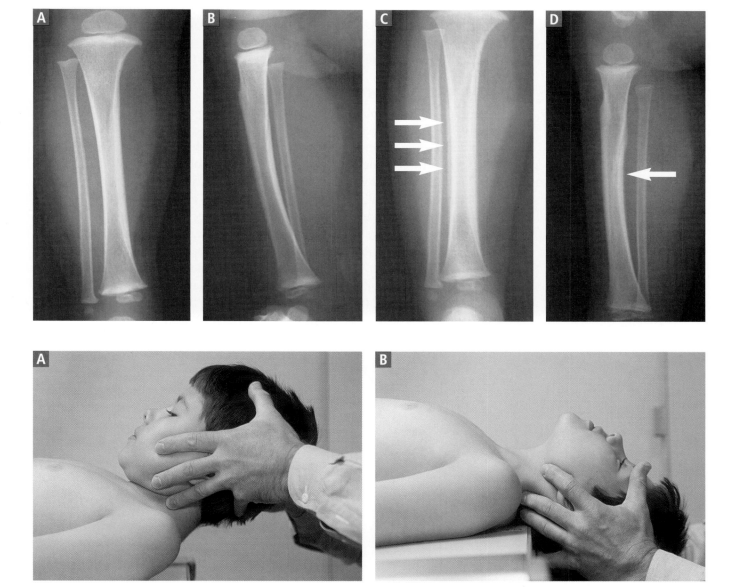

Figure 28.3 Positioning the patient for flexion-extension views of the cervical spine. Physically support the head while the patient actively **A** flexes and **B** extends the head.

In skeletally immature patients, gentle stress views under direct fluoroscopic supervision may reveal an occult physeal plate injury.

Weightbearing views may accentuate a hip subluxation not evident on a typical supine view, and use of weights may demonstrate or accentuate an acromioclavicular joint separation.

An AP clenched fist view of the wrist stresses the scapholunate ligament, accentuating a scapholunate dissociation.

Varus-valgus stressing of the thumb can be used to confirm an ulnar collateral ligament injury.

Other views

Radiographs of the chest, abdomen, and pelvis are routinely obtained following traumatic injuries to these areas. Initial imaging should include an AP view of the chest to evaluate for pneumothorax and mediastinal blood. Abdominal radiographs suggest visceral injury by the presence of pneumoperitoneum, free fluid, and bony injury. Although commonly obtained, radiographs of the skull provide very little information about the condition of the brain. Significant, acute head trauma should be evaluated by a CT scan, not radiography.

Computed Tomography

Computed tomography, or CT, results in the reformation of axial images by use of X rays combined with a sophisticated computer. Because of its versatility in imaging the entire body, it has become widely used. Costs tend to be moderate, and with newer technology, images are obtained relatively quickly.

CT is often the best way to further evaluate cortical bone after radiography. It can diagnose minimally displaced cortical fractures and provide the anatomic detail that may be necessary prior to definitive reduction. This is especially useful for small bony structures, such as the carpal and tarsal bones, or for clinically sensitive bony sites such as the spine, the physeal plate, and the articular surfaces (**Figure 28.4**). A CT scan is the image of choice in evaluating severe, acute trauma to the brain (especially in the first 3 days), spinal cord, chest, abdomen, and pelvis. It can also be used to identify the presence of nonradiopaque foreign bodies, such as wood or plastic.

With thin-slice (1- to 3-mm thick) contiguous axial images, the data can be reconstructed into two-dimensional images in other planes, or into three-dimensional images. The speed at which three-dimensional images are reconstructed depends on the sophistication of the scanner. Despite continued advances, this continues to be a time-consuming process. In selected circumstances, such as complex facial, spinal, hip, or foot injuries, three-dimensional images can provide direct visualization of complex relationships among various bony structures prior to definitive treatment (**Figure 28.5**).

The use of intravenous (IV) contrast material with a CT scan varies, depending on the differential diagnoses. Because of the potential for a serious life-threatening allergic reaction to the contrast material, which occurs in 1:100,000

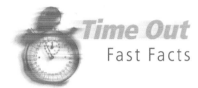

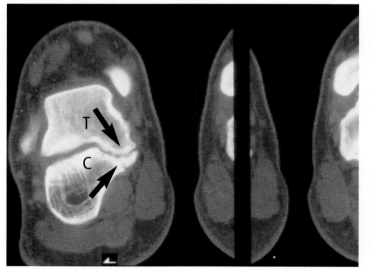

Figure 28.4 CT scan showing a bony coalition between the talus (T) and calcaneus (C).

patients, contrast material should be used only under the supervision of a radiologist and limited to valid clinical indications. Contrast material is not usually required for imaging acute skeletal and head injuries. Rather, it is typically used for imaging of acute abdominal, pelvic, or chest injuries and the evaluation of infection.

Patients with known iodine allergies can be given a nonionic contrast agent and premedicated with a combination of an antihistamine and corticosteroid, at least 12 hours prior to the study. Coordination between the radiologist and the treating physician should be considered in patients with multiple trauma in which vascular injury is also suspected. These patients may require angiography, and the total contrast agent load administered to the patient's kidneys should be considered.

Magnetic Resonance Imaging

Magnetic resonance imaging, or MRI, in its simplest form, represents the use of a magnetic field to excite protons in the body to generate images with the use of a sophisticated computer. MRI is very sensitive and can be specific when used appropriately; however, these scans are relatively expensive, and the expertise of the radiologist is variable. Because these costly machines are not widely available in some areas, patients may have to wait several days before they undergo imaging. In addition, since imaging times are significantly longer than with CT scans, patient cooperation is critical. Because of these factors and limited patient access during imaging, MRI is not commonly used in patients with acute trauma. Confused or disoriented patients or patients younger than age 8 years usually require sedation.

The strength of MRI lies in its excellent soft-tissue contrast and direct multi-planar capabilities. MRI provides exceptional evaluation of soft-tissue injuries to the spinal cord, muscles, ligaments, tendons, menisci, and articular and labral cartilage. It can be used to identify and evaluate underlying abnormalities that may contribute to various impingement syndromes, such as those to the rotator cuff or carpal canal. However, judicious use of MRI is suggested because of its cost. MRI should be limited to clinically valid situations in which the results of imaging will alter treatment. Although MRI can be used to diagnose a lateral collateral ligament injury to the ankle, it is only occasionally required to clarify a clinically confusing picture. Circumstances requiring rapid diagnosis and/or exclusion of associated injuries, such as for elite athletes who have an upcoming competition, may also be an indication for MRI.

MRI is an excellent technique for evaluating bone marrow, the "soft-tissue" component of bone (**Figure 28.6**). It is extremely sensitive in detecting radiographically occult stress fractures, bone marrow contusions, osteomyelitis, and osteonecrosis. In addition, kinematic studies of the knee can now be performed to evaluate for dynamic patellofemoral joint subluxation. Recurrent joint effusions can be evaluated for inflammatory synovitis, pigmented

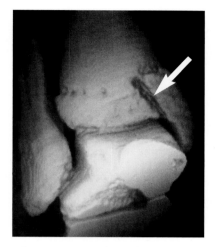

Figure 28.5 Three-dimensional reconstruction of an ankle fracture.

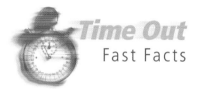

MRI provides excellent soft-tissue contrast and direct multi-planar capability. It provides exceptional evaluation of soft-tissue injuries to the spinal cord, muscles, ligaments, tendons, menisci, and articular and labral cartilage.

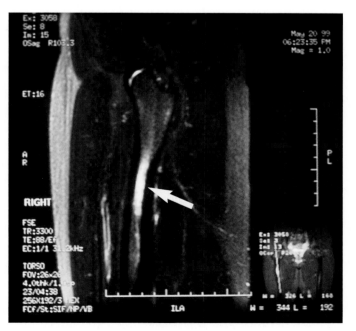

Figure 28.6 MRI scan of a stress fracture of the femur showing marrow enhancement.

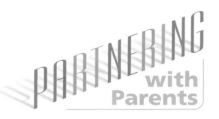

What is the difference between CT and MRI?

CT is a radiographic technique that uses x-rays in multiple planes that are then computerized and then reformatted. MRI does not use x-ray but instead a strong magnet—without any irradiation—which excites molecules in the cell that can be specifically recorded. It is excellent for providing soft tissue detail of all areas of the body.

Figure 28.7 Bone scintigraphy shows increased uptake in the mid-shaft of the tibia.

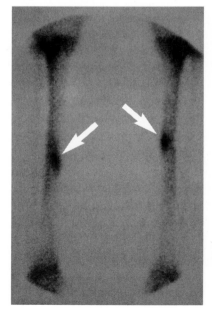

villonodular synovitis, or "internal derangement." Soft-tissue masses can be identified as cystic lesions such as soft-tissue ganglion, synovial cyst (eg, Baker's cyst, paralabral cyst, parameniscal cyst), bursitis, hematoma, or solid masses (eg, tumors, ruptured muscle fibers). In certain situations, MRI can be combined with arthrography to better delineate small intra-articular injuries such as those affecting the glenoid and acetabular labrum.

In clinically confusing cases, MRI can be used as a problem solver. Judicious use of MRI in these clinically perplexing cases can save time and money and reduce patient suffering.

Use of IV contrast material in MRI is limited primarily to evaluation of infection, soft-tissue masses, and synovitis. As with CT scans, the use of contrast material is best decided by the radiologist.

Bone Scintigraphy

Bone scintigraphy, or bone scan, is a nuclear medicine imaging technique that uses a radioactive labeled compound such as technetium methylene diphosphonate (Tc-MDP). Bone scans can evaluate the entire skeleton or be localized to an extremity; however, they are moderately expensive and are generally available only in medium- to large-sized hospitals. This imaging modality is very sensitive when used to detect bony injury, but it is relatively nonspecific. Therefore, if more detailed anatomic information is required prior to treatment, a bone scan alone may not be sufficient, and close clinical and radiographic correlation may be necessary. Indications for bone scintigraphy include evaluation of occult or stress fractures, osteomyelitis, and occasionally, reflex sympathetic dystrophy (**Figure 28.7**).

If the lesion is located in a region of complex bony anatomy, such as the spine, hip, or knee, a technique known as single proton emission computed tomography (SPECT) is suggested. SPECT images allow for separation of activity from the lesion from the adjacent or overlying bony structures. This technique improves localization of the lesion to a specific anatomic site.

Arthrography

Arthrography is a technique in which air and/or contrast medium is injected percutaneously into a joint. Arthrography is used to evaluate the synovium and the structures immediately bordering the joint space. For many years, conventional radiographic arthrography was commonly used to evaluate meniscal injury, and tears of the rotator cuff, wrist ligaments, and triangular fibrocartilage. Arthrography is relatively inexpensive and easily performed, but is gradually being replaced by MRI, which provides greater anatomic detail, as described previously. However, conventional radiographic arthrography remains valuable in the evaluation of epiphyseal fractures in skeletally immature patients.

Arthography can also be performed with more sophisticated imaging techniques, such as CT scans and MRI. Magnetic resonance (MR) arthrography has replaced CT arthrography in most situations because of its superior contrast and direct multi-planar capability. MR arthrography is most often used in the evaluation of labral tears of the shoulder and, occasionally, of the acetabulum.

Angiography

Angiography is an invasive procedure used to image the vessels of the body. Iodinated contrast agents are used with conventional angiography. The risk of severe allergic reaction is similar to that associated with a contrast-enhanced CT scan; however, additional potential complications include hemorrhage, infection, and nerve and vascular injury. Conventional angiography is occasionally indicated in the young athlete, particularly for dislocations (especially at the knee), displaced fractures with abnormal distal pulses after reduction, and severe deceleration or crush injuries to the chest (**Figure 28.8**).

Evaluation of Soft-Tissue Masses

Radiographs should be the first imaging study ordered when evaluating a soft-tissue mass, especially following trauma. Within as few as 3 weeks, these focal areas of injury may ossify, forming a radiographically characteristic lesion known as myositis ossificans (**Figure 28.9**). Radiographs are the preferred imaging technique because these lesions can mimic a soft-tissue sarcoma on MRI, and unfortunately, may also mimic osteosarcoma histologically.

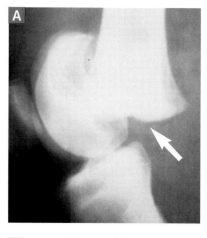

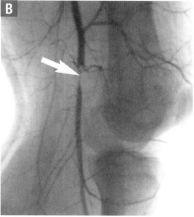

Figure 28.8 Angiography is used to image vessels in the body. **A** Radiograph of a distal femoral physeal fracture in a patient with absent pulses in the foot. **B** Post-reduction angiogram showing disruption of the popliteal artery.

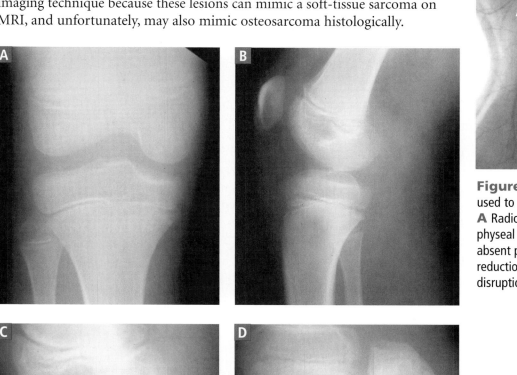

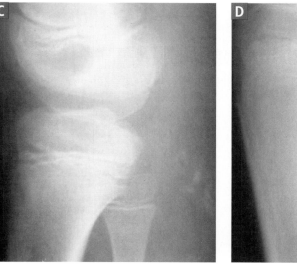

Figure 28.9 Radiographs should be ordered first after trauma. If initial images are inconclusive, follow-up images should be ordered 1 to 3 weeks later. **A,B** Normal radiographs at the time of injury. **C** Faint ossification at follow-up. **D** Mature myositis ossificans.

When the diagnosis is confirmed by radiography, clinical follow-up is necessary. Biopsy should be reserved for conditions that are not clinically compatible with this benign process on follow-up. If the initial images are not definitive, a second radiograph should be obtained 1 to 3 weeks later. If circumstances require a more urgent diagnosis, a noncontrast CT scan can be obtained to identify the typical peripheral zoning phenomenon.

FINISH LINE

As with other diagnostic tests, the value of imaging depends on the initial clinical appropriateness of the test and the proper performance and interpretation of the study. As a general rule, a study should not be performed unless there is a specific question that needs to be answered and if that answer will alter the clinical decision and treatment process. If the problem is complex or there is question regarding which imaging technique to order, direct consultation with a radiologist is recommended. If the patient is to be sent to a specialist, a phone call to that specialist may prevent unnecessary imaging or inadequate studies. The specialist may have a specific request or question that will alter the imaging approach.

For More Information

1. Collier BD Jr, Fogelman I, Rosenthail L (eds): *Skeletal Nuclear Medicine.* St Louis, MO, Mosby-Year Book, 1996, pp 46, 232, 311–332.

2. Keats TE (ed): *Atlas of Normal Roentgen Variants That May Simulate Disease,* ed 5. St Louis, MO, Mosby-Year Book, 1992.

3. Rogers LF (ed): *Radiology of Skeletal Trauma,* ed 2. New York, NY, Churchill Livingstone, 1992, p 302.

4. Stoller DW: *Magnetic Resonance Imaging in Orthopaedics and Sports Medicine,* ed 2. Philadelphia, PA, Lippincott-Raven, 1997.

5. Swischuk LE (ed): *Emergency Radiology of the Acutely Ill or Injured Child,* ed 2. Baltimore, MD, Williams and Wilkins, 1986, pp 105–116, 205–279.

Chapter 29

Principles of Rehabilitation

STEVEN J. ANDERSON, MD

Rehabilitation is a process that is designed to help athletes restore normal function following injury or illness through structured activity. Physicians provide a valuable service to athletes by identifying the functional deficits caused by injury, offering options in treatment, explaining the rehabilitation process, supervising the recovery process, and determining when function is restored adequately to permit a safe return to play. The resolution of pain is an important milestone in the recovery process, but should not be equated with full recovery. In addition to pain, injuries are associated with losses of flexibility, joint motion, muscle strength, coordination, and general fitness. These losses may persist even after pain or other symptoms have subsided. Before returning to play, these losses must be treated to avoid further injury and limitations of performance.

Rehabilitation Planning

Planning a rehabilitation program starts with an analysis of the medical needs of the injured athlete (**Table 29.1**). It is essential to establish an accurate diagnosis and identify the etiology of the problem. Without a precise diagnosis and an understanding of the natural history of the condition, it is impossible to monitor the efficacy of treatment. If treatment is going to address the cause of the problem, injury pathomechanics and relevant risk factors must also be identified.

Understanding the demands of the sport is also important in determining the potential effects of an injury on performance, the risk for further injury, the specific goals and endpoints of rehabilitation, the need to modify the activity, and the criteria for return to play. Factors such as the athlete's general health, motivation, external support systems, access to treatment resources, and time constraints also influence the rehabilitation program and its outcome. Finally, educating the athlete about his or her injury, the rationale

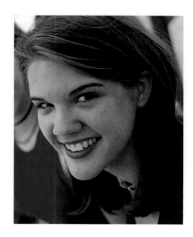

Table 29.1 *Essential Questions for Rehabilitation Planning*

1. What is the diagnosis?

2. What is the etiology of the injury or condition?

3. What are the physical demands of the sport?

4. What physical limitations are caused by the injury?

5. What are the risks of continued participation, with and without treatment?

6. What can be done to correct or ameliorate the effects of the injury?

7. What are the specific activities that the athlete can and cannot do during rehabilitation?

8. What other conditions or factors influence the treatment or outcome?

9. What resources are available to treat the injury?

10. What are the time constraints for treatment and recovery?

11. Does the athlete want to return to play?

12. Does the athlete and his or her family understand and accept the risks of returning to play, with and without treatment?

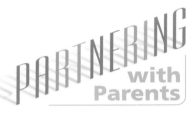

When is it best to use cold therapy?

Cold therapy should be used for almost all acute injuries that are accompanied by pain and swelling. It may also be used to decrease inflammatory changes associated with overuse injuries that may not produce significant pain or swelling.

What is the best way to apply ice?

Ice packs may be applied directly to the skin for 20 minutes every hour to every other hour.

and goals for treatment, and the risks of returning to play are all part of the rehabilitation process.

Therapeutic Modalities

Rehabilitation planning also involves identifying available treatment modalities and understanding how and when they should be used (**Table 29.2**). Therapeutic modalities include physical modalities, therapeutic exercises, and orthopaedic appliances.

Physical Modalities

Physical modalities facilitate the rehabilitation process by decreasing pain, swelling, spasm, and soft-tissue restrictions, and by preparing an injured athlete for the therapeutic exercise phase of rehabilitation. Physical modalities include therapies that use cold, heat, and electricity primarily in the initial phase of treatment to control pain, swelling, and muscle spasm.

Cold therapy

Cold therapy, or cryotherapy, is the application of cold to the injured area using ice packs, ice massage, and hydrotherapy, including ice baths and ice whirlpools to decrease pain, swelling, capillary blood flow, muscle spasm, and local metabolic activity (**Table 29.3**). Cold is the modality of choice for nearly all acute injuries that are accompanied by pain and swelling. In addition, cold therapy may be used to diminish inflammatory changes associated with overuse injuries that may not produce significant pain or swelling.

Ice packs may be applied directly to the skin for 20 minutes at a time and as frequently as once per hour. Chemical ice packs, or "blue ice," may be colder than frozen water and can cause burns if left in place too long. The use of ice packs is not recommended for athletes with cold-induced urticaria, Raynaud's disease, or when the injury is in a location that has poor circulation. In addition, ethyl chloride spray can provide rapid, superficial cooling to the skin. This modality is used primarily as a topical anesthetic.

Table 29.2 *Use of Therapeutic Modalities*

Symptoms and Physical Findings	Modalities	Exercise	Equipment	Comment
Acute swelling	• Ice • EGS	• Only in noninjured areas	• Compression • Braces and splints for immobilization	
Chronic inflammation	• Ice • Phonophoresis • Iontophoresis • NSAIDs	• Stretching • Joint mobilization • Isometric and short arc strengthening	• Tape • Soft braces • Neoprene sleeves	
Restricted joint motion with inflammation	• Ice	• Isometric strengthening • Active exercises in ROM without pain	• Compression wraps • Functional braces	Assess for intra-articular pathology
Restricted joint motion without inflammation	• Heat • Ultrasound	• Active ROM exercises • Passive ROM exercises • Active-assist ROM exercises	• Progressive splints to maintain motion • Night splints	Rule out systemic disease, RSD
Joint instability	• None, unless swelling present	• Strengthening in ROM without pain • Closed chain kinetic exercises • Proprioception exercises	• Immobilize acute injury • Functional braces later	Distinguish between static and functional instability
Muscle atrophy	• EGS	• PREs	• Weights and tubing for home exercise program	Distinguish among disuse and neurologic injuries
Muscle imbalances	• Objective measurement	• Selective strengthening exercises		Distinguish among disuse and neurologic injuries
Loss of flexibility with injury	• Ice • EGS • Ultrasound	• Static stretching • Massage • PREs	• Compression with and without immobilization	
Loss of flexibility without injury		• Active stretching, with and without assistance • Massage • Myofascial release		Address underlying cause of muscle tightness
Proprioceptive deficit		• Balance and proprioceptive exercises • Functional exercises	• Neoprene sleeve for warmth • Neoprene sleeve or wrap for tactile input • Balance board	Modified Romberg test

EGS = Electrogalvanic stimulation ROM = Range of motion
NSAIDs = Nonsteroidal anti-inflammatory drugs RSD = Reflex sympathetic dystrophy
PREs = Progressive resistive exercises

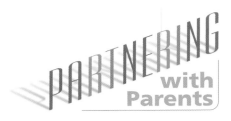

When is it best to use heat therapy?

Heat therapy is best used before exercise or in treating chronic problems in which restricted muscle or joint motion hampers recovery. Warming the muscles before stretching can enhance the positive effect of stretching exercises.

Ice massage is effective for treating injuries that cause localized areas of superficial inflammation, such as tendinitis or bursitis. With this technique, ice is rubbed over the affected area for approximately 10 minutes per session. Ice baths or ice whirlpools are used if the injured area is relatively diffuse and can be submerged. Contrast baths alternate between cold and heat and may be used to reduce edema.

Heat therapy

Heat therapy is most commonly administered with hot packs, hydrotherapy, and ultrasound. Hot packs heat the affected body part by conduction, hydrotherapy heats by convection, and ultrasound heats by transduction of mechanical sound waves to heat. Less common heating modalities use radiant heat, short-wave diathermy, paraffin baths, and fluid therapy. Analgesic ointments and sports creams can provide a perception of warmth, because they irritate the skin, but do little to elevate temperature below the skin surface.

Heat therapy can reduce pain and spasm and can increase blood flow and compliance of soft-tissue structures (**Table 29.3**). Heat has a limited role in acute injuries or in conditions where inflammation and swelling are present. The common practice of switching from cold therapy to heat therapy 48 hours after an acute injury—particularly when swelling and inflammation persist—has no basis in scientific fact. Heat therapy is best used prior to exercise or in the treatment of chronic conditions in which restricted muscle or joint motion hampers recovery. The positive effect of stretching exercises can be enhanced by warming the muscles before stretching, either actively with warm-up exercises or passively with the heating modalities mentioned above.

Heat therapy with ultrasound can penetrate deeper injuries better than the other heating modalities. Ultrasound is most helpful when heat is indicated; other modalities are unable to penetrate to the depth of the injury. Ultrasound may be used in combination with a corticosteroid cream in a technique known as phonophoresis. The ultrasound increases the permeability of the skin to allow penetration of the corticosteroid into the underlying inflamed structures. Ultrasound should be used with caution over growth plates, and it should not be used over a hollow viscus.

Therapeutic electricity

Therapeutic electricity can be delivered in the form of electrogalvanic stimulation (EGS), transcutaneous nerve stimulation (TNS), or iontophoresis.

Table 29.3 *Physical Effects of Therapeutic Heat and Cold*	Heat	Cold
Pain	Decrease	Decrease
Spasm	Decrease	Decrease
Edema	Increase	Decrease
Metabolic activity	Increase	Decrease
Capillary blood flow	Increase	Decrease
Collagen extensibility	Increase	Decrease

EGS causes small muscle contractions to produce a pumping action that mobilizes edema and reduces swelling. In addition, muscle stimulation from EGS may help decrease muscle atrophy that accompanies injury, immobilization, or disuse. TNS uses electric stimulation to block the transmission of pain impulses from musculoskeletal injury, neuritic pain, or postoperative pain. Furthermore, TNS is convenient to use because its units are portable. Iontophoresis establishes an electrical field around an injury that helps to deliver an ionized form of corticosteroid to the injured site. Both iontophoresis and phonophoresis have similar applications, but iontophoresis uses electricity rather than heat to enhance delivery of the medication.

Therapeutic Exercise

Therapeutic exercise improves joint mobility and stretches and strengthens muscles (**Table 29.4**). Therapeutic exercises can begin once swelling and spasm subside, and when the athlete can move the injured area without pain.

Joint mobilization

Deficits of joint mobility are often present after injury, and occasionally, before. Usually, a reduction of swelling and inflammation restores normal joint motion in acutely injured athletes. Occasionally, significant restrictions of joint motion persist—even after swelling resolves and mechanical barriers to joint motion have been ruled out. Returning to activity before regaining

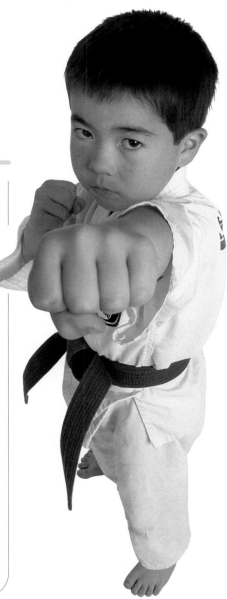

Table 29.4 *Therapeutic Exercises*

Flexibility

- Stretching exercises
    - Static stretching
    - Ballistic stretching
    - Proprioceptive neuromuscular facilitation
- Soft-tissue mobilization
    - Myofascial release
    - Massage therapy

Joint mobilization

- Active mobilization
- Passive mobilization
- Active-assist mobilization

Strengthening exercises

- Isometric exercises
- Isotonic exercises
- Isokinetic exercises
- Concentric exercises
- Eccentric exercises
- Closed kinetic chain exercises
- Functional exercises

normal joint motion can limit performance and lead to further injury. Restrictions in joint mobility that do not resolve over time or with exercise may be treated by therapists.

Details about specific techniques and their applications are not included in this chapter. The primary responsibilities of the treating physician are to assess restrictions of joint motion from muscle inflexibility, to treat or rule out mechanical restrictions to joint motion, and to prescribe therapy that can restore normal joint motion.

Techniques for improving joint mobility include active mobilization, passive mobilization, and active-assist mobilization. The first technique, active joint mobilization, requires the athlete to use his or her power to move a joint. Active joint mobilization is considered the safest and most readily available technique. The second technique, passive joint mobilization, requires an assistant, such as a therapist, to move a restricted joint. This technique can achieve motion beyond what the athlete is able or willing to perform. However, passive joint mobilization can cause or exacerbate injury, particularly when it is performed by someone who is not qualified to do so. The third method, active-assist mobilization, combines techniques of both active and passive mobilization to improve joint mobility.

Stretching

Stretching restores flexibility after an injury and corrects deficiencies in flexibility that may have contributed to the injury. The primary methods of stretching are static and ballistic stretching. With static stretching, the target muscle is stretched and held for 20 to 30 seconds. Static stretching is safe, effective, and easily performed without any equipment or assistance (**Figure 29.1**). Ballistic stretching involves rapid stretches that are often associated with bouncing motions. Muscle strains can occur with these stretches because they activate the stretch reflex that causes the muscle being stretched to contract. Therefore, ballistic stretching is not recommended for injury rehabilitation.

In general, warm muscles (achieved by either warm-up exercises or by passive heating modalities) respond better to flexibility exercises. Stretching before activity is commonly recommended; however, stretching after activity may produce greater gains in flexibility because the muscles are already warm.

Strengthening

Nearly any activity that contracts a muscle also strengthens it. With appropriate training, even pubescent and prepubescent athletes can improve strength. Strengthening exercises are categorized according to changes in length of the muscle, the amount of resistance, and the speed of contraction.

Isometric exercises With isometric exercises, a muscle contracts without changing length. Isometric strengthening is considered a safe way to resume strengthening following an injury because the athlete controls the forces generated during the exercise and performs the exercise without moving the injured joint or muscle. Isometric exercises also allow the athlete to isolate and contract single muscle groups, which aids the process of muscle reeducation. Isometric exercises do not require any special equipment or facilities.

Figure 29.1
Static stretching technique for hamstring muscles.

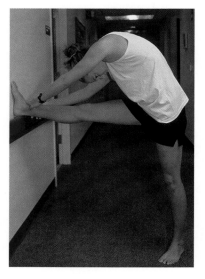

Isotonic exercises Isotonic exercises involve contracting a muscle against fixed resistance throughout its arc of motion. Most weight machines, free weights, and pulleys provide isotonic resistance. If a muscle strength is desired through the full range of motion, resistance exercises must be performed throughout the full range of motion. Isotonic strengthening should not be initiated until pain and swelling have been controlled and restrictions of flexibility and joint motion have been addressed. For an athlete to continue to gain strength, the isotonic resistance must be increased as adaptive changes occur. Progressive resistive exercises (PREs) refer to a commonly prescribed regimen of incremental strengthening.

Isokinetic exercises With isokinetic exercises, the speed of muscle contraction is constant. Typically, isokinetic machines have a lever that sets the machine to move at a predetermined number of degrees arc per second. The machine then measures the force that the athlete applies against this arm as torque. Conditioning at high speeds on isokinetic machines approximates the speed of muscle contraction during many sports activities. However, isokinetic machines are expensive to own and operate. In addition, some isokinetic exercises cause nonphysiologic loading or place abnormal shear forces on joints that may contribute to injury. With many isokinetic machines, only concentric contraction occurs.

Strengthening exercises may be further characterized as concentric, eccentric, closed kinetic chain, and functional. Clinically, these distinctions are important because each type of exercise is designed to meet the specific functional demands of different athletes and sports.

Concentric and eccentric exercises Concentric exercises contract or shorten muscles during exercise. For example, many traditional exercises for strength training such as biceps curls, bench press, and leg press are concentric exercises. Eccentric or "negative contraction" exercises oppose the forces of gravity and act to lengthen muscles. Thus, when performing a biceps curl with free weights, the flexion phase is a concentric contraction of the biceps while the extension phase is an eccentric contraction. The combination of simultaneous stretch and contraction of muscle generates high levels of tension in the

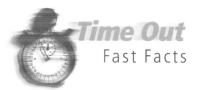

Strengthening types of exercise include isotonic, isometric, concentric and eccentric, isokinetic, closed kinetic chain, and functional.

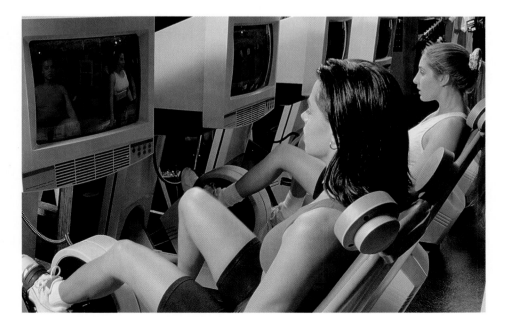

muscle-tendon unit. Since the development of strength is related to the level of tension in the muscle, significant improvements in strength are possible with eccentric exercises. Eccentric strengthening can be useful during rehabilitation to prepare an athlete to withstand the eccentric loads that lead to muscle injury. However, inappropriate use of eccentric exercises can also cause injury. For example, eccentric overload is a common cause of muscle strains.

Closed and open kinetic chain exercises With closed kinetic chain exercises, the foot or hand is fixed to the floor, such as with a squat or push-up. With open kinetic chain exercises, neither is fixed. A biceps curl or leg lift is an example of an open chain exercise. Closed chain exercises are better at improving agonist and antagonist muscle with concentric and eccentric contraction.

Functional exercises Functional exercises strengthen muscles in their position of normal use or function. Usually, functional exercises replicate movements or patterns of movement required by a sport. Unlike exercises that isolate a single muscle in a single plane of motion, functional exercises involve the integrated action of multiple muscle groups working in multiple planes of motion. Functional exercises require intact proprioception to maintain proper balance and control and can improve it, unlike isolated muscle strengthening or strengthening using weight machines.

Functional exercises are the most advanced strengthening exercises because they require mastery and integration of all the earlier types of strengthening including concentric, eccentric, closed kinetic chain, and isokinetic exercises. Usually, successful completion of a functional exercise program indicates that an athlete is ready to return to play. When functional deficits are present, more rehabilitation is needed before a safe return to play is possible.

Strength testing

Objective measures of strength provide evidence of the athlete's improvement and readiness to proceed with training. Manual muscle testing is convenient and easy to perform, although the most reliable results are obtained by a single examiner using standardized methods. The speed and ease of the exercise can easily be observed and compared with the uninjured extremity. Similarly, repetitive toe raises can test strength and endurance in the calf, and walking on the heels can test strength in ankle dorsiflexion. The strength of almost every other muscle group can be tested by having the athlete lift weights repeatedly. Lifting lighter weights multiple times also decreases the risk of injury associated with maximal lifting efforts.

Isokinetic machines assess muscle power at various speeds of contraction and at various points in the movement arc. Isokinetic machines may provide the best measurements of strength imbalances between paired muscle groups.

Functional testing examines strength and neuromuscular function and provides a last objective assessment of the success of the rehabilitation program. Functional tests can be created simply by identifying a movement performed in the sport that is likely to be affected by the injury, and then devising an exercise that tests the athlete's ability to perform that movement. For example, if a sport requires jumping and twisting, the athlete should be tested to determine if he or she can perform these movements before returning to play. More specifically, a modified Romberg test is a simple test for proprioceptive function. With this test, the athlete stands on one foot with his or her eyes closed. An athlete with a proprioceptive deficit will have difficulty maintaining balance and stability. In addition, a functional test for an athlete with an ankle sprain may be running in a zigzag pattern or sequentially jumping and rotating on the affected ankle. Functional tests support return to play decisions because the decisions are based on the functional ability of the athlete rather than arbitrary lengths of time.

Orthopaedic Appliances

Orthopaedic appliances protect an injured area and minimize the negative impact on structures that are not injured. A wide range of orthopaedic appliances are used for rehabilitation, and recommendations for their use are detailed throughout the text, and specifically in chapter 13 on injury prevention.

Usually, acute injuries that cause pain, swelling, joint instability, and/or weakness need protection and immobilization; splints, casts, braces, crutches, and slings may be used. For sprains or fractures that cause significant swelling, a splint is preferable to a cast. Splints may be prefabricated or made with casting material. Wrist splints, finger splints, knee immobilizers, and cast boots can be adjusted to allow for swelling and removed to apply ice or to repeat an examination. A splint can be converted to a cast once any swelling is controlled or if there is reason to believe that an athlete may not comply with wearing a removable splint. Also, crutches and slings may be used in conjunction with splints or casts to further protect and immobilize the injury. In addition, elastic bandages provide compression, hold ice packs in place, and remind an athlete to protect the injury during the initial phases of recovery.

When the athlete is ready to start exercising, the injured area must be protected, and a functional brace may be indicated. A functional brace allows motion within a controlled range that prevents further injury. Orthotic devices, or functional orthoses, may facilitate recovery from overuse injuries that are caused by biomechanic abnormalities.

Protective equipment such as custom pads, flak jackets, face shields, goggles, and playing casts may protect the injured area and allow the athlete to return to limited play before the injury has completely healed. Such protective equipment should be used only if the injury and the protective equipment do not significantly impair function and if the protective equipment effectively reduces the risk of further injury. An example of appropriate use of protective equipment may be a playing cast for a soccer player with a stable wrist fracture or goggles for a basketball player with a corneal abrasion. Officials for the sport must approve the protective equipment. Often, when an athlete requires equipment beyond what is normally used in the sport, the physician must submit a letter of explanation and the parents must sign a liability waiver.

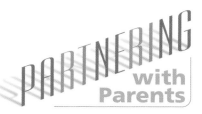

How long should my child continue therapeutic exercises following an injury?

Therapeutic exercises should be continued until motion and strength are restored in the injured extremity to a level equal to the uninjured extremity.

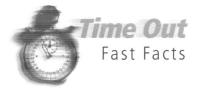

The phases of a rehabilitation program are initial, intermediate, later care, and follow-up care.

The role of equipment in causing injury must also be assessed before the athlete returns to play. Helmets, face masks, pads, and other protective equipment used in the sport may have failed to protect the athlete from injury because of faulty design, poor fit, improper maintenance, or inappropriate footwear. If the equipment contributed to the injury, procuring better equipment and teaching the athlete how to use it should be part of the rehabilitation program as well.

Phases of a Rehabilitation Program

The rehabilitation program may be roughly divided into three phases: 1) initial care that addresses the immediate effects of injury; 2) intermediate care that rebuilds normal motion and strength through activity; and 3) later care that involves more challenging exercises that facilitate the return to play (**Table 29.5**). Each phase of rehabilitation occurs sequentially and lasts approximately one third of the total time required for rehabilitation. For example, if pain and swelling resolve after 2 weeks of initial care, restoration of motion and strength during intermediate care will require 2 weeks, and fitness and function will return after another 2 weeks in later care.

The specific goals for each phase of rehabilitation are met by selecting and implementing various treatment options. In the same manner that mastery of a complex athletic skill requires mastery of fundamental skills, a successful rehabilitation outcome must also be built on a foundation of more basic steps. A well-organized rehabilitation program progresses from simple to complex, and safeguards the athlete from exposure to physical challenges that exceed his or her limits or readiness.

Table 29.5 *Phases of Rehabilitation*

Initial care
- Relative rest
- Protection and support
- Control of pain and inflammation

Intermediate care
- Resolution of residual pain and inflammation
- Restoration of joint motion
- Restoration of flexibility
- Restoration of strength
- Restoration and maintenance of fitness

Later care
- Progressive strengthening exercises
- Proprioceptive training
- Functional exercises
- Sport-specific skills

Follow-up care
- Protective equipment
- Maintenance therapy

Initial Care

Usually, initial care for an acute or overuse injury includes rest and protection from the injury-producing activity. The amount and duration of rest will depend on the nature and seriousness of the injury.

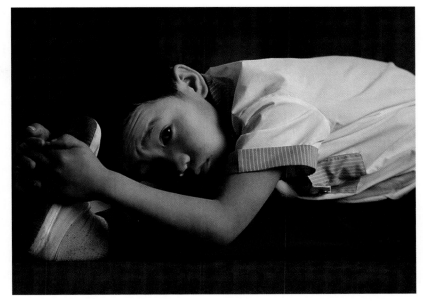

With "relative rest," the injured area is protected while the athlete continues to train to the degree possible. Athletes who have made a substantial investment in their training will want to maintain their fitness, even when they are injured. The desire of the treating physician to allow for sufficient time for healing must be balanced with the athlete's concerns about the loss of conditioning and/or fitness that result from a period of prolonged rest.

In addition to prescribing an appropriate level of rest, initial care must also address pain and inflammation. Applying ice, elevating the injured area, and applying compressive wraps are most helpful during this phase of treatment, particularly for acute injuries. For conditions with persistent inflammation, anti-inflammatory medications are an adjunct to treatment with ice, although they do not affect healing. For conditions such as tendinitis, bursitis, periostitis, and arthritis, suppression of inflammation does not interfere with healing. Anti-inflammatory medications for acute injuries such as sprains may help control pain and swelling, but their effect on long-term healing of the ligaments is not clear.

Analgesics have a limited role in the treatment of injured athletes. Athletes who need medication for pain should not play. Most pain from musculoskeletal injury can be controlled adequately with rest, immobilization, and treatment modalities. A similar caution is warranted for muscle relaxants. These medications have no direct effect on the muscle or the cause of the muscle spasm, and their side effects and addictive potential make them undesirable for use in young athletes.

Modalities such as EGS and TNS can be used for swelling and pain during initial care, but require referral to a physical therapist or athletic trainer.

Intermediate Care

The goals of intermediate care are to resolve residual pain and swelling, as well as to restore flexibility, joint motion, and strength. In general, the therapeutic exercises mentioned earlier are used in this intermediate phase of treatment.

The athlete may begin intermediate care when pain and swelling subside and the injury has had sufficient time to heal initially. By this time, the athlete should not be using any splints, casts, slings, crutches, or other devices that can prevent joint motion or muscle contraction. However, tape, elastic or neoprene sleeves, functional braces, pads, and orthotic devices may offer some protection as the athlete begins this more active phase of rehabilitation.

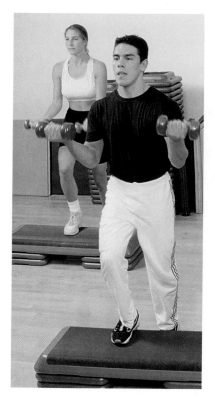

Physical therapists or athletic trainers can teach athletes exercises to restore flexibility, joint motion, and strength by demonstration and handouts. In addition to proper instruction, trained personnel can supervise the exercise to enhance compliance and the likelihood of a successful outcome. Exercises for intermediate care should not be prescribed too early in the evaluation or rehabilitation process because the athlete may not be physically or emotionally ready to participate fully. Prescription of exercises during a follow-up visit after the initial evaluation is appropriate. Usually, injured athletes will be more receptive to learning rehabilitation exercises once they have accepted their injuries and are feeling well enough to participate actively.

Therapeutic exercises should be performed only within the range of motion that does not cause pain. Initially, isometric or short-arc isotonic exercises may be the only exercises that do not cause pain. If pain or swelling develops, the exercise should be modified or curtailed. An athlete who responds favorably to strengthening exercises will be able to perform the exercises through wider ranges of motion with increasing resistance and/or more repetitions.

The endpoints for therapeutic exercise are restoration of symmetry and balance of motion and strength. The injured extremity should be equal to the uninjured extremity in motion and strength. Since muscles work in agonist and antagonistic pairs, strengthening exercises should be designed for both pairs to restore balances that are normal for the joint. Visible deficits or asymmetries warrant further attention before the athlete progresses to the later phase of rehabilitation.

During the intermediate phase of rehabilitation, the athlete can begin general conditioning exercises to maintain fitness as long as the general conditioning exercises do not overload the injured area. For example, an athlete with a knee or ankle injury may be able to tolerate swimming, whereas an athlete with a shoulder or elbow injury may be able to tolerate running, bicycling, or skating. By maintaining fitness now, the athlete will be better prepared to return to play once the injury has healed. In addition, limited activity can provide a safe outlet for the athlete's enthusiasm to return to play while rehabilitation continues.

Later Care

When the athlete regains normal joint motion, muscle flexibility, and strength, he or she is ready to advance into the last phase of rehabilitation also known as functional rehabilitation. During this phase, exercises are designed to develop more complicated, demanding, and sport-specific skills.

By the time the athlete is ready for functional exercises, there should be little need for physical modalities or medications. However, functional braces, taping, orthotics, and protective equipment may still be used. Flexibility and joint motion should be normal, but ongoing maintenance exercises can help preserve the gains made earlier.

The most significant changes during later phase rehabilitation occur with strengthening. The athlete should be pain-free while performing any of the exercises in this phase. Strengthening exercises can be expanded to include work at higher speeds of contraction, as well as exercises designed to enhance power and endurance. Closed kinetic chain exercises and functional exercises can be introduced during this later phase. Also, exercises that restore proprioception or position sense are an important element of functional rehabilitation. Balance boards or balancing exercises can be used to identify proprioceptive deficits as well as restore proprioceptive function. Training in functional exercises requires integration and coordination of multiple muscle groups and helps restore neuromuscular mechanisms that will be used in the athlete's chosen sport.

Specific requirements for muscle speed, power, endurance, and coordination will vary among the different sports. The physician can help ensure adequate functional rehabilitation by identifying the demands of a sport, assessing the deficits of the athlete, prescribing appropriate exercises, monitoring recovery, and testing functional ability prior to allowing the athlete to return to play.

Follow-up Care

Usually, once athletes successfully complete a functional rehabilitation program, they can return to play. Depending on the injury and the sport, modifications or restrictions of activity may be warranted. When an athlete has not participated in his or her sport for more than a week, a gradual resumption of activity should be advised.

When an athlete returns to practice, he or she may not have the time or need to complete the rehabilitation exercises. At this point, flexibility, strength, and fitness gained during rehabilitation may be maintained with just a few essential exercises. Integrating these maintenance exercises into the training routine for the sport is an easy way to continue rehabilitation. Maintenance exercises may be continued for the duration of the season or until the athlete has fully participated in the activity for a month without recurrent symptoms or injury.

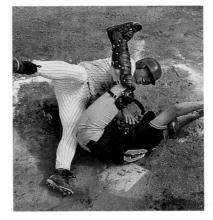

Athletes who participate in seasonal sports may develop seasonal injuries. A common example is elbow or shoulder pain that coincides with the beginning of baseball season. For athletes with these injuries, year-round maintenance exercises are impractical. Instead, selected rehabilitation exercises may be started 4 to 6 weeks before the season begins. These exercises, combined with a gradual return to activity, may prevent recurrent injury.

After discussing the type and duration of maintenance exercises, the final step of follow-up care is instructing athletes about the early warning signs of injury so that they can recognize when follow-up examination may be needed. Early intervention can prevent long-term or more serious problems.

Informed Consent

A successful rehabilitation program will help an injured athlete regain full function and return to play while minimizing the risk of further injury. However, even with the best rehabilitation plans, athletes and their parents must be informed that risks of further injury cannot be eliminated entirely. The physician should help identify and reduce the risks related to the injury and the sport and determine if the risk of further participation is disproportionately high. However, even high risks may not preclude participation, and the athlete and his or her family must determine if the risk is acceptable. Allowing an athlete to return to play is not a guarantee against further injury, and inappropriately restricting an athlete from participation is not a guarantee against liability.

FINISH LINE

Most sports injuries that affect children and adolescents can be treated effectively with rehabilitation. In fact, rehabilitation is the primary treatment for injured athletes. Furthermore, rehabilitation is necessary because the effects of injury may not disappear with rest. In addition, an active rehabilitation program reduces the incidence of long-term disability and recurrent or progressive injuries. Lastly, it encourages athletes with treatable conditions to remain active during their recovery.

For More Information

1. Kibler WB, Chandler TJ, Pace BK: Principles of rehabilitation after chronic tendon injuries. *Clin Sports Med* 1992;11:661–671.

2. Kibler WB, Lee PA, Herring SA, Press JM (eds): *Functional Rehabilitation of Sports and Musculoskeletal Injuries.* Gaithersburg, MD, Aspen Publishers, 1998.

3. Prentice WE (ed): *Rehabilitation Techniques in Sports Medicine,* ed 2. St Louis, MO, Mosby-Year Book, 1994, p 94.

4. Young JL, Press JM: The physiologic basis of sports rehabilitation. *Phys Med Rehab Clin North Am* 1994;5:9–36.

Chapter 30

Stress Fractures

DAVID A. YNGVE, MD

Astress fracture occurs as a result of repetitive stress over time in which bone remodeling is unable to keep pace with the demands placed on the bone. Today, children and adolescents have higher fitness levels and increased expectations about their sports performance. As a result, more children and adolescents are showing signs of overuse injuries of bones, tendons, and ligaments.

The primary cause of stress fractures is an increase in activity level or an abnormal repetitive stress placed on normal bone. For example, a young athlete who starts soccer practice after a summer of relative inactivity is vulnerable to stress fractures. Therefore, coaches should be advised to start training regimens gradually. A change in equipment or conditions, such as wearing different shoes or playing on a different surface, can also cause stress fractures. Stress fractures may develop even in conditioned athletes whose training regimens exceed the mechanical properties of the bones.

Adolescents are three times more susceptible to stress fractures than are children. Adolescents subject their bones to greater stresses because they are heavier, faster, and stronger. Abnormally weak bones are also susceptible to stress fractures even under normal stress. For instance, adolescents with osteopenia secondary to neuromuscular conditions or metabolic disorders (such as amenorrhea) can sustain stress fractures more easily than those whose bones are normal.

Pain is the first symptom of a stress fracture. Young athletes often ignore this pain and continue the activity. Healing will occur without complication if the athlete heeds the pain and decreases his or her activity level. However, when the pain is ignored, a stress fracture develops. In some cases, a completely displaced fracture is possible if activities are not modified. For example, a pitcher who ignores pain in the midshaft area of the humerus could sustain a displaced fracture of the humerus later.

Anatomy/Biomechanics

Compression Failure

Compression failure of bone is one cause of stress fractures. Compression failure can be caused by repeated exposure to excessive impact forces. Muscles exhausted by the forces can no longer provide dynamic support

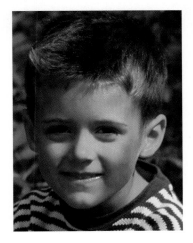

Figure 30.1 Stress fracture of the tibia. **A** AP radiograph shows fibrous cortical defect medially. Follow-up radiographs **B** AP view and **C** lateral view taken 3 weeks later show a sclerotic line across the tibia consistent with a stress fracture.

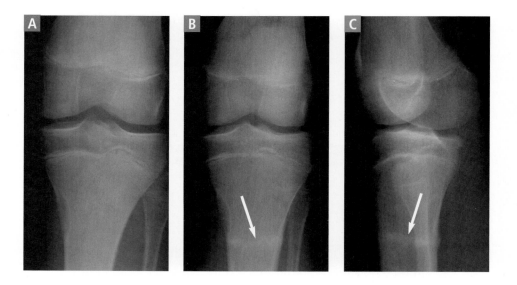

to the extremity. The physiologic response is bone resorption followed by bone formation (**Figure 30.1**). Unfortunately, bone resorption occurs more quickly and leads to increased weakness of the bone at that site. When bone formation occurs several weeks later, it may be inadequate to rebuild the area unless the impact forces have stopped. If activity is modified during this period, bone formation may exceed resorption and heal the fracture. Stress fractures can also occur from strain imposed by muscle origins or insertions.

Tension Stress Fractures

Tension stress fractures occur in the anterior cortex of the tibia, an area commonly under tension while jumping. Tension fractures heal more slowly than compression fractures because the stressing activity tends to pull the bone apart before it can heal completely.

Growth Plate Stress Fractures

Growth plate stress fractures occur when chronic stress at a cellular level occurs across the growth plate area, widening and weakening the growth plate. For example, gymnasts often experience pain when the growth plate widens at the distal radius. Although distal radial physeal stress fractures occur more frequently in gymnasts, they can occur in other athletes as well. For instance, throwing athletes can have growth plate stress fractures at the proximal humeral physis, and runners can have them in the distal tibia. Growth plate stress fractures do not affect long-term growth, but a delay in diagnosing the injury prolongs disability.

Common Sports and Related Sites of Pain

Common sports and sites of pain related to injuries in those sports are listed in **Table 30.1**. Typically, running injuries involve the tibia, but the tarsal navicular (causing pain in the medial arch of the foot), the femur, and even the sacrum can be involved. Stress fractures of the tibia are also common in basketball players and baseball players. In basketball players, the anterior cortex of the tibia is susceptible because of the stresses of jumping, and in baseball players, the stresses of running are the culprit. The stresses of throwing in these athletes also cause stress fractures of the humeral shaft or proximal humeral growth plate. Stress fractures in the lower lumbar spine (that cause low back pain) and the distal radial growth plate are common in gymnasts. The lower lumbar spine is also susceptible in football players and dancers, probably caused by hyperextension of the back. Stress fractures of the distal fibula often occur in ice skaters, especially beginners because they tend to hold their ankles in an everted position. Tennis and volleyball are associated with stress fractures in the metacarpals and ulna, respectively.

Clinical Evaluation

History

The history of a stress fracture includes pain with activity that lasts more than a week. At first, the pain occurs at the end of the activity. Then, onset becomes earlier, until the symptoms begin as soon as the activity starts and continue throughout the period of activity. Pain occurs at time of impact, for example, when the foot strikes the surface (loading response) while running.

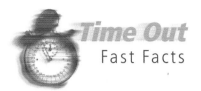

Table 30.1 **Common Sports and Sites of Pain Associated with Stress Fractures**

Sport	Sites of Pain
Baseball	Tibia
	Humerus, shaft
	Proximal humeral growth plate
Basketball	Anterior cortex of the tibia
	Tarsal navicular
Football	Lumbar spine: Pars interarticularis
Gymnastics	Lumbar spine: Pars interarticularis
	Distal radial growth plate
	Tibia
	Fibula
Ice skating	Distal fibula
Running	Proximal tibial metaphysis
	Distal tibial metaphysis
	Fibula
	Tarsal navicular
	Midshaft of femur
	Distal femur
	Femoral neck
	Sacrum
Soccer	Patella
Swimming	Proximal tibia
Tennis	Nondominant ulna (from two-handed backhand stroke)
	Dominant side metacarpal
Volleyball	Ulna
	Tibia

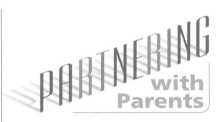

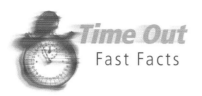

Stress fractures often develop when there is a change in activity level. In most instances, the diagnosis can be confirmed by plain radiographs at presentation or after 2 weeks of rest.

Because stress fractures often develop when there has been a change in activity level, a sports history should be obtained to determine if there has been an increase in the amount of running, a change to a new or different sport, or an increase in activity following a sedentary period. Unlike some overuse injuries that involve soft tissues, stress fractures do not resolve with short rest periods of 1 to 3 days' duration.

These fractures can also occur in conditioned athletes. For example, a well-trained athlete who participated in a series of tournaments sustained a stress fracture of the fibula at the end the season. In another example, an athlete who played multiple sports during the same season experienced a femur fracture while playing basketball and soccer.

Physical Examination

In most cases, physical examination reveals tenderness on palpation over the affected bone. However, some bones, such as the femoral neck, are too deep to palpate. Early stress reaction of bone may produce only slight tenderness that may be difficult to elicit on physical examination. Stress fractures of subcutaneous bones such as the tibia, fibula, and ulna should elicit tenderness to palpation over the area of the stress fracture. Tenderness over bone may also indicate bone contusion, tendinitis, or tumor.

Diagnostic Tests

Radiographs are the principal means to confirm a diagnosis of stress fractures. Although they are sometimes negative initially, radiographs will often show positive findings if repeated about 2 weeks later. In the cancellous bone found at the ends of bones, positive findings are often seen as cloud-like formations of new bone with a linear radiolucency that develops in subsequent weeks. Usually, stress fractures in cortical bone appear as periosteal elevations and cortical thickening with subsequent lucent fracture lines (**Figure 30.2**). If a stress fracture is suspected and the initial radiographs are negative, radiographs should be repeated in about 2 weeks. In exceptional cases that require a quick diagnosis, a bone scan may be positive before the changes are apparent on plain radiographs. Early experience with MRI indicates that it may be diagnostic, but at greater cost. These studies are helpful early in the care of athletes who require a quick diagnosis because they can delineate lesions within 10 days of the onset of symptoms. However, about 90% of athletes require only radiographs for diagnosis.

Bone scan with an injection of technetium 99m MDP is very sensitive and misses very few lesions. In fact, it detects subclinical stress reactions of bone before they become stress fractures. However, bone scans are not specific, because increased uptake occurs not only with stress fractures, but also with periosteal contusions, tumors, and tendon avulsions.

MRI is a promising tool for the diagnosis of stress fractures. Possibly as sensitive as bone scanning in detecting lesions, MRI also detects edematous soft tissue that bone scans cannot. In some cases, MRI may detect tendinitis without sign of a stress fracture. However, MRI is more expensive and generally less available than a bone scan.

Figure 30.2 Cortical thickening of the anterior cortex of the tibia consistent with a stress fracture.

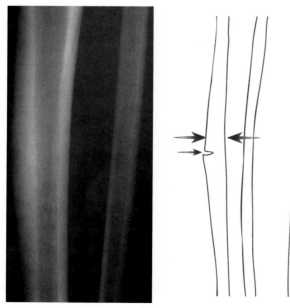

Treatment

Treatment begins with identifying the activity that is causing the abnormal stress and then decreasing that activity. Cast immobilization of the affected area or the use of crutches to redistribute body weight may be necessary if limiting the activity does not provide symptom relief. Occasionally, electrical stimulation is indicated, particularly for anterior tibial stress fractures that do not respond to other measures. Some athletes who have acute pars interarticularis defects in the lumbar spine may heal with immobilization in a thoracolumbar spinal orthosis.

Usually, surgical referral is not necessary. Occasionally, anterior tibial stress fractures that do not respond to nonoperative therapy or electrical stimulation may respond to bone grafting. However, most other pediatric stress fractures will respond to nonoperative treatment. If activity modifications do not relieve symptoms, thorough evaluation for other etiologies is necessary.

Rehabilitation

Rehabilitation of stress fractures should start with a program for maintaining general physical fitness. Activities designed to protect the injured area, but emphasize strength and cardiovascular fitness should be initiated. During rehabilitation, strengthening and flexibility of the surrounding musculature should also be addressed. After an athlete has been asymptomatic for at least 3 weeks, he or she should be allowed to slowly resume previous activities. Activity should be increased gradually every 3 weeks with the aim of returning to full activity at 9 to 12 weeks if the athlete remains asymptomatic.

Female athletes with amenorrhea or oligomenorrhea should be further evaluated and steps taken to normalize menstrual function to decrease or minimize further bone density loss.

Equipment Modification

Occasionally, modifying equipment is helpful. For example, shoes with adequate shock absorption should be recommended. In addition, running surfaces with some spring are superior to unyielding surfaces such as concrete. Also, use of a shock-absorbing wrap on the handle of a tennis racquet may help in some instances.

Prevention

The key to preventing stress fractures is skeletal conditioning. Over time, bone responds to stress by becoming stronger. Typically, increases in strength are first noticed 3 to 4 weeks after exercise begins. Although muscle size does not increase until later, effective muscle strength can increase in the first 2 weeks of training because of improved neuromuscular coordination and increased recruitment of muscle fibers. As a result, an imbalance can occur between effective muscle strength and bone strength during the first 2 weeks of increased activity. Therefore, training intensity should be gradually increased every 3 weeks.

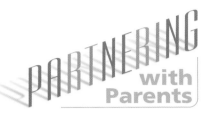

How is a stress fracture treated?

A period of rest should follow the recognition of a stress fracture. The rest period may require two weeks or longer. Generally the child may return to the same sport with few exceptions—and the return to sports should be guided by the physician, therapist and trainer. The pain usually improves immediately upon cessation of the activity. In some cases crutches may be recommended.

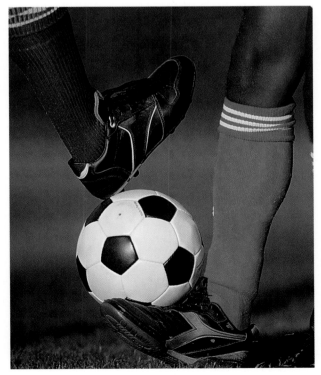

Return to Play Guidelines

With supervision, young athletes should be able to practice at full intensity for 3 to 5 days without symptoms before returning to play without restrictions. Also, repeat radiographs should demonstrate signs of healing.

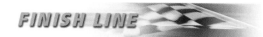

Stress fractures of bone occur when "too much is done too soon." In most patients, diagnosis is confirmed by tenderness on physical examination, plain radiographs, and response to rest. A high index of suspicion is necessary. Gradual, supervised return to activity is usually successful.

For More Information

1. Bruns BR, Yngve D: Stress reaction and stress fracture, in Grana WA (ed): *Advances in Sports Medicine and Fitness.* Chicago, IL, Year Book Medical, 1989, vol 2, pp 201–221.

2. Shin AY, Morin WD, Gorman JD, Jones SB, Lapinsky AS: The superiority of magnetic resonance imaging in differentiating the cause of hip pain in endurance athletes. *Am J Sports Med* 1996;24:168–176.

3. Walker RN, Green NE, Spindler KP: Stress fractures in skeletally immature patients. *J Pediatr Orthop* 1996;16:578–584.

4. Yngve DA: Stress fractures in the pediatric athlete, in Sullivan JA, Grana WA (eds): *The Pediatric Athlete.* Park Ridge, IL, American Academy of Orthopaedic Surgeons, 1990, pp 235–240.

Chapter 31

Spine

BROCK E. SCHNEBEL, MD

The incidence of back pain in the adult athlete is essentially the same as that in the general population. However back pain in the young athlete is a cause of concern because the potential causes differ from those in adults (**Table 31.1**). Many spinal conditions, including endplate fractures or slipped vertebral endplate, apophysitis, scoliosis, kyphosis, and spondylolisthesis are contributed to by a child's immature skeleton.

Table 31.1 Cause of Back Pain in Adolescents Compared With Adults	Adolescents	Adults
Spondylolysis (Stress fractures)	47%	5%
Discogenic back pain	11%	48%
Muscle tendon strain	6%	27%
Stenosis/Osteoarthritis	0%	10%

Anatomy/Biomechanics

The spine is a mechanical structure consisting of bones, joints, ligaments, and muscles. The thoracic spine is more stable than the lumbar or cervical spine, and therefore less mobile, because of the rib cage. The spinal column is composed of 33 vertebrae divided into five sections: cervical (7), thoracic (12), lumbar (5), sacral (5), and coccygeal (4) (**Figure 31.1**). The spinal column has five principal functions:

1. Support of the head.

2. Support of the abdominal contents and pelvic girdle.

3. Point of attachment for the thoracic cage.

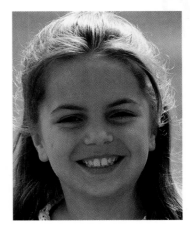

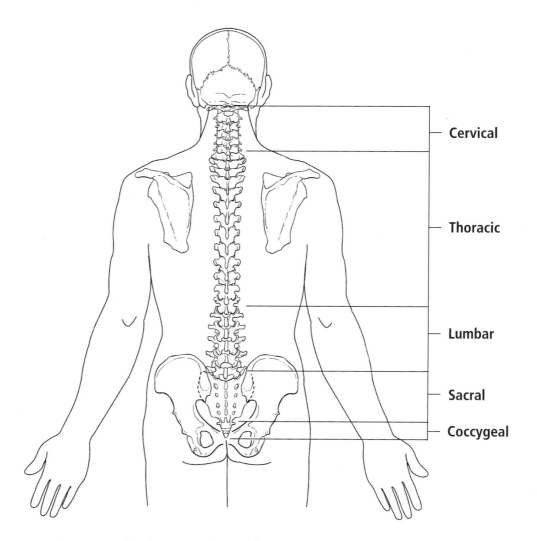

Figure 31.1 The five sections of the spine.

4. Protection of the spinal cord and the neural elements within while allowing motion.

5. Transfer of the weight and bending movements of the head and trunk to the pelvis.

Several anatomic features make the pediatric spine more flexible and therefore more susceptible to traction injuries than the adult spine. For example: the facet joints in a child's spine are more horizontal; and the soft tissues, particularly those in the neck, are more elastic than those in adults.

In an adult, each vertebra consists of an anterior body and a posterior arch that enclose the spinal canal. However, at birth, each vertebra consists of three bony parts; these assume their normal adult shape by the time a child is age 7 to 9 years. The individual vertebra are joined by joints between the bodies (disk) and the neural arches (facets). The pedicle is the portion of bone that joins the body to the arches. The part of the lamina between the upper and lower facet joints is called the pars interarticularis. It is the region of the

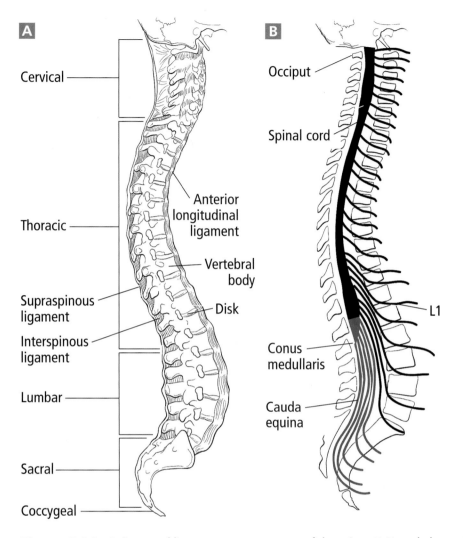

A Cervical

Thoracic

Supraspinous ligament

Interspinous ligament

Lumbar

Sacral

Coccygeal

Anterior longitudinal ligament

Vertebral body

Disk

B Occiput

Spinal cord

Conus medullaris

Cauda equina

L1

Figure 31.2   A Bony and ligamentous components of the spine. **B** Neural elements of the spine.

bone that fails, resulting in a spondylolysis or stress fracture in the adolescent or adult athlete.

The neural elements within the spinal canal are the spinal cord from the occiput to about L1, the conus medullaris or lower portion of the cord from T11 to L1, and the cauda equina from L1 to the sacrum (**Figure 31.2**).

Two major ligaments connect the vertebral bodies: the anterior longitudinal ligament and the posterior longitudinal ligament. The primary ligaments are the ligamentum flavum, the interspinous ligaments, and the supraspinous ligaments. Of course, the disk also functions as a ligament and as part of the anterior joint at each level, while the facet capsules function as ligaments at each facet joint.

The multiple segments of the spine make it flexible. The thoracic spine is less flexible than the cervical or lumbar spine because its vertebrae are attached to the rib cage, and it normally has a kyphosis (concave toward the front). The cervical and lumbar spine assume a secondary curve that is lordotic (convex toward the front).

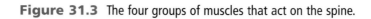

Figure 31.3 The four groups of muscles that act on the spine.

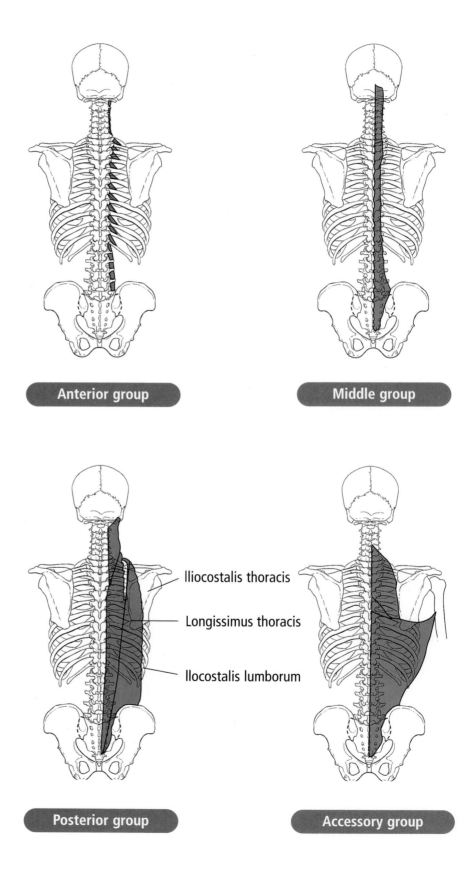

Four groups of muscles act on the spine, as follows (**Figure 31.3**):

1. *The anterior muscle group.* These lie anterior to the plane of the transverse processes.

2. *The middle muscle group.* These are attached in the plane of the transverse processes.

3. *The posterior muscle group.* These comprise the "true" back muscles known as the erector spinae. They lie posterior to the transverse processes.

4. *The accessory muscles.* These exert an effect on the spinal column without being attached directly to it.

Clinical Evaluation

History

As with all medical encounters, the information obtained in the history and physical examination is critical. The following questions about the athlete's history are particularly relevant.

1. **What is the exact location of the pain?**
   Neurologic involvement is likely when a patient perceives more pain in the leg than in the back. Associated neurologic symptoms, such as numbness or dysesthesia, weakness, or spasticity, are also important to note.

2. **When does it hurt?**
   Pain that occurs only with motion suggests a mechanical cause. Night pain or pain at rest can be more ominous.

3. **What makes the pain worse?**

4. **What makes the pain better?**

5. **When and how did your symptoms begin?**
   A gradual onset associated with low-grade stresses that occur after long periods of training suggests a stress reaction. A sudden onset during anaerobic training such as sprinting or lifting single weights may indicate a more acute injury.

6. **How do you train for your sport?**
   Specific information regarding the sport or the training technique may be useful, such as "What activities are involved in training for the sport?" and "Is the athlete involved in a resistance program that is appropriate for his or her skeletal age?" Voluntary functional restrictions of certain activities may be revealing.

Physical Examination

The physical examination must include a thorough evaluation of neurologic status. Upper motor neuron findings such as spasticity, clonus, or hyperreflexia and weakness, suggest myelopathy or spinal cord malfunction. Lower motor neuron findings such as weakness, hyporeflexia, or flaccidity, suggest nerve root or cauda equina dysfunction.

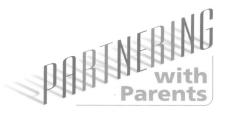

When can a young athlete return to play after a "burner" or "stinger"?

The athlete may return to play if there is no associated neurologic deficit and if the pain has subsided.

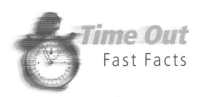

Sports-related spinal cord injuries are uncommon.

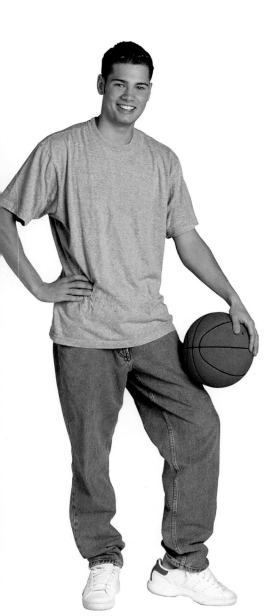

Specific motor groups must be evaluated in the context of areas of innervation. For example, an injury to the S1 nerve root may appear as motor weakness in the gastrocnemius-soleus complex, an Achilles reflex deficit, and/or a sensory distribution deficit at the lateral aspect of the foot.

Inspection and palpation of the spine is critical. The patient should be asked to attempt to touch the toes, extend, and bend to the right and left. The spine should also be examined during gait. Posture alone can suggest a diagnosis such as scoliosis, kyphosis, or a list with a herniated disk. Pain with tests that stretch nerves, such as the straight leg raise, may indicate neurologic involvement, while pain with extension of the spine may indicate a stress reaction in the pars interarticularis. Provocative tests that load the sacroiliac joint may indicate its involvement.

Diagnostic Tests

The initial studies should include a standing AP and lateral of the lumbar spine. If spondylolysis or spondylolisthesis is suspected, right and left obliques should be added. If spondylolisthesis is present, a standing spot lateral view of L5-S1 will more accurately demonstrate the L5-S1 disk and the amount of displacement. If radiographs are normal and spondylolysis is suspected, a bone scan with SPECT imaging is indicated. With spondylolisthesis, flexion-extension views will demonstrate any instability. A CT scan is used to more clearly evaluate bony lesions such as spondylolysis, congenital lesions, or bony sclerosis. An MRI is the study of choice to examine the spinal cord, nerve roots, disks, or other soft tissues.

If neurologic involvement is suspected, electromyography (EMG) and nerve conduction velocity studies might be indicated for more exact identification of the involved nerve or to differen-tiate a peripheral nerve injury from a more central lesion. Labor-atory studies can be useful in diagnosing diskitis, inflammatory spondylitis, or neoplasia, but these studies are rarely needed.

Differential Diagnosis

The differential diagnoses are discussed according to type: trauma, congenital lesions, and deformities. This does not represent a complete list of the differential diagnoses, but rather the most common. If neurologic involvement is present, consultation with a specialist is warranted.

Trauma

Physicians responsible for sideline management must be equipped to care for spinal injuries on the field. To be prepared for on-the-field decision making and emergency management of spinal injuries, several steps must take place prior to competition. An emergency plan must be in place, in which the physician must:

1. Understand the venue, its limits, and needs.

2. Prepare communications, including phone, radio, and pager.

3. Define the responsibilities of those involved and know the level of experience and training of those involved.

4. Arrange for transportation and emergency equipment.

5. Have appropriate hospital/care system referral arranged.

In an injury situation on the field, the physician must do the following:

1. Perform an initial examination.

2. Recognize the injury.

3. Provide emergency care as described below.

4. Determine if further evaluation or treatment is needed.

5. Make return to play decisions.

Sideline and On-Field Management of Trauma

Remember that a spine-injured athlete may make it to the sidelines with the ability to walk, move the extremities, and have normal sensation. However, this does not rule out a spinal injury (**Figure 31.4**). Athletes with suspected spinal injuries can be found in supine, prone, sitting or even standing positions. Regardless of the position in which the athlete is found, if a spinal injury is suspected the athlete should not be moved and full body immobilization is necessary because 10% to 15% of cervical spine fractures are associated with spine fractures at other levels. Level of consciousness should be assessed initially, as head and neck injuries may occur simultaneously. Evaluate the airway, breathing, and circulation. Leave the helmet on in football players but be prepared to remove the face mask if the airway is

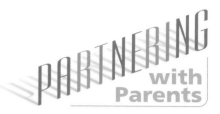

If a football player is down on the field and there is a concern about a neck injury, should the helmet be removed?

No! The athlete should not be moved unless absolutely essential to maintain airway, breathing, and circulation! When appropriate EMS help arrives at the scene, the athlete is carefully log rolled onto a back board with helmet in place.

Figure 31.4 Algorithm for evaluation of athlete with cervical injury.

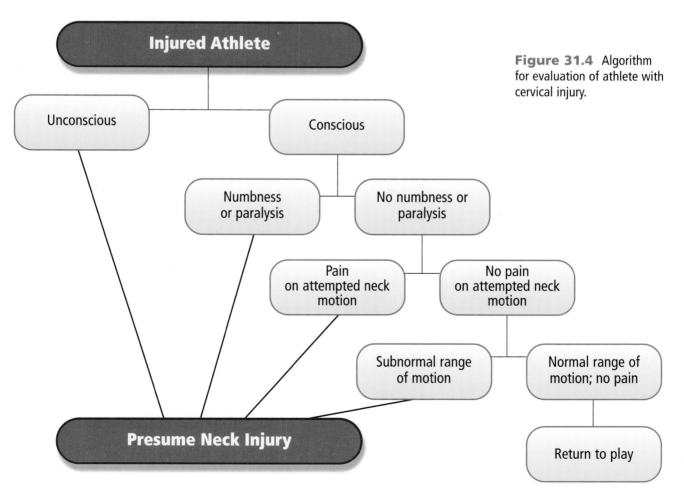

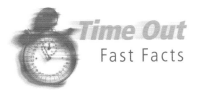

Most spinal cord injuries occur as a result of motor vehicle accidents, falls or jumps, and gunshot wounds; however, trampoline injuries are an increasing cause of spine and spinal cord injuries.

compromised. A brief neurologic evaluation should be done immediately. Be aware of injuries to the other organ systems that could be simultaneously injured. If the athlete is stable, and airway, breathing, and circulation are functioning, then wait for emergency medical services (EMS) to assist in immobilization of the athlete in preparation for transportation. **Table 31.2** summarizes guidelines developed in 1998 by the Inter-association Task Force for the Appropriate Care of the Spine-Injured Athlete.

Restoring the airway. Improper handling of a spinal injury can leave an athlete permanently paralyzed; however, without an open airway the athlete will die. If the athlete with a spinal injury has an airway obstruction, open the airway with the jaw-thrust maneuver. Do not use the head-tilt/chin-lift maneuver, as it extends the neck and may further damage the cervical spine. If the athlete is unconscious, lift or pull the tongue forward, assuring that the neck is not moved. The athlete's head should be held still, in a neutral, in-line position, until it can be fully immobilized. If the airway cannot be opened because of the position of the head and the athlete, reposition the athlete using spinal precautions and maintain alignment of the head and neck.

After the airway is open an oral airway can be inserted. If an oral airway is used the athlete should be monitored closely.

Immobilizing the cervical spine. After obtaining an open airway while using spinal precautions, the next step is to stabilize the head and trunk. Even small movements can injure the spinal cord. In-line manual stabilization of the head and neck should be initiated, ensuring that movements are gentle and that the head is moved until the athlete's eyes are looking straight ahead and the head and trunk are in line. The head should not be twisted, flexed, or extended excessively. The cervical spine should be maintained in this position until the athlete is properly secured to a backboard and the head is immobilized with a cervical collar and strapped to the board (**Figure 31.5**). EMTs typically will be responsible for packaging and transporting the athlete to the hospital.

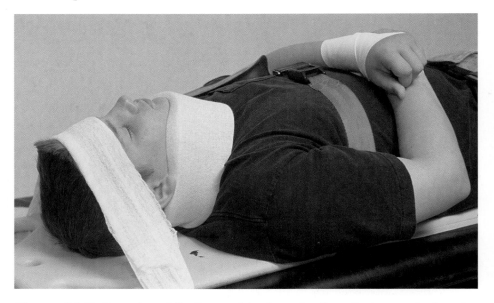

Figure 31.5 Proper immobilization consists of securing the patient on a spine board with a cervical collar in place and the head, chest, and the lower extremities secured to the board. The wrists are secured as well.

Table 31.2 *Guidelines for the Appropriate Care of the Spine-Injured Athlete* ———

General guidelines

- Any athlete suspected of having a spinal injury should not be moved and should be managed as though a spinal injury exists.

- The athlete's airway, breathing, circulation, neurologic status, and level of consciousness should be assessed.

- The athlete should not be moved unless absolutely essential to maintain airway, breathing, and circulation.

- If the athlete must be moved to maintain airway, breathing, and circulation, the athlete should be placed in a supine position while maintaining spinal immobilization.

- When moving a suspected spine-injured athlete, the head and trunk should be moved as a unit. One accepted technique is to manually splint the head to the trunk.

- The Emergency Medical Services (EMS) system should be activated.

Face mask removal

- The face mask should be removed prior to transportation, regardless of current respiratory status.

- Those involved in the prehospital care of injured football players should have the tools for face mask removal readily available.

Football helmet removal

The athletic helmet and chin strap should only be removed:

- If the helmet and chin strap do not hold the head securely, such that immobilization of the helmet does not also immobilize the head.

- If the design of the helmet and chin strap is such that even after removal of the face mask the airway cannot be controlled, or ventilation cannot be provided.

- If the face mask cannot be removed after a reasonable period of time.

- If the helmet prevents immobilization for transportation in an appropriate position.

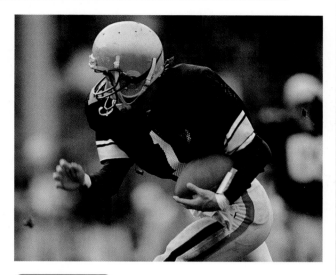

Helmet removal

- Spinal immobilization must be maintained while removing the helmet.

- Helmet removal should be frequently practiced under proper supervision.

- Specific guidelines for helmet removal need to be developed. In most circumstances, it may be helpful to remove cheek padding and/or deflate air padding prior to helmet removal.

Equipment

- Appropriate spinal alignment must be maintained.

- There needs to be a realization that the helmet and shoulder pads elevate an athlete's trunk when in the supine position.

- Should either be removed, or if only one is present, appropriate spinal alignment must be maintained.

- The front of the shoulder pads can be opened to allow access for CPR and defibrillation.

Note: The Task Force encourages the development of a local emergency care plan regarding the prehospital care of the athlete with a suspected spinal cord injury. This plan should include communication with the institution's administration and those directly involved with the assessment and transportation of the injured athlete.

All providers of prehospital care should practice and be competent in all of the skills identified in these guidelines before they are needed in an emergency situation.

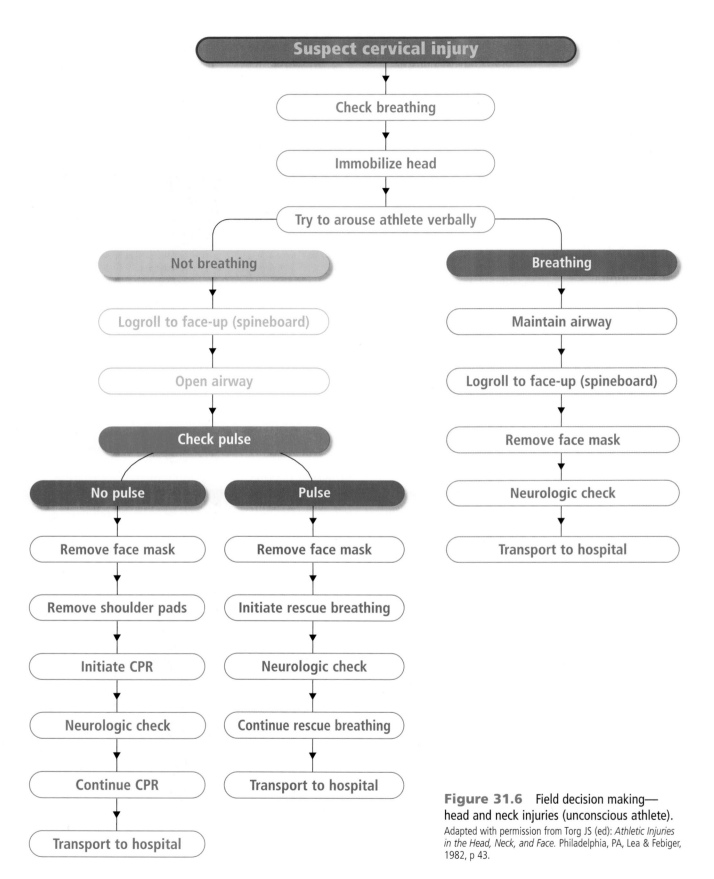

Figure 31.6 Field decision making—head and neck injuries (unconscious athlete).

Adapted with permission from Torg JS (ed): *Athletic Injuries in the Head, Neck, and Face.* Philadelphia, PA, Lea & Febiger, 1982, p 43.

In some situations, the head should not be forced into a neutral, in-line position, including the following:

1. Muscle spasms in the neck.

2. Increased pain with motion.

3. If the positioning produces numbness, tingling, or weakness.

4. If the positioning produces compromised airway or ventilations.

In these situations, the athlete should be immobilized in the position in which he or she was found.

Appropriate stabilization and transfer techniques are outlined in **Figure 31.6.**

Cervical Spine

Trauma to the cervical spine in young athletes is of great concern. Therefore, a thorough evaluation is necessary to assess the extent of an injury so that management and possible referral decisions can be made. Treatment options vary, depending on the nature of the bony or ligamentous injury. Any injury involving the spinal cord (myelopathy), whether permanent or transient, requires the involvement of a specialist.

Fractures. Fractures or dislocations can occur at any level of the cervical spine. In children younger than age 10 years, injuries tend to occur in the upper cervical spine. Injury patterns in children older than age 10 are similar to those in adults with most injuries occurring between C3 and C7. Most cervical spine fractures result from a force that axially loads the spine and forces it into flexion. These injuries occur in sports as a result of a fall on the head or by ramming the head into an opponent in a collision sport, such as football. Spinal fractures should be assumed in any athlete who has persistent neurologic complaints or limited neck motion. Return to play in these athletes is prohibited until fracture is ruled out, normal range of motion is restored, and neurologic signs and symptoms abate.

Ligamentous injuries. Ligament injuries at the C1-C2 articulation can result in widening of the atlanto-dens interval. If not identified, this ligamentous injury can lead to quadriplegia or death. Surgical stabilization may be required, regardless of sports participation. A child with torticollis (wry neck) may have an atlantoaxial rotatory subluxation. Plain radiographs or a CT scan at the C1-C2 region confirm the diagnosis (**Figure 31.7**). Pseudosubluxation and other normal variations occur in radiographs of the pediatric spine so physicians must be knowledgeable in their interpretation. Treatment of torticollis includes rest, traction, or occasionally surgery.

One type of ligamentous injury, called the hidden lesion of McSweeney, is characterized by rupture of the supraspinous ligaments, interspinal ligaments, facet capsule, ligamentum flavum, and disk. Radiographs may appear normal with this injury, but an athlete may be at extreme risk of further injury or quadriplegia if allowed to return to play. Gentle, self-administered flexion-extension radiographs confirm the diagnosis, but are indicated only if plain radiographs are normal, if the patient is conscious and able to actively flex and extend the neck, and if the patient is neurologically

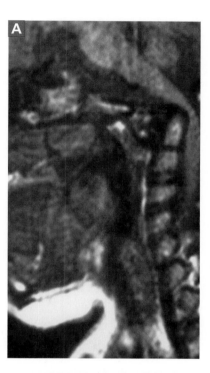
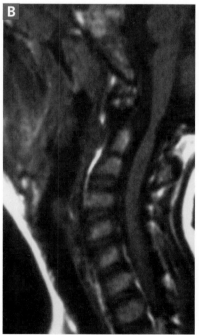

Figure 31.7 A Flexion and **B** extension MRI scans of the cervical spine showing compression of the spinal cord on the dens with flexion.

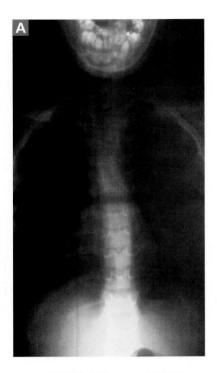

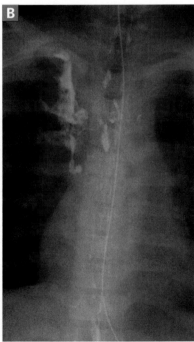

Figure 31.8 **A** Normal radiograph of a patient with T4 paraplegia, demonstrating SCIWORA. **B** Contrast myelogram shows severe spinal cord and dural damage.

intact. This diagnosis is difficult to make, but should be suspected in athletes with persistent pain or pain in excess of what is expected. Evaluation by a specialist is warranted.

Spinal cord injury can also be present without radiographic evidence of abnormality, a condition called Spinal Cord Injury Without Radiographic Abnormality syndrome (SCIWORA) (**Figure 31.8**). These children have normal imaging studies but a neurologic deficit that can range from subtle paraparesis to obvious paralysis. Evaluation by a specialist is warranted.

Burners and stingers. Cervical radiculopathy or plexopathy is commonly known to athletes as burners and stingers. Signs and symptoms include temporary paresis, paralysis, or dysesthesia caused by a neurapraxia of a nerve root of the brachial plexus. Burners and stingers can be prevented or limited with appropriate equipment such as spacers and neck collars to limit lateral bending of the cervical spine. A strengthening program may be beneficial to protect the spine from excessive bending forces. Treatment of chronic burners consists of rest and medication, including anti-inflammatory drugs and rehabilitation with strengthening exercises. Many factors are involved in return to play decisions, and a specialist should be consulted if the athlete has a persistent neurologic deficit or limited range of motion.

Transient neurapraxia of the spinal cord. This condition is a transient neurologic deficit up to and including complete paralysis with immediate or rapid recovery to normal and no identified spine or spinal cord injury. This condition requires evaluation by a specialist.

Thoracic Spine

Traumatic injuries are less common in the thoracic spine because it is relatively protected by the rib cage. However, compression fractures or endplate fractures may occur. An athlete who has pain, spasm, or guarding and no radiographic evidence of an abnormality and who fails to respond to restrictions, rest, and physical therapy may require a bone scan or SPECT. Depending on the injury, bracing may be required. Gradual return to activity can be allowed as symptoms abate.

Herniations. Thoracic disk herniations are rare.

Apophysitis. Apophysitis is caused by repetitive traction on the anterior longitudinal ligament during activities such as dance, diving, and gymnastics that involve marked flexion and extension of the thoracolumbar spine.

Athletes with apophysitis can have back pain that increases with activity and improves with rest. This entity has no distinguishing clinical features, but plain radiographs of the thoracolumbar spine will reveal irregularities of the ventral apophysis at multiple levels. Rest relieves the symptoms and should be followed by back and abdominal stretching and strengthening exercises before returning to sports. Bracing might be required in the early stages if symptoms are severe. Some athletes can be ready to return to sports within several weeks, but others might have to wait for several months until symptoms have sufficiently subsided. Walking and cycling are encouraged during the early rehabilitation program because these activities maintain muscular and cardiovascular conditioning in the athlete as well as build strength in the back and abdominal muscles without aggravating the apophysitis.

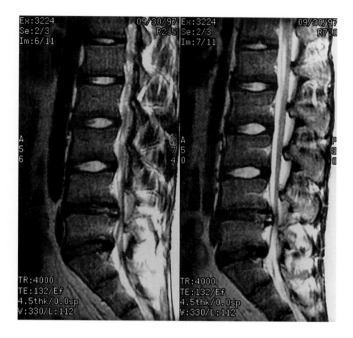

Figure 31.9 MRI scan shows narrowed spinal canal and degenerative changes at the L4-L5 and L5-S1. Disk herniation and endplate fracture at L4-5 with compression of the dural sac.

Reproduced with permission from Richards BS, McCarthy RE, Akbarnia BA: Back pain in childhood and adolescence, in Zuckerman JD (ed): *Instructional Course Lectures 48.* Rosemont, IL, American Academy of Orthopaedic Surgeons, 1999, pp 525–542.

Lumbar Spine

Soft-tissue injury to the low back is common and responds rapidly to rest. Therefore, activity limitations are usually indicated to prevent additional injury. However, an athlete should be encouraged to maintain conditioning and flexibility.

Disk herniation. This condition is not common in adolescents. When herniation occurs, it can appear as an apophyseal fracture. The outer layer of the vertebral disk (the annulus fibrosis) is stronger than the growth plate in children; therefore, a torsional bending force can result in the inner portion of the disk (the nucleus pulposus) extravasating through the apophysis, resulting in a fracture of the apophysis and herniation of the nucleus pulposus.

Apophyseal fractures differ from herniated disks in adults because in adolescents the injury also involves the bone. Despite these physiologic differences, the clinical picture is often the same even though the physical examination might not include a positive straight leg raise test as in an adult. CT, myelogram, or MRI is often needed to visualize the fracture's endplate because it is not visible on plain radiographs (**Figure 31.9**).

Treatment options are the same as for adults with a herniated disk. Nonsurgical treatments include 2 days of bed rest, medications with use of anti-inflammatory drugs, occasionally epidural steroids, physical therapy, and time. Physical therapy initially is directed at pain relief, followed by gradual mobilization and then eventual stabilization techniques to strengthen the spine. Sport-specific rehabilitation techniques can be added. Surgical intervention can be required if neurologic involvement is significant or if the condition fails to improve with nonsurgical care.

When the disk herniates through the anterior aspect of the apophysis into the vertebral body, the resulting radiographic appearance is known

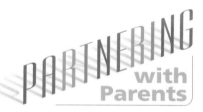

What is a "burner" or a "stinger"?

A shocklike pain going from the shoulder down the arm to the finger tips have been termed "burners" and "stingers." These occur as a result of injuries to the neck or brachial plexus particularly when the neck is bent one way and the same shoulder is depressed.

as a Schmorl's node. This finding is very common, appearing in approximately 40% to 75% of lumbar radiographs. This condition affects both athletes and non-athletes equally. Pain is possible, and temporary activity limitations may be needed.

Degenerative disk disease. The disk can also present as a pain source because of annular tears. The tears can occur as a result of a predisposition to degenerative disk disease. Degenerative disk changes are two times more commonly found in the MRI studies of gymnasts as compared with non-athletes. Because the long-term natural history of these changes is unknown, their significance is in question. The relationship between pain and degeneration in athletes is also unknown; however, the lifetime incidence and prevalence of low back pain is higher in retired wrestlers 50 years of age than in the general population.

Stress fractures. Stress reactions or stress fractures may occur in the lumbar spine, especially in the pars interarticularis region or the pedicles. These fractures can progress to a nonunion called a spondylolysis. Initially, patients can report back pain on one side that worsens with motion and running. In addition, they usually have pain with spine extension centrally and/or to that side. Plain radiographs should be ordered first. If these appear normal and the diagnosis is strongly suspected, a bone scan with SPECT may reveal increased uptake supporting the diagnosis. A CT scan and/or MRI can be used to further evaluate the continuity of the pars interarticularis.

The diagnosis of acute spondylolysis should be considered in athletes who participate in "back-intensive" sports such as dance, skating, gymnastics, diving, weight lifting, and football who have normal radiographs and a history of low back pain for more than 6 weeks that has failed to respond to nonsurgical care. The incidence of spondylolysis in female gymnasts is four times the normal population incidence. A bone scan/SPECT or MRI might be needed to identify the lesion.

Early treatment of acute stress fracture includes rest from sports activities and possible use of a brace if patients are symptomatic with activities of daily living. A "modified Boston" orthosis, which places the spine in slight flexion, may unload the stress fracture and decrease symptoms. As symptoms begin to improve, a spine stabilization exercise program is started. When symptoms improve more, the athlete can return to the sport, protected by the brace that can be used during biking, swimming, and conditioning drills that do not require marked flexion or extension of the lumbar spine. A dancer can advance from floor bar drills to bar drills to free floor exercise, whereas a skater can begin to practice figures and free skate, then slowly advance to more difficult forms.

The duration of brace protection and limitation of activities in athletes with acute pars defects has sparked much debate. Some physicians recommend bracing until there is evidence of radiographic healing, while others recommend bracing and limited activity for 3 to 6 months until the athlete is asymptomatic, has full range of motion of the spine, and excellent strength.

Pars defects or spondylolysis. This condition can develop in children between the ages of 5 and 8 years, but may not be detected until adolescence. These children may be at increased risk for associated dysplasia, such as spina bifida, at adjacent structures. Forward slipping, or spondylolisthesis, as a result of a pars defect usually occurs during the teenage years. Both spondylolysis and spondylolisthesis can be present without pain.

Spondylolysis presents an intriguing diagnostic problem in athletes. The condition can be a stress reaction resulting from repetitive hyperextension activities or it can be a developmental abnormality. Between 10% and 15% of gymnasts and dancers are affected, compared with only 5% to 6% of the general population.

In symptomatic athletes who have radiographs that show a chronic defect of the pars consistent with long-standing spondylolysis, treatment consists of temporary rest, anti-inflammatory drugs, and a well-designed strengthening program using stabilization techniques if symptoms allow. Permanent disability or slippage has not been proved, but pain may limit the athlete's participation.

Congenital Problems

Many congenital problems are compatible with sports participation, but should be evaluated by a specialist.

Cervical Spine

Congenital scoliosis. Congenital scoliosis is caused by congenital defects of the spine, such as failure of the spine to form, to segment, or a combination of both. Patients with congenital scoliosis of the cervical spine can demonstrate progressive deformity, especially if a hemivertebra is present at C7-T1. These lesions are usually stable, but further evaluation and follow up are required and activity limitations are possible.

Klippel-Feil syndrome. With this syndrome, segments of the cervical spine are autofused, possibly resulting in instability at the segments above or below the fused segment (**Figure 31.10**). The type I lesion, which is a mass fusion of cervical and upper thoracic vertebra is an absolute contraindication to participation in contact sports. Athletes who have a type II lesion, which is a fusion of one to two interspaces, can participate if they have a full range of motion, and no occipital cervical anomalies, instability, disk disease, or degenerative changes. Specialist consultation is required. Other disorders, including scoliosis, heart disease, and genitourinary abnormalities, are associated with this condition.

Atlanto-occipital fusion. Occipitalization of the atlas, which is autofusion of the atlas to the skull, is usually asymptomatic and sometimes difficult to diagnose. This condition, which can be isolated or can coexist with other abnormalities, is a contraindication to participation in contact activities.

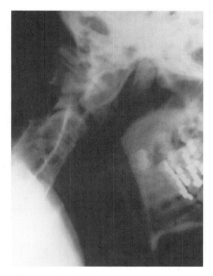

Figure 31.10 Flexion lateral radiograph shows fusion segments of the upper and lower cervical spine. Radiograph also shows instability of the unfused segment.

Reproduced with permission from Pizzutillo PD: Spinal considerations in the young athlete, in Heckman JD (ed): *Instructional Course Lectures 42.* Rosemont, IL, American Academy of Orthopaedic Surgeons, 1993, pp 463–472.

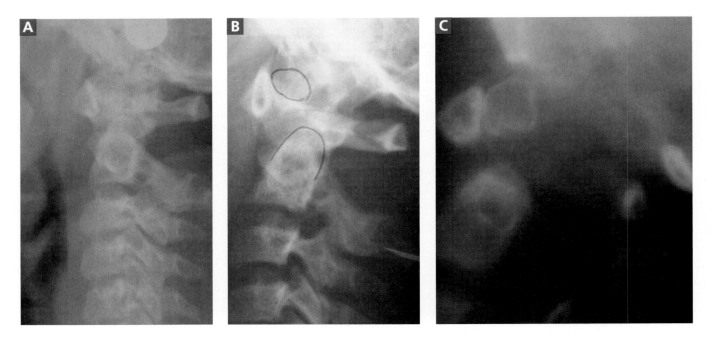

Figure 31.11
Anterior displacement of C1 and the odontoid on C2 shown on **A** anterior and **B** lateral views. **C** CT scan shows the displacement more clearly and also shows that the odontoid is a separate fragment from the body of C2.

Os odontoideum. This is a condition in which the odontoid is separated from the body of C2 (**Figure 31.11**). It can be congenital or acquired as a nonunion of a dens fracture. Os odontoideum can be detected on an open-mouth odontoid radiograph and be mistaken for an acute fracture. Therefore, flexion-extension radiographs should be ordered, and contact or collision sports should be discouraged.

Thoracic Spine

Congenital scoliosis and kyphosis result from failure of formation or failure of segmentation of the vertebral segments. These conditions can appear clinically as abnormal curvatures of the spine and can be diagnosed with plain radiographs. Both conditions can have serious consequences and require evaluation by a specialist to predict prognosis and recommend treatment. Progression in both can be slow and relentless throughout growth. Associated renal, cardiac, and cervical anomalies also need evaluation. Depending on the severity of the condition, participation in sports may have to be limited.

Spinal dysraphism, an abnormality of the spinal cord, can be associated with congenital scoliosis and kyphosis. Examples include a tethered cord or diastematomyelia. The congenital anomalies, including absence of one kidney, affect up to 20% of patients with congenital spinal anomalies. Some lesions can be compatible with athletic activity, while others may be limiting.

Lumbar Spine

Dysplastic spondylolisthesis is characterized by slippage of the vertebral bodies because the posterior elements are abnormal and do not provide the necessary stability. Progression of the deformity is likely, as are associated neurologic problems. Collision sports and sports involving hyperextension of the spine are discouraged. This type of spondylolisthesis differs from the other types discussed under the deformity section in that it can be more progressive.

Deformities

Scoliosis

Scoliosis is a lateral spinal curvature of more than 10° (**Figure 31.12**). Eighty percent of scoliosis is of unknown etiology and is called idiopathic scoliosis. Idiopathic scoliosis is more common in girls than boys. A careful history and physical examination are necessary to rule out the other causes of scoliosis, most of which are neurologic. Examination should include careful inspection from behind, noting the alignment of the posterior spinous processes. Rotation associated with this curve is revealed by having the athlete bend forward and noting the prominence of the rib cage on the convex side of the curve. If the curve is unbalanced, the pelvis might be higher on one side than the other, giving the athlete an apparent limb-length discrepancy. Neurologic examination is normal. If radiographs are ordered, make sure that standing views on a 14 × 36 cassette are ordered.

Treatment varies from observation to surgery, depending on the patient's age and the amount of curvature. Because treatments vary widely, the most appropriate treatment is best decided by a physician familiar with all options.

Most patients with idiopathic scoliosis are asymptomatic and therefore allowed to participate in sports. For curves of less than 20°, full participation in sports is reasonable followed by careful repeat examinations every 6 months. However, bracing is recommended in an athlete with a curve greater than 25° and significant skeletal growth remaining or in an athlete whose curve progression is greater than 5° in 6 months. Bracing is not a contraindication to participation, as the number of hours the athlete wears the brace varies from nighttime only to 23 hours a day. Some physicians allow patients to participate without wearing the brace. All patients require follow-up examination so that curve progression can be monitored until they stop growing.

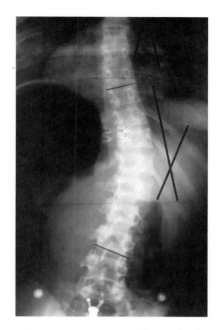

Figure 31.12 PA radiograph of the entire spine demonstrating a scoliotic deformity and the Cobb method of measuring its magnitude.

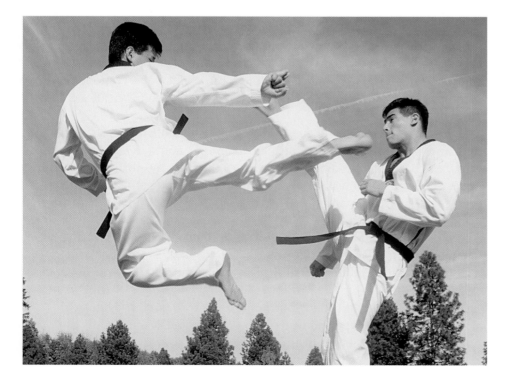

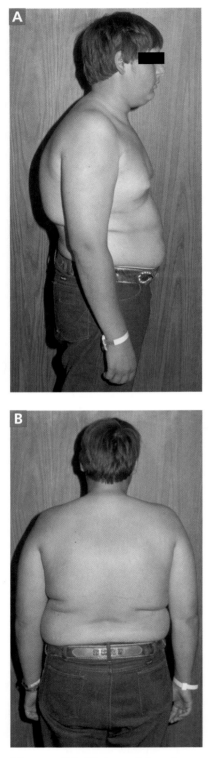

Figure 31.13 Lateral **A** and posterior **B** clinical views of Scheuermann's disease.

If surgical intervention is required, the surgeon must approve sports participation. The type of surgery done and the desired sport are clearly factors in this decision. In general, collision sports are not recommended. Following surgery, sports are permitted beginning with swimming at 6 to 12 weeks and biking after 3 months, but the decision for contact activity and running should be left up to the surgeon. Sports are usually limited for 6 months to 1 year. Athletes should be advised that fusion will limit flexibility and can alter performance in sports that demand flexibility, such as dancing, gymnastics, and skating. It is important to note that spinal fusion places additional stress on the remaining motion segments; therefore, sports that place repetitive loads on the spine, such as those that involve jumping and running, will put increased stress on adjacent spinal segments.

Kyphosis

The normal thoracic spine has a kyphosis, or forward curvature of the spine, of 25° to 45°. The most common causes of excessive kyphosis in young athletes are postural kyphosis, which results from postural habits, and Scheuermann's disease (**Figure 31.13**). Abnormal kyphosis is also associated with a variety of conditions, such as neurofibromatosis and collagen disorders.

Thoracic Scheuermann's disease. Scheuermann's disease, or juvenile kyphosis, is thought to be caused by necrosis of the ring apophysis (growth center of the vertebra), perhaps related to repetitive trauma. In fact, the incidence of Scheuermann's disease in adolescent weight lifters and rowers is high. The diagnosis is confirmed by the presence of abnormal kyphosis associated with anterior wedging of three or more adjacent vertebral bodies (**Figure 31.14**). In addition, Schmorl's nodes and endplate irregularities are usually seen on radiographs. However, the presence of Schmorl's nodes is not in itself diagnostic of Scheuermann's disease and, in fact, must be differentiated from Scheuermann's disease, which will tend to progress to a thoracic round back deformity, will have an association with vertebral wedging, and will have the radiographic appearance of undulations of the endplate.

Most patients are asymptomatic, but some report pain or fatigue. Progression of the deformity later in life is unusual. Active participation in contact sports is not prohibited. Treatment can include observation, treatment, or surgery. Referral to a specialist is recommended for treatment and participation decisions.

Lumbar Scheuermann's disease. This diagnosis is confirmed by a loss of lumbar lordosis, vertebral wedging, and Schmorl's nodes in the lumbar spine (**Figure 31.15**). This condition is seen in weight lifters, football players, and gymnasts. In weight lifters, the history usually reveals repetitive attempts to press maximal weights and high repetition training. In gymnasts, repetitive dismounts can be the cause.

Spondylolisthesis. Spondylolisthesis is a slipping of the spine. Usually, the upper body slips forward relative to the lower body, resulting in a kyphotic deformity at the level of the slippage and a reactive lordosis above (**Figure 31.16**).

Of the many types of spondylolisthesis, some are caused by abnormal anatomy (dysplastic type), some by high-velocity injuries, and some by tumors or pathologic bone. Isthmic spondylolisthesis, which is caused by a defect in the pars regions, is the most common in young athletes.

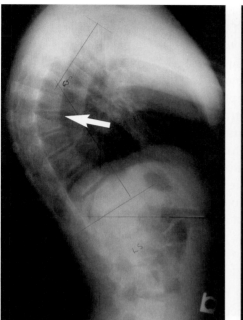

Figure 31.14 Radiograph of a patient with Scheuermann's disease showing abnormal kyphosis, vertebral wedging, and end plate irregularity.

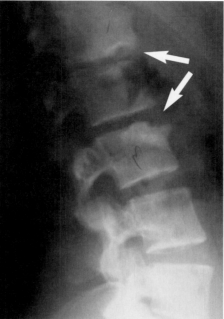

Figure 31.15 Lumbar Scheuermann's disease, with loss of lumbar lordosis, vertebral wedging, and end plate irregularity.

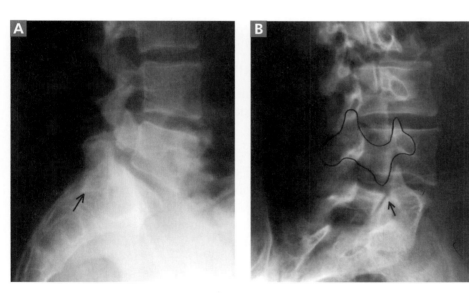

Figure 31.16 **A** Lateral radiograph of a grade 2 to 3 spondylolisthesis at the lumbosacral junction. **B** Oblique radiograph shows a normal "Scotty dog" appearance to the lamina (outlined area). In the vertebra below, the neck of the Scotty dog is broken (see arrow) and is the site of the pars interarticularis defect of spondylolisthesis.

Figure 31.17 The percentage slip of L5 on S1 is 2/A, and the grade of slippage is I to IV(A). The slip angle reflects sagittal rotation of L5, measured by intersection of lines from the posterior edge of L5 (perpendicular to the top of vertebra) and the posterior sacral line.

Reproduced with permission from Richards BS, McCarthy RE, Akbarnia BA: Back pain in childhood and adolescence, in Zuckerman JD (ed): *Instructional Course Lectures 48.* Rosemont, IL, American Academy of Orthopaedic Surgeons, 1999, pp 525–542.

Spondylolisthesis can be graded on a scale of I to V, based on the amount of forward displacement of the vertebra above on the vertebra below (**Figure 31.18**). Grade I is less than 25%, grade II less than 50%, grade III less than 75%, grade IV less than 100%, and grade V or spondyloptosis is complete displacement.

Patients with higher-grade spondylolisthesis (greater than 50%) typically cannot participate in sports because of pain and hamstring tightness. This type of spondylolisthesis is likely to progress to an even higher grade. Patients with less than 50% slippage might be able to participate in sports. An evaluation by a specialist would be helpful.

Spondylolisthesis is frequently asymptomatic; however, if an athlete has pain, it is imperative that the pain be tracked to the appropriate source, as the spondylolisthesis might not be the source. Trunk stabilization exercises might be required to keep the athlete asymptomatic and to allow participation. One treatment option is to follow the stabilization program and control symptoms by limiting sports activity. If the athlete has symptoms even with activities of daily living, surgery then becomes an option. If surgery is required, the athlete cannot participate in sports for at least a year and needs to understand that he or she may not be able to return to the previous sport, even after surgery.

Return to Play Decisions

With so many potential diagnoses that may present with spinal signs or symptoms, return to play decisions are difficult to summarize. Each of the conditions discussed in this chapter has its own criteria and may allow return to play at some but not at all levels.

The following findings may prohibit participation in contact sports:

1. Intersegmental instability on flexion-extension radiographs.

2. Anterior/posterior glide in the upper cervical spine.

3. Cervical stenosis in association with transient quadriplegia.

4. Cord impingement with myelopathy.

5. Significant neurologic impairment, or risk of neurologic impairment with a herniated disk, or obstructing lesion.

6. Limiting pain.

7. A previous spinal fusion.

Consultation with a specialist is recommended to help make return to play decisions and to discuss the advantages and disadvantages of participation with the athlete and the family. After treatment of some of these lesions athletes can be placed into risk categories, as described below, and allowed to return to play with the understanding that there is a level of risk involved (**Table 31.3**).

Minimal risk
The increase in risk is very small compared with play before injury.

Moderate risk
There is a reasonable chance that symptoms will recur, and the patient is at some risk for permanent injury.

Extreme risk
The risk that symptoms will recur and cause permanent damage is high.

Table 31.3 *Risk Classifications by Type of Spine Injury*

Minimal risk

Asymptomatic bone spurs

Certain healed facet fractures

Stingers or burners

Healed disk herniation

Healed laminar fracture

Fractured tip of the spinous process

Asymptomatic foraminal stenosis

Moderate risk

Facet fractures

Lateral mass fractures

Nondisplaced healed odontoid fractures

Nondisplaced healed ring of C1 fractures

Acute lateral disk herniations

Cervical radiculopathy caused by a foraminal spur

Extreme risk

Os odontoideum

Rupture of transverse ligament C1-2

Occipitocervical dislocation

Odontoid fracture

Total ligamentous disruption of a neuromotor segment of the lower cervical spine

Unstable fracture-dislocation

Unstable Jefferson fracture

Cervical cord anomaly

Acute large central disk herniation

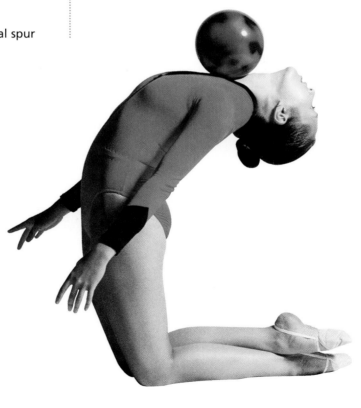

Red Flags

Consultation with a specialist is recommended for congenital lesions of the spine, lesions with neurologic involvement, and any acute trauma with a significant fracture or dislocation.

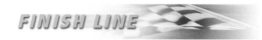

Spinal injuries can be catastrophic. Guidelines must be followed in evaluating, immobilizing, and initially treating these injuries. The equipment needed must be available. Failure to follow the necessary steps may worsen or cause injury to the neural elements.

For More Information

1. Browner BD, Jacobs LM, Poll AN (eds): American Academy of Orthopaedic Surgeons *Emergency Care and Transportation of the Sick and Injured,* ed 7. Sudbury MA, Jones and Bartlett, 1999, pp 682–713.

2. Herzenberg JE, Hensinger RN, Dedrisk DK, Phillips WA: Emergency transport and positioning of young children who have an injury of the cervical spine: The standard backboard may be hazardous. *J Bone Joint Surg* 1989;71A:15–22.

3. Jackson DW, Lohr FT: Cervical spine injuries. *Clin Sports Med* 1986; 5:373–386.

4. McGrory BJ, Klassen RA, Chao EY, Staeheli JW, Weaver AL: Acute fractures and dislocations of the cervical spine in children and adolescents. *J Bone Joint Surg* 1993;75A: 988–995.

5. Torg JS, Ramsey-Emrhein, JA: Management guidelines for participation in collision activities with congenital, developmental, or post-injury lesions involving the cervical spine. *Clin Sports Med* 1997;16:501–530.

6. Watkins RG: Neck injuries in football, in Watkins RG, Williams L, Lin P, Elrod B, Kahanovitz N (eds): *The Spine in Sports.* St. Louis, MO, Mosby Year Book, 1996, pp 314–336.

Chapter 32

Elbow and Forearm

MERVYN LETTS, MD, FRCSC
NEIL E. GREEN, MD
JOHN A. FOX, MD

Injuries to the elbow joint and forearm are a serious cause of morbidity in young athletes, with fractures about the elbow joint comprising about 10% and forearm fractures 55% of all fractures in children. The elbow is largely a ligamentous joint and has little bony stability, especially in children where the components are largely cartilaginous until the child reaches the early teens.

The immature elbow is quite vulnerable to extreme varus or valgus forces, as well as to dislocations. These forces are often applied to the elbow during gymnastics, collision sports such as hockey or football, and any of the running sports, including track and field, where a fall on the outstretched hand is common.

When a young athlete falls on an outstretched hand, the velocity of the forward momentum at the time of the fall usually determines the amount of force that will be exerted across the forearm and elbow joint, and hence the type and magnitude of the injury. Whether this occurs on the basketball court, an icy surface, or on the football or soccer field, the elbow and forearm are vulnerable to forces from the impact at the hand transmitted up the radius and ulna and interosseous membrane to the elbow joint. As the body falls over the fixed arm, valgus or varus forces may be exerted on the elbow (**Figure 32.1**). If the momentum propels the body forward or backward over the fixed hand, a hyperextension force may be exerted across the elbow joint, causing a supracondylar fracture, a dislocation of the radial head and fracture of the ulna (Monteggia fracture), or a dislocation of the elbow. The direction of these forces often predicates the type of injury that will be sustained.

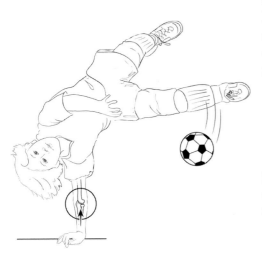

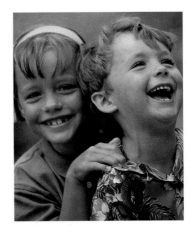

Figure 32.1 Forces exerted on the elbow in a fall on the outstretched hand resulting in fractures and dislocation.

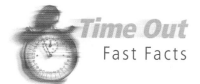

Anatomy/Biomechanics

Many injuries sustained by young athletes are related to the unique anatomy of the child's elbow. The attachments of ligaments and muscles in children are much stronger than the adjacent physes; therefore, forces exerted about the elbow joint often result in an apophyseal avulsion, such as the medial epicondylar apophyses being avulsed by the pull of the flexor tendons.

Salter-Harris types I and II physeal injuries are uncommon in the distal humeral physes but do occur through the proximal radial physes as the result of falls on the outstretched hand.

Because the elbow has very little bony stability, dislocations are much more common in young athletes than in skeletally mature athletes. In many instances, a child may simply have a swollen elbow as a result of a fall during soccer, a sign that often suggests a dislocation and spontaneous relocation of the elbow.

A child's elbow is also considerably more flexible than an adult's; therefore, it is not unusual for a child to hyperextend the elbow joint 10° or 15°. This combination of hyperflexibility and a lack of bony stability predisposes the elbow joint to increased valgus and varus strains, as well as to dislocations. The major stabilizing ligaments on the medial and lateral sides are attached to the distal humerus through apophyses, structurally weak areas that are prone to avulsion and a loss of joint integrity.

The proximal ulna and distal radius are largely cartilaginous until later in childhood. Therefore, they do not contribute as effectively to the "locking in" phenomenon in flexion or extension that occurs with a well-ossified coronoid process and olecranon that fit snugly into their respective fossa. This lack of bony stability predisposes young athletes to dislocation of the elbow.

The normal mechanics of the forearm rely on the rotation of a bowed radius around a relatively straight ulna. When the forearm is pronated, the radius and ulna are positioned such that a deformity of either bone may reduce range of motion. The articulation of the ulna and radius at their proximal and distal ends is complex, and even minor injury in these areas can cause pain and profound loss of motion. The radial and ulnar shafts are connected by an interosseous membrane and are separated by an interosseous space. Fracture displacement, angular deformity of the forearm bones, or growth deformity can narrow this space, restricting rotation of the forearm, which is the most common problem following a forearm fracture.

The radial head and neck in children are also cartilaginous, but have the same relative diameters as the radial head and neck in adults. Dislo-cation of the radial head, either as an isolated event or in association with the Monteggia fracture, is facilitated by the resiliency of the cartilaginous component and the plasticity of the radius itself. A pulled elbow, or nursemaid's elbow, is uncommon in children older than age 3 years, but occasionally occurs in 4- to 5-year-olds. The combination of generalized laxity, the large cartilaginous component, the lack of bony stability, and the presence of bony plasticity, as well as the numerous secondary centers of ossification and apophyses, all contribute to a joint vulnerable to both fractures and dislocations.

Clinical Evaluation

History

A thorough history of the mechanism of injury is often helpful in estimating the amount of force applied to the forearm and elbow. Athletes who have fallen from a height or sustained high-velocity trauma may have an associated growth arrest secondary to a fracture. Athletes in throwing sports can present with overuse injuries.

Physical Examination

Pain may be caused by direct or indirect trauma to the forearm and elbow joint. Direct trauma as a result of a fall on the outstretched hand is the most common cause of pain, but overuse can result in pain as well. Initial examination usually reveals some immediate swelling and pain with flexion or extension. Tests of active range of motion should include the following: wrist flexion, wrist extension, radial and ulnar deviation, forearm supination, forearm pronation, elbow flexion, and elbow extension. These should also be compared with the uninjured, opposite arm.

Careful examination of the skin for any associated lacerations or puncture marks is also critical as these are signs of an open fracture. Open fractures, even those with small puncture wounds, are considered surgical emergencies that require immediate diagnosis and irrigation of the wound within 8 hours of the injury. Tetanus prophylaxis and antibiotic therapy may also be required.

Deformity about the elbow and/or forearm should always be treated as a fracture. Although dislocation of the elbow or radial head will also cause deformity, the athlete will frequently have associated fractures. With a supracondylar fracture or a dislocation, the joint itself may also appear deformed. Point tenderness, crepitus and/or decreased supination and pronation about the forearm also suggests a fracture. Effusion at the elbow is often a hemarthrosis caused by dislocation or fracture; therefore, radiographs should be obtained.

An elbow contusion may draw attention to a congenital malformation of the elbow, such as a congenital dislocation of the radial head. The contour of the radial head is convex in congenital dislocation and concave when acutely dislocated (**Figure 32.2**).

Diagnostic Tests

To anyone who does not routinely read radiographs of the child's skeleton, the elbow is an enigma (no two seem alike because the child is constantly growing,

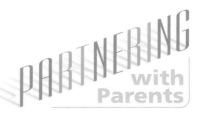

Why are elbow injuries so common in young throwing athletes?

Repetitive (valgus) stress causes compression on the lateral (outer) side and traction/stretching on the inner (medial) side, which results in the injuries known as Little Leaguer's elbow.

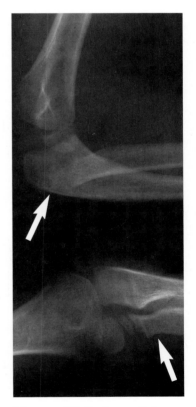

Figure 32.2 Congenital dislocation of the radial head may be detected after an acute injury and mistaken for an acute dislocation. The key is the long-standing deformity of the deformity of the radius (arrow).

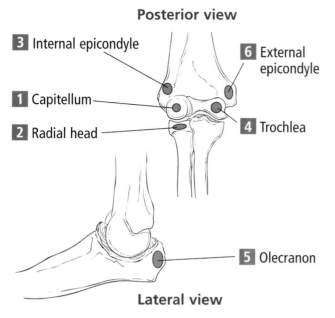

Posterior view

3 Internal epicondyle
6 External epicondyle
1 Capitellum
2 Radial head
4 Trochlea
5 Olecranon

Lateral view

Figure 32.3 Secondary ossification centers of the elbow in order of appearance.

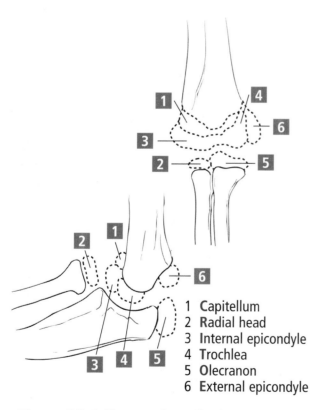

1 Capitellum
2 Radial head
3 Internal epicondyle
4 Trochlea
5 Olecranon
6 External epicondyle

Figure 32.4 Illustrates the ossification pattern about the elbow joint and the order in which the ossification centers appear. Remembered by the mnemonic CRITOE—capitellum, radial head, internal epicondyle, trochlea, olecranon, external epicondyle.

ossification centers appear and fuse at different times (**Figure 32.3**), and cartilage calcifies progressively until skeletal maturity . Therefore, a detailed discussion of how to interpret radiographs of the elbow is included here.

Although the exact age of appearance and fusion of the ossification centers is difficult to remember, the time of ossification of the various apophyses about the elbow can be remembered by the mnemonic CRITOE (**Figure 32.4**). It is helpful to remember that the ossification center of the medial epicondyle appears between ages 4 to 6 years, because this area is injured frequently. If the ossification center is absent on the radiograph of a 6-year-old child, it may be lying within the joint (**Figure 32.5**).

Anteroposterior (AP) and lateral radiographs of both the injured and uninjured wrist, forearm, and elbow should be obtained for comparison. Displaced apophyses and fracture fragments are much easier to delineate when images of the normal, unaffected elbows are available for comparison. Assessing a radiograph of the elbow requires methodical review of the anatomy. Even if the fracture or

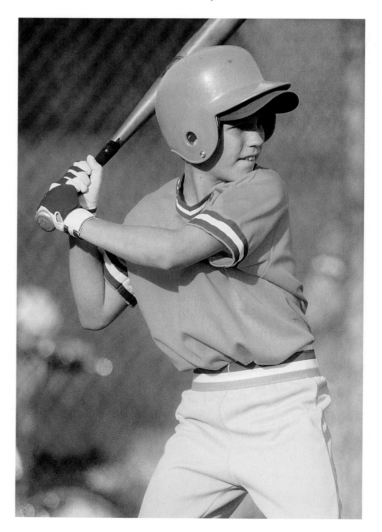

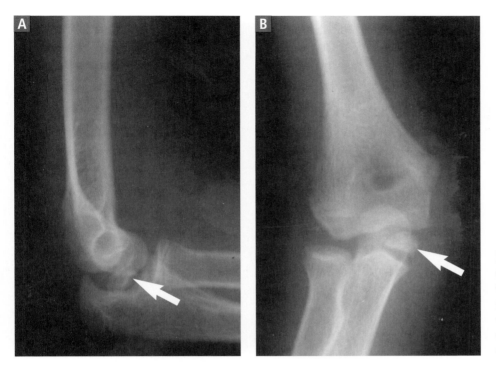

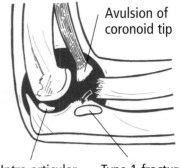

Figure 32.6 Fractures about the elbow in association with a dislocation of the elbow. The presence of these fractures usually indicates that the elbow has been dislocated even though it may be relocated at the time of examination.

Adapted with permission from Letts M: Dislocation of the child's elbow, in Morrey B (ed): *The Elbow and Its Disorders.* Philadelphia, PA, WB Saunders, 1993, pp 309–310.

Figure 32.5 Avulsion of the medial epicondyle with entrapment in the joint that occurred during dislocation of the elbow and relocation, trapping the medial epicondyle in the joint.

dislocation appears obvious, more than one fracture may be present (**Figure 32.6**). The most important fracture is often the one that is missed.

Acute Injuries

Medial Epicondyle Fracture

Assessment of the radiograph for this injury should begin on the medial side. Remember that the ossification center appears between ages 4 and 6 years. In children older than age 10 years, an imaginary line drawn along the distal medial metaphyses of the humerus should intersect the superior portion of the ossification center of the medial epicondyle. If it does not, an avulsion with slight displacement of the fragment is most likely present (**Figure 32.7**). If the medial epicondyle is absent on the AP view of the injured elbow but appears on the image of the unaffected elbow, then the medial epicondyle may be lying within the joint, hidden from view by the overlapping humerus and ulna. Careful examination of both the AP and lateral views will usually reveal the medial epicondylar fragment within the joint. After fusion of the medial epicondyle in adolescence, avulsion of the medial collateral ligament can occur.

Medial Condyle Fracture

Medial condylar fractures are uncommon in children, but do occasionally occur, especially with varus forces across the elbow joint. These fragments are large, usually displaced, type IV fractures that create a break in the

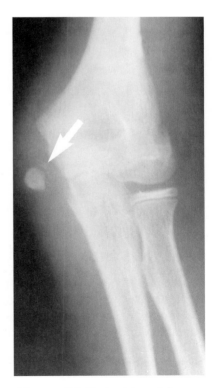

Figure 32.7 Avulsion of the medial epicondyle caused by a valgus force on the elbow.

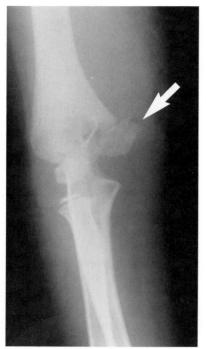

Figure 32.8 Fracture of the medial condyle of the elbow in a 5-year-old child. This fracture required an open reduction and internal fixation.

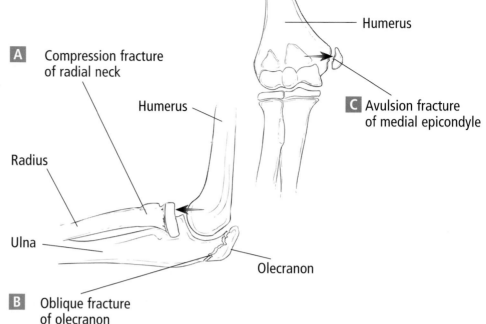

A Compression fracture of radial neck

Humerus

C Avulsion fracture of medial epicondyle

Radius

Ulna

Olecranon

B Oblique fracture of olecranon

Figure 32.9 This triad of fractures often occurs in a valgus force on the elbow in full extension, resulting in: **A** a compression fracture of the radial neck; **B** an oblique fracture of the olecranon of the ulna; and **C** an avulsion fracture of the medial epicondyle.

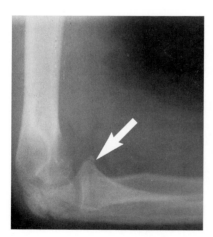

Figure 32.10 The small avulsed fragment of the coronoid process usually indicates that the elbow has been dislocated and the coronoid process has been either knocked off by impingement of the trochlea of the humerus and/or partially avulsed by the attachment of the capsule and brachialis muscle.

medial cortex (**Figure 32.8**). They frequently require open reduction because accurate reduction of the articular surface and physes is essential to the future normal growth at the elbow joint of the distal humerus.

Proximal Ulna Fracture

The proximal ulna in children usually is developed well enough that it can be examined for any transverse fractures or breaks in the cortex of the olecranon. If an extreme valgus force has been exerted on the elbow, such as a gymnast falling from a height, an associated fracture of the medial epicondyle, an oblique fracture of the proximal olecranon, and a compression fracture of the neck of the radius may be present (**Figure 32.9**). Whenever one of these fractures is present, always look for the other two.

The coronoid process of the ulna is also a common site of an avulsion fracture. Although this fracture may be seen on the AP view, it is better appreciated on the lateral view and almost always indicates that the elbow has been dislocated. As the elbow dislocates, the anterior attachment of the capsule and some fibers of the brachialis may pull off the attachment to the coronoid process; this is seen as a small fragment of bone lying just superior to the coronoid process on the lateral view (**Figure 32.10**). In children, the elbow may undergo a transitory dislocation at the moment of impact, but by the time they reach the emergency department, examination will reveal only a boggy elbow. The presence of a coronoid fracture always confirms the clinical impression that the elbow has been dislocated and spontaneously reduced.

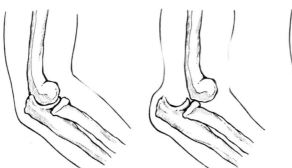

Normal anatomic position

Elbow dislocation

With reduction humerus impinges on radius, shearing off radial head

Figure 32.11 Type I fracture of the radial head may occur with a dislocation of the elbow. As the humerus relocates, it impinges on the anterior aspect of the radius and shears off the radial head that often lies within the joint.

Adapted with permission from Letts M: Dislocation of the child's elbow, in Morrey B (ed): *The Elbow and Its Disorders.* Philadelphia, PA, WB Saunders, 1993, pp 309–310.

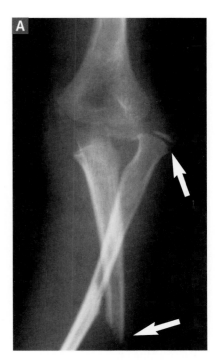

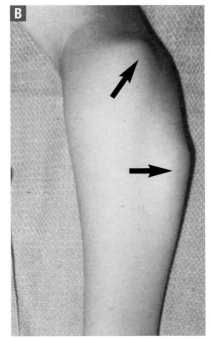

Figure 32.12 A A Monteggia fracture-dislocation with lateral displacement of the radial head and fracture of the midshaft of the ulna. **B** The dislocated radial head and the fracture of the midshaft of the ulna can be clearly seen on examination of the child's arm.

Adapted with permission from Letts M (ed): *The Management of Pediatric Fractures.* Philadelphia, PA, Churchill Livingstone, 1994, p 302.

Radial Head and Neck Fracture

Radiographs should not show any angulation of the radial head. If angulation is present, it is probably secondary to a compression fracture of the neck of the radius. Children very seldom fracture the head of the radius. A valgus force exerted on the extended elbow may result in a compression fracture of the neck, or in younger children, a type I or II fracture through the radial physis with displacement of the radial head.

Occasionally, the radial head can be displaced into the joint, which appears on radiographs as a wafer-thin area of ossification within the joint itself (**Figure 32.11**). The radial head should always align with the capitellum, and a line drawn through the neck of the radius should intersect the capitellum in any view of the elbow. If it does not, a dislocation of the radial head should be suspected. This is especially true if there is an associated fracture of the shaft of the ulna creating the Monteggia fracture-dislocation, a fracture of the ulna with a dislocation of the radial head usually anteriorly, but frequently laterally in the young athlete (**Figure 32.12**).

The joint above and below the elbow should always be assessed for associated injuries. Although uncommon, fractures of the distal radius and ulna in association with fractures of the elbow do occur because the mechanism (eg, a fall on the outstretched hand) is the same for both injuries. In addition, an associated fracture of the clavicle or the proximal humerus may also be associated with a fracture about the elbow joint.

Lateral Condyle Fracture

Lateral condylar fractures of the humerus can be very subtle in children because of the large cartilaginous component of the lateral condyle. Only a sliver of metaphyseal bone may appear separated slightly from the main

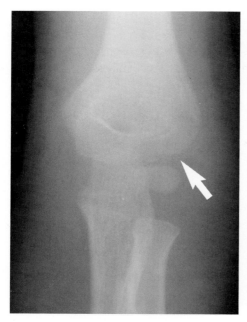

Figure 32.13 Fracture of the lateral condyle of the humerus in children can be subtle, as seen in this radiograph that shows only a small line of subchondral bone outlining a very large and mostly cartilaginous fragment and the capitellum.

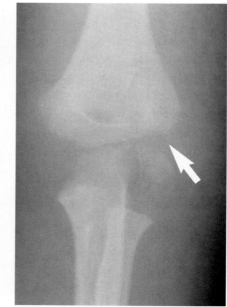

Figure 32.14 A fracture of the lateral condyle with displacement in a 10-year-old hockey player.

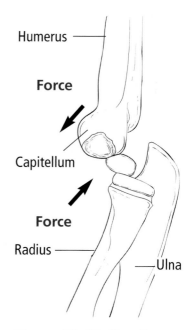

Figure 32.15 Shear fracture of the capitellum may occur with a fall on the extended outstretched arm that causes some hyperextension at the elbow.

lateral metaphyseal condyle (**Figure 32.13**). This fragment contains the entire capitellum.

In older children, lateral condylar fractures are usually more obvious because the fragment is frequently displaced, and sometimes even rotated, because of the pull of the extensor muscles of the forearm that are attached to the fragment (**Figure 32.14**). These are considered Salter-Harris type IV fractures, which are serious physeal injuries that require open reduction and internal fixation to reconstruct the articular surface as well as the physes. These fractures are the most prone to develop physeal bars and to arrest growth. Surgical supervision is required to manage these fractures. Also, shear fractures of the capitellum with direct impingement by the radial head caused by a fall on the extended elbow almost always require an open reduction (**Figure 32.15**). Shear fractures are best visualized in the lateral radiograph.

Supracondylar Fracture

Supracondylar fractures of the humerus are one of the most common injuries about the elbow, especially in children younger than age 8 years. The coronoid and olecranon fossae weaken this area of the humerus, and frequently, a hole in the distal humerus where these two fossae fuse creates an inherent weakness. This weakness makes children with reduced ossification in this area more susceptible to fractures. These fractures are usually quite obvious, especially on lateral views. Occasionally, a greenstick fracture may occur with a simple straightening of the normal forward inclination of the distal humerus on the lateral view. Also, these fractures may occasionally be

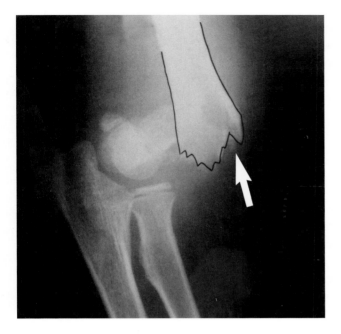

Figure 32.16 Marked displacement of a supracondylar fracture of the humerus in a 7-year-old boy who fell from his bicycle. The metaphyseal fragment has bruised the overlying skin causing a hematoma. This child also had an anterior intraosseous nerve neurapraxia.

impacted with only a slight varus or valgus tilt of the distal humerus that can usually be diagnosed when compared clinically with the uninjured side.

Supracondylar fractures of the humerus are always serious and require surgery (**Figure 32.16**). Typically, there is considerable swelling and often concomitant nerve injury, most often involving the anterior interosseous branch of the median nerve. Compartment syndrome in the forearm is a limb-threatening complication that often requires immediate fasciotomy and ongoing aggressive management, sometimes including vascular repair to salvage the limb. Assessment for the "five Ps" is key to confirming a diagnosis of compartment syndrome: 1) Pain, especially with passive extension of the finger; 2) pallor; 3) paresthesias; 4) pulselessness; and 5) paralysis. If there is any question about the diagnosis, measurements of compartment pressure should be obtained. Because of the possibility of a severe complication, supracondylar fractures should always be managed by an orthopaedic surgeon.

Chronic Injuries

Children are not prone to the overuse syndromes of the lateral epicondylar (tennis elbow) and the medial epicondylar ligaments that are common in adult tennis players and golfers, respectively. However, two conditions—Little Leaguer's elbow and osteochondritis dissecans of the capitellum—can cause significant problems for young athletes.

Little Leaguer's Elbow

Little Leaguer's elbow affects skeletally immature pitchers, those age 10 years or younger, who throw for long periods of time. Chronic elbow strain and pain over the medial and lateral epicondyles may develop in young athletes who are involved in pitching and repetitive throwing. During the acceleration phase of pitching, considerable force is exerted on the elbow that causes tension on the medial side of the elbow and compression on the lateral side.

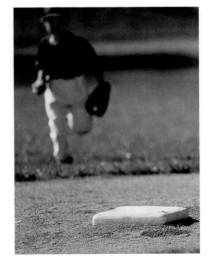

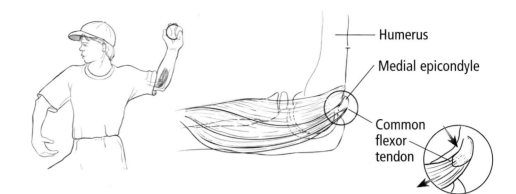

Humerus

Medial epicondyle

Common flexor tendon

Figure 32.17 Mechanism of elbow injury in Little League pitchers.

These forces are accentuated by sidearm throwing. Because young pitchers are still learning proper throwing techniques, the elbow joint is often subjected to abnormal and increased forces. It is controversial whether learning to throw a curve ball at a young age has a deleterious effect on the adolescent pitcher's elbow. However, because of the correlation between pitching frequency and repetitive traumatic injuries to the elbow, Little League pitchers should play only three to four innings per game. The total number of pitches thrown in one week, including those thrown both outside of practice and during competition, should be limited to 200 or less.

The classic injury is a repetitive valgus stress reaction of the medial epicondylar physes (**Figure 32.17**). Basically a valgus stress fracture, this injury occurs at the medial epicondylar apophyses, the weakest structure on the medial side of the elbow. Typical signs and symptoms include swelling of the medial elbow, flexion contracture, and direct pain over the medial epicondyle that is worse with pitching. Pain is also worse when valgus stress is applied to the elbow in 20° of flexion. The affected elbow may not be able to extend fully compared with the unaffected elbow. Both flexor and extensor muscle groups of the forearm may also be weak. Usually, the ulnar nerve is not affected unless the condition becomes chronic. Little Leaguer's elbow is similar to Osgood-Schlatter disease in which the patellar tendon pulls on the tibial apophyses, except that in the elbow, the pronator flexor tendons or flexor group pulls on the medial epicondylar attachment.

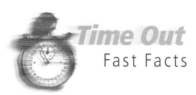

Time Out
Fast Facts

The total number of pitches thrown in one week should be limited to 200.

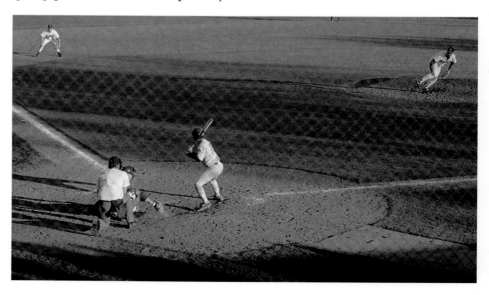

Radiographs of the elbow often appear normal. However, some will show fragmentation of the medial epicondyle with subsequent accelerated growth and associated joint changes at the radiocapitellar joint.

Treatment should consist of rest until the athlete is asymptomatic, followed by gradual stretching and muscle strengthening to regain full range of motion and normal forearm strength. Throwing should be resumed slowly, over a period of 6 to 8 weeks. Conditioning exercises for the elbow should be continued, even after the athlete returns to sports.

Occasionally, an avulsion of the medial epicondyle may occur, with the athlete either hearing or feeling a pop or the elbow giving way, followed by acute pain over the medial epicondyle. If the displacement is less than 5 mm, treatment consists of immobilizing the elbow at 90° flexion with a splint or cast for 3 weeks, followed by range of motion exercises for the elbow until full motion is regained. For displacements of greater than 5 mm, pinning of the fragment should be considered.

Osteochondritis Dissecans of the Capitellum

Osteochondritis dissecans of the capitellum affects athletes involved in any sport, but it seems to be more common in athletes who are involved in throwing sports, particularly baseball and football. Some controversy exists as to whether this condition is secondary to osteonecrosis or direct trauma, or perhaps both. Most young athletes who have osteochondritis dissecans of the capitellum are pitchers or quarterbacks who throw repetitively. Frequent valgus compressive forces may cause vascular insufficiency of the subchondral bone and result in osteochondritis dissecans (**Figure 32.18**). Usually, a young athlete who has osteochondritis dissecans of the capitellum reports pain and limited full extension of the elbow. There may be associated swelling or locking, especially if a fragment has become detached. The use of tomograms, CT arthrography, and MRI may be necessary to delineate the lesion fully. Rest and immobilization for the undisplaced lesion may allow the fragment to heal, but drilling of the lesion may be necessary and is usually curative. Loose bodies should be removed either by arthroscopy or open arthrotomy, followed by early rehabilitation and exercising.

Panner's Disease

Panner's disease involves variations in the normal ossification of the capitellum of the humerus and typically affects children between 5 and 11 years of age. It is not a pathologic condition and may be seen as an incidental radiographic finding or may be associated with low-grade elbow pain and limited motion that is either self-resolving or quickly responds to decreased activity. Radiographs of the affected elbow should be compared with views of the normal elbow. Eventually, full, symmetrical ossification of the capitellum will be seen on radiographs.

Olecranon Bursitis and Apophysitis

Chronic contusion of the elbow occurs frequently in hockey and football and may cause an olecranon bursitis. Though aggravating, chronic olecranon bursitis usually subsides with rest and avoidance of repetitive trauma. Protective elbow pads are helpful in minimizing this problem.

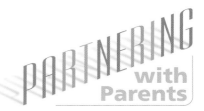

What are some specific guidelines for preventing a pitching or throwing injury?

The 10% rule is a helpful guide. For example, a young pitcher who throws 30 pitches per game 5 times a week can increase the next week to 33 pitches per game, up to 5 times a week.

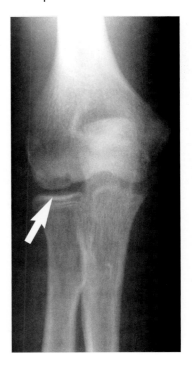

Figure 32.18 A lucent area in the capitellum associated with restriction of elbow motion and pain is characteristic of osteochondritis dissecans of the capitellum.

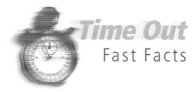

The olecranon is also subject to minor stress fractures and microavulsion of the triceps attachment, an injury similar to Osgood-Schlatter disease. Radiographs are seldom helpful; the diagnosis is best made by clinical examination. Management should consist of rest; however, the athlete should be educated about the nature of the injury and that it is usually more aggravating than serious. If the athlete cannot tolerate the discomfort, a change in activity may be appropriate for a period of 2 to 3 months. Once the cartilaginous apophysis of the ulna has ossified, the symptoms will subside.

Treatment

The treatment of traumatic injuries to the elbow and forearm begins on the field. Following initial evaluation, a sterile dressing should be placed over any wounds without any attempt to reduce exposed bone fragments. An air splint, malleable splint, or even a rolled up newspaper should be applied at this time to any suspected fracture to provide pain relief and prevent further injury. Coaches and team physicians should ensure that some form of commercial splint is available in the first aid kit. In addition, neurologic status of the affected extremity should be assessed and documented.

Radiographs of both the injured and unaffected extremities will almost always be required to delineate the true nature of the injury. Most fractures about the elbow and forearm require surgical referral because of the high rate of complications with fractures in this area. Immobilization of the elbow in a splint or cast is seldom required for longer than 4 weeks. For nondisplaced fractures of the forearm, immobilization for 3 to 5 weeks is indicated.

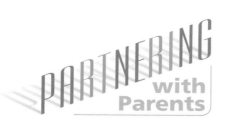

The elbow is extremely sensitive to any type of trauma, and frequently, its range of motion will be reduced for some time after the injury. Joint stiffness is also common following fractures of the forearm. As a result, rehabilitation measures should begin as soon as the athlete no longer requires immobilization—in most instances, after 3 to 4 weeks. Initial management should consist of active exercises, as early passive stretching may aggravate the pain and contracture. Occasionally, equipment designed to perform continuous passive motion will help the young athlete with a recalcitrant flexion contracture to regain motion. Athletes can return to full activity once the elbow has regained 90% of its motion and any fractures have healed satisfactorily, usually about 8 weeks from the time of injury.

Because most acute injuries are caused by a fall on the outstretched hand, the athlete must be cautioned to avoid falling again while the fracture is healing. Sometimes, acute injuries are caused by direct falls onto the elbow. Sports such as skateboarding, snowboarding, and motorbike riding pose greater risks of direct trauma. Children who participate in these sports should wear protective elbow pads. With the chronic elbow injuries, such as the ulnar bursitis, Little Leaguer's elbow, and osteochondritis dissecans, parents and coaches should be educated about the causes so they can take steps to minimize repetitive trauma to the elbow and prevent injury.

Red Flags

Complications from elbow injuries are frequent and often serious because of the close proximity of the nerves and vessels entering the forearm.

Displaced fractures and dislocations, particularly supracondylar fractures, can cause contusion and neurapraxia to any of the three major nerves, most commonly the median nerve. The risk of compartment syndrome is increased in conjunction with injury to the brachial artery. Displaced fractures and injuries require surgical referral to minimize any complications.

The most common complications include loss or limitation of motion about the elbow joint, the presence of intra-articular fragments in the elbow, physeal arrest, malunion with deformity, and myositis ossificans. In addition, incomplete healing or repeat injury may cause recurrent fractures. Loss of motion in the elbow joint is common, and frequently it may be difficult for even the young athlete to regain full motion. Parents, athletes, and coaches should be informed that several months of active exercising may be required before the last 10° or 15° of full flexion and full extension are recovered. Fortunately, full motion is usually regained rapidly in children. Myositis ossificans can be minimized by splinting the elbow immediately after injury and avoiding aggressive passive therapy by a therapist or well-meaning parent. However, active range of motion by the patient is helpful in the rehabilitation process.

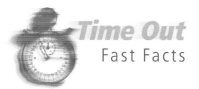

Time Out
Fast Facts

The constellation of injuries at the elbow with Little Leaguer's elbow include: osteochondritis dissecans of the capitellum and radial head; fragmentation of the medial epicondyle; micro tears of the flexor pronator group; avulsion fracture of the medial epiphysis; ulnar neuritis; and loose bodies in the elbow joint.

FINISH LINE

Injuries about the elbow and forearm in skeletally immature athletes are potentially serious because of the tremendous growth potential and the intricate articular mechanism of the bones in this area. Because of the myriad of growth plates and apophyses to which large muscle groups attach, sports-related injuries to the elbow are often difficult to interpret. Frequently, surgical referral is required.

Radiographs should be obtained to rule out a physeal injury or dislocation for any child who has pain, swelling, or deformity about the forearm and elbow. Certain sports, such as baseball and gymnastics, predispose the elbow joint to injury because of the nature of the activity and the stress it places on the elbow joint. Fortunately, when recognized early and treated promptly, these injuries can usually be treated successfully, and the child can return to play in 2 to 3 months.

The young athlete's elbow requires periodic maintenance and rest during periods of constant activity, especially highly repetitive activities such as pitching or throwing a football. Any sign or symptom that indicates a problem with the smooth functioning of the articular motion must be thoroughly investigated by proper imaging studies to ensure that treatment is timely, effective, and curative.

For More Information

1. Morrey BF (ed): *The Elbow and Its Disorders,* ed 2. Philadelphia, PA, WB Saunders, 1993, p 181.

2. DaSilva MF, Williams JS, Fadale PD, Hulstyn MJ, Ehrlich MG: Pediatric throwing injuries about the elbow. *Am J Orthop* 1998;27:90–96.

3. Gill TJ IV, Micheli LJ: The immature athlete: Common injuries and overuse syndromes of the elbow and wrist. *Clin Sports Med* 1996;15:401–423.

4. Green NE: Fractures and dislocations about the elbow, in Green NE, Swiontkowski MF (eds): *Skeletal Trauma in Children Vol. 3.* Philadelphia, PA, WB Saunders, 1994, pp 127–211, 213–256.

5. McIntyre WM, Sullivan JA, Huurmann W, Blasier, RD: Section 3: Fractures of the elbow in children, in Letts RM (ed): *Management of Pediatric Fractures.* New York, NY, Churchill Livingstone, 1994, pp 167–282.

6. Wilkens KE: Fractures and dislocations of the elbow region, in Rockwood CA Jr, Wilkins KE, Beatey JH (eds): *Fractures in Children,* ed 4. Philadelphia, PA, Lippincott-Raven, 1996, vol 3, pp 653–821.

Chapter 33

Shoulder

CHARLES B. PASQUE, MD
DONALD W. MCGINNIS, MD
LETHA YURKO-GRIFFIN, MD, PHD

N ormal shoulder function is critical to young athletes partici-pating in almost any sport. The need for proper upper extremity function ranges from the obvious stresses encountered during throwing or overhead sports to the very physical collision sports. Even lower extremity-dominated sports such as running or soccer require good shoulder function for balance and locomotion. Therefore, any shoulder injury or dysfunction can significantly limit optimal performance.

Shoulder problems can be caused by acute direct or indirect traumatic events or by repetitive overuse that gradually and ultimately causes tissue failure. Acute traumatic injuries can occur in any sport, with the highest incidence occurring in collision sports such as football and hockey. Chronic overuse injuries usually occur in sports that require repetitive throwing or overhead activity, but they can also occur in sports that rely heavily on shoulder motion and strength, such as wrestling and gymnastics. To properly recognize and treat young athletes with shoulder injuries, physicians must be able to: 1) understand the basic anatomy and biomechanics of the shoulder; 2) perform a proper screening history and physical examination; and 3) recognize common shoulder injuries. Understanding and implementing these measures will result in more informed decisions regarding return to play or deciding when specialty evaluation is needed.

Anatomy/Biomechanics

The shoulder is a complex structure, which is more easily understood by dividing it into the involved bones, cartilage, ligaments, and musculo-tendinous units. The interaction of these individual structures allows the shoulder to provide a wide range of motion with good functional stability. Injury results when the extremes of shoulder motion are exceeded, or more commonly, when the individual structures themselves are overloaded.

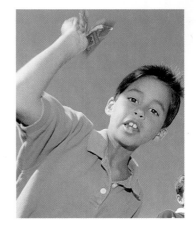

Focusing on these individual structures as part of the evaluation of injuries will provide a more complete clinical picture.

Bones

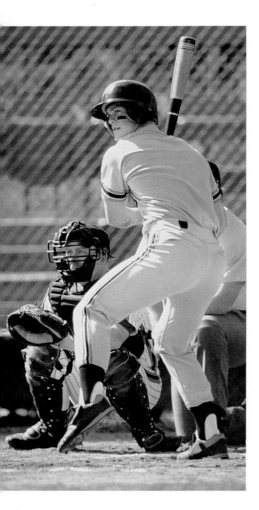

The four principal bones of the shoulder are the humerus (arm bone or "ball"), scapula (shoulder bone or "socket"), clavicle (collar bone), and the thorax (rib cage). Together, these bones form four articulations (junction between two or more bones): the glenohumeral articulation, the acromioclavicular articulation, the sternoclavicular articulation, and the scapulothoracic articulation. All of these articulations have little inherent bony stability and rely almost entirely on the surrounding soft tissues for support.

The glenohumeral articulation is the main joint of the shoulder. The proximal humerus consists of a ball-shaped head covered almost completely with articular cartilage. The humeral head surrounds the articular cartilage and serves as an attachment site for the capsular ligaments and musculotendinous units known as the rotator cuff. The lateral scapula articulating region is called the glenoid. It consists of a shallow, concave area that encompasses less than 20% of the surface of the humeral head. The peripheral margins of the glenoid rim are deepened by the labrum and serve as attachment sites for the capsular ligaments and the long head of the biceps tendon. The labrum contributes to joint stability as well as contact force distribution. Together, the humeral head and the glenoid of the scapula form the main joint contributing to the wide range of motion of the shoulder. These motions include flexion/extension, abduction/adduction, and internal/external rotation.

The acromioclavicular articulation, or AC joint, is considered the second main joint of the shoulder and has distinctly different anatomy and function. The acromion is the lateral "roof" area of the scapula whose medial border forms the lateral side of the AC joint. The lateral end of the clavicle forms the medial side of the AC joint. The joint itself is filled with a fibrocartilaginous disk with surrounding ligaments that stabilize the two bones. The AC joint stabilizes the scapula to the chest wall while allowing for slight rotation with flexion and extension of the glenohumeral joint. The acromion and clavicle also serve as important attachment sites for the external shoulder muscles.

The sternoclavicular articulation, or SC joint, is on the medial end of the clavicle. The medial end of the clavicle forms the lateral side of the SC joint, and the sternum, or "breastbone," forms the medial side. The SC joint has a fibrocartilaginous disk that improves articular congruency between the medial edge of the clavicle and the sternum. This joint also has a surrounding capsule and ligaments that provide excellent stability. Like the AC joint, the SC joint also stabilizes the scapula to the chest wall while allowing for slight rotation with flexion and extension of the glenohumeral joint. The clavicle and sternum also protect the underlying great vessels from trauma.

The scapulothoracic articulation is one of the most important and overlooked areas of the shoulder. The large, thin anterior body of the scapula forms one side of the articulation. The superior lateral and superior posterior thoracic cavity forms the other side of the scapulothoracic articulation. The two bones are mainly stabilized by the surrounding muscles with small contributions from ligaments. The main function of the scapulothoracic articulation is to stabilize the scapula to the chest wall and to allow proper positioning and rotation of the scapula. This allows the glenoid to face the proper direction with enough stability to maximize glenohumeral joint function. The scapula also protects the posterior thorax from penetrating injury.

The immature skeleton of young athletes has additional anatomic and bio-mechanic factors that require consideration. Open physes are at increased risk of injury because of their rapid cell proliferation and relatively weak resistance to significant stress. The principal physis in the shoulder is located in the distal clavicle and is important because it does not close until early adulthood. Because this physis remains open, a fracture through the distal clavicular physis can be misdiagnosed as a ligamentous disruption through the AC joint. Another area of potential misdiagnosis in the shoulder involves the multiple centers of ossification of the acromion. These ossification centers often do not fuse until early adulthood and sometimes do not completely fuse at all. Incomplete fusion can result in a bony separation known as an os acromiale, which is frequently not recognized, but can be misdiagnosed as an acromial fracture.

Cartilage

The two main types of cartilage in the shoulder are articular cartilage and fibrocartilage. Articular cartilage is the shiny white hyaline cartilage that covers the ends of the humeral head and glenoid fossa. Its main function is to provide a smooth gliding articulating surface between the humerus and the scapula; it also serves as a shock absorber for the underlying bone when axi-ally loaded. Fibrocartilage is the thick tissue found in the AC and SC joints. The fibrocartilage serves as a disk or "spacer" between the bone ends, and as a shock absorber to axial, rotational, and shear loads. In addition, the fibrocarti-lage helps increase joint stability.

Ligaments

Ligaments attach bone to bone and serve primarily to provide static stability to a joint. Shoulder ligaments can be classified by the individual joints they support.

The glenohumeral joint relies heavily on the surrounding ligaments and muscles for stability. The glenohumeral joint is analogous to a golf ball on a tee. The articular surface of the humeral head and glenoid provide very little bony stability. The glenoid fossa is deepened by a thick ring of tissue called the labrum that distributes contact forces about the glenohumeral articulation and provides some restraint to translation of the humeral head on the gle-noid. The glenohumeral ligaments provide most of the static stability to the joint. The anterior and posterior inferior glenohumeral ligaments act like a hammock around the humeral head and function mainly when the shoulder is in an abducted position to prevent anterior, inferior, and posterior transla-tion. The superior and middle glenohumeral ligaments and the coraco-humeral ligament act primarily when the arm is at the side in an adducted position. These ligaments prevent anterior superior and anterior posterior translation with contributions to inferior stability. Anterior and superior stability is also supported by the coracoacromial ligament, which can cause impingement anteriorly when abnormal rotator cuff function exists.

The AC joint is supported by two sets of ligaments. The coracoclavicular ligaments (conoid and trapezoid) provide the primary superior stability for the AC joint. The superior and inferior AC ligaments and surrounding joint

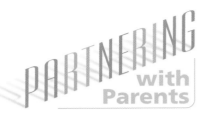

Is a rotator cuff tear common in young athletes?

No. The young athlete is more likely to sustain bruises or strains of the rotator cuff caused by acute or chronic injuries. Chronic overuse injuries are very common in overhead sports such as swimming, throwing, and racket sports. Rest, ice, NSAIDs, and rehabilitation are generally successful in resolving the problem.

capsule also reinforce superior stability, but are important primarily in preventing anterior/posterior and medial/lateral translation. The specific ligaments injured help define the severity of an AC separation and will be discussed later in the chapter.

The sternoclavicular joint is supported by anterior and posterior ligaments that provide good stability and minimize the potential for subluxation or dislocation. The posterior ligament is the most critical for overall joint stability. The joint is also supported by a surrounding capsule and a fibrocartilaginous disk.

Musculoskeletal Units

The muscles of the shoulder are critical to its overall function due to the wide range of motions and activities required both in sports as well as in daily activities (**Figure 33.1**). The various muscle groups involved are the rotator cuff muscles, the biceps tendon complex, the scapulothoracic muscles, and the external shoulder muscles.

Rotator cuff

The rotator cuff muscles are the primary dynamic stabilizers of the glenohumeral joint. The term rotator cuff refers collectively to the subscapularis, supraspinatus, infraspinatus, and teres minor muscles. All of the muscles arise from the scapula and insert on the lateral side of the humeral head. The main function of the rotator cuff is to keep the humeral head centered within the glenoid fossa. This provides the shoulder with a stable range of motion and prevents impingement on the surrounding structures. The rotator cuff, as its name implies, also provides important rotational strength to the glenohumeral joint.

Figure 33.1 Anatomy of the shoulder.

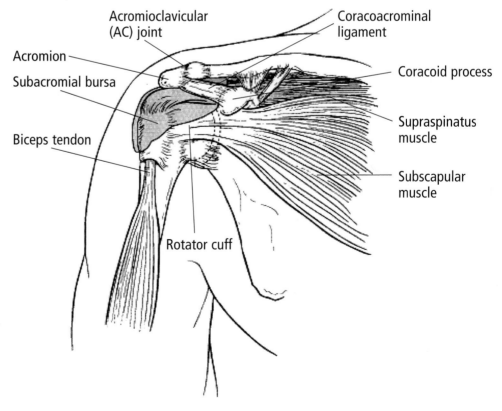

Biceps tendon complex

The biceps tendon complex consists of the long head of the biceps and its associated superior glenoid capsulolabral attachment and the short head of the biceps that attaches to the coracoid. Its main function is to help keep the humeral head depressed and centered in the glenoid fossa. It also contributes to superior stability of the glenohumeral joint as well as arm flexion and supination.

Scapulothoracic muscles

The scapulothoracic muscles consist of the levator scapulae, the rhomboid major and minor, and the serratus anterior. All arise from the thorax or spine and insert on the scapula. These muscles work together to stabilize the scapula to the thoracic wall, allowing for increased strength and stability to the shoulder. They also rotate the scapula on the thoracic wall, improving overall motion and placing the shoulder in more efficient positions for various tasks.

External muscles of the shoulder

The external muscles of the shoulder consist of the deltoid, trapezius and pectoralis major, and each contribute important strength-related shoulder functions. The deltoid is the large muscle that covers the rotator cuff muscles. It arises from the clavicle and scapular spine and inserts on the deltoid tuberosity of the humerus. The deltoid has anterior, middle, and posterior muscle fiber groups that each contribute to shoulder abduction and flexion/extension. The trapezius is a large muscle extending from the cervical and thoracic spinous processes to the scapular spine and lateral clavicle region. It serves mainly to stabilize the shoulder to the chest wall, and it contributes to elevation and slight rotation. The pectoralis major muscle is a powerful muscle over the anterior chest and shoulder. It arises from the medial clavicle, sternum, and abdominal wall and inserts on the humerus near the deltoid tuberosity. It serves mainly in adduction and internal rotation.

Clinical Evaluation

History

A thorough but focused history is vital to correctly diagnosing shoulder injuries. Learning to ask the right questions comes with experience but can be learned rapidly if a systematic approach is taken. A minimum history should include the following questions: Is the problem acute or chronic; what was the mechanism of injury, including whether the symptoms began with a specific event or repetitive activity; what is the sport and position played; what is the location and type of pain and swelling; and what are the mechanical symptoms (eg, locking, popping, catching), instability symptoms, and functional limitations. Information about previous injuries, especially similar injuries, and previous evaluations and treatments are helpful, including notes from the physician and/or athletic trainer, radiographs, and any special diagnostic studies. Videotapes or eyewitnesses can also provide key information about the mechanism of acute injuries such as the direction of force and position of the arm at the time of injury.

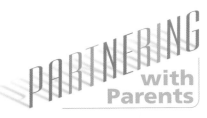

What is shoulder instability?

Shoulder instability refers to abnormal motion of the ball-and-socket joint of the shoulder and can be caused by acute traumatic shoulder dislocation or subluxation (partial dislocation) or chronic instability from muscle imbalance or overuse injuries. The most common instability pattern is anterior in acute injuries and multi-directional in chronic injuries without a severe trauma injury. Many symptomatic athletes with a history of an acute dislocation have recurrent problems and may require surgical repair. Athletes with chronic subtle instability usually can be treated with a stretching and strengthening program.

Physical Examination

Consistent use of a systematic shoulder examination is critical to evaluate shoulder injuries properly and to prevent missing important clinical findings. Even though an on-field examination differs from an office or clinic visit, a thorough examination can be performed rapidly if done consistently and systematically. Team physicians, athletic trainers, and coaches should be able to perform the basic physical examination. When possible, this examination should be performed in a quiet, isolated area, away from distractions from the crowd and other athletes.

Cervical spine disorders, such as fractures or ligamentous injuries, can cause pain referred to the upper extremity, especially the shoulder. Similarly, elbow, wrist, and hand injuries can occur in conjunction with acute shoulder injuries. *Therefore, the neck and the remainder of the upper extremity should be examined in any young athlete with shoulder pain.*

Observation

The shoulder should be exposed from the neck to the hand. Depending on the environment, this may require removing jerseys, padding, or other sports equipment. The first step is to assess the overall position of the limb, noting any gross deformities that suggest fractures or dislocations. Comparison with the contralateral extremity for muscle atrophy and overall limb alignment is also important, especially in chronic injuries. The next step is to closely inspect for skin and soft-tissue abnormalities, such as redness, swelling, ecchymosis, and abrasions or lacerations. The final step, when possible, is to observe the athlete performing tasks with the shoulder, such as throwing

Table 33.1 *Key Palpation Landmarks*

Site of tenderness	Possible injury
Acromium	Os acromiale
	Deltoid detachment
Scapula	Fractures
	Trigger points
Clavicle	Fracture (crepitus), contusion
AC joint	Fracture, separation, inflammation
SC joint	Fracture, separation, inflammation
Biceps groove	Biceps tendinitis,
	Biceps instability
Greater tuberosity	Rotator cuff tendinitis,
	Proximal humeral epiphysitis
	(Little Leaguer's shoulder),
	Impingement syndrome
Coracoid	Fracture, short head biceps injury, or tendinitis
Posterior shoulder at the glenohumeral joint	Posterior capsular tear, Posterior labral tear

or lifting. This part of the examination can be modified to fit sport-specific activities. An athlete who cannot perform basic sport-specific activities should be kept out of competition until able to do so.

Palpation

Systematic palpation of key bony and soft-tissue landmarks is essential to localizing areas of injury (**Table 33.1**) (**Figure 33.2**). Although swelling and pain can be diffuse, point tenderness can be elicited in most areas of injury. This examination is best done with the athlete in a sitting position with the arms resting comfortably across the lap. An alternative position is to have the athlete lie supine on the ground or examining table. Begin by palpating the bony structures for possible fracture because these findings will significantly affect any decisions regarding the need for splinting and on-field return to play. Bony palpation should include the sternoclavicular joint, the entire clavicle, the AC joint, the acromion, and the scapular spine. The sternoclavicular joint and AC joint should be palpated for tenderness, crepitus, and instability. The remaining structures are palpated primarily to identify areas of tenderness and gross deformity. Any areas of exquisite tenderness should be of concern and warrant immobilizing the arm against the athlete's side, followed by careful transportation off the playing field. Further evaluation should include plain radiographs and specialty referral, if needed.

The soft tissues should then be palpated. The arm should be in a relaxed position during this part of the examination. The lateral neck muscles and anterior and posterior chest muscles on the affected side should be palpated first, followed by the anterior, lateral, and posterior rotator cuff muscles. This examination can be facilitated by slightly extending the shoulder to help

Figure 33.2 Anterior and posterior views of the scapula.

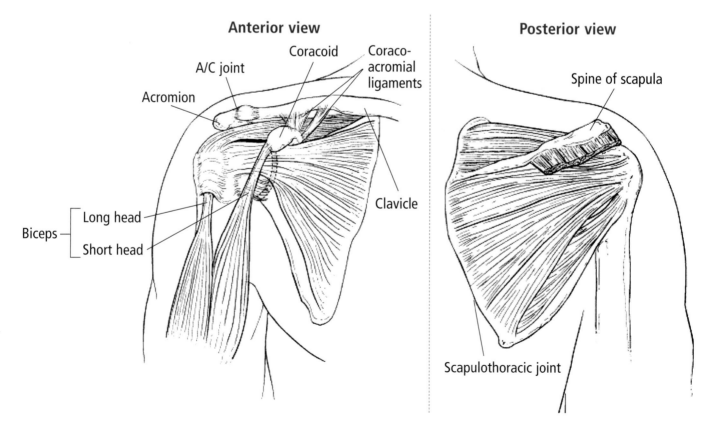

uncover the anterior and lateral cuff muscles. Finally, the external shoulder muscles including the deltoid, pectoralis major, and trapezius should be palpated. The biceps and triceps should be evaluated if indicated. The order and extent of soft-tissue examination can be altered depending on the situation. Suspected areas of tenderness can be examined last to be more comfortable for the patient.

Range of motion

Range of motion is also a vital factor in the shoulder examination, especially regarding return to play decisions. Any athlete with an abnormal passive or active range of motion should be held out of competition until full motion is achieved or the cause is determined. Range of motion of the glenohumeral joint should be assessed and compared with that of the opposite, uninjured extremity for symmetry. The extent of range of motion can be evaluated by having the athlete actively move the shoulder in full flexion and extension, abduction, and internal/external rotation at 0° and 90° of abduction. If there is a major deficit in active motion, further evaluation with passive motion should be performed. This additional evaluation helps determine if there is a true mechanical block or if motion is limited by pain or weakness. The shoulder should be palpated for crepitus as range of motion is assessed. If the athlete appears very apprehensive or experiences pain, place him or her in a supine position during the examination. Severe mechanical blocks to abduction or internal/external rotation should raise concern for a possible fracture or shoulder subluxation or dislocation. Many athletes with limited findings are unwilling to move their shoulder because of apprehension. If a fracture or subluxation/dislocation has been ruled out, the athlete should be placed in an arm sling with swelling control measures and then reexamined when the shoulder symptoms have improved and the athlete has calmed down.

Strength testing

Strength testing is important for determining the etiology of the shoulder problem and whether the athlete can return to play. Any major strength deficits usually need to be corrected before the athlete can return to competition to ensure that he or she can protect the extremity. The strength examination is best performed with the examiner standing in front of the seated athlete. With the athlete's arms at the side and the elbows flexed to 90°, the examiner should resist the athlete's clinched fists in all directions, noting any asymmetry with the opposite side. The shoulders can then be resisted in flexion/extension and abduction/adduction. Specific tests for rotator cuff and biceps injuries will be discussed in later sections. Shoulder strength should be graded to document increases and decreases in muscle function and to allow communication with other health care providers (**Table 33.2**).

Glenohumeral stability evaluation

Ligamentous stability can be assessed with the athlete in either the sitting or supine position. The sitting position can be used for a relaxed patient and is usually satisfactory for all tests except some of the provocative maneuvers such as the fulcrum or relocation tests. The supine position is often more comfortable for the patient and is preferred for performing all of the required testing. The examiner should be positioned behind and to the side of the

Grade	Strength
5	Normal strength through complete range of motion with maximum resistance
4	Complete range of motion with some (moderate) resistance
3	Complete range of motion against gravity
2	Joint motion with gravity eliminated
1	Evidence of slight contraction, but no joint motion
0	No contraction

Table 33.2 *Strength Testing*

athlete. When examining the right shoulder, the examiner should gently but firmly grasp the glenohumeral region with the left hand. The joint should be palpated with the examiner's thumb positioned posteriorly and the index and long fingers anteriorly. The right hand should be used to position the athlete's arm by grasping either the elbow or wrist region. The opposite should be done for the left shoulder. It should be noted during any of the testing maneuvers whether abnormal subluxation or dislocation is voluntary or involuntary.

Glenohumeral translation. This maneuver is performed to test the surrounding ligamentous complexes. When evaluating the integrity of the anterior-inferior and posterior-inferior glenohumeral ligaments, the shoulder should be abducted to approximately 80° to 90°. The humeral head should first be centered in the glenoid fossa by axial loading, followed by gentle manipulation in all directions. The arm should be in external rotation during anterior-inferior testing and in flexion and internal rotation during posterior-inferior testing. An attempt should be made to quantify the amount of translation of the humeral head on the glenoid in the anterior, anterior-inferior, posterior-inferior, and posterior directions (**Figure 33.3**). The arm can then be adducted to the side for testing in the anterior-superior and posterior-superior directions. Measurements should always be compared with those on the opposite side and can be graded as normal, increased translation without subluxation, increased translation with subluxation, or increased translation with dislocation. An example of a common grading system is as follows: grade 1 = no increased translation; grade 2 = translation up to the glenoid rim; grade 3 = translation onto the glenoid rim (subluxation); and grade 4 = translation over the glenoid rim (dislocation).

The anterior and posterior apprehension tests. These tests are similar to translational testing and should be performed on any athlete believed to have glenohumeral instability or impingement. An anterior apprehension test is performed by abducting the shoulder to 90°, and then slowly externally rotating the shoulder toward 90°. An athlete with anterior or anterior-inferior instability will usually become "apprehensive" either verbally or with distressing facial expressions. A posterior

Figure 33.3 Glenohumeral translation test. This test may be performed more easily with the patient supine.

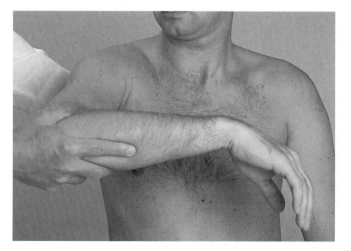

Figure 33.4 Apprehension test.

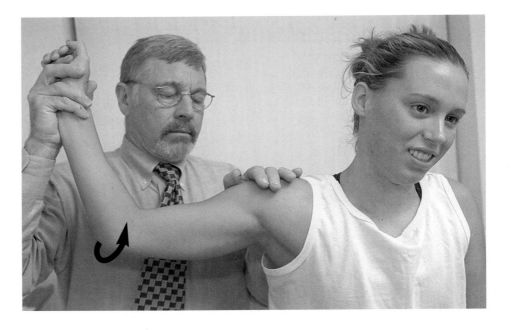

apprehension test is performed by flexing the glenohumeral joint to 90°
and then internally rotating the shoulder while applying a posterior stress
(**Figure 33.4**).

The relocation and fulcrum tests. These tests are additional provocative maneuvers for evaluating anterior and anterior-inferior shoulder instability. Both are
most easily performed with the athlete in a supine position. The relocation test
should be done in conjunction with the anterior apprehension test. It is performed by applying pressure with a hand over the anterior proximal humerus
region while abducting and externally rotating the arm (**Figure 33.5**). The posteriorly directed pressure on the arm will decrease the anterior translation of
the humeral head and usually reduce the apprehension symptoms in an athlete
with anterior shoulder instability. Sudden release of the pressure on the arm
will often cause a return of the athlete's apprehension and further confirm a
diagnosis of anterior-inferior instability.

The fulcrum test is performed with the athlete supine and the arm abducted
and externally rotated 90°. The examiner then places a clenched fist or solid
object under the posterior midhumerus region. The other hand is used to
apply an anterior to posterior levering force at the distal humerus or elbow
region (**Figure 33.6**). The applied force levers the humerus over the examiner's fist or object (the fulcrum), causing anterior translation of the humeral
head on the glenoid. The test is considered positive when the patient's symptoms are reproduced, often causing similar discomfort to the apprehension
test. The fulcrum test can also be performed by grasping the midhumerus
with both hands and applying pressure in a posterior to anterior direction
while simultaneously abducting and externally rotating the shoulder to 90°.

The sulcus test. The primary purpose of this test is to evaluate inferior stability. It is usually easier to perform this test with the athlete sitting, but it can
also be done with the athlete supine. The athlete should be in a relaxed position with the arm at the side. The examiner should grasp just above the elbow
and apply straight distal traction on the arm (**Figure 33.7**). The test is considered positive when a dimple or gap appears over the lateral shoulder because

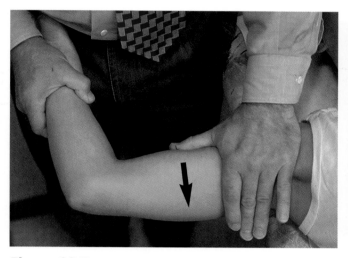

Figure 33.5 Relocation test.

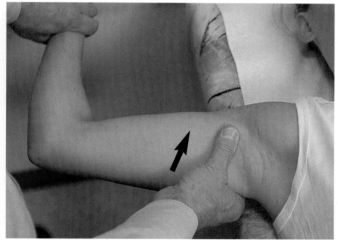

Figure 33.6 Fulcrum test.

of increased distance between the lateral edge of the acromion and the greater tuberosity of the humerus. This represents inferior translation of the humeral head on the glenoid. The rotator cuff interval is the main area being tested with the arm at the side. The test should be repeated with the arm in 70° to 90° of abduction because this position is believed to better represent pathologic increases in inferior translation caused by a redundant inferior capsule. The amount of inferior translation can be estimated by findings based on direct observation or more accurately by direct palpation. This evaluation is done by placing a thumb at the inferior edge of the lateral acromion while applying distal traction on the arm. Knowing the exact width of the examiner's thumbnail helps make more precise measurements. The measurements should always be compared with those on the opposite side and can be graded as follows: grade 1 = translation up to 1 cm;

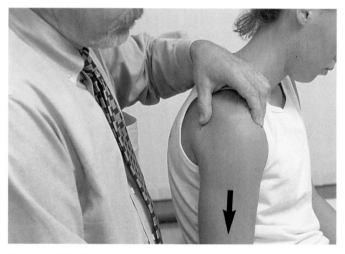

Figure 33.7 Sulcus test.

grade 2 = translation up to 2 cm; and grade 3 = translation up to 3 cm. Some grading systems also add half-centimeter translations such as 1.5 cm and 2.5 cm. Any athlete with large bilateral and symmetric increases in inferior translation requires additional testing for generalized ligamentous laxity.

Generalized ligamentous laxity evaluation. This test should be performed on any athlete with significant instability or impingement symptoms. Although the cause, significance, and diagnostic testing used for this finding are controversial, a simple and rapid evaluation can be performed anywhere using six standardized tests: 1) thumb to forearm; 2) small finger metacarpophalangeal joint hyperextension of greater than 90°; 3) elbow hyperextension of greater than 10°; 4) knee hyperextension of greater than 10°; 5) ankle hyperextension of greater than 45°; and 6) palms to floor (with the knees straight). The palms to floor test is sometimes excluded since many believe it only represents an athlete's flexibility. Excessive patella mobility can also be used, but is often

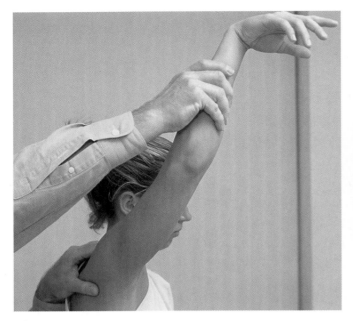

Figure 33.8 Neer impingement test.

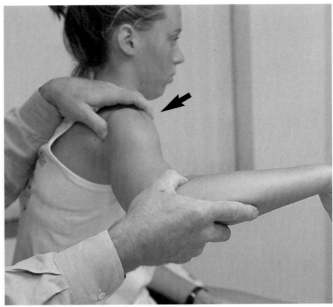

Figure 33.9 Hawkin's impingement test.

hard to quantify. Any athlete exhibiting more than two of these signs can be considered to potentially have generalized ligamentous laxity. This finding has implications regarding encouraging nonsurgical treatment because of the perception that surgical treatment is less successful in these individuals.

Glenohumeral impingement evaluation

Impingement tests are performed with the athlete in a sitting position and the examiner standing to the side or behind the affected shoulder. The Neer impingement sign is performed by stabilizing the scapula with one hand and passively forward flexing the arm with the other hand (**Figure 33.8**). An athlete with anterior impingement of the humerus on the acromion will report pain with this maneuver. The flexion angle at which the pain occurs should be noted because a positive sign at 90° can represent more advanced symptoms than a positive sign at 180°. The test can also be done actively by having the athlete flex the arm forward independently. The Hawkins impingement sign is performed by stabilizing the scapula with one hand and passively forward flexing and internally rotating the arm, causing the humeral head to roll under the acromion (**Figure 33.9**). A positive sign is when the patient has pain with terminal internal rotation.

An impingement test can be performed by injecting 3 to 5 mL of a local anesthetic into the subacromial bursa at the site of impingement. After the anesthetic takes effect, impingement signs are performed again with straight flexion and flexion with internal rotation. A positive test occurs when the athlete reports decreased pain with these maneuvers. The amount of relief should be noted because concomitant conditions can exist. Additional diagnostic anesthetic injections can also be performed in the AC and SC joints. These tests provide an excellent means of differentiating complex problems of the shoulder. Specialty referral is suggested if the examining physician is unfamiliar with these injection techniques.

AC and SC joint evaluation

The AC and SC joints are easily accessible because of their subcutaneous location. Each joint should be palpated for tenderness, crepitus, or prominence of the bony structures. Any gross abnormalities should be further evaluated by radiographs to delineate any clavicular fractures or joint separations. Both joints can be stressed by performing an adduction crossover test. This test can be performed by stabilizing the scapula with one hand and passively flexing and adducting the arm with the other hand (**Figure 33.10**). Any pain or crepitus noted at either joint may represent an injury. The AC joint can be further stressed by placing the shoulder in 90° of forward flexion and either a neutral or adducted position. The athlete then attempts to abduct the shoulder against resistance applied by the

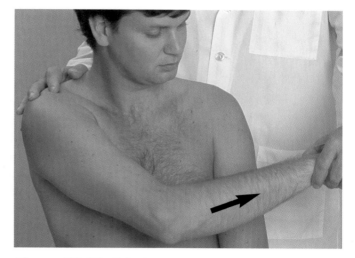

Figure 33.10 Abduction crossover test.

examiner. Athletes with AC joint injuries will report pain with this maneuver. Diagnostic lidocaine injections can be performed in the AC and SC joints to help confirm the diagnosis. These joints are more difficult to inject than the subacromial space because of their tighter spaces and joint angulation. Specialty referral is suggested if the examining physician is unfamiliar with these injection techniques.

Scapulothoracic evaluation

The scapulothoracic articulation is often overlooked during routine shoulder evaluation. The athlete's upper extremity should be exposed to observe both scapulae for any asymmetry caused by congenital malformation (Sprengel's deformity) or muscle weakness. Any scapular winging or elevation at rest may be a sign of a severe neurologic injury. The levator scapula and rhomboid muscles should then be palpated along the medial border of the scapula for tenderness and atrophy. The scapular stabilizers should then be evaluated with provocative maneuvers such as wall push-ups, seated push-ups, or having the athlete press his or her hands together in front of the body.

Neurovascular evaluation

The physical examination is not complete without a proper neurovascular evaluation of the involved extremity. Most instances of shoulder trauma do not require an extensive neurovascular examination, but documentation of grossly intact extremity circulation and motor and sensory function should be included at a minimum. A more thorough examination should be performed in athletes with high-energy injuries that have resulted in extensive soft-tissue damage as well as any fractures or dislocations. This examination should include documentation of lateral shoulder (axillary nerve) and lateral forearm (musculocutaneous nerve) sensation, as well as a thorough motor function examination. In addition, any athlete with a traumatic injury that could potentially result in severe swelling or bleeding leading to a compartment syndrome requires a more thorough neurovascular examination. Any acute neurologic symptoms or signs persisting for more than 15 minutes may represent a cervical or brachial plexus injury and should be evaluated further in the emergency department or by a specialist. Athletes with more chronic conditions should also be inspected for signs of muscle atrophy such as the deltoid or supraspinatus and infraspinatus fossas. Marked atrophy may suggest a severe neurologic injury that requires further evaluation.

Diagnostic Tests

Plain radiographs are indicated in any athlete with physical findings of severe bone tenderness or deformity. These can also be helpful in athletes with persistent shoulder problems that do not respond to routine nonsurgical treatment to help differentiate injuries from other conditions such as bone cysts, tumors, or infections.

Routine views include an anteroposterior (AP) view in the scapular plane with the humerus internally and externally rotated and an axillary lateral. Y scapular lateral views are also sometimes obtained, especially if the athlete is too uncomfortable for an axillary view or if acromial roof morphology requires more precise definition. The AP views are useful in evaluating proximal humeral physeal injuries or other fractures. When a physeal injury is a concern, comparison radiographs of the opposite shoulder are helpful. Athletes with a history of an acute anterior dislocation can also exhibit a Hill-Sachs lesion, which is a posterolateral impression defect of the humeral head seen on the AP internal rotation view. The axillary and Y scapular lateral views are important in determining if the glenohumeral joint is reduced. The axillary view is also helpful in determining glenoid defects or deficiencies.

Numerous ossification centers exist in the shoulder and can make radiographic interpretation difficult in the skeletally immature athlete. When complex bony involvement is present, CT scans may help. MRI can also provide significant information about injuries to the growth plates as well as soft-tissue injuries. An MRI with contrast material within the glenohumeral joint (arthrogram) is an excellent diagnostic tool for intra-articular pathology such as labral tears in athletes with acute instability injuries.

Treatment—General Guidelines

Most shoulder injuries result in self-limited abrasions, bruises, muscle strains, and mild ligament sprains that rarely affect sports participation for extended periods of time. Acute traumatic injuries generally are not difficult to differentiate from chronic overuse injuries. Fractures or dislocations should be strongly considered if the athlete has a history of a sudden traumatic event with acute swelling, deformity, or restricted motion. These injuries should be evaluated with radiographs, and if additional treatment is needed, referred to a specialist. Extra-articular injuries with no gross evidence of fracture or ligamentous instability can be safely treated with rest, ice, compression, and elevation (RICE). Most of these injuries will resolve in 1 to 6 weeks, depending on their severity. Athletes and their parents should be instructed to contact their physician or proceed to the emergency department if the athlete reports any acute increases in pain, swelling, or neurovascular symptoms. Initially, the athlete should be examined weekly to monitor swelling, motion, and pain. Athletic trainers, physical therapists, and coaches also are helpful in monitoring the athlete's progress while at school.

Usually within the first few weeks after the injury the pain and swelling will begin to resolve. Exercises to improve motion and general strength should be initiated as soon as possible. As the pain and swelling subside and shoulder motion returns, sport-specific rehabilitation activities should begin in a controlled environment and include activities to improve agility, coordination, and endurance. Specialty consultation is indicated if these initial phases of management fail. When possible, the consultation should occur before other diagnostic tests are ordered, such as an MRI, because tests can delay evaluation and treatment, are often expensive, and are often not needed.

Differential Diagnosis

Fractures of the Clavicle

Clavicle fractures are a common pediatric shoulder injury in young athletes. The mechanism of injury is usually blunt trauma to the anterior shoulder or a fall onto the point of the shoulder. Most clavicle fractures occur in the middle third of the bone and are usually minimally displaced (**Figure 33.11**). Examination typically reveals tenderness, deformity, swelling, and crepitus at the fracture site. Management should focus on pain relief with analgesics or nonsteroidal anti-inflammatory drugs (NSAIDs) until the fracture stabilizes itself with healing callus within the first few weeks. Additional comfort can be provided with the use of an arm sling or a figure-of-8 bandage. Neither of these measures has been shown to significantly affect fracture alignment, but can be very helpful in providing comfort. If a figure-of-8 bandage is used, the parents should be advised to avoid fastening the bandage too tight because this can result in skin ulcers or neurovascular compromise within the axilla region. Immobilization and activity restriction for 3 to 6 weeks are usually sufficient but vary with the age of the patient. Most children will discard any form of immobilization after the first few weeks due to marked improvements in pain. Parents should be assured that the large bump that usually develops is part of the healing process and will often disappear completely as remodeling occurs over the next year. Surgical treatment is rarely indicated, but may be necessary in open fractures or severely displaced fractures. Return to play will depend on the sport. Athletes can usually resume any noncontact sport or sports not requiring repetitive throwing as soon as the pain has subsided. Return to football or any sport that is likely to stress the clavicle requires a minimum of 6 to 8 weeks.

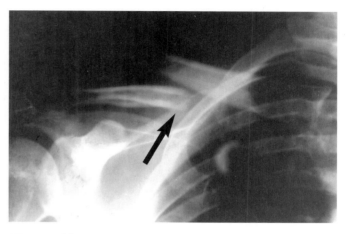

Figure 33.11 Displaced midshaft clavicle fracture.

Time Out
Fast Facts

The medial physis/epiphysis of the clavicle is the last physis in the body to close at age 22 years.

AC and SC Joint Physeal Fractures of the Clavicle

The lateral and medial clavicular physes usually remain open through late adolescence and often into early adulthood. Downward blows to these areas or falls onto the point of the shoulder usually cause physeal fractures rather than AC or SC joint separations. In the AC joint, the strong coracoclavicular ligaments usually remain attached to the periosteum of the undersurface of the clavicle. This provides good stability and allows for excellent healing and remodeling. In the SC joint, the anterior and posterior sternoclavicular ligaments similarly provide good stability and healing potential. AC and SC joint physeal fractures can usually be treated nonoperatively with a simple sling and swathe or a figure-of-8 bandage. The swathe is discontinued as soon as pain subsides. Pendulum exercises should be initiated 2 to 3 weeks after the injury. The sling is discontinued after 3 to 4 weeks, and return to play is allowed as soon as the athlete is pain-free and has normal range of motion. Return to play varies depending on the sport's demands on the shoulder.

AC Separations and SC Dislocations

AC and SC joint dislocations are rare but can occur in a young athlete. These injuries usually have similar presentations to physeal fractures and can also usually be treated nonoperatively. Dislocations or separations of the AC joint are classified as grades I through III, with grades I and II considered subluxations and grade III considered a complete separation. Radiographs confirm the diagnosis and help differentiate a suspected separation from a fracture. Stress radiographs with and without 5 to 10 lb of traction in the athlete's hands may accentuate the AC separation deformity. Dislocations of the SC joint are classified as either anterior or posterior. The diagnosis can sometimes be confirmed on plain radiographs such as an AP chest or apical lordotic view, but may require CT for a definitive diagnosis. Management typically includes attempted closed reduction, either anterior or posterior to the sternum, by hyperextending the shoulders with careful manipulation of the medial clavicle. Even if closed manipulation is unsuccessful, surgical treatment is rarely indicated unless the dislocation is posterior and causing neurocirculatory compromise. Care should be taken to confirm a fracture does not exist prior to any attempts at closed reductions. Specialty referral is indicated if there is any question about whether a physeal fracture or dislocation exists, or if there is marked displacement of the joint region.

Fractures of the Scapula

Scapula fractures are extremely rare in young athletes, but occasionally occur in collision sports such as football or ice hockey. They are more commonly seen as the result of high-energy trauma in adults such as motor vehicle accidents or falls from heights. Associated injuries are common, including neurovascular injuries to the shoulder region or head and chest trauma. Physical examination usually reveals severe bony tenderness at the fracture site and should guide the radiographic evaluation because most fractures are minimally displaced and difficult to see on plain radiographs. Fractures can be divided into body, glenoid, coracoid, and acromion. With fractures of the acromion, a pre-existing os acromiale should be suspected. Os acromiale is a failure or delay in the fusion of the ossification centers. Treatment of scapula fractures is usually nonoperative, consisting of an arm sling, unless the athlete has an open injury or severe fracture displacement, especially near the glenoid. Specialty referral is usually required so that associated injuries can be identified.

Fractures of the Humerus

Fractures of the proximal half of the humerus are classified as either physeal fractures or shaft fractures. Physeal fractures are usually the result of a severe blow or fall on the shoulder and are characterized by pain over the anterior and anterolateral aspect of the shoulder. Radiographs can show mild physeal widening to complete displacement. The proximal humerus physis is variable in appearance and can often be mistaken for a fracture. Comparison AP

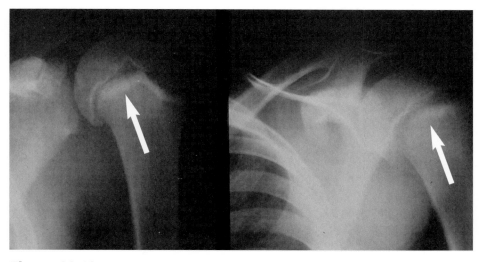

Figure 33.12 Mildly displaced fracture of the proximal humeral physis.

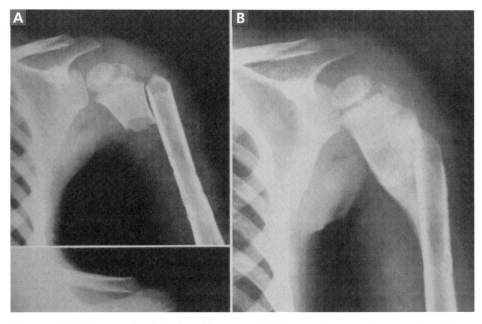

Figure 33.13 Completely displaced fracture and follow-up. **A** Proximal humeral physeal fracture immobilized in bayonet apposition. **B** Subsequent healing and remodeling.

radiographs of the opposite shoulder can be helpful in evaluating these injuries. Salter-Harris type I separations of the proximal humerus typically occur before the age of 5 years and are therefore rare in young athletes. Between the ages of 5 to 11 years, fractures in the proximal humerus occur in the metaphysis. In adolescence, Salter-Harris type II fractures are the most common because the physis of the proximal humerus is one of the last to close (**Figure 33.12**). These injuries are almost always treated nonoperatively with a sling for 4 to 6 weeks. Even completely displaced fractures in skeletally immature athletes have an incredible capacity for healing and remodeling because 80% of humeral growth occurs at the proximal humerus (**Figure 33.13**). Any fractures with severe displacement of more than 50% or possible shaft incarceration in the deltoid require specialty consultation, as do any fractures through lytic areas

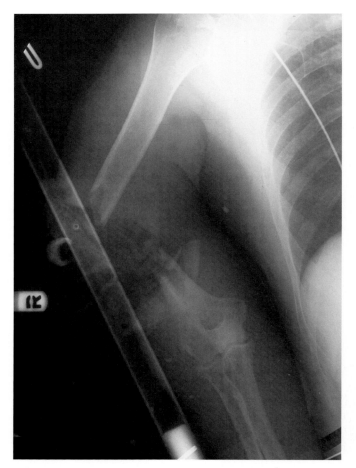

Figure 33.14 Fracture of the mid-diaphysis of the humerus.

of the proximal humerus. The latter usually represent simple bone cysts that will likely require additional treatment.

Fractures of the humeral shaft are much less common than other fractures about the shoulder (**Figure 33.14**). Radial nerve function (eg, wrist extension, first web space sensation) requires careful evaluation because of its close proximity as it winds around the middle portion of the humeral shaft. Most of these fractures are managed using coaptation splints, fracture braces, and a sling for approximately 4 to 8 weeks (**Figure 33.15**). Fracture braces can be used for treatment and then for protection with return to play. Specialty referral is indicated if proper splinting or bracing is not available or if a nerve injury or severe fracture displacement exists.

Little Leaguer's Shoulder

Proximal humeral epiphysitis, or Little Leaguer's shoulder, is most commonly a result of overuse in throwing sports such as baseball, but occasionally occurs in racket sports such as tennis. Physical examination usually reveals pain in the lateral aspect of the proximal humerus, palpable tenderness, and swelling over the anterior and lateral shoulder. Weakness with resisted abduction and external rotation of the shoulder are also possible. Routine radiographs reveal classic widening of the proximal humeral physis in the affected arm (**Figure 33.16**). Views of the opposite, uninjured shoulder are useful to confirm subtle physeal widening.

Treatment is almost always nonsurgical and focused on resting the irritated physis. Local measures include wet heat and adequate warm-up prior to activity, and ice and rest after activity. NSAIDs can help with acute pain. Physical therapy should focus on progressive stretching and strengthening of the rotator cuff with light weights and high repetitions. The coach, athlete, and parents also should be involved in making proper modifications in throwing technique, intensity, and frequency. Many athletes benefit from temporary changes to other less strenuous positions such as first or second base or decreasing their involvement in two leagues at the same time. Racket sport athletes require similar changes in playing intensity and frequency, as well as changing to rackets with smaller grips and faces. The length of activity modifications varies but should continue until the athlete can perform sport-specific activity without pain.

Acute Traumatic Anterior Shoulder Instability

Acute shoulder dislocations can be a very frightening experience for an athlete. Knowing how to recognize these injuries can help alleviate unnecessary fears and facilitate proper treatment. Most athletic shoulder dislocations are anterior and are caused by indirect trauma to the upper extremity. The mechanism of injury is usually a violent force applied to the abducted and externally rotated shoulder, resulting in anterior inferior dislocation of the humeral head.

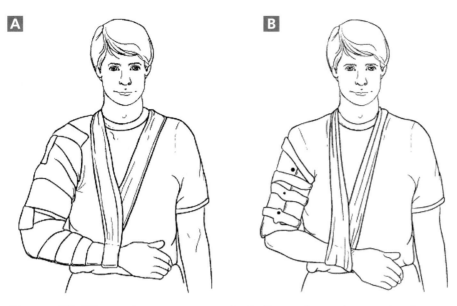

Figure 33.15 Most fractures are managed with slings, or fracture braces and a sling.
A Coaptation splint and sling. **B** Fracture orthosis and sling.

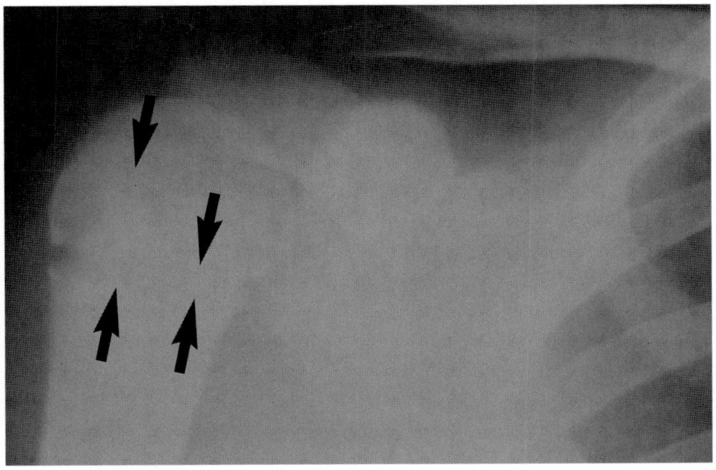

The shoulder can appear "squared off" due to the prominence of the lateral acromion without the humeral head. The athlete's arm is usually held in a slightly abducted and externally rotated position with severe pain and mechanical blocking to any movement. The mechanical block to movement of the shoulder is often key in distinguishing these injuries from brachial plexus stingers, as described in chapter 31, and shoulder subluxations or dislocations that spontaneously reduce ("dead arm" sensation). Axillary nerve damage can occur with acute shoulder dislocation but is difficult to detect clinically. Some athletes report numbness and tingling in the ulnar digits. The athlete's arm should be immobilized or supported in a position of comfort for transport from the playing field. Forceful internal or external rotation should be avoided to prevent potential fracture of the humerus. If the physician has experience recognizing and treating these injuries, an attempt to reduce the shoulder can be made prior to the onset of muscle spasm. However, if the athlete is believed to have a fracture or if no one on site is experienced in this technique, the athlete should be transported to the emergency department for radiographic evaluation and sedation before reduction is attempted.

Treatment after reduction of a glenohumeral dislocation in young athletes remains controversial. Initial management should include immobilization in an arm sling with ice and rest for the first 1 to 2 weeks. Gentle passive range of motion exercises with a physical therapist or athletic trainer should be initiated as soon as the acute phase of the injury has passed. Because of the high incidence of labral (Bankart lesions) and capsular injuries and the high probability of recurrent instability in young athletes, early specialty referral is recommended to discuss treatment options.

Figure 33.16 Little Leaguer shoulder. Radiograph demonstrates widening of the physis.

Table 33.3 *Classification of Shoulder Instability*

1. Degree of Instability
   a. Dislocation
   b. Subluxation

2. Chronology of Instability
   a. Congenital
   b. Acute
   c. Recurrent
   d. Locked/fixed

3. Cause
   a. Traumatic
   b. Atraumatic
      i. Voluntary
      ii. Involuntary

4. Direction
   a. Anterior
   b. Posterior
   c. Inferior (luxatio erecta)
   d. Multi-Directional

Plain radiographs that reveal a bony Bankart lesion (inferior glenoid avulsion) or an MRI/MRI arthrogram that reveals significant labral detachment can support early surgical treatment. Other important factors are the amount of force causing the dislocation, the severity of instability on examination after the acute phase and the future athletic demands that will be placed on the shoulder. Initial dislocations are still widely managed with nonoperative measures until recurrent instability becomes a problem. Nonoperative management plans vary, but should include a 4- to 6-week period of immobilization and gentle passive motion exercises, followed by a 2- to 4-month period of progressive shoulder strengthening and sport-specific training. Strengthening should focus on scapular stabilization and the anterior rotator cuff. Return to play averages 3 to 4 months or longer after the injury, depending on the severity of injury, success of physical therapy, and sport-specific demands on the shoulder. Athletes in collision sports may benefit from shoulder harnesses that limit extreme abduction, flexion, and external rotation of the shoulder.

Acute Traumatic Posterior Shoulder Instability

Posterior shoulder dislocations are rare in young athletes but can occur in collision sports such as football and hockey. Many times these dislocations reduce spontaneously and remain unrecognized, described as "shoulder strains." The mechanism of injury usually is a posteriorly directed force on a forward flexed extremity, such as when a football offensive lineman is blocking an opponent. The arm is usually held in a forward flexed, adducted, and internally rotated position with a mechanical block to any movement. Any attempts at forceful internal or external rotation of the arm should be avoided. As with anterior shoulder dislocations, if the physician has experience with posterior shoulder dislocations, an attempt to reduce the shoulder can be made at the site of the injury prior to the onset of muscle spasm. If the athlete is believed to have a fracture or if no one on site is experienced in closed reduction techniques, the athlete should be transported to the emergency department for radiographic evaluation and sedation before reduction is attempted.

Because posterior glenohumeral dislocations occur so infrequently, there is even less consensus on the treatment after reduction. Therefore, early specialty referral is indicated. Initial dislocations are more likely to be treated nonoperatively because of the current variable success rates associated with posterior shoulder stabilization procedures. Nonoperative management should include immobilization in an arm sling in an abducted, externally rotated position with ice and rest for the first 1 to 2 weeks. Gentle passive range of motion exercises with a physical therapist or athletic trainer should be initiated as soon as the acute phase of the injury has passed. Two to 4 months of progressive strengthening exercises should follow with the emphasis on scapular stabilization and the posterior rotator cuff. Use of a shoulder harness for posterior dislocations is less successful but may be worth trying.

Chronic Traumatic Shoulder Instability

Chronic or recurrent traumatic shoulder instability can affect athletes with persistent symptoms following a traumatic injury or activity that caused their initial symptoms. These athletes can be very difficult to treat. A careful history is important to identify the mechanism of injury, direction of instability if known, associated symptoms, and previous treatment. All athletes will benefit from a formal shoulder stretching and strengthening program if they have not previously had one. Any athlete who does not respond to physical therapy or who has symptoms of instability with minimal activity requires specialty referral for possible surgical stabilization. A specialist should also evaluate any athlete with persistent neurologic symptoms. In athletes with voluntary subluxation and a traumatic etiology, appropriate psychiatric consultation may be indicated.

Atraumatic Multidirectional Shoulder Instability

Multidirectional shoulder instability (MDI) is a condition that affects athletes who lack a significant history of traumatic episodes but report a "shifting" sensation in their shoulder. Symptoms of subluxation generally occur in activities in which the shoulder is repetitively abducted and externally rotated, such as in swimming, throwing a ball, or swinging a racket. Anterior shoulder impingement symptoms are also common, but are often missed as a sign of underlying instability. Athletes commonly report that their shoulder "dislocates all the time" but then reduces spontaneously without medical attention. Physical examination may reveal anterior or posterior shoulder tenderness with associated impingement signs or muscular weakness. Ligamentous examinations usually reveal increased glenohumeral translation in more than one direction, most commonly anterior and inferior or posterior and inferior. Examination for signs of generalized ligamentous laxity is important in these athletes due to its potential association with MDI. Diagnostic studies, including plain radiographs, CT, and MRI are usually unremarkable. Initial treatment should focus on stabilizing the humeral head in the glenoid fossa. In reference to the earlier analogy of a golf ball on a tee, it is just as important to keep the ball on the tee as it is to center the tee under the ball. Physical therapy should thus emphasize scapulothoracic mobility, strength, and endurance, as well as glenohumeral rehabilitation. NSAIDs, wet heat prior

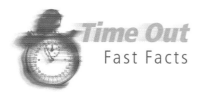

to activity, and ice after activity will help with acute exacerbations of pain that are usually caused by rotator cuff tendinitis. Athletes, parents, and coaches must be patient and ensure that the physical therapy program is followed to facilitate resolution of symptoms. Return to play is based on the athlete achieving good motion and strength with no symptoms of pain or instability with sport-specific activity. If nonoperative measures fail, the athlete requires specialty evaluation for possible surgical stabilization.

Shoulder Impingement Syndrome/Rotator Cuff Tendinitis

Shoulder impingement symptoms are common in young athletes, especially those involved in sports that require repetitive overhead motions. Impingement occurs when there is an imbalance or injury of the shoulder muscles, ligaments, and capsule that results in the inability to keep the humeral head properly positioned within the glenoid fossa. This improper positioning causes pain from irritation of the rotator cuff muscles as a result of the humeral head impinging on the anterior acromion when the arm is flexed forward and internally rotated. Impingement symptoms have many causes and should warrant a careful history. Athletes should be questioned about any acute episodes that may have initiated their symptoms, such as contusions, lifting strains or possible shoulder subluxations or dislocations. Training errors should be identified and corrected including poor technique, increased activity intensity and frequency, or poor equipment use. Associated neurologic symptoms may signal some type of shoulder instability, brachial plexus stretch, or cervical problem. Of particular diagnostic challenge is the athlete with voluntary instability that may be associated with emotional or psychological problems.

Athletes with impingement usually report pain over the anterior and lateral shoulder with overhead activities such as throwing or swimming. The pain is often insidious in onset and progressively worsens, especially if the shoulder is not allowed to rest or the underlying cause is not corrected. Physical examination usually reveals localized tenderness over the anterior and lateral rotator cuff with the shoulder slightly extended to uncover the muscles. Range of motion may be limited, especially due to posterior capsular tightness. A thorough strength testing examination will often reveal muscle weakness imbalances that can be corrected with physical therapy. Provocative maneuvers such as the Neer or Hawkins impingement signs are usually positive. Impingement tests performed with subacromial lidocaine injections can also be helpful. The temptation is to stop the examination at this point and treat the athlete as an adult. However, additional examination for increased joint laxity in all directions is needed to identify any potential instability patterns. Global shoulder laxity may result in an increased incidence of overuse injuries secondary to impingement from the humeral head not being firmly contained in the glenoid or from frank episodes of shoulder subluxation. Generalized ligamentous laxity testing should also be performed since this is often present in adolescents with impingement symptoms. Plain radiographs are usually unremarkable except in the rare young athlete with a type III acromion. MRI is usually unnecessary, but may reveal partial-thickness rotator cuff tears or a labral detachment caused by instability.

Treatment of young athletes with impingement should focus on correcting the underlying cause, but this rarely requires specialty referral for the sole purpose of performing a subacromial decompression. Most cases of impingement are caused by shoulder motion or strength problems resulting from underlying instability. These problems can usually be corrected with a well-structured physical therapy program, including rest from the sports activity. Progressive strengthening exercises that build endurance along with sport-specific activities are the key to return to play without recurrence. The speed at which the athlete progresses through the phases of treatment depends on the nature of the injury, the duration of the injury, and the correction of underlying factors such as poor technique or muscle imbalances. Athletes who do not respond to rest and rehabilitation require specialty referral. Surgical treatment should be aimed at correcting underlying instability.

Biceps Tendinitis

Injury to the biceps tendon complex is very rare in young athletes. Mechanisms of injury can include acute flexion or abduction forces, but injuries are more commonly caused by repetitive overhead activity. Symptoms can include pain with overhead activity and occasionally pain with arm flexion or supination activity. Athletes occasionally report a painful snapping sensation over the anterolateral aspect of the shoulder. Physical examination is similar to that of athletes with impingement. Additional findings can include localized tenderness in the bicipital groove of the proximal humerus and pain with resisted flexion of the outstretched forward flexed arm (**Figure 33.17**). Athletes with subluxation of the long head of the biceps have a palpable snapping of the tendon near the bicipital groove with resisted internal and external rotation of the shoulder. Plain radiographs are unremarkable. MRI can reveal abnormal signal at the site of the long head attachment to the superior glenoid, possibly suggesting a superior labrum, anterior/posterior (SLAP) lesion, which is a partial or complete detachment of the biceps tendon complex. This lesion is very rare in young athletes but has been reported in adolescents. Treatment is usually non-operative in this age group, consisting of rest, stretching, and progressive strengthening. Exercises should focus on correcting strength deficits that may have been the initial cause of the problem. Early specialty referral is warranted if the condition is identified.

Equipment

Most sports do not allow any type of external shoulder bracing or taping, which leaves the injured athlete unprotected or out of the sport until fully recovered. Collision sports such as football and hockey require protective shoulder pads that are very effective in preventing most injuries. Shoulder harnesses are also available that can help prevent excessive abduction, flexion, and external rotation in injured or susceptible shoulders. In addition, custom plastic braces are available to protect the humerus after fracture.

Prevention

The majority of both acute and chronic athletic injuries of the shoulder can be prevented or decreased with proper conditioning and technique. This is especially true in young athletes who are not only developing physically and mentally, but who also are learning how to play their individual sports. Most conditioning and technique training are usually provided by coaches who,

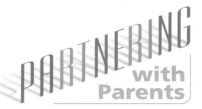

What are some other injuries of the shoulder that are unique to the young athlete?

Physeal or growth plate fractures of the ends of the clavicle are common. Proximal humeral epiphysitis or Little Leaguer's shoulder is also common in the throwing athlete.

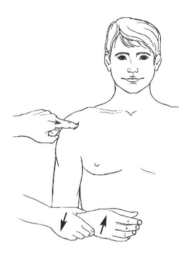

Figure 33.17 The patient is asked to flex the elbow against resistance. The biceps tendon is then palpated.

unfortunately, have variable experience in this area. Therefore, it is beneficial for physicians, physical therapists, and athletic trainers to be proactive in teaching this information when the situation allows.

Conditioning should include stretching, strengthening, and sport-specific activities. A good stretching program should include stretches for flexion/extension, abduction/adduction and internal/external rotation. Strengthening programs should be supervised and should emphasize scapular stabilization and rotator cuff exercises. Light weights with high repetitions should be used initially with slow progression to moderate weights and high repetitions. Heavy weights should be avoided in young athletes. Low back and lower extremity strengthening is also important, especially in throwing or overhead racket sports. Sport-specific activities should include repetitive exercises that mimic common situations for the individual sport, such as throwing or swimming motions. These activities should be well structured, with gradual progression and avoidance of rapid changes. These exercises are good for developing agility, coordination, and overall conditioning that improve performance and hopefully prevent injury.

Proper technique is obviously individualized to each sport. The main goal is to prevent errors in training and competition that overstress muscles or joints or place the athlete in a high-risk position for injury. Common errors include rapid increases in the duration, frequency, or intensity of a certain activity such as throwing a baseball or swinging a racket. Rapid changes result in muscle fatigue that can decrease performance and increase the chance of injury. For example, many athletes who participate in overhead throwing sports are either taught or allowed to continue with poor throwing techniques. Young baseball pitchers who throw with a sidearm motion or who try to throw too many curve balls will have an increased incidence of shoulder and elbow problems. Another example is young football players who tackle with their arms only, resulting in increased shoulder subluxations and rotator cuff strains.

Return to Play Guidelines

Parents are quick to ask when their child can return to play. This question may be difficult to answer because clear return to play guidelines do not exist. As a general rule, athletes may return to play when the following occurs: 1) absence of localized tenderness or swelling; 2) full range of motion and symmetric strength in representative muscle groups; 3) stable ligaments about the shoulder; and 4) the ability to perform representative sports activities without recurrent injury. When any doubt exists about an athlete's readiness to play, proceed with a course that is safest for the athlete.

Pitching Recommendations for Young Baseball Players

	Amount of Pitching	
Age	Maximum Pitches Per Game	Maximum Games Per Week
8–10	52 ± 15	2 ± 0.6
11–12	68 ± 18	2 ± 0.6
13–14	76 ± 16	2 ± 0.4
15–16	91 ± 16	2 ± 0.6
17–18	106 ± 16	2 ± 0.6

The American Academy of Orthopaedic Surgeons recommends limiting the number of innings that young baseball pitchers play to a maximum of 4 to 10 a week. While there is no concrete guideline for the number of pitches allowed, reasonable limits are 80 to 100 pitches in a game and 30 to 40 pitches in a single practice session. Any persistent pain, weakness, or loss of motion should disqualify a child from playing until these findings resolve or are evaluated by a physician.

Red Flags

Any athlete with severe bony tenderness or deformity about the shoulder after an injury should be evaluated with radiographs. Acute loss of motion in the shoulder that is felt to be caused by a mechanical block suggests a fracture or dislocation, and the athlete requires radiographs and specialty evaluation. Athletes should be asymptomatic with full motion and strength prior to return to play. Athletes with persistent symptoms should be referred for specialist evaluation.

Any young athlete who sustains a suspected shoulder injury should have careful neurologic examination performed. Shoulder subluxations can occasionally present as "dead arms" or stingers, but may also represent cervical or brachial plexus injuries. Any athlete with acute neurologic symptoms lasting longer than 15 minutes should be referred to an emergency department for further evaluation.

FINISH LINE

The shoulder depends on muscles and tendons for its stability. Recurrent shoulder instability after an acute dislocation is a major problem in the adolescent athlete. Chronic overuse injuries occur in sports involving overhead throwing or activities.

For More Information

1. Ireland ML, Hutchinson MR: Upper extremity injuries in young athletes. *Clin Sports Med* 1995;14:533–569.

2. Andrish JT: Upper extremity injuries in the skeletally immature athlete, in Nicholas JA, Hershman EB, Posner M (eds): *The Upper Extremity in Sports Medicine,* ed 2. St Louis, MO, Mosby-Year Book, 1995, pp 649–662.

Chapter 34

Hand and Wrist

CARLOS A. GARCIA-MORAL, MD
NEIL E. GREEN, MD
JOHN A. FOX, MD

Several factors influence the type, location, and extent of sports-related injuries to the hand and wrist, such as the athlete's age and ability, the sport, and the playing environment. Fractures occur more frequently in the hand than in any other anatomic region of the upper extremity, and approximately 25% of hand fractures and up to 9% of wrist injuries are sports-related. The incidence of hand injuries tends to be lower in children under age 12 years, but gradually increases during the early teenage years, the time at which many children begin participating in sports. Most of these injuries are closed and involve the muscles, tendons, and ligaments, neurovascular disturbances, and/or fractures and dislocations.

Fractures of the phalanges are among the most common sports-related injuries, followed by fractures of the metacarpal and scaphoid. Hand fractures are distributed as follows: 45% to 50% in the distal phalanges, 30% to 35% in the metacarpals, 15% to 20% in the proximal phalanges, and 8% to 12% in the middle phalanges. In addition, one third of these hand fractures are intra-articular fractures. If improperly treated, fractures may cause residual stiffness, pain, and loss of normal function. The long-term prognosis is directly related to the severity of the initial trauma, associated tissue injury, initial treatment, and rehabilitation.

The three most common tendon injuries in sports are the boutonnière deformity, the mallet finger deformity, and avulsion of the flexor digitorum profundus tendon at its insertion in the distal phalanx. Injuries to the proximal interphalangeal (PIP) and distal interphalangeal (DIP) joints can involve a loss of the functional continuity of the extensor tendon. Other tendon injuries include recurrent dislocation of the extensor carpi ulnaris tendon, longitudinal tears of the sagittal bands over the metacarpophalangeal joint, and avulsion of the flexor digitorum sublimis tendon.

Wrist injuries account for up to 9% of all sports-related injuries. In young athletes, acute fractures of the wrist are most common, whereas in adoles-

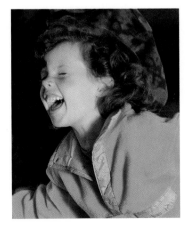

cents, overuse injuries are more common. Most wrist injuries occur as the result of compressive loading of the joint with the wrist in an extended position, such as a fall on an outstretched hand. Ultimately, injuries of the hand and wrist may affect the athlete's future ability to compete, and residual functional impairment may even influence the choice of a future career.

Anatomy/Biomechanics

Hand

The bony architecture of the hand is arranged into three arches, one longitudinal and two transverse (**Figure 34.1**). The longitudinal arch consists of the digits and the apex of the metacarpophalangeal joint. The proximal transverse arch passes through the carpal bones with its center at the capitate, and the distal transverse arch is located at the metacarpal heads with its center at the head of the third metacarpal. In addition, the fourth and fifth digital rays (digits and corresponding metacarpi) offer mobility on the ulnar aspect of the hand, while the second and third metacarpal rays provide stability. Stiffness, deformity, or structural damage to these functional units will disturb function.

Each digit has one long extensor tendon and two long flexor tendons. The small intrinsic muscles of the hand insert into the extensor mechanism. The anatomy of the extensor apparatus of the fingers is very complex, and injury to any element of this apparatus will produce an imbalance with subsequent deformity.

Wrist

The carpal bones in the wrist undergo progressive ossification during development. In children, the osteochondral composition of the immature wrist protects it from injury, and the elasticity of their tissues protects the ligamentous structures. As a result, ligamentous injury to the wrist is very uncommon in children.

Figure 34.1 Bony anatomy of the hand and wrist.

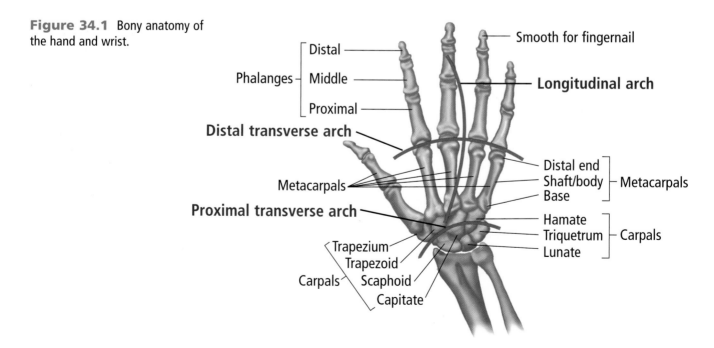

Deforming Forces

The intrinsic-extrinsic muscle tendon units of the hand maintain a delicate balance during digital function, but in the presence of a fracture, there is a possibility of additional angulation, depending on the site (**Figure 34.2**).

Rotational deformities are usually encountered in spiral fractures (**Figure 34.3**). The direction of the fingernails can indicate rotational deformities. Because fingers rotate slightly around the middle metacarpophalangeal axis and converge toward the scaphoid, the fracture must be realigned according to this convergence. If they are not, overlapping will then occur when the child makes a fist (**Figure 34.4**). Even 5° of rotation will cause the digits to overlap during flexion.

Fractures of the distal phalanx occur more frequently than other fractures. Dorsal articular fractures, in which a fragment of the bone from the side of the extensor insertion is avulsed, cause mallet finger deformities. Shortening deformities are usually the result of comminuted fractures, segmental bone loss, or oblique fragments.

Knowledge of physeal centers is important in evaluation. The growth plates in the fingers are located in the proximal aspect of the phalanges, whereas in the second through fifth metacarpals, they are located distally. The first metacarpal epiphysis is located proximally. The epiphysis appears in the phalanges and metacarpals between the ages of 1 to 4 years in boys and 10 months to 3 years in girls. The completion of the bone growth center of the fingers and metacarpals occurs by age 17 years in boys and age 16 years in girls.

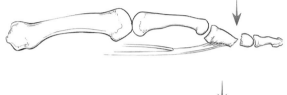

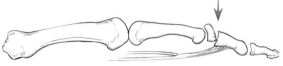

Figure 34.2 Angulation of the midphalanx (top). Angulation from a physeal injury (bottom).

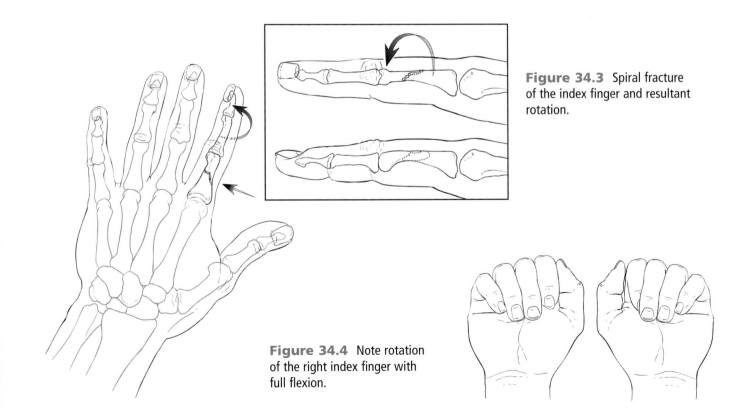

Figure 34.3 Spiral fracture of the index finger and resultant rotation.

Figure 34.4 Note rotation of the right index finger with full flexion.

Clinical Evaluation

History

History should include the time and mechanism of injury. Any attempt at treatment, such as realignment, by the player or coach which may have reduced a dislocation is sought.

Physical Examination

Adequate examination, anatomic reduction, effective immobilization, and rehabilitation are the keys to successful treatment. Each area of the hand and wrist requires specific physical examination. Likewise, specific injuries require different examination techniques. In general, examination should include inspection of the alignment of the hand and fingers and for any swelling. Range of motion is tested actively and passively. Joint instability is tested.

Diagnostic Tests

Anteroposterior (AP), true lateral, and oblique radiographs provide sufficient information for most hand and wrist conditions.

Hand Injuries

Fracture of the base of the first metacarpal

With fractures of the base of the thumb metacarpal, the volar (palmar) fragment remains connected to the trapezium by the volar ligament. As a result, the abductor pollicis longus pulls the unstable metacarpal and causes its proximal subluxation. Radiographic examination of fractures of the base of the first metacarpal distinguishes four types of fractures by location (**Figure 34.5**). Surgery is typically required.

Figure 34.5 A Fracture-dislocation of the base of the thumb metacarpal (Bennett's fracture). **B** Radiograph showing the same.

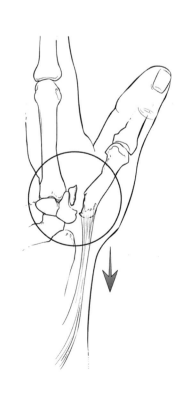
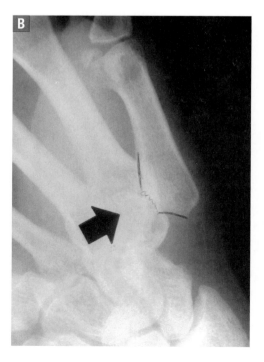

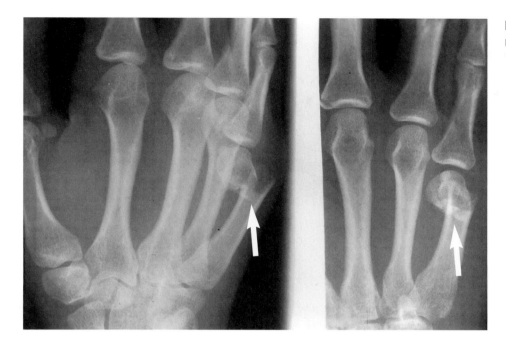

Figure 34.6 Fracture of the fifth metacarpal neck, also called a "boxer's fracture."

Fracture of the Metacarpal Neck

The most common metacarpal fracture, Boxer's fracture, involves the neck of the fifth metacarpal (**Figure 34.6**). The volar cortex becomes comminuted, and the metacarpal head is flexed. Correction of the deformity with closed reduction is difficult, but should be attempted by flexing the metacarpal and PIP joint to 90° and then pushing the metacarpal head into position. Afterward, the injury can be immobilized in a well-molded plaster gutter splint to maintain the arches of the hand. After 3 weeks, the athlete may begin moving and gently exercising the hand, with additional splint protection for another 2 weeks.

Up to about 35° of volar angular deformity is acceptable because there is no loss of function; however, there is a cosmetic loss of the knuckle prominence. Excessive angulation causes pain during forceful grasping and the perception of having a poor grip. The fourth metacarpal has much less motion in the carpometacarpal joint, and volar displacement must be minimal or the athlete will experience problems with grip. Any volar angulation in the first and second metacarpals impairs function and is not acceptable.

Fracture of the Metacarpal Shaft

Fractures of the metacarpal shaft commonly occur in the fourth and fifth metacarpals, where they cause dorsal angulation. The mechanism of injury involves longitudinal compression, torsion, or direct impact.

Management of a stable fracture without displacement or rotation should consist of 3 to 4 weeks of immobilization in a plaster cast that is molded to conform to the transverse and longitudinal metacarpal arch, followed by active motion and protection with a splint. Spiral or short oblique metacarpal fractures are unstable and usually associated with rotational deformity. For these fractures and for transverse fractures, surgery is the treatment of choice. In general, angulation of up to 20° does not cause functional impairment. Acceptable angulation should be less than 10° in the second and third metacarpals.

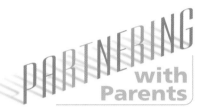

What is buddy taping?

Taping the injured finger to the adjacent preferably longer, uninjured finger.

Physeal injuries of the metacarpal are usually seen in older children and are the result of a direct longitudinal force directed to the flexed metacarpophalangeal joints. More commonly seen are the Salter-Harris type II fractures with a metaphyseal fracture proximal to the physis, the counterpart to the Boxer's fracture seen in adults. Remodeling of the volar angulation is expected in the young athlete and is acceptable to 50° in the ring and little fingers, with no more than 30° of angulation in the index and middle fingers. Again, any degree of rotation is unacceptable and requires either manipulation or surgery to correct the malalignment.

Fracture of the Phalanges

Stable nondisplaced fractures of the proximal and middle phalanges may be treated simply by splinting or immobilizing the hand in a plaster gutter splint. The adjacent uninjured fingers should also be immobilized to support the injured finger and control its alignment and rotation. Taping the injured finger to the adjacent digit protects it and allows the athlete to begin moving the finger early in treatment. Displaced fractures of the proximal phalanx are unusually stable following reduction.

Usually, unstable proximal and middle phalangeal fractures require surgery. An athlete with multiple phalangeal fractures may need surgery to be able to move the fingers early in treatment and to regain function of the extremity.

Intra-articular fractures of the head of the proximal or middle phalanx are common sports-related injuries. AP, lateral, and oblique radiographs are necessary to properly assess the fracture. Usually, these condylar fractures require surgery.

Fractures of the phalangeal neck typically occur in children between ages 5 and 10 years, most commonly in the proximal phalanx. Accurate diagnosis of this injury is important. One hallmark sign is the 90° rotation of the distal fragment (**Figure 34.7**). Usually, this type of fracture requires surgical correction.

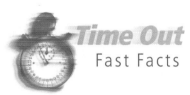

Time Out
Fast Facts

A jammed finger is a joint sprain without a fracture—it usually involves the PIP joint.

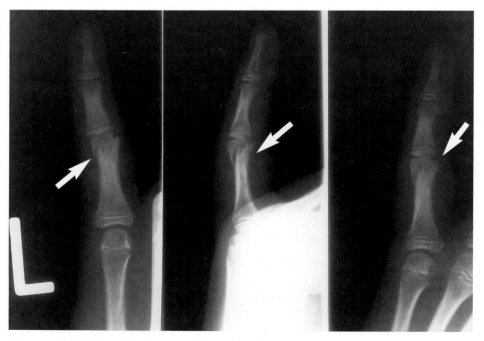

Figure 34.7 Unstable fracture of the neck of the proximal phalanx with rotation.

Physeal Injuries

Injuries of the distal phalanx

Physeal injuries of the distal phalanx are common, and the type of fracture depends on the mechanism of the injury and the age of the patient. Distal phalangeal injury involves the epiphyseal plate, nail, and surrounding soft tissue. Management consists of closed reduction and splinting.

Injuries of the Middle Phalanx

Physeal injuries of the middle phalanx are uncommon. The collateral ligaments at the interphalangeal joints extend beyond the growth plates and attach to the periosteum of the metaphysis to stabilize the physis to a much greater extent than the metacarpophalangeal joints. Clinical alignment and rotation may be restored. Management should consist of immobilizing the finger by taping or splinting it to the adjacent digits in a position between 10° and full extension and applying a short arm cast that extends to the tip of the fingers. Salter-Harris type III fractures also may be seen at the PIP joint associated with an avulsion of the dorsal lip of the epiphysis by the central slip of the extensor tendon. These fractures require surgical correction.

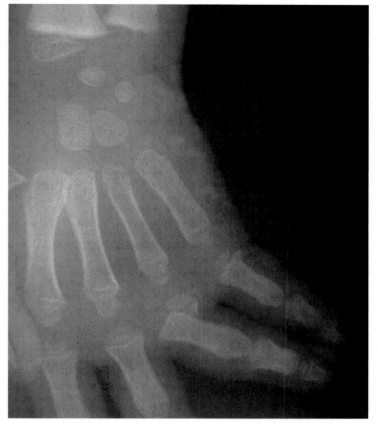

Figure 34.8 Physeal fracture of the proximal fourth and fifth phalanges.

Fracture of the Proximal Phalanx

Fractures of the proximal phalanx are probably one of the most common physeal injuries in the fingers, accounting for about one half of all hand fractures (**Figure 34.8**). Salter-Harris type II fractures involving the index, ring, or little fingers are the most common, caused by forced rotation and angulation. Unless there is a soft-tissue interposition, reduction is relatively simple by flexing the metacarpophalangeal joint and then adducting the finger to realign the proximal phalanx. A pencil may be placed in the web space to act as a fulcrum between the fractured finger and the uninjured finger on the radial side. Any degree of rotation should be corrected since it will not remodel independently.

Fracture of the Thumb

Salter-Harris type III fractures are often seen in the thumb and are analogous to avulsion injuries of the ulnar or radial collateral ligaments in adults. Usually, these injuries involve small fragments, and immobilization will allow adequate healing without loss of stability. However, if fragments are large and rotated, or if a significant portion of the joint is involved, surgical correction is required.

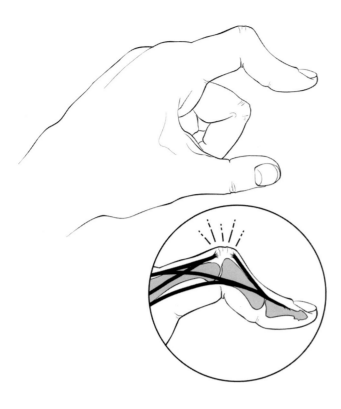

Figure 34.9 Boutonnière deformity of the index finger with rupture of the central slip.

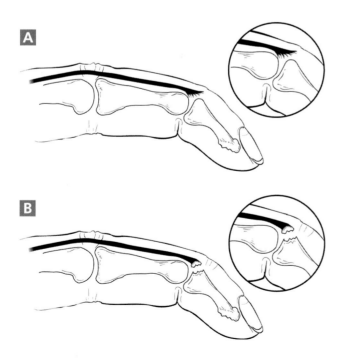

Figure 34.10 Mallet finger deformity. **A** Deformity from tendon rupture. **B** Deformity from bony avulsion.

Tendon Injuries

Boutonnière deformity

Boutonnière deformity is caused by an injury to the central slip of the extensor tendon (**Figure 34.9**). This deformity affects the middle finger most often, followed by the little and index fingers, and occurs in sports that use balls such as volleyball, basketball, handball, baseball, and soccer.

Initial examination may reveal swelling over the dorsum of the PIP joint, pain, and limited active finger extension. Making the initial diagnosis can be quite difficult because the lack of extension can be minimal and is often masked by the swelling and pain. Weak extension of the PIP joint against resistance suggests an injury to the central slip of the extensor tendon. The DIP joint may be in neutral extension, but later becomes hyperextended.

If left untreated, the deformity may progress, leading to chronic contracture of the PIP joint and hyperextension of the DIP joint. With prompt treatment, good functional range of motion will be restored, preventing progression of the deformity. For all acute closed injuries, treatment includes splinting of the PIP joint in a neutral position for a minimum of 6 weeks. Internal or external splinting immobilizes the PIP joint in extension. The DIP joint is left unsupported, and the child should be encouraged to flex the joint periodically. After 6 weeks, gradual and gentle exercises can begin, and the splint may be removed gradually during the day. Splints should be worn at night for an additional 4 weeks. An avulsion of the central slip of the extensor by a bone fragment requires surgery. Deformity that persists for more than 4 to 6 weeks will probably require referral to a hand surgeon.

Return to play in contact sports without hand protection should not be permitted until the PIP joint has at least 45° of active flexion and full active extension. Protective splinting or taping of the PIP joint is recommended for an additional 6 weeks.

Mallet Finger Deformity

A longitudinal force directed to the distal phalanx of a finger can produce an extensor tendon rupture, avulsion fracture, or fracture subluxation of the DIP joint with subsequent mallet finger deformity (**Figure 34.10**). This type of injury is more common in the ulnar fingers and rarely occurs in the thumb.

The DIP joint usually demonstrates full passive extension, but lacks full active extension. The extent of the deformity may vary from a few degrees to a complete extension lag.

Table 34.1	*Injuries that Cause Mallet Finger Deformity*

Type	Injury
1A	Extensor tendon rupture or attenuation
1B	Avulsion fracture of the dorsal phalangeal lip
1C	Open tendon lacerations
2A	Intra-articular fracture without subluxation of the palm (10% to 30% of the articular surface)
2B	Intra-articular fracture with subluxation of the palm (shear fracture of greater than 33% of the articular surface)
3A	Epiphyseal plate injury

AP and lateral radiographs of the DIP joint are useful in identifying whether a bone fragment is attached to the avulsed extensor tendon.

Table 34.1 summarizes the types of mallet finger deformities based on examination and radiologic findings. In types 1A, 1B, and 2A injuries, a longitudinal force flexes the dorsal phalanx while the middle joint is held in extension. In children, either flexion or extension forces directed to the distal phalanx can cause type 3A injuries to the physeal plate, typically a Salter-Harris type II or III physeal injury. The physeal plate of the distal phalanx usually remains open until age 15 years. To assess this injury in children, lateral views of both the injured finger and the opposite, uninjured finger can provide a helpful comparison. Physeal injuries will be apparent on the radiograph.

For most mallet finger deformities, splinting with the DIP joint in neutral extension is the most effective treatment. The splint should be worn continuously for 8 weeks, followed by gentle, progressive exercises until motion has reached 35° to 40° of flexion and full extension. At that point, the splint may be discontinued. Physeal injuries are also typically splinted. Surgery is rarely indicated for a mallet finger deformity, except for those associated with open tendon lacerations or physeal fractures with avulsions of the nail from the matrix. The latter requires surgery. Surgery is also required for type 2B injuries with volar subluxation of the distal fragment.

Athletes may participate in sports while a mallet finger deformity is healing, depending on the sport. With sports that require the use of the hands, an appropriate protective immobilization splint should be worn.

Avulsion of the Flexor Digitorum Profundus Tendon

Avulsion of the flexor digitorum profundus tendon at its insertion point in the distal phalanx is a fairly common injury. Commonly called a "jersey finger," this injury most often occurs when an athlete grabs an opponent's uniform while playing rugby, football, or soccer (**Figure 34.11**). Approximately 75% of avulsion injuries occur in the ring finger.

Physical examination reveals pain and swelling of the injured finger or palm, along with an inability to actively flex the distal phalanx.

Lateral radiographs of the finger are typically normal, although a small fleck of bone may be detected along the course of the flexor tendon.

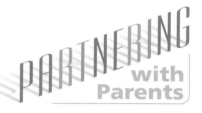

What is mallet finger?

This is an injury to the DIP joint (farthest joint) of the finger usually when hit by a softball where the finger incurs severe/forced flexion. The tendon pulls off the bone—or in the case of a child—the growth plate. It requires uninterrupted splinting for 6 weeks.

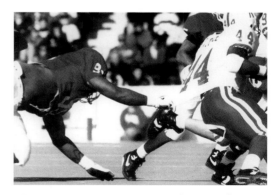

Figure 34.11 Common mechanism of injury of flexor profundus avulsion "jersey finger."

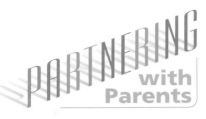

with Parents

What is a jersey finger?

This is an avulsion of the long flexor of a finger when it is caught in another player's jersey and extended forcefully. Surgical repair by a specialist in hand surgery is required.

After an acute injury is diagnosed, the hand must be protected in a splint, and the athlete should not participate in sports until treatment decisions are made. The extent of soft-tissue trauma influences the prognosis. An avulsion caused by something other than violent pulling may be associated with only moderate soft-tissue trauma and edema. Prompt surgical repair of this tendon is indicated to protect the vascular supply to the hand and provide the best prognosis.

Recurrent Dislocation of the Extensor Carpi Ulnaris Tendon

The extensor carpi ulnaris tendon inserts into the dorsal aspect of the base of the fifth metacarpal. It plays an important role in stabilizing the distal ulna and prevents dorsal subluxation in pronation. Forced pronation against resistance may disrupt or stretch the retinacular fibers and allow subluxation of the tendon at the level of the distal ulna. Injury to this tendon is commonly seen in racquet sports, baseball, and golf.

Diagnosis is not difficult. On examination, a snapping sensation can be palpated on the ulnar aspect by placing the wrist in flexion, ulnar deviation, and supination.

Nonsurgical treatment, typically immobilization or a temporary decrease in activities, usually is not successful. With symptomatic recurrent dislocations, surgical reconstruction of the dorsal extensor compartment is the treatment of choice.

Ligamentous Injuries

Collateral ligament of the thumb

The metacarpophalangeal (MP) joint of the thumb has a more limited arc of motion than the MP joint of the fingers that allows it to remain stable when forces are applied to it during pinching and grasping. The less spherical shape of the metacarpal head, the adductor and abductor aponeurotic expansions, and the collateral ligaments contribute to the anatomic stability of the MP joint of the thumb.

Acute injuries to the ulnar collateral ligament frequently occur in downhill skiing, football, baseball, and wrestling. The athlete may report a forcible abduction of the thumb or a combination of abduction with hyperextension. Injuries to the radial collateral ligament are less common, but with complete tears, surgical repair is recommended. Tears of the collateral ligament of the thumb in children are usually Salter-Harris type III epiphyseal injuries and almost always require surgery if there is any displacement present.

Examination reveals pain, swelling in the ulnar MP joint, and weakness of the thumb-index lateral pinch, a motion similar to when you are pinching a key. The joint should be examined with the MP joint in full extension and in 20° to 30° of flexion. In full extension, the accessory collateral ligament is tight and the collateral ligament is relaxed. The reverse occurs when the MP joint is flexed. Compare the injured thumb with the opposite, unaffected thumb to identify excessive instability. In some cases, infiltration of a local anesthetic into the area of the collateral ligament will facilitate this examination. Tenderness over the volar or dorsal aspect of the joint indicates a more severe injury to the adductor aponeurosis and/or volar plate.

AP, lateral, and stress views of both thumbs should be obtained for comparison. Displacement of 30% or more of the proximal phalanx and a lateral laxity of 30° or more (when compared with the opposite thumb) indicate a complete disruption of the ulnar collateral ligament (**Figure 34.12**). Usually, the ulnar collateral ligament is avulsed from the proximal phalanx, and in 75% of patients, the ligament folds back on itself, and healing is impaired by interposition of the adductor pollicis tendon.

Management of incomplete tears without joint instability consists of functional bracing or immobilization with a thumb spica cast for 4 weeks. At the end of this period, active range of motion with protection may be allowed. Complete disruption of the ulnar collateral ligament or displaced intra-articular avulsion fractures are managed by early surgical repair. The thumb should be protected for an additional 6 to 8 weeks with a molded splint or by taping the thumb during activities.

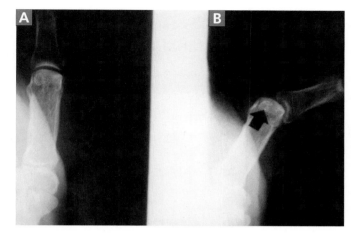

Figure 34.12 MP joint of the thumb. **A** Relaxed view. **B** Stress view showing complete rupture of the ulnar collateral ligament.

Collateral Ligament of the PIP Joint

The PIP joint is vulnerable to the hyperextension and lateral forces produced in ball sports. The most common injuries at this joint are caused by partial tears of the collateral ligament without compromise of the joint stability. In addition to the collateral ligament tear, hyperextension forces may produce an avulsion of the volar plate that is accompanied by a fracture of the volar surface of the middle phalanx.

Physical and radiographic examination may reveal tears associated with increasing disruption of the ligamentous complex of the joint, instability, subluxation, or even dislocation. Immobilization of the joint in extension for 3 weeks, followed by protective taping to the adjacent finger is usually sufficient for partial tears of the collateral ligament. Complete tears with joint stability on active motion may also be managed nonsurgically with immobilization. For these injuries, surgery is indicated to repair ligaments and help ensure recovery of the functional arc of motion.

Wrist Injuries

Fracture of the scaphoid

The scaphoid bone is the bone most frequently fractured in the wrist. After falling on an outstretched hand, an athlete may report pain along the dorsal radial aspect of the wrist.

Initial examination usually does not demonstrate gross deformity; however, the anatomic snuffbox, the area between the extensor pollicis longus and brevis, may be tender (**Figure 34.13**). Range of motion may also be decreased, and pain is elicited on radial deviation of the wrist.

Radiographic evaluation must include four views: posteroanterior (PA) wrist, true lateral wrist, 45° pronation PA, and ulnar deviation PA. Despite thorough examination, many scaphoid fractures are often

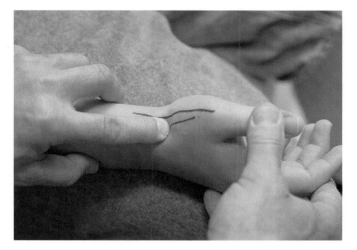

Figure 34.13 The extensor pollicis longus on one side and the abductor pollicis longus and extensor pollicis longus on the other.

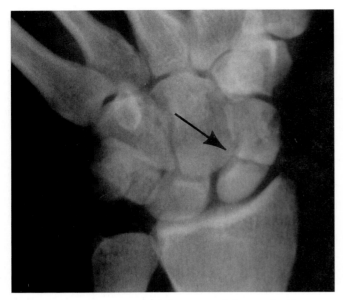

Figure 34.14 Fracture of the waist of the scaphoid.

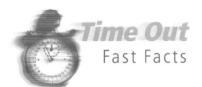

Fast Facts

The "position of function" is used to immobilize fingers and hands to prevent stiffness and contracture following an injury. The MP joints are flexed 90° and fingers extended. The wrist is slightly dorsiflexed.

not evident on initial radiographs. If an injury is suspected, but the radiographs appear normal, immobilization in a thumb spica cast is indicated. Follow-up examination and radiographs should be performed 10 to 14 days following injury if a fracture is present, revealing the previously undetected fracture (**Figure 34.14**).

Management of nondisplaced fractures includes cast immobilization; however, the type of cast that should be used is controversial. One approach advocates the use of a long arm-thumb spica cast for 6 weeks to prevent pronation and supination, followed by a short arm-thumb spica cast until radiographs show evidence of healing. The other approach advocates use of a short arm-thumb spica cast as initial treatment.

Most scaphoid fractures heal within 6 to 10 weeks of immobilization. Delay in the diagnosis of fracture displacement can lead to delayed union or nonunion. If union is not achieved or if the initial fracture is displaced, surgery may be indicated.

Fracture of the Hamate

Hamate fractures are rare in the general population, but more common in young athletes who participate in racquet sports, baseball, golf, or hockey. When the athlete swings, force is directly transferred to the prominent "hook" of the hamate.

With a hamate fracture, the athlete typically reports missing a swing or striking a stationary object, then immediately feeling a sharp pain on the ulnar aspect of the wrist. Later, this pain becomes a dull, ill-defined discomfort during sports activity, but not during daily activities. Examination reveals point tenderness along the ulnar aspect of the hand, just distal to the flexion crease.

Radiographs should include a carpal tunnel view and a 45° supination oblique view if there is a suspicion of a hamate fracture. Also, a CT scan can be very useful in defining this injury.

Initial management includes application of a short arm cast that immobilizes the base of the thumb and holds the fourth and fifth MP joints in a flexed position. If the fracture has not healed after 6 weeks of immobilization, surgical excision of the fracture fragment is recommended.

Other Fractures of the Wrist

Fractures of the other wrist bones are exceedingly rare, but have been reported, sometimes in combination with other wrist injuries. In general, immobilization and treatment of symptoms are considered adequate management. Diagnosis of these injuries is typically the most challenging aspect of care, since they are rare and often difficult to detect on routine radiographs.

Soft-Tissue Injuries

Acute injuries of the soft tissues about the wrist are rare in children. However, ligamentous injuries and wrist instability may occur in adolescents and are usually associated with a distal radial physeal injury. Ligamentous laxity and joint hypermobility may predispose the child to ligamentous injury with tension loading and to joint injury with repetitive stress.

Overuse Injuries

Several overuse injuries of the wrist are common in young athletes. For example, tendinitis or tenosynovitis occurs in athletes who perform repetitive motions with the wrist. Tenosynovitis of the first dorsal compartment of the hand, or deQuervain's disease, frequently occurs in activities that require hyperabduction of the thumb, such as golf and racquet sports.

An inflammatory condition called "intersection syndrome" can develop in athletes who row or train with weights. This condition is named for the anatomic point at which the abductor pollicis longus, the extensor pollicis brevis, and the wrist extensors intersect and where pain and tenderness are localized.

Tendinitis is also seen in the extensor carpi ulnaris of athletes who participate in racquet sports and rowing. With tendinitis, pain is localized over the dorsal ulnar aspect of the wrist and exacerbated by wrist extension against resistance.

Repetitive stress can also injure the distal physis of the radius and cause a growth disturbance. This type of injury is common in gymnasts-found in up to 10% of female gymnasts-and is most likely caused by the repetitive compression forces associated with load bearing on the upper extremity. Athletes may describe wrist pain, particularly with dorsiflexion and axial loading. Radiographs may reveal widening and irregularity of the physis that can cause growth inhibition or premature growth arrest (**Figure 34.15**). The relative overgrowth of the ulna may result in "positive ulnar variance" in which the ulna is equal to or longer than the radius. As a result, the ulna and radius do not appropriately share the stress loads at the wrist articulation. Also, positive ulnar variance can cause other secondary injuries, including ulnar impingement syndrome and tears of the triangular fibrocartilage complex. Initial management should include rest, along with the use of topical and oral anti-inflammatory drugs. After the acute phase resolves, a gradual return to play should include exercises to strengthen the wrist flexors and bracing or taping to control wrist dorsiflexion. If symptoms recur, modification of grip techniques or quitting the activity may be necessary. Regular radiographic examination may be justified in high-risk athletes.

Overuse injuries are often difficult to treat. At times, parents and coaches place significant pressure on the child to return to play, despite a need for the child to rest and heal. In general, anti-inflammatory medications, rest, and short-term immobilization are helpful in treating these conditions. A supervised, gradual return to play can often prevent symptoms from recurring.

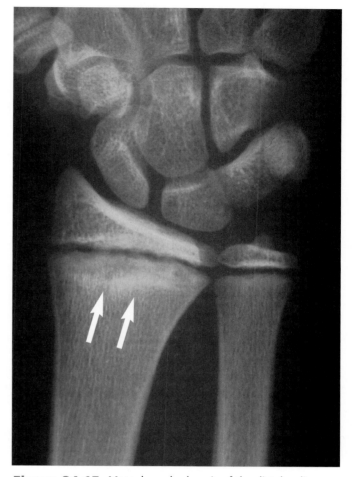

Figure 34.15 Metaphyseal sclerosis of the distal radius consistent with radial epiphysitis.

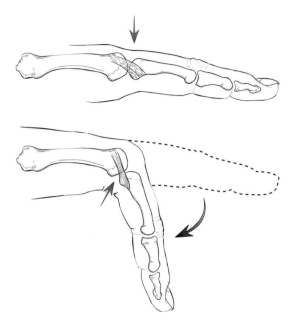

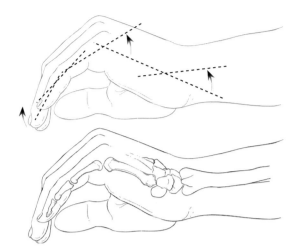

Figure 34.16 Immobilization of the MP joint in flexion (bottom) prevents shortening of the collateral ligaments.

Figure 34.17 Intrinsic plus position with the PIP joint flexed 15°.

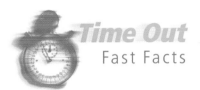
Fast Facts

Aluminum and foam finger splints are most comfortably worn on the dorsum of the hand. They can be pre bent using the uninjured side as a model or template.

Rehabilitation

Immobilization of fractures for 4 to 6 weeks is usually sufficient. However, splinting should be continued until symptoms disappear.

The well-known "position of function" is not necessarily the ideal position in which to immobilize the hand during rehabilitation. The concept of an "ideal position" is based on the anatomic configuration of the collateral ligaments of the MP and PIP joints. The ligamentous system of the digit is arranged to provide stability during flexion. At the level of the MP joint, the collateral ligaments are lax during extension and tight during flexion. Therefore, immobilizing the MP joint in a flexed position will prevent shortening of the collateral ligaments and restrict motion of the MP joint (**Figure 34.16**).

Likewise, the PIP joint has an ideal position for immobilization. The greatest tension of the collateral ligament occurs at approximately 15° of flexion. Therefore, the intrinsic plus position is the position in which contracture of the joint is least likely to occur (**Figure 34.17**). The hand should be immobilized with the wrist in 30° of dorsiflexion, the MP joints in 40° to 60° of flexion, and the interphalangeal joint in neutral to 15° of flexion.

Return to Play

Several factors need to be considered before the injured athlete is allowed to return to play: type of fracture, reduction stability, use of the hand in the sport involved, and whether or not the injured part can be protected from further damage. Rigid external immobilization by cast, splints, and silicone rubber compounds may protect the hand and should be safe for all athletes.

Red Flags

Numerous complications of hand fractures can occur. Joint stiffness is probably the most common. In addition, flexion and intrinsic contracture, chronic edema, flexor and extensor tendon adhesions, and malrotation caused by nonunion or malunion all affect the outcome and function of the hand. Also, reflex sympathetic dystrophy, infection, residual pain, and weakness are other possible sequelae that should be considered during treatment.

FINISH LINE

Sports activities by young people have increased in all school levels and community programs. Therefore, coaches, trainers, parents, and team physicians share the responsibility to care for and develop the young athlete. Because coaches and trainers are often the first to recognize injuries, they must know how to protect the athlete and prevent further injuries. Hand injuries can result in significant impairment if not recognized and treated appropriately. Because of the unique function of the hand, alignment of fractures must be more exact. The position of immobilization is often crucial and should not be prolonged beyond what is necessary. Rehabilitation is very important.

For More Information

1. Mosher JF: Flexor and extensor tendon injuries, in Pettrone FA (ed): *American Academy of Orthopaedic Surgeons: Symposium on Upper Extremity Injuries in Athletes.* St Louis, MO, CV Mosby, 1986, pp 114–121.

2. Leddy JP, Packer JW: Avulsion of the profundus tendon insertion in athletes. *J Hand Surg* 1977;2A:66–69.

3. Hastings H II, Simmons BP: Hand fractures in children: A statistical analysis. *Clin Orthop* 1984;188:120–130.

4. Simmons BP, Lovallo JL: Hand and wrist injuries in children. *Clin Sports Med* 1988;7:495–512.

5. Dixon GL Jr, Moon NF: Rotational supracondylar fractures of the proximal phalanx in children. *Clin Orthop* 1972;83:151–156.

6. McCue FC III, Hakala MW, Andrews JR, Gieck JH: Ulnar collateral ligament injuries of the thumb in athletes. *J Sports Med* 1975;2:70–80.

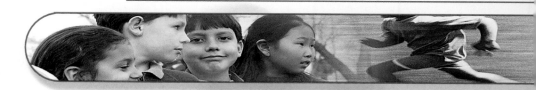

C h a p t e r   3 5

Hip, Pelvis, and Thigh

J A M E S   H .   B E A T Y ,   M D

njuries to the pelvis, hip, or thigh in a young athlete can be caused
by acute trauma or by subacute, repetitive trauma, as in overuse
injuries. Several anatomic factors unique to children make them susceptible to sports-related injuries. For instance, the cartilage of the physes
and apophyses is vulnerable to shear forces and, because of its relative
weakness, it is more likely to be injured than the stronger adjacent ligaments. As a result, a child or adolescent is more likely to sustain a physeal
fracture from a force that would cause only a ligament or muscle strain in
an adult. In addition, the soft tissues lengthen to accommodate growing
bone, but during growth spurts lengthening of the muscles and tendons
may lag behind skeletal growth. This disparity causes tightness and loss
of flexibility, which increases the likelihood of injury. Also, alignment problems of the lower extremities or spine can increase the risk of injury.

Anatomy/Biomechanics

Hip

The secondary ossification centers of the proximal femur appear at different
ages in a child—the femoral head at age 4 to 6 months, the greater trochanter
at age 2 to 5 years, and the lesser trochanter at age 8 to 12 years—but all fuse
at about age 16 to 18 years. The femur changes in shape and alignment during
growth. The neck-shaft angle decreases from 155° to 130° at skeletal maturity,
and femoral anteversion gradually decreases from approximately 40° to 10° in
men and from 40° to 15° in women.

The muscles surrounding the hip joint allow flexion, extension, abduction,
adduction, circumduction, and rotation. The primary hip flexors are the iliopsoas, sartorius, rectus femoris, and adductor muscles. The primary extensors
are the gluteus maximus and hamstrings. Adduction is mediated primarily by
the adductors and medial hamstring, while abduction is mediated by the
tensor fascia lata and gluteus minimus and medius muscles. Internal rotators
are the gluteus medius and minimus, tensor fascia lata, adductors, and iliopsoas. External rotators include the gluteus maximus, piriformis, obturator,
and gemellus muscles.

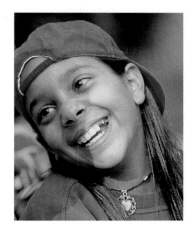

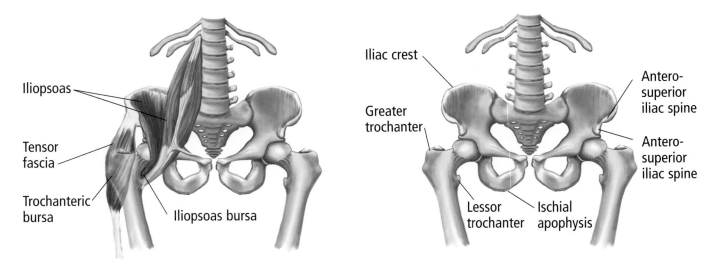

Figure 35.1 Trochanteric and iliopsoas bursae.

Figure 35.2 Sites at which avulsion fractures can occur.

Although numerous bursae surround the hip joint, the two most important are the trochanteric bursa, located just behind the greater trochanter and deep to the gluteus maximus and tensor fascia lata muscles, and the iliopsoas bursa, located between the capsule and iliopsoas muscle anteriorly (**Figure 35.1**).

Pelvis

The pelvis develops from three primary ossification centers: the ilium, ischium, and pubis. Secondary centers of ossification—the iliac crest, ischial apophysis, anteroinferior and anterosuperior iliac spines, pubic tubercle, angle of the pubis, ischial spine, and lateral wing of the sacrum—appear during puberty and fuse at varying intervals. It is important to be aware of these ossification centers so that they are not confused with avulsion fractures (**Figure 35.2**).

The pelvis is the origin for a number of large paraspinous, abdominal, and thigh muscles, including the sartorius, quadriceps, rectus femoris, adductor longus and brevis, and hamstrings (**Figure 35.3**). These muscles place strong functional forces on the cartilaginous and bony structures.

Several important anatomic differences distinguish a child's pelvis from an adult's. A child's pelvis is more malleable because of its cartilaginous structures, and the joints (sacroiliac, symphysis) are more elastic. Avulsion fractures of the apophyses are more common in children and adolescents than in adults because cartilage is weaker than bone. Injuries to the pelvis that damage the physeal cartilage can result in growth arrest, leg-length discrepancy, and faulty development.

Thigh

The thigh contains four major groups of muscles: flexors, extensors, abductors, and adductors. The knee extensors, or quadriceps, are the strongest group on the anterior aspect. On the posterior aspect, the hamstrings are strong flexors of the knee and major extensors of the hip. The thigh muscles are covered and divided into groups by the fascia, a heavy fibrous sheath.

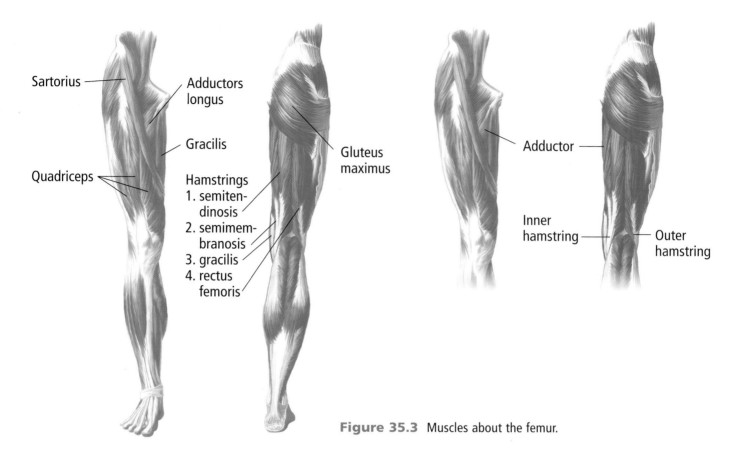

Sartorius

Adductors longus

Gracilis

Quadriceps

Hamstrings
1. semiten-
   dinosis
2. semimem-
   branosis
3. gracilis
4. rectus
   femoris

Gluteus maximus

Adductor

Inner hamstring

Outer hamstring

Figure 35.3 Muscles about the femur.

Clinical Evaluation

History

A careful history is essential to an accurate diagnosis and appropriate treatment. If the injury is acute, the athlete may be able to recall a single motion or traumatic event that caused the injury. If the injury is chronic and the history reveals persistent pain that restricts participation or decreases performance, the quality, location, duration, and severity of the symptoms must be determined. Also the sport in which the injury occurred and the equipment used may offer diagnostic clues.

Physical Examination

A complete physical examination should include an evaluation of the spine, knees, feet, and overall alignment of the lower extremity. Areas of local tenderness, limitations of range of motion, changes in gait, alterations in muscle strength, and muscle atrophy should be identified. Loss of internal rotation and/or abduction is crucial because it is often present in disorders of the hip such as slipped capital femoral epiphysis and Legg-Calvé-Perthes disease.

Diagnostic Tests

Initial radiographic examination includes standard anteroposterior (AP) and lateral views of the hip and pelvis. Special views, such as oblique or inlet-outlet pelvic views may be necessary. Full-length standing views of the lower extremities help detect malalignment problems or knee pathology that may cause referred pain to the hip or pelvic area. Bone scans are useful to confirm a suspected stress fracture, pathologic lesion, or apophysitis. A CT scan will confirm adequate reduction of a hip dislocation and rule out the presence of an intra-articular fragment. MRI may be helpful in detecting early osteonecrosis of the femoral head and in evaluating soft-tissue injuries. Indications for special imaging techniques are described in the context of specific injuries.

Acute Injuries

Apophyseal Avulsions

Avulsion injuries most commonly occur in children and adolescents who participate in strenuous athletic endeavors; they account for 14% to 40% of pelvic fractures in children and adolescents. Many "pulled muscles" may, in fact, be avulsion fractures that are undetected if radiographs are not obtained. Acute separations of the apophyses can occur with sudden contractions or stretching of the hamstrings, adductors, or other muscles that originate from or insert into the pelvis and proximal femur. Occasionally, direct trauma also may cause an avulsion fracture. Sites of possible apophyseal avulsion include the iliac crest, anterosuperior and anteroinferior iliac spines, ischial tuberosity, and greater and lesser trochanters (**Figure 35.2**).

Treatment varies somewhat depending on the fracture site and the muscular forces acting across the physis, but most can be treated nonoperatively. A five-stage progressive rehabilitation program for all apophyseal avulsion injuries is shown in **Table 35.1**. In stage I, rest, ice, analgesics, and limb positioning are

Table 35.1 *Nonoperative Treatment of Pelvic Apophyseal Avulsions**

Treatment phase	Days after injury	Subjective pain	Pain on palpation	Range of motion	Muscle strength	Level of activity	Radiographic appearance
I	0 to 7	Moderate	Moderate to severe	Very limited	Poor	None, protected gait	Osseous separation
II	7 to 20	Minimal	Moderate	Improving with guided exercise	Fair	Protected gait, guided exercise	Osseous separation
III	14 to 30	Minimal with stress	Moderate	Improving with gentle stretchings	Good	Guided exercise, resistance	Early callus formation
IV	30 to 60	None	Minimal	Normal	Normal to good	Limited athletic activity	Maturing callus
V	60 to return	None	None	Normal	Normal	Normal	Maturing callus

*Modified from Metzmaker JN, Pappas AM: Avulsion fractures of the pelvis. *Am J Sports Med* 1985;13:349–358.

used to relieve tension on the involved muscle group. In stage II, when acute pain subsides, active and passive motion may be increased gradually. A comprehensive progressive resistance exercise program may begin when full active range of motion is possible in stage III. Stage IV begins when approximately 50% of the anticipated strength has been restored. In this stage, limited return to activity is permitted. The final stage, stage V, includes sport-specific training and return to play. **Table 35-2** summarizes the types of apophyseal avulsions and their treatment.

Because of the frequency of persistent symptoms and continuing functional disability after nonoperative treatment of avulsion fractures, some authors recommend surgical treatment, especially for displaced avulsions of the ischial tuberosity. However, surgery is rarely indicated for hamstring injuries in adolescent athletes. The only indication might be an acute, large bony avulsion from the ischial tuberosity that is displaced more than 3 cm.

In the healing phase, a large amount of heterotopic bone and callus can mimic a neoplasm. A careful history will differentiate the two, and, if necessary, MRI can confirm the diagnosis.

Hip Fractures and Dislocations

Sports-related fractures of the head and neck of the femur are rare. However, when they do occur, they usually are caused by high-energy trauma. Fractures through the capital femoral physis may be one extreme of the spectrum of slipped capital femoral epiphysis. Hip fractures may be associated with a pathologic lesion, such as a unicameral bone cyst or fibrous dysplasia, or with a systemic condition, such as renal osteodystrophy or hypothyroidism. Plain radiographs are usually diagnostic (**Figure 35.4**). Most hip fractures, especially those in adolescent athletes, are best treated surgically. Complications of hip fractures include osteonecrosis and nonunion.

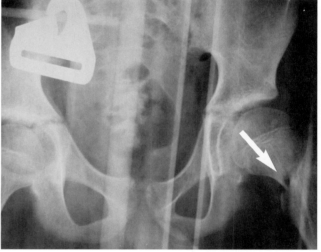

Figure 35.4 Fracture of the base of the left femoral neck.

Hip dislocations are more common than hip fractures in children and young adolescents. Most hip dislocations occur posteriorly, causing the athlete to hold the leg in flexion, adduction, and internal rotation. With an anterior dislocation, the leg is extended, abducted, and externally rotated. Radiographs identify the direction of the dislocation and the presence of any fracture fragments or acetabular fracture. A CT scan can help detect fracture fragments or interposed tissue within the hip joint and can evaluate nonconcentric reduction or associated pelvic fracture.

A hip dislocation is a true orthopaedic emergency, and immediate treatment is necessary. Closed reduction usually is possible, and concentric reduction should be confirmed with radiographs or CT scans. After concentric closed reduction, light skin traction is used for 3 to 7 days, followed by non-weightbearing crutch ambulation for 3 weeks. Progressive weightbearing is then begun, and activities are restricted for 3 more weeks. Full return to activity is allowed when full strength, motion, and agility have been regained. If closed reduction is impossible because of an inverted limbus, interposed capsule, or osteochondral fragments, or if the hip is unstable after closed reduction, open reduction is required.

Table 35.2	Types of Apophyseal Avulsions

Site	Mechanism of injury	Type of sports activity	Physical findings
Iliac crest	• Sudden contracture of abdominal muscles • Direct trauma • Overuse	• Runner makes an abrupt change in direction • Football • Runners	• Pain over injury site • Gluteus medius lurch during gait • Localized tenderness over anterior aspect of iliac crest • Limited active range of motion
"Hip pointer" or contusion to iliac crest	• Direct trauma	• Football	• Pain over injury site
Antero-superior iliac spine	• Forceful pull of sartorius, with hip extended and knee flexed	• Sprinters, hurdlers, and runners	• Snap or pop at time of injury • Acute pain over injury site • Pain on passive extension or active flexion of hip • Possible to palpate fragment
Antero-inferior iliac spine	• Violent contraction of the rectus femoris • Hyperextension of hip and flexion of knee in kicking sports	• Sprinter's fracture, when coming out of starting block • Kicking sports	• Acute pain over groin region • Localized tenderness over site • Increased tenderness with hyperextension or resisted hip flexion • Pain on full weightbearing • Antalgic gait
Greater trochanter (uncommon)	• Forceful contractions of the hip abductors	• "Cutting" maneuvers	• Tenderness over site of injury • Hip held in slight flexion • No active hip abduction • Inability to stand alone on affected leg (positive Trendelenburg's sign)
Lesser trochanter	• Violent contraction of iliopsoas	• Kicking, sprinting, jumping	• Sudden pain in groin or anterior hip • Sudden snap at time of injury • Inability to walk or walk with antalgic gait • Hip in slight adduction or internal rotation • Inability to actively flex the hip while seated (positive Ludloff sign)
Ischial tuberosity (most common)	• Violent contraction of hamstrings • Direct trauma	• Hurdlers, long jumpers, athletes who perform the splits (gymnasts, cheerleaders)	• Pain in buttock at gluteal fold • Pain can radiate along proximal hamstrings • Stretching of hamstrings increases tenderness on palpation • Inability to walk or walk with antalgic gait
Symphysis pubis	• Pull of adductor muscles	• Kicking across the body (cross kicking) or doing the splits	• Pain in medial groin area • Pain can radiate to perineal region or along adductor region of thigh • Increased tenderness on passive abduction or resisted adduction of hip

Imaging	Treatment	Average return to play
• Radiographs show avulsion and possible displacement of fragment	• Crutch ambulation, with gradual increase in activities	4 wks
• Radiographs, eventually, to rule out acute fracture	• Symptomatic, with modifications or additional equipment	
• Plain radiographs show inferior, lateral displacement of fragment • Oblique or lateral views confirm defect of the ilium	• Activity restrictions • Crutch ambulation	3 to 4 wks 6 to 10 wks to pain free
• Plain radiographs differentiate avulsion from hematoma or inguinal hernia • Radiographs of opposite side to distinguish from os acetabuli	• Bed rest for a few days with hip and knees flexed • Crutch ambulation • Gradual return to activities	6 wks
• Plain radiographs show extent of injury • Radiographs of opposite side to confirm a questionable diagnosis	• Bed rest for a few days. Hip spica cast/orthotics for 10 to 14 days. • Gradual return to activities	
	• Decreased activity • Crutch ambulation • Bed rest with hip mildly flexed	12 wks
• Radiographs show separation of crescent-shaped apophysis from ischial tuberosity	• Bed rest for a few days with minor (less than 2-cm displaced) fractures. (Note: Fractures greater than 2 cm probably need surgery.) • Activity restrictions • Crutch ambulation • Gradual return to activities	6 to 12 wks
• Radiographs may not show any abnormalities	• Activity restrictions • Crutch ambulation • Surgery may be needed if nonsurgical treatment does not relieve pain	

Fractures of the Femur

The femur is the largest bone in the body and the muscle mass of the thigh the strongest. Fractures of the femur should be managed by an orthopaedic surgeon. In children ages 6 to 12 years, treatment can consist of traction and spica casting, external fixation, or internal fixation. Adolescents usually are treated as adults, typically with internal fixation.

Contusions, Sprains, and Strains

Contusions, sprains, and strains are the most common injuries in athletes. Most contusions and sprains are self-limited and can be treated with rest, ice, compression, elevation (RICE), and a gradual return to play.

Muscle strains, also called pulls or tears, are common in athletes who run, jump, or kick. Strains can range in severity from mild first-degree strains to severe third-degree tears of the muscles. Hamstring strains are especially troublesome because they are functionally disabling and they tend to recur. Several factors may predispose certain athletes to muscle strains: muscle imbalance (eg, when the quadriceps are stronger than the hamstrings), poor posture, inflexibility, fatigue, and poor coordination.

Athletes with hamstring strains usually report immediate localized pain in the posterior thigh that occurs while they walk in full stride. Palpation or any attempt to stretch the hamstring elicits local tenderness and pain. An athlete with a third-degree strain will be unable to walk. Frequently, hamstring tears cause profuse hemorrhaging and ecchymosis that becomes evident a few days after the injury. Immediate treatment consists of RICE and crutch ambulation, if needed. Gradual active stretching and progressive exercises can be started as soon as pain subsides. The athlete should not be allowed to return to play until flexibility, strength, and muscle balance are regained, a process that may take 10 days to 3 weeks for a mild strain, and 2 to 6 months for a severe strain.

Myositis Ossificans

Intramuscular hemorrhage occasionally results in posttraumatic myositis ossificans. The process of bone deposition into muscle typically begins within 1 to 2 weeks after a severe contusion, and the new bone can be palpated as a hard mass within the soft tissue within 3 to 4 weeks of injury. Radiographs taken at this time show fluffy, immature bone in the muscle tissue. Over a period of months, the bone matures to typical cortical-type bone.

Myositis ossificans is self-limited if the muscle is not irritated by active exercise or vigorous massage. A series of radiographs follow the progress of the lesion until the calcium deposit matures, typically in 6 to 12 months. Usually, the bony mass is not painful, and no treatment is required other than padding the area. Most of the mass will be resorbed in time. The mature bony mass can be excised if it causes functional disability or pain, although this usually is not necessary nor recommended because if the mass is removed before it matures, it is likely to recur.

Chronic Injuries

Overuse can produce stress fractures in bone, tendinitis, and bursitis at bone-tendon junctions. Often chronic injuries require longer periods of rehabilitation than acute injuries.

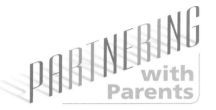

How is a quadriceps contusion treated?

The quadriceps is rested by using crutches. As pain subsides, gentle motion is begun. Full return to sports is allowed when there is a normal range of pain-free knee motion.

Several simple measures can decrease the risk of overuse injuries, as follows:

1. Shoe inserts or orthotics for mild leg-length discrepancies or pronation

2. Improved flexibility to prevent injuries caused by muscle-tendon tightness

3. Proper design and supervision of muscle-strengthening programs to help correct muscle imbalances

4. Appropriate equipment, including shoes, for the sport and for the age and size of the athlete

Many overuse injuries can be avoided by appropriate conditioning and gradually increasing the intensity of training by approximately 10% per week. Young athletes should not be asked to do too much too soon or too often.

Stress Fractures

Femur

Stress fractures of the femoral neck are rare in children, but tend to affect older adolescents who participate in track and field events. Persistent groin pain that increases with activity is the most common symptom. Examination may also reveal increased pain as the hip is moved through its range of motion. Initial radiographs may be negative, but a bone scan with technetium-99 or an MRI may show early signs of a stress fracture. Treatment of stress or compression fractures of the inferior femoral neck should consist of protected weightbearing until radiographs reveal evidence of healing. Range of motion exercises and nonimpact conditioning, such as bicycling or swimming, can be continued. A stress or tension fracture of the superior femoral neck requires surgical fixation.

Pelvis

Stress fractures of the pelvis are uncommon in young athletes, except in runners. Pain is typically localized to the inguinal, perineal, or adductor region and is relived by rest and increased by activity. Tenderness to palpation may be localized to the pubic ramus. The hip may be moved through its entire range of motion without pain, but typically the patient is unable to stand on the affected leg without support. Radiographs can be negative for 2 to 3 weeks, but bone scans will be positive earlier. Treatment includes protected weightbearing, use of oral analgesics, flexibility exercises, and a gradual return to play, often over a period of 3 to 4 months.

Apophysitis

Apophysitis is caused by a chronic traction stress that is not forceful enough to cause an actual avulsion. The most common sites of apophysitis are the iliac crest and ischial tuberosity. Iliac crest apophysitis is most common in runners, but has been reported in hockey, lacrosse, and football players as well (**Figure 35.5**). Usually, modification of activities, such as changing the running surface or decreasing the intensity and frequency of activity for 3 to 4 weeks, using nonsteroidal anti-inflammatory drugs, and stretching exercises allow return to full activity within 4 to 6 weeks.

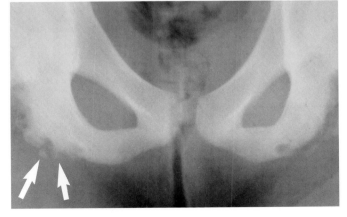

Figure 35.5 Chronic apophysitis of the ischial tuberosity.

Snapping Hip Syndrome and Iliotibial Band Syndrome

Snapping hip syndrome is rarely painful, but may cause an annoying snapping sensation with certain motions of the hip. This syndrome has two principal causes: tenosynovitis of the iliopsoas tendon near its insertion at the lesser trochanter and "catching" of the tendon as is passes over the iliopectineal eminence. Irritation of the greater trochanteric bursa by the overriding iliotibial band can also cause a snapping hip and an underlying trochanteric bursitis. Usually, rest, anti-inflammatory drugs, and stretching of the iliopsoas and iliotibial band, especially in hip abduction and external rotation, usually are sufficient treatment. Surgical treatment, including lengthening of the ilopsoas lengthening or surgical release of the iliotibial band, is rarely indicated.

Bursitis

The trochanteric and iliopsoas bursae can become inflamed from overuse, as may happen as a result of jogging or long-distance running. If the trochanteric bursa is involved, athletes typically report pain and aching after running. Discomfort is localized laterally over the greater trochanter and can be elicited by palpation. If the iliopsoas bursa is involved, pain is more medial and anterior in the groin, and discomfort can be elicited by passive rotary motion of the hip. Treatment includes rest of the hip joint, application of ice packs to the affected area, and the use of nonsteroidal anti-inflammatory drugs.

Synovitis

Synovitis is a generalized, nonspecific inflammation of the lining of a joint. In the hip joint, synovitis can be caused by a direct injury, by overuse, or occasionally by a bacterial infection. Hip joint pain may radiate down the medial aspect of the thigh to the knee. Patients usually hold the hip slightly flexed and externally rotated, and any type of motion causes pain. Athletes with suspected synovitis should undergo a full orthopaedic examination, including radiographs and aspiration of the hip joint, to determine the cause so that appropriate treatment can be initiated.

Figure 35.6 Slipped capital femoral epiphysis of the right hip.

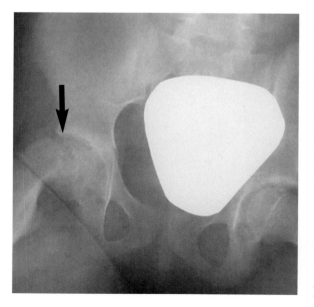

Acquired Conditions

Slipped Capital Femoral Epiphysis and Legg-Calvé-Perthes Disease

Slipped capital femoral epiphysis (SCFE) and Legg-Calvé-Perthes disease (LCPD) should be considered in the evaluation of a young athlete with hip, pelvic, or knee pain. SCFE is the most common hip disorder in adolescents and should be considered in any athlete with hip pain, which may be referred to the knee or anteromedial thigh. Acute SCFE can cause dramatic onset of symptoms, including severe hip pain and inability to bear weight. Chronic SCFE can limit athletic performance because of chronic pain in the groin, thigh, or knee. Pertinent physical findings include loss of internal rotation of the hip and compensatory external rotation with flexion. A standard AP radiograph of the pelvis and a lateral view of the hip will identify the slipped epiphysis (**Figure 35.6**).

Legg-Calvé-Perthes disease is more frequent in children younger than age 8 years, but has been reported in adolescents as well. Most patients with LCPD experience an insidious onset of mild hip or knee pain or limp over several months. Physical findings include loss of internal rotation and hip abduction. Radiographic findings depend on the stage of the disease and may include a small, radiodense femoral ossific nucleus, crescent sign, fragmentation of the epiphysis, reossification with alteration of the shape of the femoral head, or residual deformity in late stages (**Figure 35.7**). Both SCFE and LCPD often require surgical correction. Almost all patients with SCFE and some with LCPD require surgical treatment.

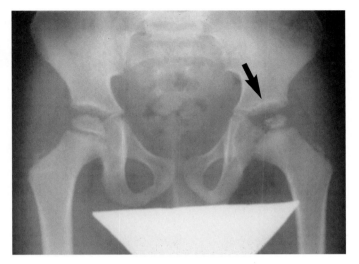

Figure 35.7 AP radiograph of the pelvis shows an irregular ossific nucleus of the left hip consistent with LCPD.

Meralgia Paresthetica

Meralgia paresthetica is an entrapment syndrome of the lateral femoral cutaneous nerve, manifested by sensory loss or pain in the distribution of the nerve, or both. Although this condition is considered rare, a report of 30 such lesions in children and adolescents suggests that it is more common and often unrecognized or misdiagnosed. The principal symptom is pain, often severe, in the anterior or lateral region of the thigh. Palpation of the lateral femoral cutaneous nerve, just inferomedial to the anterosuperior iliac spine, reproduces symptoms in the distribution of the nerve. Pain increases with extension of the hip with the patient prone and the knee flexed 90° because this maneuver stretches the sartorius tendon and the adjacent nerve. Temporary relief of pain after local injection of lidocaine confirms the diagnosis. Open decompression of the nerve may be required for persistent pain.

FINISH LINE

Most sports-related injuries to the structures within the hip, thigh, and groin in young athletes can be treated effectively with a 2- to 4-week period of rest, followed by a gradual return to play as symptoms subside. Some fractures and dislocations require surgical treatment. Dislocations of the hip are considered true orthopaedic emergencies that require immediate treatment.

For More Information

1. Paletta GA Jr, Andrish JT: Injuries about the hip and pelvis in the young athlete. *Clin Sports Med* 1995;14:591–628.

2. Sundar M, Carty H: Avulsion fractures of the pelvis in children: A report of 32 fractures and their outcome. *Skeletal Radiol* 1994;23:85–90.

3. Metzmaker JN, Pappas AM: Avulsion fractures of the pelvis. *Am J Sports Med* 1985;13:349–358.

4. Outerbridge AR, Micheli LJ: Overuse injuries in the young athlete. *Clin Sports Med* 1995;14:503–516.

5. Walker RN, Green NE, Spindler KP: Stress fractures in skeletally immature patients. *J Pediatr Orthop* 1996;16:578–584.

6. Edelson R, Stevens P: Meralgia paresthetica in children. *J Bone Joint Surg* 1994;76A:993–999.

Chapter 36

Knee

C H A R L E S   B .   P A S Q U E ,   M D
D O N A L D   W .   M C G I N N I S ,   M D

K nee injuries are some of the most common problems encountered in young athletes. Sports activities can subject the knee joint to severe stresses that increase the risk of both acute traumatic injuries and chronic overuse injuries. Most knee injuries are self-limiting, such as abrasions, bruises, and muscle strains. More serious and potentially debilitating injuries can also occur and must be evaluated properly to prevent further injury and to maximize the chances for full recovery. Therefore, it is essential for anyone caring for athletes with these injuries to: 1) understand the basic anatomy and biomechanics of the knee; 2) perform a proper screening history and physical examination; and 3) recognize common knee injuries. Understanding and implementing these measures will result in more informed decisions regarding return to play or deciding when further evaluation by a specialist is needed.

Anatomy/Biomechanics

The knee is a complex structure that is more easily understood if it is considered by its components: the involved bones, cartilage, ligaments, and musculotendinous units. The interaction of these structures allows the knee to perform amazing movements in many different directions with good functional stability. Injury occurs when the extremes of knee motion are exceeded or the individual structures are overloaded. Focusing on these individual structures during evaluation of injuries will likely result in a correct diagnosis.

Bones

The three main bones of the knee are the femur (thigh bone), tibia (shin bone), and patella (knee cap) (**Figure 36.1**). Together these bones form the tibiofemoral articulation and the patellofemoral articulation. Both articulations have little inherent bony stability and rely almost entirely on the surrounding soft tissues for support.

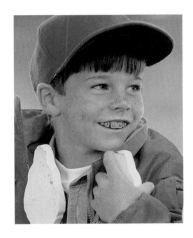

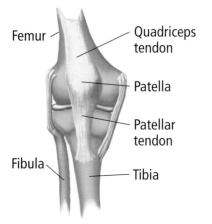

Femur
Quadriceps tendon
Patella
Patellar tendon
Fibula
Tibia

Figure 36.1 Principal structures of the knee.

The tibiofemoral articulation is the principal joint of the knee. The distal femur has medial and lateral convex condyles with a central tunnel, or intercondylar notch region, for the anterior and posterior cruciate ligaments. The proximal tibia has opposing medial and lateral plateau regions that articulate with the femoral condyles and a tibial spine or eminence that protrudes slightly into the intercondylar notch region. Together, the tibia and femur contribute mainly to the complex motions required during knee flexion and extension. Mild anterior/posterior translation, medial/lateral translation, varus/valgus rotation and internal/external rotation occurs throughout a full range of motion.

The patellofemoral articulation can be considered a second joint in the knee that has distinctly different anatomy and function. The underside of the patella consists of the lateral facet, central ridge, and medial facet. A smaller "odd" facet is also located on the extreme medial side of the medial facet. The patella normally articulates or glides with the underlying femoral trochlea or groove during knee flexion and extension. The depth of the femoral trochlea or the prominence of the patellar central ridge provides some mild inherent stability to medial/lateral motion. When this groove or the patella are flattened, the patella loses some of its bony restraint and becomes more susceptible to subluxation or dislocation. During normal knee motion, the inferior pole of the patella articulates with the superior femoral trochlea when the knee is in full extension or is straight. As the knee flexes, the area of patella contact migrates superiorly and the area of femoral contact migrates distally. Knowing what degree the knee was flexed during an injury or at what degree the athlete reports pain can help identify the location of the damage on the patella or femoral trochlea. The patella acts to increase the lever arm effect of the quadriceps mechanism to increase its power and efficiency. It also protects the underlying knee joint during blunt trauma.

The immature skeleton in young athletes adds additional anatomic and biomechanical factors that must be considered during examination. Open physes are at increased risk of injury because they are areas of rapid cell proliferation and are relatively weak in resisting significant stress. Both the distal femoral and proximal tibia physes can be injured with excessive loads of compression, tension, sheer, or rotation. The distal femoral physis is more commonly injured by high-energy forces and can result in residual growth disturbances. Proximal tibial physeal injuries are more commonly seen in athletic environments and are usually manifested by tibial eminence avulsions.

Cartilage

Articular and meniscal cartilage are the two principal types of cartilage in the knee. Articular cartilage is a shiny white hyaline cartilage that covers the ends of the distal femur and proximal tibia. It functions primarily as a smooth gliding articulating surface between the femur and the tibia, as well as a shock absorber for the underlying bone when axially loaded. Meniscal cartilage is a C-shaped structure on both the medial and lateral tibial plateaus. It also serves as a shock absorber to axial loads by distributing contact forces to wider areas on articular cartilage surfaces. In addition, the menisci help increase knee stability by resisting translation of the tibiofemoral joint during weight bearing.

Ligaments

Ligaments attach bone to bone and serve primarily to provide static stability to a joint. The four main ligaments in the knee joint are the anterior cruciate (ACL), the posterior cruciate (PCL), the medial collateral (MCL), and the lateral collateral (LCL) (**Figure 36.2**). Several smaller ligamentous structures also contribute knee stability and are discussed briefly.

The ACL and PCL are located in the center of the tibial-femoral articulation in the intercondylar notch region. The ACL extends from the anterior aspect of the tibial eminence to the inner posterior lateral femoral condyle. It is the primary restraint to anterior tibial translation on the femur at 30° with important contributions to valgus and internal/external rotational stability. The PCL extends from the central aspect of the proximal posterior tibia to the inner anterior medial femoral condyle. It is the primary restraint to posterior tibial translation on the femur at 90° with important contributions to varus and external rotational stability. Together, the ACL and PCL help maintain a functional moving center of knee rotation by allowing the femur to naturally roll back on the tibia during progressive knee flexion. This movement allows a greater range of motion, which is less constrained compared with the static hinge-type motion found in other joints.

The MCL and LCL are located outside the tibiofemoral articulation on the medial and lateral sides, respectively. The MCL consists of two bands: superficial and deep. The superficial band attaches at the medial epicondyle and traverses extra-articularly to a fairly long attachment on the proximal medial tibia. It is a very wide and thick ligament and serves as the primary restraint to valgus rotation at 20° to 30° of knee flexion. The deep MCL band lies beneath the superficial band and is much shorter. It extends from the distal medial femur to the central margin of the medial meniscus, thickening the capsule, then attaching to the proximal portion of the medial tibia. It serves mainly as a stabilizer of the medial meniscus. The LCL is also extra-articular and extends from the lateral femoral epicondyle to the proximal aspect of the fibular head. It is a much thinner ligament than the LCL and is the primary restraint to varus rotation at 20° to 30° of knee flexion. Together, the MCL and LCL also make important contributions to anterior/posterior translation and internal/external rotation stability.

Several other ligaments contribute to knee stability. The medial and lateral patellofemoral ligaments lie within their respective retinaculum and extend from the central borders of the patella to the adjacent femoral condyle regions. They act primarily to maintain the patella centered in the underlying femoral trochlear groove during knee flexion, and they resist severe medial or lateral stress to the patella. The popliteofibular ligament (PFL) extends from the posterior fibular head to the popliteus tendon near the joint line. The PFL, the posterolateral capsule, and the popliteus tendon help form the posterolateral complex, a structure that contributes to external rotation and varus rotation stability. The meniscofemoral ligaments extend from the posterior femoral condyles and capsule to the posterior edges of the meniscus. Their function is controversial but is felt principally to be meniscal stability with important contributions to posterior translation stability.

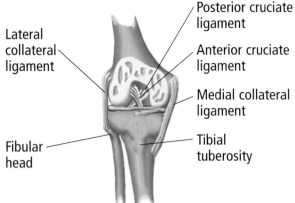

Figure 36.2 Principal ligaments of the knee.

Figure 36.3 Musculature of the knee.

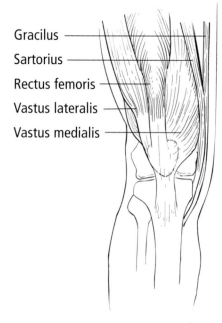
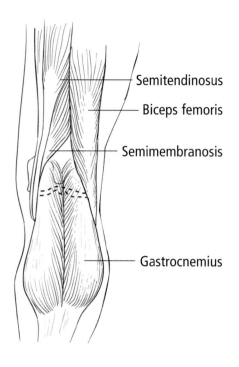

Gracilus

Sartorius

Rectus femoris

Vastus lateralis

Vastus medialis

Semitendinosus

Biceps femoris

Semimembranosis

Gastrocnemius

Anterior   **Posterior**

Figure 36.4 **A** Genu varus or bowlegs. **B** Genu valgus or knock-knee.

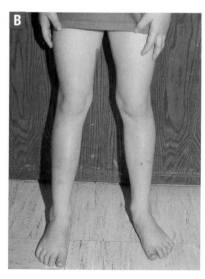

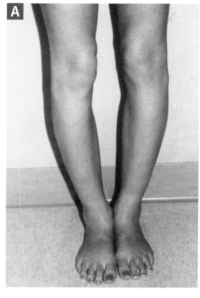

Musculotendinous Units

The musculotendinous units around the knee provide important dynamic stability during activity (**Figure 36.3**). Anteriorly, the quadriceps helps support the PCL by preventing excessive posterior tibial translation. The medial quadriceps, or vastus medialis obliquus (VMO), helps prevent lateral patellar translation. Posteriorly, the medial and lateral hamstring muscles and the gastrocnemius (calf) muscles help support the ACL by preventing excessive anterior tibial translation or internal/external rotation. Medially, the MCL and capsular structures are further supported by the medial hamstrings, consisting of the semimembranosus, semitendinosus, gracilis, and sartorius. Laterally, the LCL and capsular structures are supported by the iliotibial band and lateral hamstring or biceps femoris. The synchronous dynamic function of each of these musculotendinous units is vital for the overall function and stability of the knee. Injury or weakness in any individual or group of muscles can result in poor knee function or possibly further injury.

Lower Extremity Alignment

Overall alignment of the lower extremity is another important factor in predisposing an athlete to injury or causing abnormal function. Excessive genu varum (bow leg), genu valgum (knock-knee), recurvatum (knee hyperextension) or internal/external rotation can be caused by multiple factors throughout the extremity (**Figure 36.4**). Increased femoral anteversion (femoral head and neck point forward more than normal) can cause the athlete to compensate by internally rotating the extremity at the level of the knee or ankle/foot. Slipped capital femoral epiphysis or Legg-Calvé-Perthes disease can result in limited hip motion, with compensations made at the level of the knee or ankle/foot region.

Abnormal femoral or tibial bowing from development or prior injury can result in excessive varus or valgus alignment with resultant increased stresses on the medial or lateral compartments of the tibiofemoral joint. Ankle/foot deformities such as clubfeet or Achilles tendon contractures can also cause similar abnormal stresses at the level of the knee joint. The patellofemoral joint is especially sensitive to abnormal extremity alignment. Excessive valgus alignment at the knee joint, external rotation of the proximal tibia, or internal rotation of the femur decreases the stability of the patella. These abnormalities increase the risk of injury from uneven distribution of forces to the lateral patella facet or can result in actual lateral patella subluxation or dislocation. Thus, a thorough knowledge of the anatomy of the entire extremity can help identify the cause of knee problems or prevent the wrong diagnosis.

Clinical Evaluation

History

A thorough but focused history is vital to making the correct diagnosis. Learning to ask the right questions comes with experience but can be learned rapidly if a systematic approach is taken. Specific questions will be discussed in later sections on common injuries, but a minimum history should include at least the following: whether the problem is acute or chronic; the mechanism of injury, including whether the symptoms began with a specific event or repetitive activity; the location and type of pain; swelling; mechanical symptoms (locking, popping, catching); instability symptoms, and any functional limitations. Information about previous injuries, especially similar injuries, and previous evaluations and treatments are helpful, including notes from the physician and/or athletic trainer, radiographs and any special diagnostic studies. Videotapes or eye witnesses can also provide key information about the mechanism of injury such as the direction of force and position of the leg at the time of injury.

Physical Examination

Learning to perform a systematic knee examination is critical in the proper evaluation of knee injuries to prevent missing important findings. Even though an on-field examination will differ from an office or clinic visit, a thorough examination can be performed rapidly if it is done consistently and systematically. Physical examination within the first hours of injury is recommended, because once the knee begins to swell, examination becomes more difficult. The initial adrenaline rush may mask pain, making examination easier. As a result, team physicians, athletic trainers, and even coaches should be able to perform the basic physical examination. When possible, this examination should be performed in a quiet, isolated area, away from distractions from the crowd and other athletes.

Proximal femoral disorders, such as Legg-Calvé-Perthes disease, slipped capital femoral epiphysis, and tumors, can cause referred pain to the knee or malalignment that causes knee pain. Similarly, foot and ankle problems such as internal tibial torsion, hyper-pronation, and pes planus can cause malalignment problems with resultant knee pain. Therefore, both the hip and the ankle/foot regions must be examined in any young athlete with knee pain.

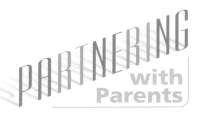

When should radiographs be ordered for a child with knee pain or following a knee injury?

If pain is present for more than two days or if swelling is observed, radiographs should be obtained.

Observation

The knee should be exposed from at least the middle of the tibia to the middle of the upper thigh. Depending on the environment, this may require removing pants, padding, or other sports equipment. The first step is to assess the overall position of the limb and note any gross deformities that might suggest a fracture or dislocation. Comparison with the contralateral extremity for muscle atrophy and overall limb alignment is also important, especially in chronic injuries. The next step should be closer inspection for skin and soft-tissue abnormalities such as redness, swelling, ecchymosis, and abrasions or lacerations. The final step of the examination, when possible, should be to observe the athlete ambulating. If an athlete cannot walk without significant difficulty, he or she should be kept out of competition until able to do so.

Palpation

Systematic palpation of key bony and soft-tissue landmarks is essential to localizing areas of injury (**Table 36.1**) (**Figure 36.5**). Although swelling and pain may be diffuse, point tenderness can be elicited in most areas of injury. This examination is best done with the athlete lying supine with the knee in a relaxed position. Begin by palpating the bone structures for possible fracture as this finding significantly affects any decisions regarding the need for splinting and on-field return to play. Bony palpation should include the distal femur, proximal tibia, and the entire patella. Some areas, such as the femoral epicondyles and the distal femoral growth plate, are close in proximity and

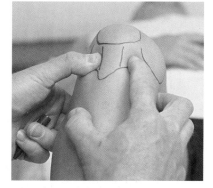

Figure 36.5 Palpation of the medial joint line (index finger) and lateral joint line (thumb).

Table 36.1	Key Palpation Landmarks
Site of tenderness	**Possible injury**
Tibial tubercle	Fracture
	Osgood-Schlatter disease
Patellar tendon	Patellar tendinitis
Patella	Fracture
	Bipartite patella
Inferior pole	Sinding-Larsen-Johansson disease
Superior pole	Quadriceps tendinitis
Medial joint line	Medial meniscal tear
	Pes anserinus bursitis
Lateral joint line	Lateral meniscal tear
Medial epicondyle	MCL tear
	Physeal injury
Lateral epicondyle	LCL tear
	Physeal injury
	Iliotibial band syndrome
Fibular head	LCL tear
	Biceps femoris tendinitis
Medial retinaculum	Patellar subluxation and/or dislocation
	Medial plica

can be difficult to differentiate, especially in a swollen knee (**Figure 36.6**). Any areas of exquisite tenderness should be of concern and warrant splinting and careful transport from the playing field. Further evaluation should include plain radiographs and specialty referral if needed.

The soft tissues should then be inspected. It is often helpful to flex the knee to at least 30° to 90° for this part of the examination. Begin by palpating the extensor mechanism, including the peripatellar soft tissues, inferior patella, the patellar tendon and the tibial tubercle. Next, palpate the step-off between the tibia and femur on the anterior medial and lateral sides of the knee. This step helps identify the joint lines, which can then be palpated circumferentially toward the posterior aspect of the knee on each side. Next, palpate the proximal and distal aspects of the medial and lateral collateral ligaments. The order and extent of soft-tissue examination can be altered depending on the situation. Suspected tender areas can be examined last to make the examination more comfortable for the athlete.

Knee effusion, which is the collection of fluid in the joint space, is an important indicator of intra-articular pathology. Knee effusion differs from soft-tissue swelling outside of the knee joint and can be differentiated with a careful examination. The athlete should relax the knee in full extension on the floor or examining table. Place the thumb and fingers of one hand on opposite sides of the patella while applying gentle superior and posterior compression. Form an upside down V with the opposite hand and place it on the distal anterior thigh while applying gentle posterior and inferior compression. "Milk" any fluid in the knee from proximal to distal. Any fluid in the knee will then be felt with the fingers in the peripatellar or suprapatellar regions. The patella will also be ballottable or "float" in the fluid with either anterior/posterior palpation or medial/lateral palpation. If the athlete has only soft-tissue swelling with no underlying fluid, the soft tissue usually feels thick with these maneuvers. When in doubt, the knee can be sterile prepped, draped, and aspirated. Most traumatic hemarthrosis (bloody effusion), whether acute or chronic, are usually a sign of intra-articular pathology and require specialty referral for further evaluation. In the young athlete, the most common cause of a hemarthrosis is an ACL injury, followed by patellar subluxation or dislocation. Other possible causes of traumatic effusions include meniscal injuries, osteochondral fractures, or fragmentation of the articular cartilage surfaces.

Range of motion

Range of motion is also a vital factor in the knee examination, especially when regarding return to play decisions. Any athlete with an abnormal passive or active range of motion should be held out of competition until full motion is achieved or the cause is determined. Range of motion of the tibiofemoral articulation should be assessed and compared with that of the opposite, uninjured extremity for symmetry. This evaluation is done with the athlete squatting from the standing position or from a supine position on the floor or examining table. If a quadriceps injury or tightness is suspected, knee flexion in both extremities should be compared with the athlete in a prone position with both hips on the ground. Limitations to passive full extension can be caused by any condition causing a knee effusion such as an ACL tear, displaced meniscal tear, or osteochondral loose body. Limitations to active full extension are less common and are usually caused by disruptions of the

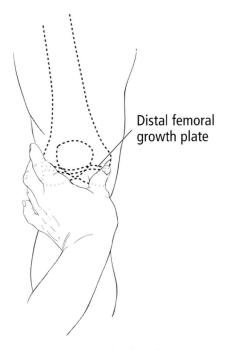

Distal femoral growth plate

Figure 36.6 Palpation of the distal femoral physis.

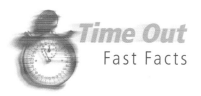

A bipartite patella is an interesting radiographic curiosity requiring no treatment. It may be mistaken for a fracture.

extensor mechanism. Many athletes with limited findings are unwilling to straighten their knee due to apprehension. In these instances, the athlete should be placed on crutches with swelling control measures and reexamined at a later time.

Patellofemoral evaluation

The patellofemoral joint should be evaluated simultaneously during range of motion testing to identify any abnormal patellar tracking, tilting, or crepitus. The patella is normally in a central position within the femoral trochlear groove at 30° to 40° of knee flexion. Lateral patellar tracking noted on examination can be the result of abnormal limb alignment (increased Q angle, abnormal bony constraints (shallow trochlear groove or deficient patellar facets), tight lateral restraints (lateral retinaculum), or insufficient medial restraints (VMO, medial retinaculum). Lateral patellar tilting during early knee flexion is usually caused by tight lateral restraints. Medial patellar tracking is extremely rare and is usually due to iatrogenic causes.

Evaluation of patellar crepitus should begin with the knee in full extension and the quadriceps relaxed. The patella should be gently compressed to the underlying femoral trochlea to feel for any rough areas on the patella. Palpation for crepitus through a complete range of motion should then be done both passively with the athlete in a supine position and actively, when possible, with the athlete moving from standing to a squatting position. Any areas of abnormal clicking or crepitus should be noted.

Inferior patellar cartilage lesions are usually palpated during early knee flexion and superior lesions during terminal flexion. If a medial plica band is suspected, a palpable snapping sensation will be felt medial to the patella on the femoral condyle during midknee flexion.

The patellofemoral compression test should be reserved for last. This test can be performed by applying gentle but firm compression to the superior patella while the athlete performs an active quadriceps contraction. Severe anterior knee pain can suggest patellofemoral articular pathology. Anterior knee pain with similar compression over the inferior patellar region is more suggestive of fat pad irritation.

Patella stability can be assessed by applying medial and lateral stresses with the knee at or near full extension. Normal lateral translation averages 25% of the width of the patella, and normal medial translation averages approximately 10 mm. Significant apprehension, pain, or subluxation with lateral stressing suggests lateral patellar instability (**Figure 36.7**).

Figure 36.7 The fingers are forcing the patella laterally. Check for translation and an apprehension or panic sign.

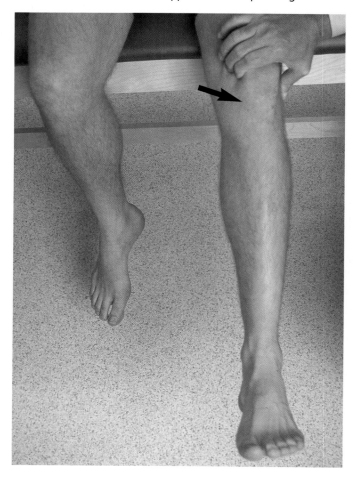

Meniscal evaluation

Evaluation of the meniscus should begin with palpation of the joint lines with the knee in 90° of flexion.

This examination slightly uncovers the joint lines by pulling the soft tissues posteriorly. Isolated localized pain in the anterior meniscus usually does not indicate meniscus pathology. Pain in the middle or posterior meniscus region is usually more suggestive of pathology. Comparing the amount of tenderness in the areas just above and below the joint line help differentiate a meniscus tear from a collateral ligament injury, muscle strain, or bursitis. Palpation for meniscal cysts is also necessary, especially along the posterior medial and lateral central regions of the knee. In older adolescents with a history of trauma, cysts can be a sign of meniscal pathology.

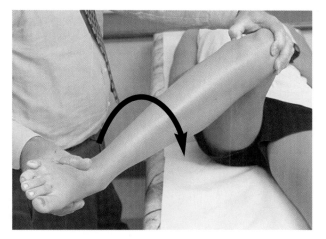

Figure 36.8 Pivot shift test.

Provocative maneuvers for meniscal tears are plentiful, but not always accurate or necessary. The principal goal of the evaluation is to position the knee in such a way that tests the integrity of the meniscus by pinching or subluxating it in the tibiofemoral joint. This is best done by performing some variation of the McMurray test. With the athlete in a supine position, the knee should be maximally flexed and then the tibia gently rotated internally and externally while a slight varus or valgus stress is applied (**Figure 36.8**). With slow extension of the knee, external rotation can load the medial meniscus and internal rotation the lateral meniscus. With meniscal tears, the athlete may report discomfort along the joint line of the meniscus in question and the examiner may hear or feel a pop. Many athletes report pain anteriorly during these maneuvers, primarily due to quadriceps tightness or pathology in the patellofemoral region, and not a meniscus tear.

ACL evaluation

The ability to identify an ACL injury on physical examination is especially important when caring for young athletes. All tests for ACL insufficiency should be compared with the opposite uninjured extremity because tibiofemoral translation varies widely among individuals. ACL insufficiency is best evaluated with the Lachman test performed with the knee flexed at 20° to 30º (**Figure 36.9**). First, stabilize the distal femur with one hand and then apply an anterior translation stress to the proximal tibia with the other hand. An alternative technique can be used when the examiner's hands are too small or the patient's leg is too large. The examiner should rest the patient's slightly flexed knee on top of his or her flexed knee. The distal femur should then be stabilized by pushing it down against the examiner's thigh with one hand and manipulating the tibia with the other hand. This maneuver is also extremely helpful in helping an anxious patient to relax the leg for a proper examination. Increased tibial translation in relation to the femur without a solid endpoint is diagnostic for ACL insufficiency. In the young athlete, the insufficiency can be caused by an ACL tear or a tibial spine avulsion and should be evaluated further with plain radiographs. Grading systems are variable but include mild increases of 3 to 5 mm (grade I), moderate increases of 5 to 10 mm (grade II), and severe increases of greater than 10 mm (grade III).

Other tests used for evaluation of ACL insufficiency include the pivot shift test, flexion rotation drawer test, and the anterior drawer test. A positive pivot shift test or flexion rotation drawer test can be pathognomic for ACL insufficiency but requires that the athlete be relaxed. These tests are also somewhat

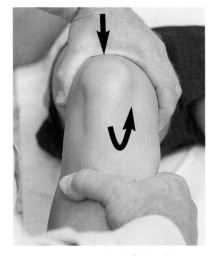

Figure 36.9 The left hand stabilizes the femur while the right applies an anterior translational force. The knee is relaxed and flexed 20° to 30°.

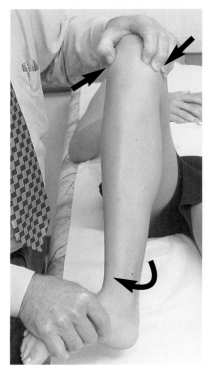

Figure 36.10 The McMurray test.

difficult to learn. The athlete should lie supine while the examiner abducts the affected lower extremity and slightly flexes the hip.

Pivot shift test. The pivot shift test is performed by gently internally rotating the tibia with the athlete's knee in flexion and extension (**Figure 36.10**). In an athlete with an insufficient ACL, a shift or "clunk" will be noted as the knee is moved toward full extension (subluxated position) or toward 30° to 40° of flexion (reduced position).

Flexion rotation drawer test. This test is performed by grasping the medial and lateral proximal tibia with each hand with the index fingers in a position to palpate the joint line. The knee is then gently manipulated back and forth between full flexion and extension. In a knee with an insufficient ACL, a shift or "clunk" of the proximal tibia will be felt and seen as the knee is moved toward full extension (subluxated position) or toward 30° to 40° of flexion (reduced position).

Anterior drawer test. This test used to be the standard in evaluating the ACL but is now reserved primarily for PCL testing. It is performed with the athlete supine, the knee flexed 90°, and the foot stabilized. An anterior translational force is then applied to the proximal tibia with both hands (**Figure 36.11**). Increased tibial translation on the femur may be a sign of ACL insufficiency. Palpation of an anterior solid endpoint is not as consistent as with the Lachman test.

PCL evaluation

Evaluation of PCL integrity should begin while palpating the anterior tibiofemoral step-off during routine joint line and meniscus evaluation. With the athlete supine, the knee flexed to 90°, and the foot stabilized, the edges of the medial and lateral tibial plateaus normally extend up to 10 mm anterior to the medial and lateral femoral condyles. Absence of this normal step-off is an immediate indication of a possible PCL injury. The tibiofemoral step-off can be evaluated further by looking for a sag sign. The sag sign is seen in PCL deficient knees because the tibia sags posterior to the femur, causing an indentation over the anterior joint line and patellar tendon region. This finding can be made more pronounced by flexing both the hips and knees to 90° while supporting the ankle regions. The increased force of gravity on a

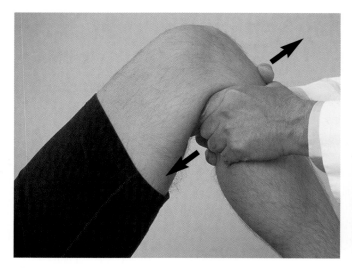

Figure 36.11 Anterior drawer test.

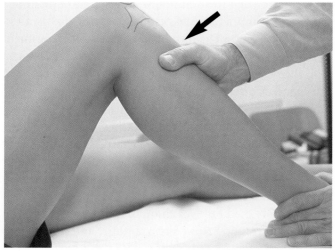

Figure 36.12 Posterior drawer test.

PCL deficient knee will make the sag more evident, especially when comparing it to the contralateral extremity.

Posterior drawer test This test is the most reliable and reproducible evaluation for PCL insufficiency (**Figure 36.12**). It is also performed with the athlete supine, the knee flexed 90°, and the foot stabilized. A posterior translational force is then applied to the proximal tibia with both hands while the thumbs palpate the anterior joint line. The amount of posterior tibial translation relative to the femur is determined, as well as whether there is a solid or soft endpoint. With a PCL injury, the amount of posterior translation of the tibia on the femur will increase. In addition, a soft endpoint will be felt rather than the normal solid stop. Grading systems are variable but include mild increases up to 5 mm (grade I), moderate increases of 5 to 10 mm (grade II), and severe increases of greater than 10 mm (grade III). In severe injuries, the anterior edge of the tibia moves posterior to the edge of the femoral condyle. This measurement should be compared with that of the opposite knee.

MCL, LCL, and posterior lateral complex evaluation

The MCL and LCL should be evaluated in conjunction with the ACL because of the similar positioning of the leg required for both evaluations. Because it is more difficult to control the leg during varus and valgus stressing as opposed to anterior/posterior stressing, the distal femur should be stabilized against a solid object. This test can be performed with the athlete's knee gently flexed over the examiner's thigh or by pressing the distal femur onto the examining table with the rest of the leg hanging over the edge. Gently flex and extend the knee to find the most neutral zone to begin the examination. Apply a varus or valgus stress to the knee at both 0° and 30° with one hand while palpating the joint line that is placed under tension with the other hand (**Figure 36.13**). Important information includes the amount of joint line opening (estimated in mm), the degree of pain, and the quality of the endpoint (soft or firm). A grade I injury is an increase of 0 to 5 mm, grade II is 5 to 10 mm, and grade III is 10 to 15 mm. Any increased opening, especially at 0°, or failure to reach an endpoint signifies a severe injury or a possible fracture. Palpating the joint line with the distal femur stabilized also helps distinguish between collateral ligament injuries and physeal fractures. Physeal fractures should not cause an increase in joint line opening unless there is severe intra-articular involvement. In addition, these fractures usually are associated with marked pain to any attempts at manipulation of the leg.

Posterolateral complex (PLC) evaluation is often overlooked in the young athlete because injuries to this region are rare in this age group. The PLC should be evaluated with the ACL, MCL, and LCL because of the similar positioning required for testing these structures. One hand should stabilize the distal femur to the table or the examiner's thigh while palpating the anterior medial and lateral joint lines. The other hand should grab the ankle and apply an external rotation stress to the leg at 30° of flexion while observing the tibial tubercle (not the foot) for rotation. Note the amount of increased external

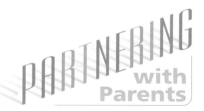

Figure 36.13 A Valgus stress applied in 0° extension. **B** Valgus stress applied in 30° flexion.

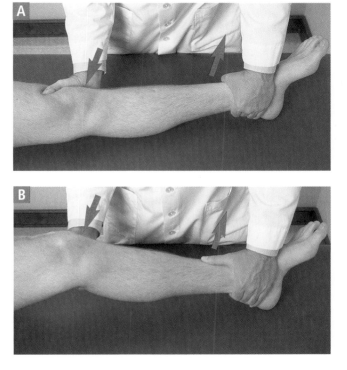

rotation, the degree of pain, and the quality of the endpoint (soft or firm). Increased external rotation at 30° that remains the same at 90° is consistent with an isolated PLC injury. Increased external rotation at 30° with a larger increase at 90° is consistent with a combined PLC and PCL injury. In athletes with increased external rotation, the structure that is actually allowing the rotation should be noted. In PLC injuries, the anterior lateral tibial plateau should rotate posteriorly. If the anterior lateral tibial plateau remains stable and the medial tibial plateau rotates anteriorly, the PLC can be intact and an ACL and posterior medial capsule injury should be suspected. PLC testing can also be performed by placing the athlete prone and then comparing thigh-foot angles at both 30° and 90°.

Neurovascular Evaluation

The physical examination is not complete without a proper neurovascular evaluation of the involved extremity. Most knee trauma does not require an extensive neurovascular examination but should include as a minimum the documentation of grossly intact foot circulation and motor and sensory function. A more thorough examination should be performed in instances of high-energy injuries that result in extensive soft-tissue damage, fractures, or dislocations. In addition, any athlete with a traumatic injury that could result in swelling or bleeding severe enough to cause a compartment syndrome of the leg or thigh should undergo a more thorough neurovascular examination.

Diagnostic Testing

Any injuries that produce severe pain, swelling, or marked bony tenderness or deformity on examination require radiographs or specialty referral. In addition, any injury that results in symptoms that persist for longer than a week also warrant further evaluation. Standard radiographic views should include an anteroposterior (AP), a standing (when possible) 45° bent-knee posteroanterior (PA), lateral, and patella Merchant views. If osteochondral injuries are suspected, a notch or tunnel view can be added. Varus and valgus stress radiographs can be performed for suspected ligamentous or physeal injuries but should be done under the supervision of a specialist. If hip involvement is suspected, such as a slipped capital femoral epiphysis or Legg-Calvé-Perthes disease, AP and frog lateral pelvis radiographs should be obtained. Technetium bone scans usually are not necessary but can be helpful in identifying stress fractures and possibly the healing potential of osteochondritis dissecans. When information about bony configuration is needed, CT may be helpful. MRI has become an increasingly popular method for evaluating ligamentous and soft-tissue injuries about the knee, as well as osteochondral injuries, physeal fractures, and stress fractures. Although MRI can be helpful in these cases, it is rarely necessary for diagnostic purposes. A specialist should be consulted before ordering these expensive tests.

Treatment—General Guidelines

Most knee injuries result in self-limited abrasions, bruises, muscle strains, and mild ligament sprains. Extra-articular injuries with no evidence of fracture or gross ligamentous instability can be safely treated with rest, ice, compression, and elevation (RICE). Most of these injuries will resolve in 1 to 6 weeks, depending on their severity. Athletes and their parents should be given strict

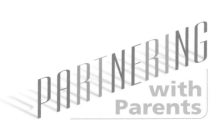

I hear a lot about MRIs being ordered for professional athletes with knee injuries. Why is that?

The MRI is an excellent noninvasive imaging method. The MRI study allows the assessment of subtle and not-so-subtle injuries ranging from bruises/contusions to complex ligament tears, meniscal and cartilage lesions.

instructions to contact their physician provider or go to the emergency department if there are any acute increases in pain, swelling, or neurovascular symptoms. Weekly examinations are recommended initially to monitor swelling, motion, and pain. Athletic trainers, physical therapists, and coaches also are helpful in monitoring the athlete's progress while at school.

Usually within the first few weeks after the injury, the swelling and pain begin to resolve. Exercises to improve motion, weight bearing, and general strength should be initiated as soon as possible. Once the pain and swelling subside and knee motion returns, sport-specific rehabilitation activities should begin in a controlled environment and include activities to improve agility, coordination, and knee loading. A young athlete who does not progress steadily through these phases of recovery should be reevaluated for more significant or unsuspected injuries.

Specialty consultation is indicated if nonoperative therapy fails or if there is evidence of internal derangement and effusion with or without ligamentous laxity. When possible, the consultation should occur before other diagnostic tests, such as an MRI, are ordered. These tests can delay evaluation and treatment, are often expensive, and are often not needed.

Differential Diagnosis

Osgood-Schlatter Disease

Osgood-Schlatter disease (or condition) is one of the most common knee problems in children between ages 10 and 15 years. It is thought to be caused by repetitive overuse injuries to the tibial tubercle apophysis, but it might also involve distal patellar tendinitis. Athletes usually report intermittent aching pain made worse with activity. Examination reveals a tender and enlarged tibial tubercle region, often bilaterally. The remainder of the knee examination is usually normal but may reveal patellar tendon and peripatellar tenderness with tight quadriceps during prone flexion testing. Radiographs usually are not necessary, but occasionally will show fragmentation of the tibial tubercle or a separate, discrete ossicle (**Figure 36.14**).

Pain control is the main focus of management because the condition typically resolves spontaneously within 6 to 18 months. Identifying training errors and recommending an overall decrease in the frequency and intensity of activity will help decrease the intensity of symptoms. Hamstring and quadriceps stretching prior to sports participation and icing of the tubercle afterwards also may help. Use of nonsteroidal anti-inflammatory drugs (NSAIDs) has not been shown to have a significant long-term effect but may prove helpful during acute exacerbations. Steroid injections should be avoided. Although pain can persist, Osgood-Schlatter disease is not an absolute contraindication to sports participation. Tibial tubercle avulsions are rare but can occur in athletes in jumping sports who report persistent pain not associated with a loose ossicle. After skeletal maturity, a large ossicle and bursa occasionally remain and can be excised in those who continue to have symptoms with activity or direct pressure.

Figure 36.14
Lateral knee radiograph showing fragmentation of the tibial tubercle (Osgood-Schlatter's disease).

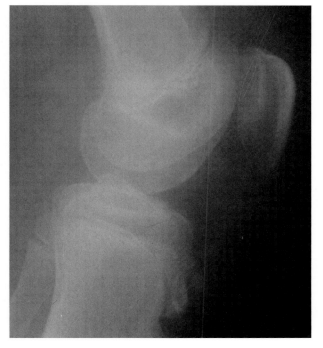

Fracture of the Tibial Tubercle

A fracture of the tibial tubercle typically affects adolescents from the ages of 12 to 16 years when the tubercle apophysis is still open, but the proximal tibial physis is near closure. The mechanism of injury varies, but usually involves a violent contraction of the extensor mechanism during a jumping or take-off maneuver. Physical examination reveals severe tenderness, swelling, and sometimes a prominence of the tibial tubercle region depending on the amount of fracture displacement. A hemarthrosis can be present secondary to intra-articular extension of the fracture or other associated injuries such as a meniscus or ACL tear. The athlete also may be unable to fully extend the knee because of the hemarthrosis, pain, and loss of an intact extensor mechanism. Radiographs show either partial or complete avulsion of the tibial tubercle with the fracture line sometimes extending into the articular surface. Treatment consists of aspiration and injection of the knee hemarthrosis, followed by casting in 0° to 15° of flexion for at least 4 to 6 weeks. Failure to reduce the fracture in this manner requires specialty consultation for possible surgical treatment.

Sinding-Larsen-Johansson Condition

Sinding-Larsen-Johansson condition is most commonly seen in active 10- to 12-year-old boys. It is thought to be caused by repetitive stress injuries to the junction of the developing patella and patellar tendon. Running or jumping sports participation, climbing stairs, or kneeling may make the pain worse. Athletes complain of anterior knee pain and usually have tenderness at the distal pole of the patella on examination. Radiographs show fragmentation of the distal pole of the patella or small calcifications in the proximal patellar tendon (**Figure 36.15**).

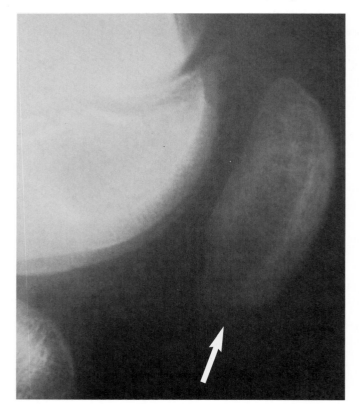

Figure 36.15 Fragmentation of the distal pole of the patella (Sinding-Larsen-Johansson condition).

Several conditions can mimic this condition and must be ruled out. Acute sleeve fractures of the patella usually are associated with an acute traumatic event and require specialty referral for surgical repair. A type I bipartite patella (inferior pole) can have similar radiographic findings but is usually asymptomatic. Jumper's knee typically is seen in older adolescents with presentations similar to adult proximal patellar tendinitis.

Management is similar to Osgood-Schlatter's disease and focuses on pain control, stretching the quadriceps, and icing the area after activity. Restriction of sports participation is necessary only if the athlete is unwilling or unable to tolerate the symptoms.

Jumper's Knee

Jumper's knee affects older adolescents and refers to a partial tear of the deep layers of the patellar tendon just distal to the distal pole of the patella. The history and physical examination are usually more chronic in nature but otherwise very similar to Sinding-Larsen-Johansson condition. Radiographs can be unremarkable but may reveal marked osteopenia in the distal pole of the patella secondary to hyperemia in the area of injury. As with other overuse injuries of the extensor mechanism, treatment should focus on pain control, stretching, and icing of the area after activity. Steroid injections should be avoided. Modification of activity is usually necessary; athletes with persistent symptoms sometimes require surgical debridement.

Sleeve Fracture of the Patella

Sleeve fractures of the patella can occur in younger athletes between 9 and 12 years old. The fracture is often an acute isolated event or is an acute event in an athlete with preexisting chronic pain in this region. The mechanism of injury usually involves a forceful contracture of the quadriceps from a rapid hyperflexion or deceleration motion. Athletes usually are unable to actively extend the knee, and examination reveals swelling over the distal pole of the patella with a palpable gap. Radiographs reveal a small rim of bone separated from the patella and a high riding patella (**Figure 36.16**). A thorough physical examination is important because radiographs may be unremarkable because of the cartilaginous nature of the inferior pole during development. An accurate diagnosis is essential because this injury usually requires surgical repair.

Bipartite Patella

A bipartite patella can be diagnosed at any age and is caused by the failure of one or more of the secondary ossification centers to fuse to the main body of the patella. The most common location is the superior lateral quadrant (type III), followed by the lateral margin (type II) and inferior pole (type I). Most patients are asymptomatic and require no treatment. Its importance lies in the fact that bipartite patella is often an incidental finding during routine radiography and mistaken for a fracture (**Figure 36.17**). If the patient is symptomatic and the pain is well localized over that portion of the patella, immobilization in a knee immobilizer or a cast for 3 to 4 weeks may be

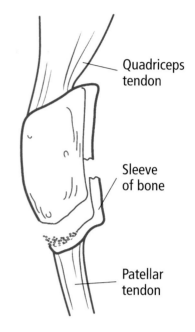

Figure 36.16 A "sleeve" of bone is displaced from the patella with the patellar tendon.

Figure 36.17 A Lateral and **B** AP views of the knee showing a type III bipartite patella.

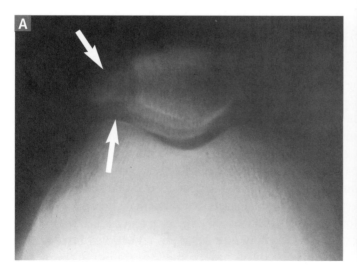
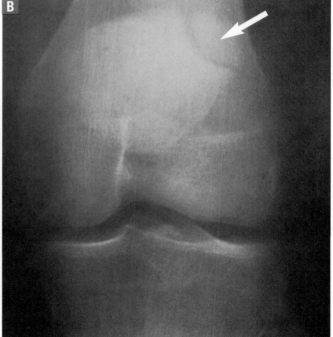

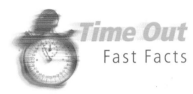

indicated. In rare instances, nonoperative treatment fails, and referral is necessary for surgical excision of the fragment and repair of the extensor mechanism.

Anterior Knee Pain

Anterior knee pain in young athletes has been called the low back pain of sports medicine because it is so common and it lacks adequate treatment. This combination of factors, along with the absence of a clear etiology, has resulted in extreme frustration for many athletes, parents, coaches, and physicians. To further add to the confusion, anterior knee pain that is not attributed to a specific cause has continued to be inappropriately labeled as chondromalacia patella or the vague patellofemoral pain syndrome. This imprecise approach to diagnosis has propagated poor treatment protocols and prevented proper scientific communication on the subject. Therefore, when treating the young athlete with this presentation, the first course of action is to rule out any specific identifiable causes of knee pain. If a readily identifiable cause is not found, it is then helpful to have a systematic evaluation and treatment approach for athletes with anterior knee pain.

Anterior knee pain is most commonly seen in adolescent female athletes. The athlete typically reports a vague, aching pain over the anterior knee with occasional popping and giving way sensations that are caused by a quadriceps inhibition reflex. Symptoms are usually made worse with sports activity but can also occur after prolonged sitting with the knee flexed (movie sign) or while resting at night. Common treatable causes include training errors, so athletes should be questioned about any recent changes in the duration, frequency, or intensity of their activity. Any alterations in equipment or playing surfaces should also be noted. Identifying specific aggravating activities (eg, stair climbing, jumping) or positions (eg, prolonged sitting, squatting) is also important so they can be corrected.

Examination usually is unremarkable for most athletes with anterior knee pain. There usually is no effusion or soft-tissue swelling. Tenderness in the peripatellar region is possible and can sometimes be exacerbated with patellar compression testing. The athlete typically has full range of motion with occasional crepitus and sometimes anterior pain at the extremes of flexion. Lower extremity alignment is a critical part of the examination because malalignment problems are common, treatable causes of anterior knee pain. The alignment of the quadriceps, the patella, and the tibial tubercle should be evaluated, both actively and passively. The quadriceps vector runs from the anterior superior spine to the center of the patella. The distal vector runs from the center of the patella to the tibial tuberosity. The relationship of the quadriceps and patellar vectors is called the quadriceps or Q angle. The Q angle formed by these landmarks can depend on the patient's height, the width of the pelvis, and the amount of knee valgus. With an increase in this angle of greater than 20°, the patella tends to track laterally, causing increased stress on the lateral patella and femoral trochlea. To track properly, the lateral patellar soft tissues and the pull of the vastus medialis must be balanced. Pressure directed laterally on the medial aspect of the patella determines whether there is subluxation, or stimulates an apprehension sign as the athlete attempts to prevent subluxation. Some athletes report only pain while others feel subluxation, or in some cases, actual dislocation of the patella. Examination should also include an estimation of femoral anteversion and the degree of external tibial torsion. The athlete must also be checked for tightness of the heel cords and pronated feet. Initial routine radiographs should be obtained. Further diagnostic testing such as patellofemoral CT or MRI should be delayed until after specialty evaluation.

Treatment of anterior knee pain is controversial but should focus on any identifiable causes. All training errors should be corrected when possible, such as decreasing the frequency, duration, and intensity of training. The simplest but often most difficult treatment involves avoiding any activities that aggravate the pain. Athletes are often unwilling to stop any type of training or competition during the season until the pain becomes debilitating. With this condition, cross training is vital to proper rehabilitation. Providing creative alternatives for training to help maintain fitness, but rest the knee, is key to the athlete's well-being. Water aerobics or bicycle training are good examples for low-impact cross-training activity. Exercises should emphasize lower extremity stretching, including the quadriceps, hamstrings, and hips. Isometric quadriceps and hamstring strengthening should be started, followed by progressive resisted exercises. Closed chain exercises, such as wall squats and leg presses, are preferred. A graded running program with sport-specific activities is introduced when the athlete demonstrates good lower extremity strength and coordination. The final phase of reconditioning focuses on preventing recurrence with maintenance stretching and warm-up exercises before all athletic activities. A patellar stabilizing knee brace or Neoprene knee sleeve may be helpful, but these usually are worn only during athletic activity. Icing after activity and the judicious use of NSAIDs can provide some symptomatic relief. Failure of this program, especially in an athlete with a correctable malalignment problem, is an indication for specialty referral.

Acute Patellar Instability

Most patients with acute patellar dislocation have underlying pathology similar to that described above. The greater incidence of this condition in female athletes is believed to be related to the higher incidence of lower extremity malalignment in women. The mechanism of injury is typically a flexion twisting injury with the foot planted. In those instances in which the patella does not spontaneously reduce, the athlete usually is found on the ground in extreme pain while clutching a flexed knee. Examination reveals an obvious deformity of the laterally displaced patella and prominence of the femoral condyles (**Figure 36.18**). If the athlete is seen immediately, the patella usually can be easily reduced by applying lateral to medial pressure on the patella while slowly straightening the knee. Sometimes the athlete is in too much pain with too much muscle spasm. In these instances, the athlete should be transported to the emergency department for proper sedation and closed reduction.

Many acute patellar dislocations reduce spontaneously on the playing field and are mistaken for an ACL injury. The athlete can usually describe in vivid detail seeing or feeling their knee cap "off" to the lateral side temporarily,

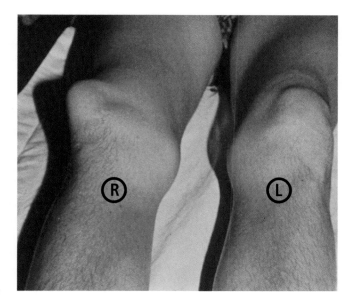

Figure 36.18 Clinical photo of lateral dislocation of the right patella.

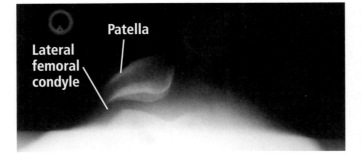

Figure 36.19 Sunrise radiograph demonstrating lateral subluxation of the patella.

although some athletes have difficulty accurately describing the problem. In the latter cases, a physical examination is essential to make the diagnosis. Physical examination will reveal a large effusion with severe tenderness over the medial retinaculum, the medial patellofemoral ligament (palpate down to the adductor tubercle above the medial epicondyle), and the medial patella as a result of extensive soft-tissue damage. The lateral side of the lateral femoral condyle usually is tender as well, especially if there has been an osteochondral injury. Note that athletes typically are extremely apprehensive with any medial to lateral pressure on the patella or any attempts at flexing the knee. However, a complete knee examination is necessary to confirm the diagnosis and to rule out associated injuries.

Routine radiographs, including a Merchant or sunrise view, should be obtained to confirm satisfactory patellar reduction and to rule out obvious osteochondral injuries (**Figure 36.19**). The latter usually appear as ossifications lateral to the lateral femoral condyle or avulsions from the medial patella or medial femoral condyle. Lateral subluxation or tilting of the patella can appear on the Merchant view.

Treatment of acute patellar dislocations is controversial. Many physicians advocate early surgical repair of an initial dislocation because the risk of recurrence is 10% to 20%. Surgical intervention can be especially helpful if initial radiographs reveal a large osteochondral fracture. However, nonoperative management is sufficient for most asymptomatic patients after an initial episode, with repair reserved for the recurrent dislocations.

Treatment after reduction should consist of immobilization in a commercial knee immobilizer or a nonweightbearing cast for at least the first 2 weeks. Most physicians now prefer an immobilizer as it allows for earlier rehabilitation. Casting is reserved for potentially noncompliant athletes. The extremity should be iced and elevated with aspiration of the hemarthrosis as needed for patient comfort or to facilitate rehabilitation.

Rehabilitation can begin in the immobilizer with isometric quadriceps exercises such as quadriceps setting and straight-leg raises. Use of the immobilizer can be gradually discontinued after 3 to 6 weeks and replaced with a patellar stabilizing brace or taping. A formal rehabilitation program consisting of exercises to achieve full range of motion and quadriceps strength and coordination should follow. Exercises may then progress to aerobic activity such as bicycling and jogging. Activities such as cutting maneuvers should be delayed until strength and motion have been regained.

Chronic Patellar Instability

Athletes with recurrent patella subluxations or dislocations typically report that they feel their patella shift to the lateral side and then their knee give way, almost always when the involved foot is planted. Examination should focus first on checking for lower extremity malalignment problems. Knee examination often reveals proximal and distal extensor mechanism causes for the instability. Proximally there may be deficient medial restraints such as a weak VMO or torn medial retinaculum and a tight lateral retinaculum. Distally there may be posterior lateral positioning of the tibial tubercle as a result of tibial anatomy or overall extremity malalignment. The combination of insufficient proximal and distal malalignment results in an increased Q angle and easy lateral subluxation of the patella both passively and actively. This may be seen by observing a "J" sign when the patella subluxates laterally during terminal active knee extension. Apprehension signs can vary in cases of chronic lateral instability and should not be the sole determinant of diagnosis and treatment. Examination for generalized ligamentous laxity is necessary, such as observing for bilateral patella hypermobility, knee or elbow hyperextension, fifth metacarpophalangeal joint hyperextension, and positive thumb-to-forearm testing. Radiographs can appear normal, but can also reveal lateral patellar subluxation and/or a shallow femoral trochlear groove or deficient patella facets.

Initial management should be nonoperative, especially for athletes with generalized ligamentous laxity and otherwise no gross anatomic abnormalities. A vigorous quadriceps rehabilitation program should be instituted with or without patella stabilizing bracing or taping. Athletes who do not respond to nonoperative management require surgical evaluation.

Plicae

Plicae refers to normal synovial folds in the knee that are believed to be remnants of embryologic development. The most commonly involved plicae in knee pain is the medial patellar plicae, which extends from the superior or midpatella to the medial patellar fat pad. Other less commonly involved plicae are the suprapatellar, lateral, and infrapatellar, also known as the ligamentum mucosum.

The diagnosis of a plicae as the source of pain or popping should be a diagnosis of exclusion as most are asymptomatic. Sometimes a plicae may become a source of anterior medial knee pain caused by either acute blunt trauma or repetitive knee flexion trauma. Athletes may also report a popping sensation in this region in midflexion that causes their knee to give way. Physical examination is unremarkable except for tenderness in the area of the plicae, usually anterior and medially. A palpable snapping sensation may be felt, especially when the leg is actively loaded during stance from 30° to 60° of knee flexion. Lateral patellar instability may be present and cause increased tension on the plicae.

Treatment should be focused on removing or modifying any offending exercises or activities. Strength or flexibility imbalances should be corrected. Ice after activity and NSAIDs can be helpful. Steroid injections directly into the offending plicae can prove effective in persistent cases and are one of the few indications for their use in children. Direct pressure from any braces should be avoided. Athletes who do not respond to nonoperative management require specialty evaluation.

Osteochondritis Dissecans

Osteochondritis dissecans is a condition of unknown etiology that results in the separation of areas of articular cartilage with or without the underlying subchondral bone. It typically affects boys between the ages of 9 and 18 years and most commonly involves the lateral aspect of the medial femoral condyle. The diagnosis is often confirmed in asymptomatic children as the result of

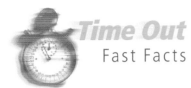

Osteochondritis of the knee is like a "bruise on an apple." In younger children with growth remaining, it generally heals without surgery. In older children with little or no remaining growth, surgery is often necessary.

Figure 36.20 A Notch or tunnel view and **B** lateral view of the knee showing osteochondritis dissecans.

incidental findings on knee radiographs. Therefore, the history and examination must correlate with the radiographic findings before treatment is initiated. In the early stages, athletes report vague knee pain associated with activity but the results of physical examination are unremarkable. In the later stages, athletes report activity-related pain with intermittent episodes of swelling and limited motion. Physical findings can include tenderness to palpation directly over the involved femoral condyle with the knee in maximal flexion. A mechanical block to terminal extension is rare but may occur with a detached or loose fragment.

Osteochondritis dissecans lesions can be missed on routine radiographs. Therefore, the lateral view should be supplemented with a notch or tunnel view, as these usually reveal the lesion. Most clinically important lesions of the medial femoral condyle are located anterior to the posterior border of the femoral shaft on lateral radiographs, while irregularities in ossification usually occur posterior to this border. Advanced or large lesions will also be apparent on the standard AP view. Typical lesions reveal a zone of radiolucency surrounding a thin linear bone fragment (**Figure 36.20**). The fragment can appear attached, partially detached with most of the articular cartilage intact, or free within the joint. Increased radiodensity or sclerosis around the margin of the lesion is a sign of chronicity and poor healing potential.

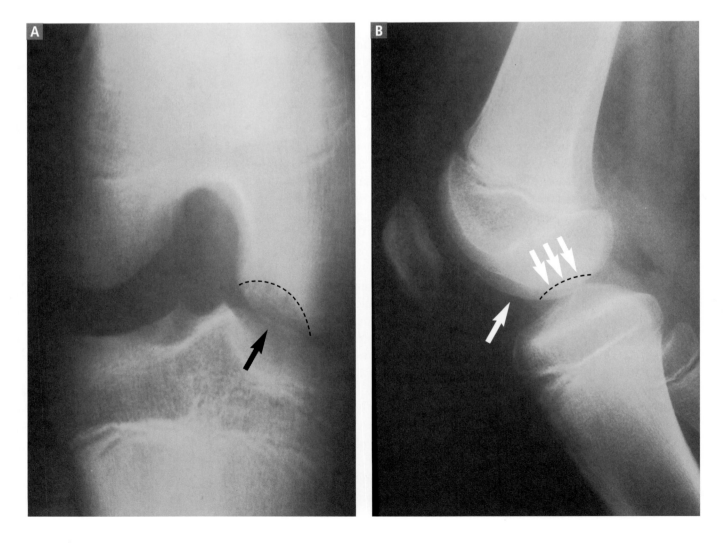

Note that radiographs may not clearly delineate the condition of the articular surface or distinguish diseased areas from areas of irregular ossification that are not clinically significant. MRI can be helpful in these situations, especially in determining the stability of the overlying articular cartilage. T2-weighted images reveal fluid within the subchondral bone underlying the osteochondritic fragment if the articular cartilage has been violated. Serial technetium bone scans are occasionally used to help determine healing potential of fragments.

Treatment is very controversial and ranges from periodic observation with radiographs to surgical fixation. No treatment or activity limitations are necessary for asymptomatic athletes with a grossly intact lesion. This is especially true in younger athletes who are felt to have a better chance for spontaneous healing. These athletes require follow-up examinations and radiographs at 6- to 12-month intervals. In symptomatic athletes in the early stages with an intact lesion, a period of activity restriction with or without limited weight bearing on crutches is felt to be helpful. Range of motion and strengthening exercises are believed to be beneficial to cartilage healing. Any type of cast or splint immobilization should be short in duration (4 to 6 weeks) and reserved for very symptomatic lesions in noncompliant patients.

Sports participation should be prohibited until the athlete is pain-free and has evidence of healing on examination and radiographs. Full rehabilitative function should be obtained before the athlete is allowed to gradually return to sports activity. If symptoms recur, or a recurrent effusion is present, specialty referral is recommended. Other indications for referral include older symptomatic athletes or any individual in the later stages with partially or completely detached lesions.

Meniscal Cartilage Tears

Most meniscal tears in young athletes occur as a result of tears of the cruciate ligaments or a discoid lateral meniscus. Athletes typically report feeling a twisting or hyperflexion motion at the knee, but rarely report hearing or feeling a pop at the time of injury. Isolated meniscal tears usually cause localized pain at the site with delayed or minimal effusion. Meniscal tears with associated ACL injuries cause diffuse knee pain followed by rapid development of an effusion and limited ability to bear weight. Displaced tears limit the athlete's ability to straighten the knee.

Examination usually reveals an effusion with tenderness along the joint line of the involved meniscus, usually just posterior to the adjacent collateral ligament. A mechanical block to full extension may be present and should be differentiated from other causes of extension loss, such as a large hemarthrosis or an extensor mechanism injury. Provocative testing for a meniscal tear should include some variation of the McMurray test. Hyperflexion of the knee with internal and external rotation of the tibia will elicit pain and possibly popping at the site of the tear posteriorly. Performing this maneuver while bringing the knee into extension may elicit a painful click in the medial or lateral joint line. Anterior knee pain during these motions is usually caused by patellofemoral symptoms, not a meniscal tear. A complete knee examination is necessary to identify possible associated ligamentous injuries.

Radiographs are usually normal. MRI is very valuable in identifying meniscal tears but usually is not necessary if a thorough clinical examination is performed.

Treatment should be individualized. Isolated tears with no associated ligamentous injuries and no mechanical blocks to full extension generally can be treated symptomatically the first 4 to 6 weeks. This initial treatment should also include a period of rest on crutches with ice, compression, and elevation. Exercises for range of motion should be initiated immediately, with progression of strengthening exercises as tolerated. Active flexion should be avoided during the first month, and turning or twisting activity should be avoided for at least 2 months. Any athlete who fails to improve with these measures, or has associated ligamentous injury or a mechanical block to full extension, requires specialty evaluation.

Discoid Meniscus

A discoid meniscus is characterized by meniscal tissue covering the entire tibial plateau with variable peripheral attachments. This condition most commonly affects the lateral side of the knee and is asymptomatic in most individuals. Athletes with this condition report a history similar to that of a meniscal tear, including catching, popping, and occasional swelling. Examination typically reveals tenderness over the entire lateral joint line, and at times, a palpable pop as the knee moves through a full range of motion. A mechanical block to full extension may exist. Radiographs usually are normal but can show slight widening and flattening of the lateral joint space. Discoid meniscus usually is mistaken for a routine meniscus tear and rarely diagnosed without surgery unless an MRI is obtained. No treatment is indicated for asymptomatic athletes, but those with symptoms should be treated in the same way as athletes with routine meniscal tears.

Popliteal Cyst

A popliteal, or Baker's, cyst is a fluid-filled sac located at the medial border of the popliteal fossa of the knee. Young athletes typically do not report symptoms, but parents often notice a mass on the posterior aspect of the child's knee and seek medical attention. Cysts in children differ from those in adults because they are not typically associated with intra-articular pathology such as meniscus tears.

Examination should consist of palpation of both popliteal fossa for comparison, first with the child prone and then supine with the knee flexed. The mass should be cystic in nature and will usually transilluminate with a light. Radiographs are normal, and additional diagnostic studies are not indicated unless the mass is suspicious for a tumor. If an MRI is ordered, it will show a homogenous mass in this region (**Figure 36.21**). Advise the parents that these cysts usually resolve spontaneously without treatment and can be followed with periodic examination. If the cyst enlarges or becomes painful, specialty referral is recommended.

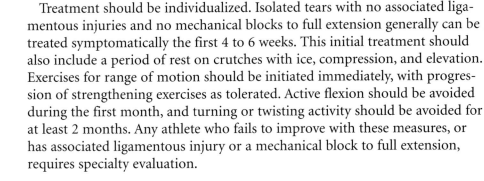

Time Out
Fast Facts

A popliteal (Baker's) cyst in a child rarely requires treatment, in contradistinction to adults.

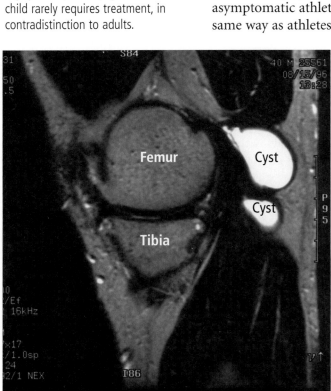

Figure 36.21 Lateral MRI of a popliteal (Baker's) cyst of the knee.

Tibial Eminence Avulsion Fracture

ACL injuries in young athletes usually are the result of tibial eminence avulsion fractures. Athletes nearing skeletal maturity are more likely to sustain intrasubstance injuries similar to those found in adults. Falling off a bike is a common mechanism of injury. Athletes usually report a noncontact, valgus, external rotation twisting injury or a hyperextension injury. Some may report an associated pop with severe pain and inability to bear weight subsequently. A large effusion secondary to hemarthosis usually develops within a few hours. Pain usually is diffuse but can be localized to regions of associated meniscal or collateral ligament injuries.

Examination results vary, depending on the time that has elapsed since the injury. Acute injuries are often easier to examine than injuries that occurred hours or days ago because of the subsequent onset of severe pain, swelling, and muscle spasm. Tenderness usually is localized to the joint lines or collateral ligaments secondary to associated injuries, compared with that of a patellar dislocation in which the tenderness is located in the peripatellar region. A large effusion is often noticeable with the knee resting in a slightly flexed position. Range of motion is uncomfortable, and there may be a block to full extension as a result of displacement of the eminence fracture into the notch. A Lachman test usually is positive, while pivot shift or flexion rotation drawer testing is more difficult in the acute phase secondary to pain but can be diagnostic when the knee is more relaxed.

Radiographs reveal eminence fractures that are nondisplaced (type I), minimally displaced (type II), completely displaced (type III), or completely displaced and rotated (type III+) (**Figure 36.22**). Additional diagnostic testing with CT or MRI usually is not necessary, but can be used to document adequacy of reduction in fractures treated with closed or arthroscopic reduction.

Athletes with tibial eminence fractures usually require specialty evaluation, especially if there is associated meniscal or collateral ligament injury. Treatment of type I and II fractures consists of closed reduction with hyperextension of the knee and subsequent immobilization for 4 to 6 weeks in neutral or slight knee flexion. If an anatomic reduction is not obtained, referral for surgical evaluation is recommended. Residual ACL laxity following closed or surgical treatment has been reported and is believed to be caused by partial ligament failure prior to the avulsion fracture. Current short-term follow-up studies report no correlation with functional complaints and the level of increased ACL laxity on examination. Long-term studies are needed to determine if there are later increases in functional instability.

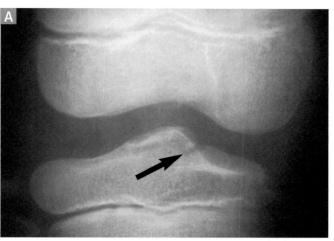

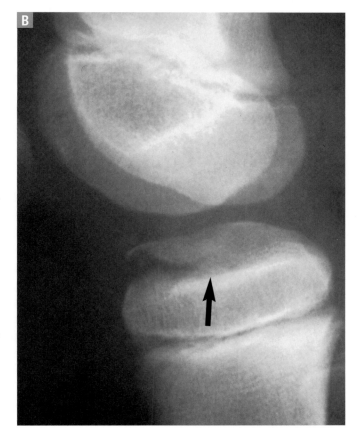

Figure 36.22 A AP and **B** lateral radiographs of a minimally displaced fracture of the tibial eminence.

ACL Injuries

Intrasubstance ACL tears are more common in young athletes nearing skeletal maturity, but have been found in children as young as age 7 years. The clinical presentation is very similar to tibial eminence fractures except often there are no radiographic findings. In chronic cases, a careful history and examination are important to identify the true cause of episodes of "giving way." ACL deficient knees sustain true pivoting episodes compared to patellofemoral pain that causes a "giving way" sensation resulting from a quadriceps inhibition reflex. Distal femoral physeal injuries should be ruled out. MRI usually is not necessary but can prove valuable in revealing associated meniscal and collateral ligament damage and any unrecognized osteochondral injuries.

Initial treatment consists of rest, ice, compression, and elevation to "calm" the knee. Early aspiration and injection of the knee may prove beneficial for patient comfort and facilitate the rehabilitation process. Range of motion and strengthening exercises should be started as soon as possible, with activity restrictions for a minimum of 4 to 6 weeks. Return to sports without surgical intervention is controversial. Some physicians still recommend a trial of nonoperative treatment with ACL bracing, especially in athletes with solid secondary restraints or who may be in the middle of a season. However, most physicians agree that recurrent instability is likely in this young, more active population. Most athletes will experience additional episodes of pivoting that can increase their risk of associated meniscal and articular cartilage damage. Many of these cartilage injuries are irreversible and support the need for early specialist evaluation.

MCL Injuries

MCL injuries frequently occur, both as isolated injuries and in association with cruciate injuries. The mechanism of injury usually is a noncontact, valgus, external rotation force on a planted foot. Valgus contact injuries still occur but are much less common with the initiation of rule changes in collision and contact sports. Athletes report severe pain localized to the medial side of the knee with any knee flexion or rotation.

Physical examination sometimes reveals an effusion, depending on the severity of the MCL injury and associated injuries. Tenderness to palpation often localizes the site of the primary tear to the femur, joint line, or proximal tibia. Distal femoral physeal injuries must be suspected in patients with severe femoral tenderness. Valgus stress testing should be done at both 0° and 30°, noting the degree of opening and the quality of the end point. Most MCL injuries will be stable at 0° and reveal a mildly increased opening only at 30°. Any abnormal increased opening at 0° signifies a severe MCL injury and probable cruciate and posterior capsule injury. Grading of injuries varies, but usually includes mild 0 to 5 mm (grade I), moderate 5 to 10 mm (grade II), and severe greater than 10 mm (grade III).

Radiographs are usually unremarkable but can reveal bony avulsions from the distal medial femur or proximal tibia. Stress radiographs can be used to differentiate MCL injuries from distal femoral physeal injuries. MRI usually is not indicated but can be helpful in identifying associated meniscal and cruciate pathology.

Treatment is usually nonoperative and consists of rest, ice, compression, and elevation, followed by immobilization in extension for the first 3 to 5 days. Weight bearing as tolerated is encouraged with no turning and twisting activity. Early protected range of motion in a brace is initiated, followed by progressive quadriceps and hamstring strengthening as tolerated. A functional brace can be used once motion and strength are recovered, and a solid end-point is felt on examination. Straight-ahead running is allowed in the brace when the athlete is pain-free and can walk without a limp. Sport-specific functional activities, including cutting, are allowed only when full protective strength and coordination are achieved. Return to activity averages 2 to 3 weeks for mild injuries (grades I and II). More severe injuries can take 4 to 6 weeks or longer for a full return. Associated meniscal and cruciate injuries must be ruled out in these type of injuries because they will determine the final overall treatment and return to play guidelines.

LCL and Posterolateral Complex Injuries

Isolated injuries to the LCL and posterolateral complex (PLC) structures are very uncommon in young athletes. However, associated cruciate or meniscus injuries are common. Mechanisms of injury typically include violent contact blows to the anterior medial tibia or noncontact hyperextension and varus stress injuries. Patients report lateral and posterior lateral pain occasionally associated with a pop caused by an LCL avulsion fracture or concomitant cruciate injury.

Examination reveals diffuse tenderness and swelling on the lateral side of the knee, depending on the severity of injury. Range of motion testing often reveals hyperextension greater than that in the opposite, uninjured knee. Varus stress testing at both 0° and 30° is important, noting the degree of opening and the quality of the end point. Any abnormal increased opening at 0° signifies a severe LCL injury and probable cruciate and posterior lateral complex injuries. Most isolated LCL injuries will be stable at 0° and reveal mild increased opening only at 30°. Grading of injuries includes mild 0 to 5 mm (grade I), moderate 5 to 10 mm (grade II), and severe greater than 10 mm (grade III). External rotation testing should be done at 30° and 90°. Increased external rotation at 30° that stays the same at 90° is consistent with an isolated PLC injury. Increased external rotation at 30° with a larger increase at 90° is consistent with a combination PLC and PCL injury. Observation of the athlete's gait may reveal a varus "thrust" to the outside during the stance phase. A thorough neurovascular examination is important because of the frequent incidence of peroneal nerve and popliteal artery injuries.

Radiographs are usually unremarkable but may reveal bony avulsions from the distal lateral femur or proximal fibula. Stress radiographs can differentiate LCL/PLC injuries from distal femoral physeal injuries. MRI can be helpful because of the higher incidence of associated meniscal and cruciate pathology.

Treatment of mild grade I LCL/PLC injuries is nonoperative and very similar to treatment of MCL injuries. Moderate or severe injuries (grades II and III) have less healing potential and a higher propensity for residual varus and external rotation deficiency. Therefore, more severe injuries, especially those associated with cruciate or neurovascular injuries, require immediate specialty evaluation.

Protective Equipment

Lightweight knee pads or support devices can be useful for many different situations. Knee pads help protect the knee from direct blows or compressive forces in sports such as football, volleyball, wrestling, and softball. This protection can be especially helpful when pre-existing pathology such as a painful Osgood-Schlatter disease exists. Numerous knee support devices are available, ranging from the inexpensive elastic bandage wrap to the more sophisticated Neoprene sleeves. Elastic wraps provide mild support and compression after acute injury. Neoprene sleeves can provide some proprioceptive feedback in an injured knee, but do not provide significant ligamentous support. Some knee sleeves can increase swelling by retaining heat about the knee or by obstructing venous return and should be worn only during sports activity.

In athletes with an unstable patella, the use of taping and patellar stabilizing braces occasionally can relieve symptoms. However, these modalities should not be routinely used in athletes with patellofemoral symptoms without instability because they can apply increased stress to the lateral aspect of the patella.

Hinged knee braces can provide protection from varus or valgus stresses to the knee in an athlete with an acutely injured collateral ligament. Injuries to the lateral ligament require specialty evaluation prior to return to play. Routine use of hinged braces to prevent collateral ligament injury during athletic activity is widely practiced at all levels of competition, but it is not supported by the current literature.

Off-the-shelf and custom braces are available for athletes with ACL or PCL injuries. ACL braces may be effective in preventing hyperextension, but they are very poor at controlling translational or rotational forces. These braces frequently are used to "protect" surgically reconstructed knees. However, they usually simply serve to improve an athlete's peace of mind, even though they may slow down the athlete's activity level. Conversely, athletes who undergo nonoperative treatment for instability are at an increased risk of subluxating or shifting, despite the use of braces. Each subluxation increases the risk for further meniscal and chondral injury. Thus, athletes with ACL or PCL insufficient knees who continue to participate in activities that require pivoting should be advised that they are at risk for further injury, even when wearing a brace.

Prevention

Proper stretching, warm up, and strengthening exercises are the cornerstone to preventing injury. Preseason training activities should begin slowly, especially in school-age athletes who quickly change or overlap their different sports seasons. Training errors involving duration, frequency, and intensity should be corrected to prevent overuse injuries. Proper equipment such as footwear and playing surfaces also should be used to minimize the forces transmitted to the knee through the lower extremity. Coaching of proper technique can prove vital, especially in kicking and running sports. Good officiating can prevent severe injuries in collision sports such as football and hockey. Despite all of these efforts, nothing can prevent an athletic injury that occurs in the heat of competition. In these cases, immediate medical care should be made available to address any injuries that do arise.

Return to Play Guidelines

Parents are quick to ask when their child can return to play. This question may be difficult to answer because clear return to play guidelines do not exist. As a general rule, athletes may return to play when the following are present: 1) full range of motion and symmetric strength in representative muscle groups; 2) absence of joint effusion; 3) stable ligaments about the knee; and 4) the ability to perform representative sports activities without recurrent injury. When any doubt exists about an athlete's readiness to play, proceed with a course that is safest for the athlete.

Red Flags

When a young athlete sustains a knee injury, the hip joint should always be evaluated. Any loss of motion-especially internal rotation-warrants further investigation. Knee joint effusion is a sign of internal derangement of the knee and generally requires further investigation. An athlete who is unable to completely extend or flex the knee or bear weight needs further evaluation. Remember, at the knee as well as other anatomic sites, an athlete with open physes is more likely to sustain a physeal fracture than a ligament injury. The findings of a physeal fracture may be subtle on a plain radiograph, but the injury can be detected by a careful physical examination and a radiograph obtained with the knee under stress (**Figure 36.23**).

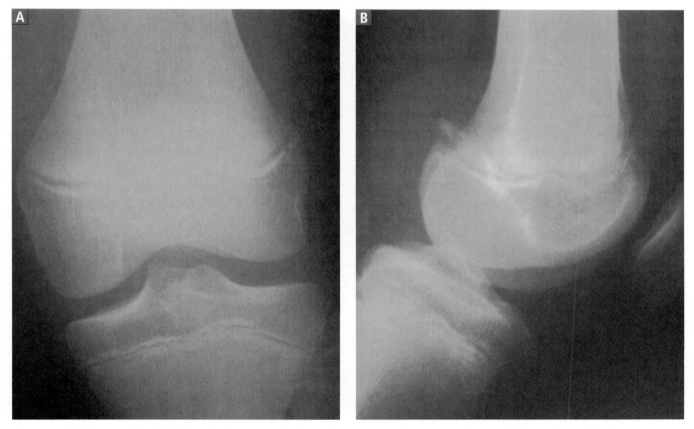

Figure 36.23 A AP and **B** lateral radiograph of a knee. There was tenderness over the medial femoral condyle. There is very subtle widening of the distal femoral physis consistent with distal femoral physeal separation. An AP radiograph taken with a valgus stress would confirm the injury by showing the opening of the physis.

FINISH LINE

Knee injuries are common in young athletes and require a thorough history and examination to make the correct diagnosis. The examination must include the hip and the ankle/foot regions along with the knee because of the many associated conditions that cause knee pain. Most knee injuries are self-limited abrasions, bruises, muscle strains, and ligament strains that can be treated nonsurgically and typically resolve within 1 to 6 weeks. However, patients with acute increases in pain, swelling, or neurovascular symptoms require immediate evaluation in the emergency department. Specialty consultation is indicated if nonsurgical therapy fails or if there is evidence of internal derangement and effusion with or without ligamentous laxity. Proper stretching, warm up, and strengthening exercises are key to preventing injury.

For More Information

1. Smith AD, Tao SS: Knee injuries in young athletes. *Clin Sports Med* 1995;14:629–650.

2. Stanitski CL: Pediatric and adolescent sports injuries. *Clin Sports Med* 1997;16:613–633.

3. Micheli LJ, Foster TE: Acute knee injuries in the immature athlete, in Heckman JD (ed): *Instructional Course Lectures 42*. Rosemont, IL, American Academy of Orthopaedic Surgeons, 1993, pp 473–481.

4. Stanitski CL: Knee overuse disorders in the pediatric and adolescent athlete, in Heckman JD (ed): *Instructional Course Lectures 42*. Rosemont, IL, American Academy of Orthopaedic Surgeons, 1993, pp 483–495.

5. McCarroll JR, Shelbourne KD, Patel DV: Anterior cruciate ligament injuries in young athletes: Recommendations for treatment and rehabilitation. *Sports Med* 1995;20:117–127.

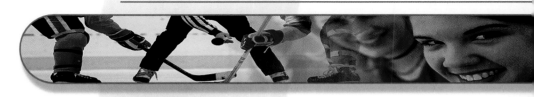

Chapter 37

Lower Leg

CURTIS R. GRUEL, MD

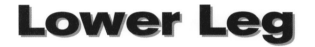

Common injuries and lower leg problems in the young athlete include acute fractures of the tibia and/or fibula, stress fractures, medial tibial stress syndrome (shin splints), and exertional compartment syndromes. Stress fractures are not caused by acute injury, but occur insidiously over time from general overuse. A more detailed discussion of stress fractures is provided in chapter 30.

Anatomy/Biomechanics

The lower leg has two bones, the tibia and fibula, that are linked by the interosseous membrane and by strong ligaments at both ends (**Figure 37.1**). Usually, when one bone fractures, the other bone fractures as well or becomes plastically deformed. Alternatively, the tibiofibular syndesmosis may be disrupted. However, the tibia or fibula may also fracture independently. In some places, the bones are closer to the surface of the skin where they are not protected by intervening muscle. Therefore, these places are more prone to open fractures.

The leg is divided into four muscle compartments: anterior, lateral, superficial posterior, and deep posterior. All four compartments are enclosed within the crural fascia, a relatively tough and unyielding structure. In addition, the compartments are separated by several structures: the tibia and fibula, the interosseous membrane, and the intermuscular septae. Each compartment contains a major nerve to the foot. Knowledge of the anatomic relationships can facilitate evaluation of each compartment and recognition of other problems, such as nerve compression injuries.

Clinical Evaluation

History

Identifying the mechanism of injury is critical. The athlete should be asked about the mechanism of injury: whether the foot was planted, and/or if a pop or snap occurred. A fracture should be highly suspected if an athlete reports a sudden, severe force, pain, or the inability to bear weight. In children, incomplete, stable fractures can occur because of the porosity and pliability of their bones and thick periosteum and can mimic sprains. Typically,

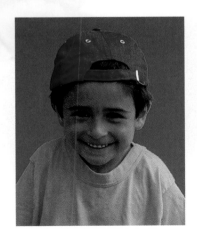

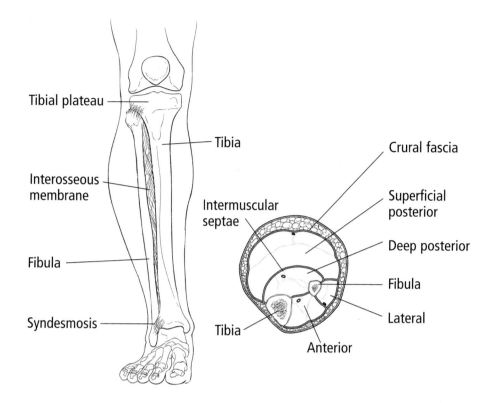

Figure 37.1 The area between the knee and ankle has four major muscle compartments: anterior, lateral, superficial posterior, and deep posterior.

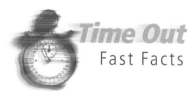

Inability to bear weight is a useful screening question in the initial history. A fracture should be highly suspected.

torus (or buckle) fractures resemble sprains, but even these fractures will usually have a history of an acute event with a sudden onset of pain.

Pain that is characterized by an insidious onset, but unrelated to any particular event suggests an overuse syndrome, stress fracture, medial tibial stress syndrome, or exertional compartment syndrome. These injuries usually develop gradually, and the athlete may have difficulty relating the onset of symptoms to any particular incident. However, the history may reveal a change in activity level, the start of a new sports activity, or a change in training regimen.

The location of the pain can suggest its source. Usually, stress fractures cause pain over the involved area of the bone, typically the proximal tibia or distal fibula. In general, a compartment syndrome causes pain over the involved muscle compartment. Medial tibial stress syndromes typically produce pain along the medial or posteromedial tibia. Radiating pain suggests a radiculopathy or nerve compression.

The timing of the pain can also provide useful information. In general, overuse syndromes produce pain during activity. With activity, stress fractures cause pain that subsides with rest. With continued activity, both overuse syndromes and stress fractures cause pain that begins earlier in the workout and lasts longer. Often, exertional compartment syndromes will produce pain after a certain period of activity. Although this pain also subsides, it requires longer periods of rest. The pain associated with medial tibial stress syndromes is typically relieved by rest, but can occur between workouts as well.

Fever, swelling, inflammation, or other constitutional symptoms can be helpful clues in identifying an underlying disease process such as osteomyelitis or neoplasm. Approximately 40% of patients with acute lymphocytic leukemia visit an orthopaedist because of bone pain.

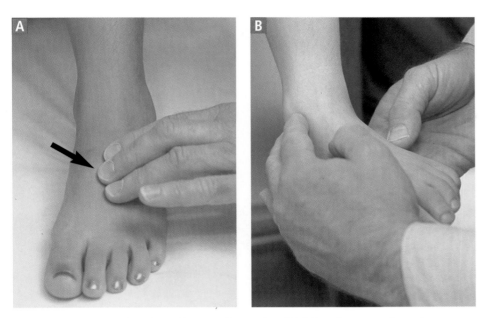

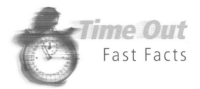

Point of maximal tenderness (PMT) is a useful clinical sign that suggests the source and location of the injury.

Figure 37.2 The dorsalis pedis **A** and posterior tibial **B** pulses are palpated to evaluate vascular status.

Physical Examination

The vascular status of the limb should be evaluated by palpating for pulses (**Figure 37.2**). Pulselessness is a limb-threatening emergency, although reduction of the fracture or even simple realignment of the extremity will usually restore circulation.

An acute compartment syndrome, a devastating complication that differs from exertional compartment syndrome, is potentially crippling. The former should be suspected when the pain seems disproportionate to the magnitude of the injury, when severe swelling occurs, and when the leg feels tense with a firmness similar to that of a grapefruit. The compartment is also tender to palpation. Usually, pulses are maintained even in severe compartment syndromes. Muscle is most susceptible to ischemia, and active contraction or passive stretch of the muscle will produce pain with this condition. The nerves are more resistant to ischemia, so sensory changes, when they become apparent, indicate an advanced problem.

Palpation is very helpful in distinguishing the overuse syndromes. In general, stress fractures are tender over the affected part of the bone, and if the fracture has been present for a while, a callus may be palpable. Swelling may also be observed. Tenderness is typically not associated with exertional compartment syndromes, but if there is tenderness, it is usually elicited over the involved muscle compartment. Athletes with medial tibial stress syndromes tend to report diffuse tenderness along the medial or posteromedial tibial shaft.

Diagnostic Tests

Anteroposterior (AP) and lateral radiographs of the extremity, including the joint above and below the injury site, should be obtained for all athletes with suspected fractures. Plain radiographs should be ordered first for athletes with potential overuse syndromes because stress fractures must always be ruled out.

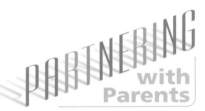

My child is experiencing leg pain during high school track training sessions. Should she be evaluated?

These symptoms could be caused by a relatively unimportant overuse problem such as shin splints, but they could also be caused by a stress fracture. If your child wishes to continue participating in sports and cannot "rest" the legs for a time, she should be examined.

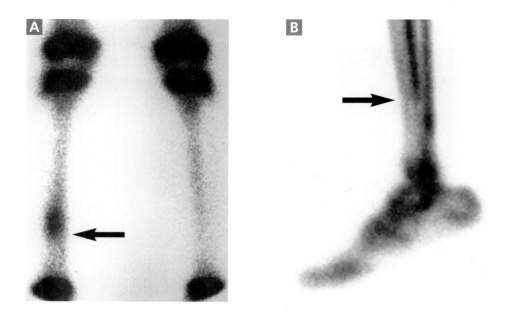

Figure 37.3 Bone scan of **A** stress fracture with focal uptake and **B** medial tibial stress syndrome with more diffuse uptake along the posteromedial shaft of the tibia.

If radiographs appear normal and a rapid diagnosis is required, a bone scan should be ordered. A bone scan will identify a stress fracture before it is visible on plain radiographs. On a bone scan, medial tibial stress syndrome may show increased uptake along the posteromedial shaft of the tibia, whereas exertional compartment syndromes show no changes (**Figure 37.3**). Also, a bone scan will demonstrate increased activity with osteomyelitis or osteoid osteoma.

Exertional compartment syndromes are typically confirmed by measuring compartment pressures during exercise with a wick catheter technique. A needle or plastic catheter designed to prevent occlusion is inserted into the muscle compartment and pressures measured during and after activity. While the exact pressures that define a compartment syndrome are controversial, the resting compartment pressure should be no more than 15 mm Hg. This pressure typically increases with exercise, but rapidly decreases to the normal value with rest. This test should not require more than a few minutes. Pressures that remain high after exercise or that return to normal slowly suggest a compartment syndrome.

Acute Injuries

Fractures of the Tibia and Fibula

Acute fractures commonly occur when bones are subjected to significant forces such as twisting forces, angular stresses, or direct blows. Deformity may be obvious if a fracture is present. In fact, deformity is the best indication of rotational malalignment. However, an undisplaced, stable fracture can be difficult to distinguish from a severe contusion or sprain. In most athletes, the second toe should align with the patella. Comparing the injured extremity with the opposite, uninjured extremity with the foot in a similar position will reveal any malalignment. Rotational alignment is often more apparent clinically than on radiographs (**Figure 37.4**).

Open fractures are usually obvious, but they can be difficult to detect if there is only a small puncture wound or a wound that occurs away from the fracture. As a general rule, a fracture associated with any type of wound should be considered an open fracture until a complete assessment is performed, and the wound clearly does not communicate with the fracture.

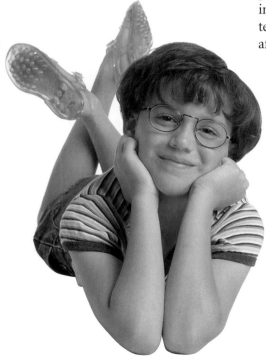

If an underlying condition weakens the bone, less force will be required to produce a fracture; this is known as a pathologic fracture. Pathologic fractures occur in children when weakening of the bone is caused by benign conditions such as nonossifying fibromas or bone cysts.

Properly treated, fractures of the tibia and fibula heal well with few sequelae. Most sports-related fractures are caused by forces of less energy than forces associated with motor vehicle accidents; greater forces produce more soft-tissue trauma. However, even with the smaller forces, an acute compartment syndrome can still develop. A seemingly benign fracture can cause permanent rotational or angular deformity.

All open fractures, which include any small wounds on the leg, require surgical debridement. The administration of antibiotics, typically a first-generation cephalosporin, and tetanus prophylaxis, if indicated, is also appropriate.

Physical therapy may be required so that the athlete regains mobility and strengthens the muscles, particularly the calf muscles. Physical therapy may not be necessary for younger children, who tend to recover well even without it.

Osteomyelitis and Neoplasms

Osteomyelitis and neoplasms, especially osteoid osteoma, cause a gradual onset of pain in the lower leg. These conditions tend to produce constant pain without the typical association of symptoms with activities. Typically, the pain from osteoid osteomas responds dramatically to nonsteroidal anti-inflammatory drugs; this response can be useful in making the diagnosis. Malignancies can also cause a gradual onset of pain with activity, but usually progress to night pain. In children and adolescents, the two most common malignancies are osteogenic sarcoma and Ewing's sarcoma.

Plain radiographs usually identify malignant tumors that show bony destruction and periosteal elevation (**Figure 37.5**). However, osteomyelitis can have the same radiographic appearance and, in fact, is often confused with Ewing's sarcoma. Discernible changes on radiographs may not appear for the first 2 to 3

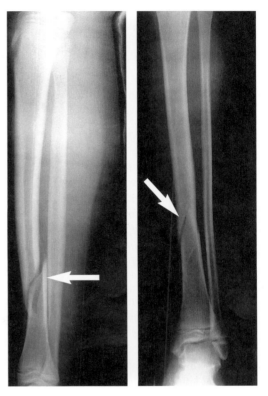

Figure 37.4 AP and lateral views, including the joint above and below, should be obtained to evaluate a fracture. A fracture with acceptable alignment in these views can still have an unappreciated rotational malalignment.

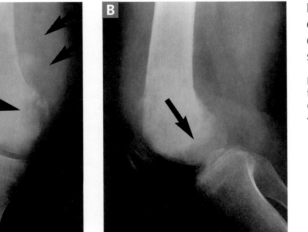

Figure 37.5 AP **A** and lateral **B** radiographs of the knee in a patient with osteosarcoma of the distal femur. Note lysis, sclerosis, and soft-tissue extension of the lesion.

Reproduced with permission from Ward WG: Orthopaedic oncology for the nononcologist orthopaedist: Introduction and common errors to avoid, in Zuckerman JD (ed): *Instructional Course Lectures 48*. Rosemont, IL, American Academy of Orthopaedic Surgeons, 1999, p 578.

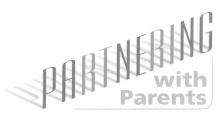

with Parents

My child has been diagnosed with a stress fracture of the fibula, based on a bone scan and radiographs. In our discussions with the doctor, a brief mention was made regarding an unlikely malignancy on the differential diagnosis list. Should we be concerned?

A healing stress fracture demonstrates periosteal new bone formation on radiographs that mimics more serious lesions such as osteosarcoma and Ewing's sarcoma. A history of overuse consistent with the timing of injury and close follow-up with radiographs demonstrating resolution over time will rule out these more serious possible causes.

Figure 37.6 Lateral tomography reveals a thickened cortex of the tibia consistent with osteoid osteoma. A lucent nidus was visible on another cut.

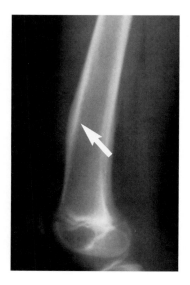

weeks. A bone scan will reveal increased uptake, and MRI will show edema. Stress fractures often show periosteal new bone and/or cortical thickening, but not bony destruction. Classically, osteoid osteomas have a thickened cortex and a radiolucent area (nidus) in the center of the lesion, but this is often not evident on plain radiographs (**Figure 37.6**). Bone scans can be helpful in differentiating osteoid osteomas, and a CT scan can be especially helpful in showing the nidus.

Chronic Conditions
Medial Tibial Stress Syndrome

Medial tibial stress syndrome, or shin splints, is a fairly common but poorly understood injury of the lower leg. Athletes with flat feet and athletes who run on their toes seem to be more prone to this injury, but other factors have not yet been clearly defined. Usually found in running athletes, this syndrome occurs most often at the beginning of the season when athletes increase their training regimen rapidly after a period of relative inactivity. Training errors, such as trying to do too much too soon, are typically to blame. Therefore, all athletes are at risk. Medial tibial stress syndrome is almost always benign and self-limited. However, it can be very difficult to distinguish from stress fractures, osteomyelitis, or neoplasms. These last three conditions are potentially much more serious.

Athletes with medial tibial stress syndrome may benefit from stretching and strengthening of the tibialis posterior muscle. Use of a longitudinal arch support also may help. Athletic shoes specifically designed for pronators are also appropriate for these athletes. These shoes have a good longitudinal arch support and an extended medial heel counter which resists pronation.

Exertional Compartment Syndrome

Although exertional compartment syndrome can affect any running athlete, adolescents sustain this injury most often. This syndrome occurs during running and resolves with rest. Unlike acute compartment syndrome, exertional compartment syndrome is not a dangerous condition in general, but it can be disabling over the long term.

Unfortunately, there may be no good nonoperative treatment for athletes with exertional compartment syndrome. Symptoms of this syndrome tend to recur when athletes resume running. Often, athletes may have to choose between a fasciotomy or giving up running altogether.

Blount's Disease

Blount's disease, or tibia vara, causes excessive bowing in the growing lower leg. Its cause is still unknown, but it may be related to excessive weightbearing forces. Varus deformity of the knee develops because forces directed at the medial side of the proximal tibial growth plate inhibit growth in the medial direction, but growth in the lateral direction continues. Blount's disease may be confused with persistent internal tibial torsion, either bilaterally or unilaterally. Internal tibial torsion will likely improve spontaneously. Radiographs of the lower leg will reveal progressive depression of the medial epiphysis, growth plate, and metaphysis, with increasing sclerosis of the medial cortex of the tibial shaft (**Figure 37.7**). Treatment of progressive deformity requires surgery.

In teenagers, unilateral depression of the medial tibial epiphysis, growth plate, and metaphysis may be noted. Radiographs of the knee may show a bone bridge across the medial growth plate that will permanently tether growth and increase the deformity. Usually, affected children are obese. As the varus deformity increases, laxity of the ligament complex of the lateral knee will develop. Bracing is ineffective in adolescents with Blount's disease. When deformity is significant clinically, osteotomy of the proximal tibia and fibula are indicated.

Treatment

Splinting is the initial treatment of choice for a minimally displaced tibial fracture, followed by specialty referral within the next day or two. Casting is almost always sufficient definitive treatment for children, but complications such as rotational malalignment can develop. Surgery is rarely necessary unless there is any question of neurovascular compromise, acute compartment syndrome, or if the fracture is completely displaced.

Initial treatment of overuse syndromes, including medial tibial stress syndrome, exertional compartment syndrome, or stress fracture, is rest, particularly from the activity that caused the injury, if known. Often, symptoms will resolve and allow the athlete to return to play gradually without further evaluation. When symptoms subside, the athlete may begin rehabilitation, or even resume activity if the symptoms were mild or if the period of disability was brief. The key to recovery, though, is rest.

Prevention

In most sports, tibial fractures are unusual because improvements in equipment have prevented many injuries. For example, modifications in ski boots for snow skiing and in shin guards for soccer have undoubtedly prevented many tibial fractures.

For all overuse problems, the best prevention is maintaining a high level of conditioning year-round. If year-round training is not possible, athletes should be encouraged to train gradually before the season starts to achieve the level of conditioning required for their sport. In younger children who may not be motivated to train, coaches should be advised to modify their conditioning programs to safely involve the less-conditioned athletes at the beginning of the season.

Return to Play Guidelines

Healing of tibial fractures should be documented by radiographic and clinical examination before athletes are allowed to return to play. Radiographs should show a bridging callus and return of trabeculation across the fracture site. On examination, there should be no tenderness on palpation, stress, and compression. In addition, full range of motion in adjacent joints and normal strength in the muscles should be regained.

Athletes with overuse problems should be pain-free and achieve a level of conditioning sufficient for safe participation in their sport before they resume their previous activity. A gradual return to sports participation should be stressed to the athlete. After a period of inactivity, athletes are especially vulnerable to overuse problems, and the extremity needs time to adjust to the increased demands. A running calendar may be useful for scheduling activities. Rules based on common sense help. First, the athlete

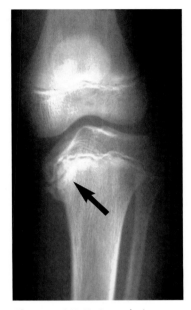

Figure 37.7 Irregularity of the medial tibial metaphysis, a finding typical of Blount's disease.

should not participate in the activity on consecutive days. A day of rest between activities is important so that the tissues can recover. Second, activity level should be increased in small increments, beginning in 25% increments. The point is to not double the stress in a day. Third, athletes should maintain the same level of activity for at least three sessions to prepare adequately for the next level. Finally, the athlete should not experience pain during the activity. If pain occurs, the athlete should return to the last level of activity that did not cause pain.

Red Flags

Wounds near the tibia and signs and symptoms of compartment syndrome are serious matters. Worsening pain or pain that is out of proportion to the injury suggests an acute compartment syndrome. Symptoms that become worse, despite rest, may indicate a cause other than overuse, such as osteomyelitis or neoplasm. Other warning signs include local swelling or inflammation or constitutional symptoms such as fever or weight loss.

FINISH LINE

Most leg pain in young athletes is caused by innocuous overuse problems such as shin splints. However, stress fractures, exertional compartment syndrome, and neoplasms also need to be considered. The key to treatment typically is rest from the inciting activity, followed by gradual return to activity. Conditioning is the key to preventing overuse problems.

For More Information

1. Abramowitz AJ, Schepsis AA: Chronic exertional compartment syndrome of the lower leg. *Orthop Rev* 1994;23:219–225.

2. Batt ME: Shin splints: A review of terminology. *Clin J Sport Med* 1995;5:53–57.

3. Eisele SA, Sammarco GJ: Chronic exertional compartment syndrome, in Heckman JD (ed): *Instructional Course Lectures 42.* Rosemont, IL, American Academy of Orthopaedic Surgeons, 1993, pp 213–217.

4. Thompson GH, Behrens F: Fractures of the tibia and fibula, in Green NE, Swiontkowski MF (eds): *Skeletal Trauma in Children,* ed 2. Philadelphia, PA, WB Saunders, 1998, vol 3, pp 459–503.

Chapter 38

Ankle

STEVEN J. ANDERSON, MD
J. ANDY SULLIVAN, MD

Acute ankle injuries are common in young athletes. Many of these injuries are diagnosed as sprains. However, with open growth plates, the possibility of physeal injuries should be considered in every skeletally immature patient. Fractures and growth-related conditions are also an important part of the differential diagnosis. To properly diagnose and manage these conditions, physicians should be familiar with ankle anatomy and how anatomy dictates specific injury patterns. When the injury pattern points to a lateral ligament sprain, a conservative approach to diagnosis and treatment is effective. However, when the injury pattern suggests a diagnosis other than a sprain, bony or growth plate pathology is more likely, as is the need for radiographs and surgical treatment.

Anatomy/Biomechanics

Bones, ligaments, and muscles stabilize the ankle. The distal tibia, the fibula, and the talus form the bony portion of the ankle joint (**Figure 38.1**). The tibia and fibula are held together by the anterior and posterior tibiofibular ligament as well as the interosseous membrane. The medial and lateral malleoli are extensions from the distal tibia and fibula, respectively. In children, an open physis separates the malleoli from the shaft of the tibia and fibula. The physis is weaker than the surrounding ligaments; therefore, skeletally immature patients are uniquely susceptible to injury here. The bony elements form a box-like joint called the mortise. The talus articulates in the mortise to form the ankle joint.

The primary ligamentous support for the ankle includes the three-part lateral ligament complex and the five-part medial or deltoid ligament complex. The three lateral ligaments include the anterior talofibular ligament (ATFL),

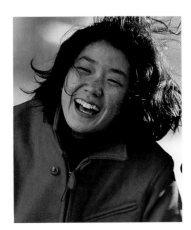

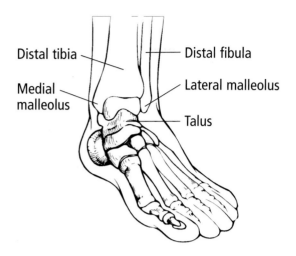

Figure 38.1 Bony anatomy of the ankle.

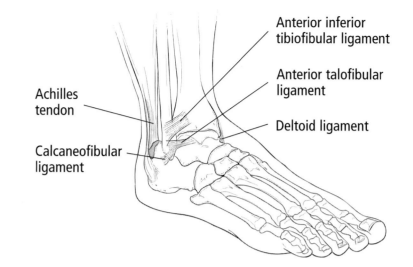

Figure 38.2 Major ligaments of the ankle and the Achilles tendon.

the calcaneofibular ligament (CFL), and the posterior talofibular ligament (PTFL) (**Figure 38.2**).

Musculotendinous structures provide additional stability to the bony and ligamentous structures. The peroneal muscles laterally provide resistance to inversion stress, and on the medial aspect of the ankle, the posterior tibialis muscle provides resistance to eversion stresses.

Mechanisms of Injury

Ligament sprains in the ankle tend to occur when the joint is in a position that provides little bony stability. For the ankle, the position of least bony stability occurs with plantar flexion and inversion. An ankle in plantar flexion has less bony stability than an ankle in dorsiflexion because the talus is narrower posteriorly than anteriorly. When the narrower posterior portion of the talus is in the ankle mortise, the space around the bony structures in the joint increases. With dorsiflexion, the wider anterior portion of the talus engages the ankle mortise with a tighter fit that increases bony stability.

Inversion is a less stable position for the ankle than eversion because the lengths of the medial and lateral malleoli differ. Compared with the medial malleolus, the lateral malleolus extends farther distally and blocks the talus from moving laterally. As the result of the shape of the talar dome and the different lengths of the malleoli, the ankle is least stable when the ankle is plantar flexed and inverted. In this position of low bony stability, the ligamentous structures must play a greater role in stabilizing the joint. Therefore, ligamentous injuries are most likely to occur when the ankle is in a plantar flexed and inverted position.

When the ankle is plantar flexed and inverted, the ATFL assumes a vertical orientation and becomes the primary lateral stabilizer for the ankle. If the ATFL is injured or fails, the CFL is subjected to inversion stresses. If both the ATFL and CFL fail, the PTFL may be injured. The anatomy of the ankle establishes a predictable pattern of injury in which the lateral ligaments are at risk in descending order from anterior to posterior. Because of anatomically determined susceptibilities, it is difficult to injure the CFL or the PTFL without first injuring the ATFL. Injuries to the medial ligaments are less common because of more prominent bony barriers to eversion. When the mechanism of injury or physical findings deviate from the typical sprain pattern, fractures or other diagnoses should be considered. For example, if an injury occurs in a ligament that is normally protected by bony structures, a bony injury should be suspected.

Clinical Evaluation

History

A history of the mechanism of injury is extremely helpful in establishing the differential diagnosis. It is important to determine the position of the foot and how the force was applied. The patient may be able to recall whether his or her foot was planted and which way his or her body twisted. The history should also include reports of the location of pain, swelling, functional restrictions, and any previous injuries, as well as questions about instability, stiffness, weakness, pain at rest, concurrent injury, and other musculoskeletal problems.

Determining the location of pain and swelling is more useful clinically than its severity. Inversion sprains should have pain and swelling that is most pronounced over the ATFL and CFL. Findings that suggest a diagnosis other than sprain include pain and/or swelling that is more pronounced medially or posteriorly rather than anteriorly or laterally. Pain and/or swelling in the midfoot, forefoot, or upper leg may indicate another type of injury.

Functional restrictions tend to be more reliable indicators of the severity of injury than the magnitude of pain, and may include the inability to run, jump or pivot, stand, walk, or bear weight.

Finally, a sports history should be obtained as part of the evaluation. An understanding of the demands of the athlete's sport will help determine specific rehabilitation goals and his or her readiness to return to play.

Physical Examination

The physical examination consists of inspection, palpation, and tests for ligament stability. The physical examination should always begin with a baseline evaluation of the uninjured ankle.

Inspection

Inspection can identify swelling, ecchymosis, and deformity. Swelling is localized over the injured structure initially, but becomes more diffuse over time. Swelling and bruising around the heel, forefoot, or between the toes may appear later with an ankle sprain or fracture.

Palpation

Bones and soft tissue to be palpated are the medial and lateral malleoli, the talus, and the calcaneus. To enhance patient cooperation, palpation should begin in the least painful areas.

Important ligaments to palpate include the ATFL, CFL, PTFL, anterior tibiofibular ligament, and deltoid ligament (**Figure 38.3**). Tenderness over the anterior joint line or anterior tibiofibular ligament warrants a more detailed evaluation for tenderness in the syndesmosis or interosseous membrane.

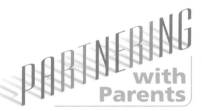

Is rehabilitation helpful following an ankle sprain?

Yes. After acute pain and swelling has been treated early exercises for mobility followed by balance, coordination and then sports specific activities begins. Rehabilitation enables the athlete to return sooner to sport with a lowered risk of recurrent injury.

Figure 38.3 Palpation of the lateral ankle ligaments. The most common injury occurs at the anterior talofibular ligament (top thumb).

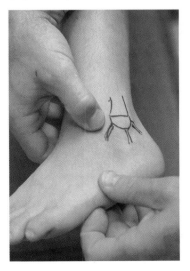

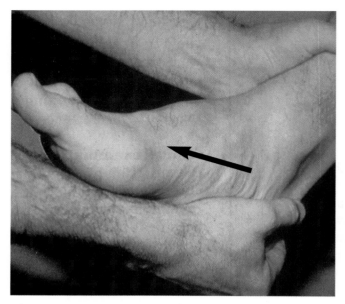

Figure 38.4 Anterior drawer test.

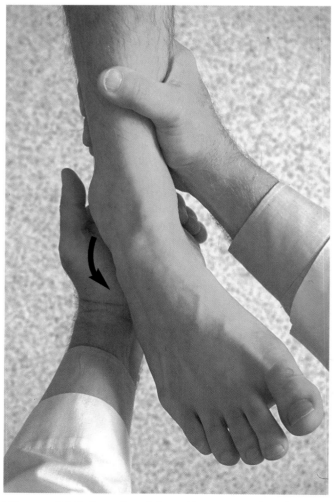

Figure 38.5 Inversion of the ankle to stress of the lateral ligaments.

Also, the peroneal tendon and Achilles tendon should be evaluated for signs of injury. Any positive findings should be analyzed for consistency with the mechanism of injury and the typical pattern for ligament sprains. The identification of the structures that are most tender on palpation is more relevant to diagnosis and treatment than the degree of tenderness.

Ligament testing

Swelling and guarding often limit tests for ligament stability, but injuries to the ATFL can be assessed reliably, even in the acute phase. To perform the anterior drawer test, hold the ankle in a neutral (90°) position with one hand stabilizing the heel and the other hand stabilizing the distal tibia and fibula. Then, pull the heel forward and assess the degree of excursion (**Figure 38.4**).

The talar tilt test is performed by first grasping the heel and stabilizing the tibia, and then inverting and everting the ankle (**Figure 38.5**). Laxity is compared with the uninjured ankle. However, the talar tilt test is often limited by pain and guarding. Fortunately, the diagnosis and initial management of ankle injuries is less dependent on talar tilt than on other factors such as the mechanism of injury, the location of maximal swelling and tenderness, and the presence of bony tenderness.

Additional testing

The benefits of strength testing in the acutely injured ankle are limited because of pain and guarding. However, athletes with chronic instability or recurrent injury may have calf or peroneal weakness. Pain or subluxation of the peroneal tendon with eversion may indicate injury to the peroneal tendon.

A modified Romberg test can identify proprioceptive deficits commonly seen with sprains (**Figure 38.6**). To perform the test, the athlete stands and balances on one foot with his or her eyes closed. The balance on the affected foot is typically impaired, even after the initial pain, swelling, and weakness have resolved.

Diagnostic Tests

Radiographic evaluation of acute ankle injuries should include anterior, lateral, and mortise views. Bony tenderness over the foot or upper leg should be evaluated with additional views. Tenderness or radiographic irregularities over a physis warrant close scrutiny of the radiograph for physeal widening, usually of the fibula. If suspicious, these should be treated as a fracture.

Determining when to obtain radiographs is a greater challenge than determining which views to order. In general, radiographs are most useful when bony injuries are probable. Common indications of possible bony injury include the following:

- Tenderness over the medial or lateral physes

- Tenderness over the medial malleolus

- Bony tenderness beyond the ligament attachment sites

- Swelling beyond that expected with a sprain

Anteroposterior (AP), lateral, and oblique radiographs should be obtained if an ankle fracture is suspected.

While not all patients with ankle injuries need radiographic evaluation, it is better to err on the side of obtaining the radiograph rather than missing a fracture. Stress radiographs, bone scans, arthrography, and MRI do not have a role in the initial evaluation or treatment of a sprained ankle.

Ankle Injuries

Sprains

Acute ankle injuries that occur with plantar flexion and inversion are most likely ligament sprains. Athletes with inversion injuries and posterolateral tenderness should be evaluated for peroneal tendon strains or subluxation. An athlete with an injury caused by dorsiflexion with or without rotation may sprain the interosseous membrane with a "high" ankle sprain. This same mechanism may disrupt the syndesmosis and cause a proximal fibular (Maisonneuve's) fracture (**Figure 38.7**).

Some injuries that are initially diagnosed as sprains are characterized by persistent pain, swelling, and/or instability, despite treatment. Under these circumstances, alternate diagnoses should be considered, including talar dome

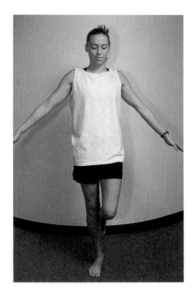

Figure 38.6 Modified Rhomberg test.

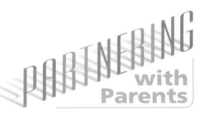

Do overuse injuries in children occur at the ankle joint?

Overuse injuries of the ankle generally are rare. Tendinitis, heel pain, and stress fractures of the tarsals and metatarsals are much more common.

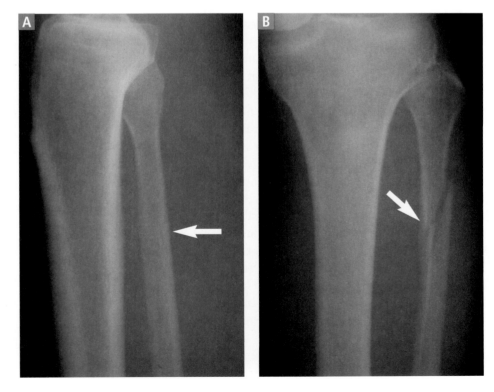

Figure 38.7
Maissoneuve fractures of the fibula.

Table 38.1 *Phases of Rehabilitation for Ankle Sprains*

Phase I

- Rest, protection (brace, wrap, splint, cast, crutches)
- Control inflammation (ice, compression, elevation)
- Early weightbearing as tolerated

Phase II

- Reduce residual swelling
- Restore flexibility and joint range of motion
- Restore strength (emphasis on peroneals and calf)
- Resume low-impact aerobic training

Phase III

- Restore proprioception
- Functional progression (running, sprinting, cutting, jumping; sport-specific skills)
- Gradual return to play
- Maintenance exercises and protection

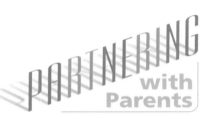

What is more common in children—ankle sprains or physeal injuries?

Ankle sprains are more common, but careful evaluation is necessary to avoid missing fractures of the distal fibular physis.

fracture, tibial plafond fracture, or an unstable ankle mortise. In these patients, repeat radiographs are indicated. Persistent pain and dysfunction in association with vasomotor changes may indicate reflex sympathetic dystrophy. Finally, tarsal coalitions and/or osteochondritis dissecans of the talus may cause the ankle to become painful or functionally unstable without commensurate degrees of ligament instability.

Effective treatment of ankle sprains depends on an accurate diagnosis. Once other diagnoses have been ruled out, ankle sprains—regardless of their severity—can be treated in three phases (**Table 38.1**). More severe sprains require additional time in each phase. The phases of treatment should follow sequentially; each successive phase of treatment depends on the successful completion of the previous phase.

Phase I treatment involves resting and protecting the ankle to permit healing, to prevent further injury, and to control pain and swelling. The use of casts, braces, and/or crutches depends on the severity of injury and the comfort level of the patient. More severe sprains may require the use of splints and/or crutches. Commercial immobilization devices are available. A mild sprain may require only an elastic bandage or ankle brace for protection.

If other diagnoses such as fracture or syndesmosis sprain have been ruled out, early weightbearing is permitted as tolerated and encouraged. Elevation, ice, and compression can be used to control swelling and pain. Heat has no role in the initial treatment of acute ligament injuries. Anti-inflammatory drugs can help reduce swelling and pain, but may not promote ligamentous healing.

Phase II treatment begins once pain and swelling have subsided to the point where the athlete can comfortably bear weight and ambulate. In this phase, active exercises are initiated to help restore range of motion and strength that was lost as the result of injury and immobilization. Range of motion and exercises using elastic tubing can help restore strength to the muscles. Exercises to strengthen the calf include toe raises, with or without added weight, and toe raises on the edge of a step. For more severe sprains, the athlete may work with an athletic trainer or a physical therapist.

Most athletes in phase II can resume some alternate form of exercise to maintain fitness while the ankle heals. Upper body exercises, such as weight lifting, may be tolerated as well as low-impact or nonimpact aerobic exercises such as swimming, pool running, cycling, stair climbing, ski machines, and/or rowing machines.

Phase III treatment focuses on restoring ankle function and sport-specific skills. This phase begins once the athlete has regained joint motion and strength and tolerates low-impact aerobic activities. During this phase of rehabilitation, exercises are designed to restore balance, agility, coordination, and proprioception. Exercises to restore proprioception are performed on a balance board, wobble board, or mini-trampoline, or by simply standing on one leg. As proprioception improves, agility exercises can be added, including jumping forward, backward, and/or laterally with one or both feet.

When the athlete recovers adequate proprioception, he or she is ready for sport-specific activities. Usually, functional progression starts with jogging or running straight ahead on an flat surface, progresses to sprinting and then to cutting. During the functional progression, an ankle brace or tape can be used to provide extra support, even if extra support is no longer required for daily activity.

Once an athlete completes the functional exercise program, sport-specific drills (eg, passing, dribbling a soccer ball, running backwards) may be started, with gradual return to practice and competition. Rehabilitation exercises should be continued until the athlete has been symptom-free with full activities for at least 1 month.

Nonoperative therapy is effective for most ankle sprains. Even with pronounced ligamentous laxity, most athletes can return to play with exercises and the use of braces and tape. Referral to a specialist is indicated for fractures of the malleolus, growth plate, fibula, or talar dome, and any injury that disrupts the integrity of the ankle mortise, including a syndesmosis sprain. Likewise, recurrent peroneal tendon dislocations and severe ligamentous laxity with chronic instability that does not respond to nonoperative treatment may also require specialty evaluation.

Fractures

Salter-Harris type I and II fractures of the fibula are caused by an inversion force. If the patient has tenderness and swelling over the distal fibula, the physician should carefully examine the radiograph for widening of the fibular physis (**Figure 38.8**). Signs of this injury can be subtle and hard to detect. If there is any indication of physeal separation, the leg should be immobilized in a short leg walking cast for 3 to 4 weeks.

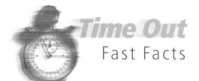

Fractures around the ankle in children that involve the joint (articular) surface often require surgery.

Figure 38.8 Careful clinical examination will localize tenderness over the fibular malleolus rather than the ligaments. **A** Maximal tenderness and swelling over the distal fibular physis. **B** Radiograph shows widening of the fibular physis.

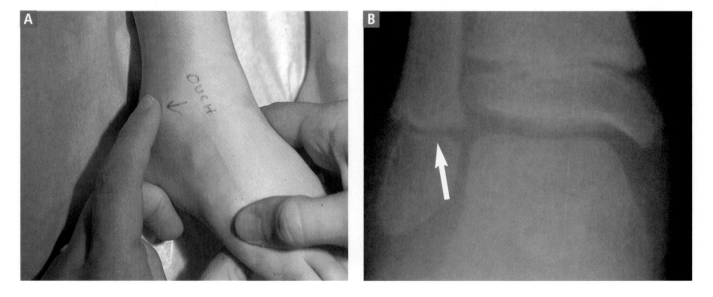

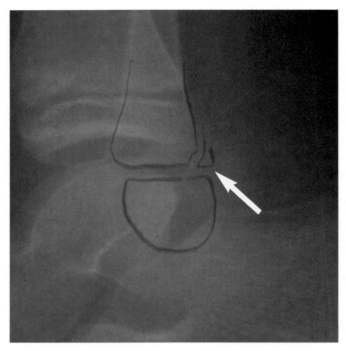

Figure 38.9 Salter-Harris type II fracture of the distal fibular physis.

Salter-Harris type II fractures of the tibia are caused by an abduction external rotation force, and are accompanied by an associated fracture of the fibula above the level of the syndesmosis. Examination will reveal gross displacement, and the metaphyseal fragment may be tenting the skin medially. Radiographs will show displacement of the distal tibial physis and an associated metaphyseal fragment (**Figure 38.9**).

Triplane fractures

As the athlete approaches skeletal maturity, the physes begin to close and the injury pattern changes. The distal tibial physis closes first medially. Fractures occur through the lateral aspect of the physis and propagate proximally through the physis and/or distally through the articular surface. This produces the triplane and Tillaux fractures.

The key to diagnosis of a triplane injury is that it will appear as a Salter-Harris type III fracture on the AP radiograph, while on the lateral radiograph, it will appear as a Salter-Harris type II fracture (**Figure 38.10**). In a Tillaux fracture, the lateral aspect of the distal tibial physis is avulsed. The syndesmosis may be disrupted as

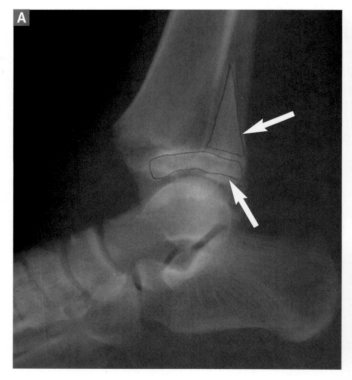

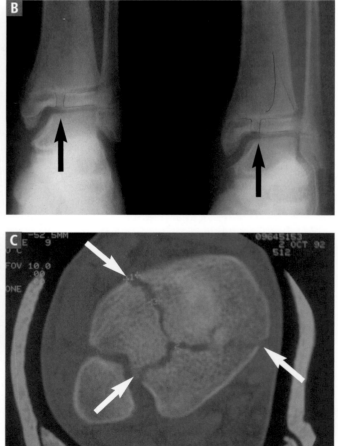

Figure 38.10 Triplane fracture. **A** On the lateral view, the entire epiphysis appears displaced with the metaphyseal fragment. **B** On the AP view, the epiphysis is fractured into at least two fragments, and the joint surface is involved. **C** A CT scan shows at least three fracture lines through the epiphysis.

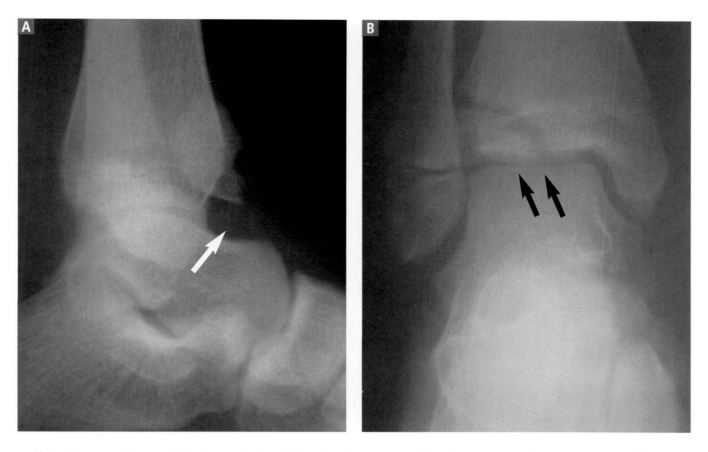

well. A CT scan will most likely be needed to define the fragments and to plan treatment, which is usually surgical (**Figure 38.11**). The goal of treatment is to restore the articular alignment and prevent traumatic arthritis. Angular deformity and leg-length inequality are unlikely.

Treatment

Most fractures can be reduced in the emergency department. The two most common types of displacement are posterior and lateral. Management of a posteriorly displaced fracture consists of sedating the patient, then grasping the heel and pulling forward. Laterally displaced fractures may require a medially directed force to realign the tibia. If examination after reduction reveals a continued widening between the medial tibial metaphysis and the physeal line, the periosteum is most likely interposed and surgery is required. Immobilization in a long leg bent-knee cast is indicated for the first 2 weeks, after which time a short leg walking cast can be used.

Most Salter-Harris type II fractures will heal and resume normal growth; however, in some, the physis will close and cause angular deformity or leg-length inequality. Therefore, AP radiographs should be obtained 3 to 6 months after the injury to detect an irregular Harris growth arrest line (**Figure 38.12**). Salter-Harris type II fractures of the ankle should be observed for at least 2 years, or until physeal closure to rule out growth arrest.

Salter-Harris type III and IV fractures are associated with a higher complication rate, including premature closure of the physis, angular deformity, and leg-length discrepancy. Because these fractures involve the articular surface and cross the growth plate, surgery is required to achieve anatomic or near anatomic

Figure 38.11 A Tillaux fracture with anterior displacement of the fragment and **B** disruption of the joint surface.

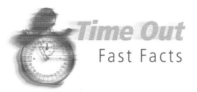

Triplane and Tillaux fractures are names of common growth plate fractures that occur during adolescence as the growth plate is beginning to close.

Figure 38.12 Salter-Harris type II fracture. **A,B** Initial radiographs show fracture of the medial malleolus. **C** AP view of both ankles at follow-up. Note overgrowth of the fibula on the right ankle and the irregular distal fibial physis.

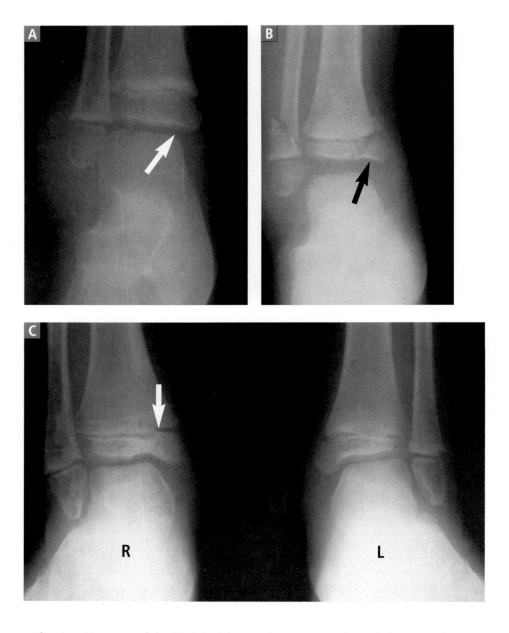

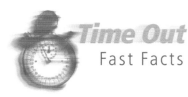

Time Out

Fast Facts

Taping and bracing are commonly used to reduce ankle sprains and injuries, but the effectiveness has not been proven scientifically.

reduction. Because of the high incidence of premature physeal closure, a fracture of the medial malleolus must be closely monitored (**Figure 38.13**).

Most tibial and fibular physeal injuries heal sufficiently in 6 weeks, and immobilization can be discontinued at that time. Rehabilitation should consist of a gradual return to activity that begins with walking, followed by jogging prior to beginning cutting exercises. Athletes at a high level of competition or those anxious to return to play may benefit from a more structured rehabilitation program, as detailed earlier in this chapter. A full return to play is possible 2 months after injury.

Prevention

The use of tape, braces, and high-top shoes has been recommended to prevent ankle sprains. However, no studies have proven that ankle braces are effective in preventing sprains or physeal separations. They may be more effective for chronic ankle instability or for prevention of recurrent sprains. Taping is considered the most secure means of ankle immobilization following a fracture or sprain, but even with the best taping, the tape will become loose during play. To ensure that the ankle remains immobilized, retaping may be necessary at least once if the athlete is participating in a prolonged athletic event. Many ankle sprains are recurrent, and proper treatment and rehabilitation of previous ankle sprains—including the use of proprioceptive exercises—reduces the risk of recurrent injury.

Return to Play Guidelines

The first thing an injured athlete usually asks is when he or she can return to play. Their desire to return to play should be weighed against the risk of complications or further injury. Recommendations for rest should be determined individually, not based on strict, often arbitrary, guidelines. Some athletes with severe injuries may recover faster than others with mild injuries. Remember that return to play also depends on the demands of the sport, the history of prior or concurrent injury, the availability and use of therapy, and the response to rehabilitation.

Functional testing may help to determine readiness to return to play. Functional testing is based on the functions the ankle performs in a given activity or sport. In most sports, a minimal level of joint motion and strength is required to allow the athlete to run, jump, or pivot. The successful completion of functional tasks minimizes the risk of further injury and a premature return to play. If the ankle is still swollen, stiff, or weak, the athlete should not be allowed to run or jump, even if he or she reports no pain. If the progression to a more demanding exercise increases symptoms, the athlete should progress more slowly or be reevaluated.

Athletes should be informed about the phases of rehabilitation so that they will know what to expect and take responsibility to participate in the recovery process. Each of the three phases of rehabilitation will require about the same amount of time to complete. For example, if an ankle injury requires 2 weeks to progress through the first phase, it is likely that the next two phases will each last 2 weeks as well.

Red Flags

Simple ankle sprains follow a particular pattern for mechanisms of injury, physical findings, and good responses to nonoperative treatment. Any ankle pain that does not follow the predictable pattern of a sprain should be evaluated for other causes. Injuries that occur in dorsiflexion or eversion are much more likely to involve fractures. Also, tenderness over the growth plates, syndesmosis, proximal fibula, or fifth metatarsal indicates an injury other than a sprain. Because of the risk of angular deformity or leg-length discrepancy in physeal injuries, care must be taken to look diligently for physeal arrest.

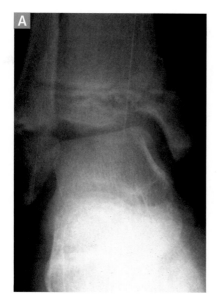

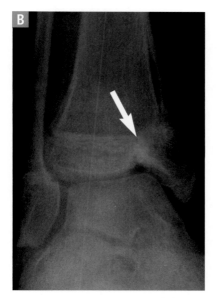

Figure 38.13 Fracture of the medial malleolus. **A** AP view of the acute fracture. **B** Follow-up radiograph showing partial closure on the medial side of the tibial physis with varus deformity at the ankle.

FINISH LINE

Acute ankle injuries are among the most common musculoskeletal problems seen in young athletes. Many such injuries are inversion sprains, which are characterized by a predictable pattern of symptoms, physical findings, and response to nonoperative treatment. Injuries that do not follow this pattern are more likely to be fractures, physeal injuries, or growth-related conditions. Careful clinical evaluation and judicious use of radiographic studies can facilitate an early, accurate diagnosis. The sooner the right course of treatment is initiated, the sooner the athlete will be ready to return to play.

For More Information

1. Anderson SJ: Evaluation and treatment of ankle sprains. *Compr Ther* 1996;22:30–38.

2. Ashworth A, Hedden D: Fractures of the ankle, in Letts RM (ed): *Management of Pediatric Fractures.* New York, NY, Churchill Livingstone, 1994, pp 713–734.

3. Jarvis JG: Tibial triplane fractures, in Letts RM (ed): *Management of Pediatric Fractures.* New York, NY, Churchill Livingstone, 1994, pp 735–749.

4. Carroll N: Fractures and dislocations of the tarsal bones, in Letts RM (ed): *Management of Pediatric Fractures.* New York, NY, Churchill Livingstone, 1994, pp 751–766.

5. Baxter MP: Fractures and dislocations of the metatarsals and phalanges of the foot, in Letts RM (ed): *Management of Pediatric Fractures.* New York, NY, Churchill Livingstone, 1994, pp 767–788.

6. Sullivan JA: Ankle and foot fractures in the pediatric athlete, in Stanitski CL, DeLee JC, Drez DD Jr (eds): *Pediatric Orthopaedic Sports Medicine.* Philadelphia, PA, WB Saunders, 1994, pp 441–445.

7. Crawford AH: Fractures and dislocations of the foot and ankle, in Green NE, Swiontkowski MF (eds): *Skeletal Trauma in Children,* Philadelphia, PA, WB Saunders, 1994, vol 3, pp 449–516.

Chapter 39

Foot

J. ANDY SULLIVAN, MD

Most fractures and sprains of the foot are easily managed, but some, although rare, are associated with serious consequences. Nontraumatic conditions in the foot, in which deformity and pain are the most common presenting symptoms, are common in young athletes.

Anatomy/Biomechanics

The foot consists of seven tarsals, five metatarsals, and 14 phalanges (**Figure 39.1**). The physes of the four lateral metatarsals occur distally, while the first is located proximally. The talus and calcaneus are called the hindfoot. The subtalar joint is responsible for side-to-side heel motion and is important in walking on uneven ground. The talus, calcaneus, navicular, and cuboid act in concert in walking. The navicular, cuboid, and cuneiforms are called the midfoot. The remainder is called the forefoot. The arch of the foot is formed by the hindfoot, midfoot, and metatarsals. The bones of the foot, along with their ligaments, have inherent stability. Muscles add dynamic support.

A number of specific terms are used to describe foot deformities. Varus is a deformity of the forefoot or heel toward the midline. Valgus is away from the midline. Adduction is a motion drawing the foot toward the midline, and abduction is drawing the foot away from the midline. Adductus describes a deformity of the distal portion of the foot toward the midline. Equinus indicates that either the forefoot or the heel is plantar flexed. A plantigrade gait describes an individual who is walking on the full sole of the foot.

Clinical Evaluation

History

The history should include information about the onset of pain, the relationship of pain to activity, and the mechanism of injury, if applicable. The athlete should also be asked about any recent changes in shoe wear or type of playing surface. History of recurrent injury or ankle sprains should also be elicited.

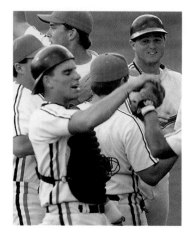

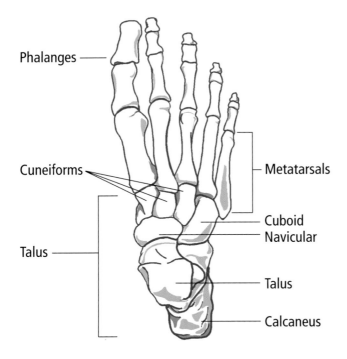

Figure 39.1 Bony anatomy of the foot.

Phalanges

Cuneiforms

Talus

Metatarsals

Cuboid

Navicular

Talus

Calcaneus

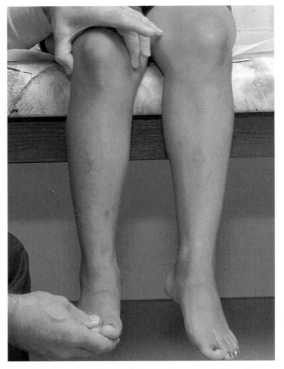

Figure 39.2 Physical examination of the alignment of the knee, ankle, and foot.

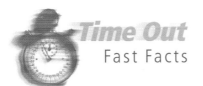

Time Out
Fast Facts

The Jones fracture (fracture of the proximal diaphysis of the fifth metatarsal) may require surgery whereas an avulsion fracture of the base of the fifth metatarsal will not.

Physical Examination

The foot should be examined initially while the athlete is seated to test the mobility of the subtalar joint. This is tested by grasping the heel and rocking it from side to side. Range of motion in the ankle and flexibility of the forefoot should also be measured. To test motor function, the athlete should plantar flex, dorsiflex, invert, and evert the foot against resistance. Any areas of pain on palpation should be noted, as should any bony prominences. The alignment of the ankle and knee should be assessed with the knee and ankle flexed 90° (**Figure 39.2**). The athlete should be asked to stand, noting what happens to the arch, then stand on tiptoe, on the heels, and finally on the lateral borders of the foot. The last part of the examination is to observe the foot during gait.

Children are born with a minimal longitudinal arch, but an arch appears in most children by age 4 years. It is also important to remember that normal gait and bony conformation do not develop until a child is about age 7 years. Before that time, children progress through genu varus, genu valgus, and an internal rotation gait. Metatarsus adductus is also common and resolves without treatment.

Diagnostic Tests

Weightbearing radiographs should be obtained whenever possible, as these maintain the foot in its normal functional position. Nonweightbearing radiographs do not demonstrate the position of function, which is shown while the patient is standing. If the athlete is unable to stand, weightbearing can be simulated by placing the ankle at 90° to the tibia. Initially, only anteroposterior (AP) and lateral views are necessary. The AP radiograph should be obtained with the central beam angle 15° toward the heel to eliminate overlap of the leg and ankle. Other special imaging techniques are discussed with specific conditions.

Acute Injuries

Fractures and dislocations are typically associated with a history of direct trauma, particularly to the metatarsals; therefore, physical examination is often limited by pain. Nonweightbearing radiographs should be ordered. Most fractures of the metatarsal shafts can be satisfactorily treated in a short leg walking cast for 4 to 6 weeks.

Metatarsal Fractures

Fractures of the base of the fifth metatarsal are troublesome because of the potential for avulsion injuries. The apophysis on the base of the fifth metatarsal is the point of attachment of the peroneus brevis tendon. An inversion injury may avulse this apophysis. Physical examination reveals tenderness at the base of the fifth metatarsal, pain with attempted eversion against resistance, and swelling. Radiographs may show widening of the apophysis. Most of these fractures heal uneventfully, but nonunion can occur in some. Immobilization, with crutches and an elastic bandage, until pain subsides is usually satisfactory. Ambulation in a short leg walking cast for 2 to 3 weeks can also produce satisfactory results.

Less predictable is the Jones fracture; this fracture at the proximal diaphysis of the fifth metatarsal is less common in skeletally immature patients than in adults (**Figure 39.3**). Management should begin with a trial of immobilization in a short leg walking cast. If delayed union or nonunion occur, surgical treatment is recommended.

Fractures of the toes occur and can be treated by taping to the adjacent toe. The only surgical indication in children would be a Salter-Harris type III or IV fracture of the proximal phalanx of the great toe. However, these fractures are rarely displaced and rarely require surgical treatment.

Stress Fractures

Stress fractures occur in children as the result of a sudden increase in training, change of training surface, or change of shoes. These can occur in athletes competing in multiple sports who change to a different sport, such as changing from football to cross-country or track. Stress fractures can also occur in association with tournaments in which multiple games are played over a weekend, such as in soccer or basketball, and in skaters and dancers.

Stress fractures most commonly affect the metatarsals, but can affect in the navicular and the medial sesamoid. In most instances, the training error is trying to do too much, too soon. Diagnosis requires vigilance and a high index of suspicion for stress fracture. A bone scan is not necessary unless the patient is an elite athlete who must return to his or her event. In most instances, immobilization in a short leg walking cast for 2 to 3 weeks and repeat radiographs will show periosteal new bone, confirming the diagnosis. Be aware that the initial radiograph may be normal in more than half of patients.

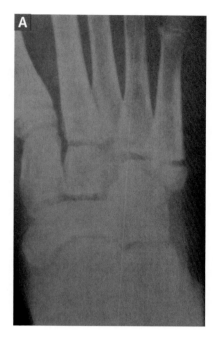

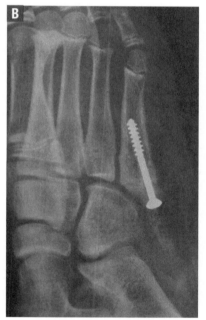

Figure 39.3 A Fracture of the proximal diaphysis of the fifth metatarsal that failed to heal with immobilization. **B** Result after operative repair.

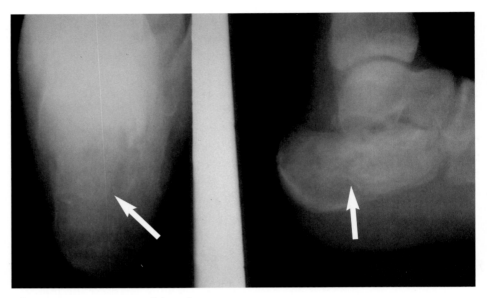

Figure 39.4 Fracture of the calcaneus.

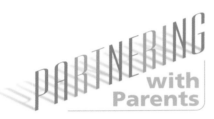

Fractures of the Calcaneus

Fractures of the calcaneus are much less common in young athletes than in their adult counterparts. Most occur as children near skeletal maturity. These fractures are often associated with other injuries, such as fractures of the lumbar spine or injuries to the pelvis. Most involve the tuberosity or the posterior portion of the calcaneus and will heal uneventfully with either nonweightbearing, or weightbearing, as tolerated (**Figure 39.4**). Most calcaneal fractures do not involve the articular surface, but those that do often require surgical management. Minimally displaced or nondisplaced fractures can be treated nonoperatively with nonweightbearing until the fracture is healed in about 6 weeks.

Fractures of the Talus

Fractures of the talus are rare in children, usually occurring as a result of forced dorsiflexion and involving the body or the neck of the talus. The dome of the talus can also be injured with significant trauma. It is critical to identify subchondral lucency on radiographs, as this indicates loss of circulation and viability of the talus. Specialty care is required for all of these fractures because of the potential for osteonecrosis, a serious complication. Osteochondral fractures of the talus can occur as young athletes approach skeletal maturity, and these require surgical treatment.

Lisfranc Fractures

The Lisfranc fracture is a fracture-dislocation of the tarsometatarsal joints, caused by severe dorsiflexion in the midfoot. The massive swelling and subtle radiographic findings associated with this fracture make it difficult to diagnose. Surgical correction is required for this fracture.

Chronic Conditions
Freiberg's Infraction

Freiberg's infraction is characterized by collapse of the articular surface and underlying bone of the involved metatarsal head. The second metatarsal head is affected most often, followed by the third and fourth metatarsal heads. Girls between ages 12 to 15 years are more commonly affected than boys.

Avascular bone at the involved sites is thought to be caused by increased stresses on the metatarsal head that occur during normal walking, dancing, or other athletic activities. Athletes are especially prone to this type of injury because the second metatarsal head is subject to increased weightbearing stresses.

Athletes often report dull, aching pain of insidious onset in the forefoot. Marked local tenderness is found on palpation of the involved metatarsal head, particularly on the plantar surface. In advanced stages, swelling and warmth about the metatarsal head may be found as well.

AP, lateral, and oblique views of the foot are needed to confirm the diagnosis. Early radiographic changes may show increased density of the involved metatarsal head with a suggestion of mild flattening of the second metatarsal head (**Figure 39.5**). As the process evolves, fragmentation of the metatarsal head is noted with gradual and progressive healing of the avascular bone.

In most young athletes, management is nonoperative. Relieving the weight-bearing pressure on the involved metatarsal will resolve the pain and allow the fragment to heal. An orthotic device with a properly molded metatarsal pad or a short leg cast with a metatarsal relieving mold can displace pressure behind and away from the involved head. Management consists of casting for 6 weeks, followed by use of an orthotic device for 1 year. Recurrence is not expected. Referral to a specialist is recommended if management fails to relieve the pain.

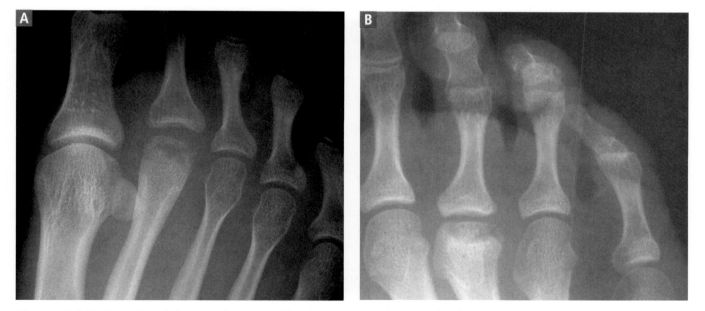

Figure 39.5 Flattening of the second metatarsal head consistent with Frieberg's infraction.

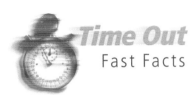

Occasionally, a small section of articular cartilage and underlying dead bone will separate from the head as a free osteochondral fragment. Symptoms that persist despite nonoperative management are most likely caused by continued instability and failure of the loose fragment to heal. In these instances, definitive treatment requires surgical excision of the loose fragment.

Flexible Flatfoot

A child with a flexible flatfoot has little or no longitudinal arch while standing. Common public opinion is that a flatfoot is undesirable. However, in most instances, this is a normal finding that does not affect sports participation nor cause disability later in life. Flatfeet are classified as flexible or rigid, and painful or not painful. Most patients with flatfeet have the flexible, nonpainful type. Those who report pain typically have rigid flatfeet and require specialty evaluation for the cause.

Physical examination should include inspection for an arch while the patient is sitting, standing normally, and standing on tiptoe. It is important to note whether the arch disappears with normal standing and whether the arch is apparent when the patient stands on tiptoe. When most patients stand on tiptoe, the posterior tibialis tendon will reconstitute the arch, and the heel will invert; this indicates that the foot is normal (**Figure 39.6**).

Treatment is not indicated in most instances, as flatfeet are usually asymptomatic and will not cause any disability. The biggest challenge of management is convincing the family that no treatment is necessary. Corrective shoes, inserts, and orthotics have not been proven to affect the natural history of a flatfoot. Radiographs obtained of children with and without these devices show no difference in the bony architecture of the foot. However, if the patient is symptomatic, reports fatigue in the foot, or is found to have a flexible flatfoot, use of inserts or orthotics, such as those that can be obtained from shoe stores, may relieve symptoms.

Patients with a rigid or painful flatfoot require specialty evaluation to identify the source of pain, such as tarsal coalition. Additional indications for specialty referral include abnormal shoe wear or failure to respond to inserts or orthotics. The role of orthotics and shoes to control pronation and supination of the foot in adolescents is still controversial.

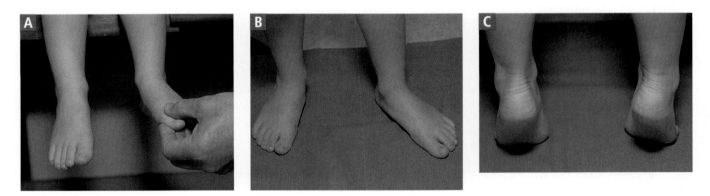

Figure 39.6 Physical examination for flexible flatfoot. **A** The arch is present while the patient is seated. **B** Standing obliterates the arch. **C** Tiptoe, standing reconstitutes the arch and inverts the heel.

Tarsal Coalition

Tarsal coalition is a fibrous bony connection of two or more of the tarsal bones that limits motion in some of the tarsal joints. The result is altered biomechanics that can lead to pain and arthritis. Coalitions are present at birth and gradually ossify, often becoming symptomatic during the second decade. Some patients have symptoms during adolescence, but are asymptomatic as adults. The true incidence of tarsal coalition is unknown, but it is often bilateral and is commonly found in other family members.

Athletes often report a history of vague, aching pain in the medial or lateral aspect of the foot over the subtalar joint that increases with activity. A history of frequent ankle sprains is also common. Walking over uneven ground or participating in athletic events that stress hindfoot tarsal joints, such as running, may precipitate pain. Physical examination may reveal a flatfoot, hindfoot valgus, loss of subtalar motion, and occasionally eversion of the foot. Attempts at inverting the foot may be met with resistance and produce pain; however, any condition involving the subtalar joint, such as rheumatoid arthritis or infection, can produce similar findings.

In addition to AP and lateral views, a 45° oblique view of the foot should be ordered, as it usually confirms the diagnosis of calcaneonavicular coalition (**Figure 39.7**). This coalition occasionally can be seen on the lateral view as a prolonged lateral aspect of the calcaneus approaching the navicular.

Diagnosing coalitions has become much easier with CT scans, as the subtalar joint is very difficult to evaluate with plain radiographs. If the oblique view does not reveal a coalition, then a CT scan should be ordered to identify coalitions between the talus and calcaneus (**Figure 39.8**). For the CT scan, the patient should be positioned with the hips and knees flexed and the soles of the feet on the table. Both feet should be imaged with 3- to 4-mm cuts. Other imaging techniques have been suggested for diagnosing tarsal coalitions, but the CT scan is simple, noninvasive, and accurate. It precisely defines the coalition and helps in planning treatment.

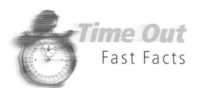

Time Out
Fast Facts

With accessory (tarsal) navicular, pain at the arch of the foot with shoe wear is often a problem.

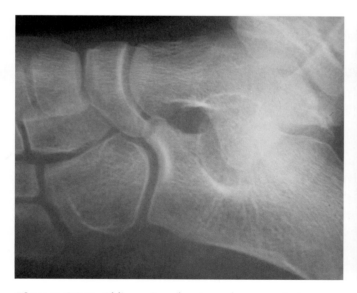

Figure 39.7 Oblique view showing calcaneonavicular coalition.

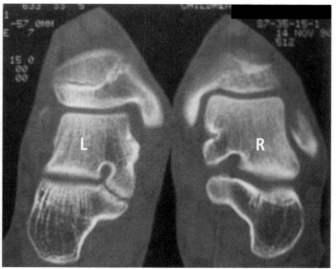

Figure 39.8 CT scan showing talocalcaneal coalition of the left foot.

Figure 39.9 A A large cornuate navicular with a small accessory ossicle. **B** A large accessory navicular. **C** An accessory navicular with a synchondrosis.

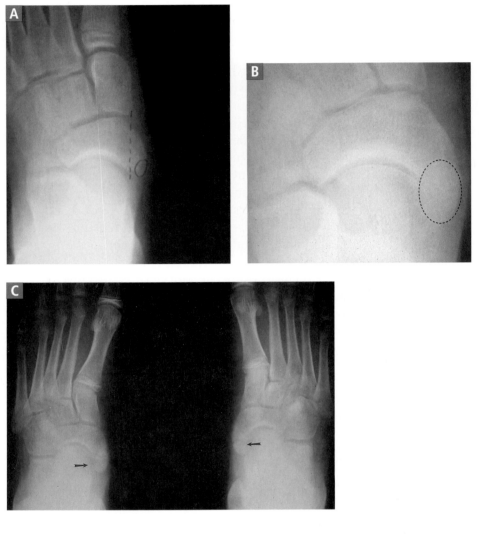

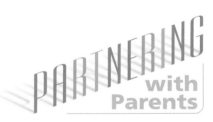

What is a cause of recurrent ankle sprains and subtalar stiffness?

Tarsal coalition—of which there are two main types—is the common cause of these complaints. Tarsal coalition is usually associated with foot and ankle pain and often requires surgery.

Surgery offers patients with symptomatic coalition the possibility of restoring motion to the tarsal joints, providing pain relief, and preventing arthritis in adjacent tarsal joints. The only nonsurgical treatment for tarsal coalition is immobilization with a cast or orthotics. The natural history is that some patients are asymptomatic as adutls. Because coalitions are often bilateral and more than one coalition can exist, a CT scan is recommended for all patients being considered for surgery.

Accessory Tarsal Navicular

The foot may have multiple accessory bones, the most common of which is the accessory navicular. This is about the only one of the accessory bones that causes problems. Athletes report a history of pain over the prominence on the medial aspect of the foot. Shoe wear is a problem. Physical examination reveals a prominence over the medial aspect of the foot at the distal end of the talus. Often, there is a bursa and erythema over the prominence. Inversion against stress will demonstrate that the posterior tibialis tendon is attached to the bony prominence. An AP or 45° eversion oblique view is recommended. Radiographically, the accessory navicular can appear as a small pea-shaped bone or as a large protrusion of the navicular (**Figure 39.9**).

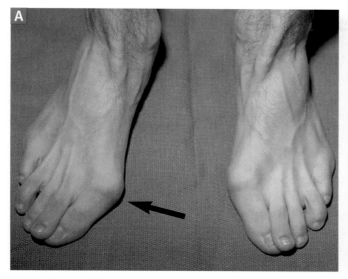

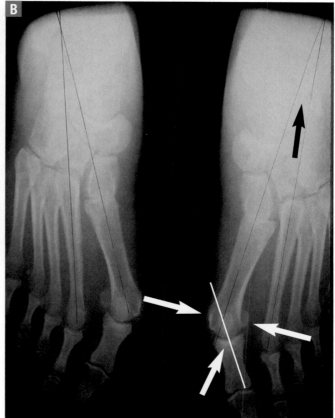

Figure 39.10 A Bilateral bunion. **B** Radiograph shows increased intermetatarsal and metatarsophalangeal angles and subluxation of the sesamoids.

Many athletes are asymptomatic or can be managed by stretching the shoes or benign neglect Simple excision is the treatment of choice for patients who are symptomatic. Return to play is possible 6 weeks after surgery.

Adolescent Bunion

Adolescent bunion is a prominence of the medial head of the first metatarsal, usually associated with hallux valgus (deviation of the great toe toward the lateral border of the foot) (**Figure 39.10**). Most patients seek medical attention because of the pain, the prominence, and difficulty with shoe wear. Unlike adults with this condition, adolescents usually have normal range of motion in the metatarsophalangeal joint. Girls between ages 10 to 15 years are more commonly affected than boys, and there is an increased familial incidence of this condition. The only restriction to play is that imposed by pain and difficulty with shoe wear.

Many patients require no treatment other than stretching the shoes and/or wearing wider shoes. Shoes wider than size D may need to be specially ordered. Patients who do not respond to nonoperative measures require surgical evaluation. However, surgical treatment of adolescent bunions is controversial, particularly with regard to the age of the patient and the type of procedure selected. Multiple surgical procedures are used, and the outcomes are variable. Many studies reveal a high recurrence rate following surgery.

A bunion can also occur over the head of the fifth metatarsal, a condition called a tailor bunion, or bunionette. Most often, stretching the shoes or buying wider shoes is all that is needed. Surgical excision is usually not necessary.

PARTNERING with Parents

Is a flatfoot in a child athlete a cause for concern?

Generally, no.

There are three types of flatfoot: flexible flatfoot with normal motion—this will require no treatment and will not be a source of pain or limitation in the future. It is the most common type of flat foot. Flexible flat foot with tight heel cord: This may require physical therapy and/or casting before restoring normal motion. It will not be a source of pain or limitation in the future. Rigid flat foot: this requires evaluation. The most common cause is tarsal coalition. Tarsal coalition often requires surgical intervention.

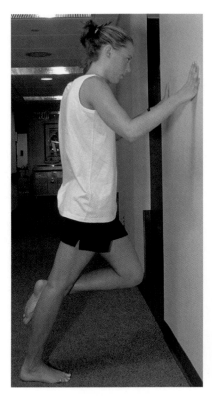

Figure 39.11 A simple technique that can be used to stretch the heel cord. The foot must be flat and the knee straight as a pushup is performed against the wall.

Heel Pain

Heel pain in young athletes is a frequent problem and can be difficult to manage. These athletes often report participation in multiple sports, but because of the pain, cannot participate in any sport. Athletes with heel pain should be asked about the type of shoes they wear and the type of surface on which they play. Cleated shoes or hard-surfaced playing fields are often the cause of the pain. However, pain can also be associated with a change in training technique or sport.

Physical examination should include assessment of subtalar joint motion and palpation over the insertion of the Achilles tendon, the plantar surface of the heel, and the plantar fascia to localize areas of tenderness. Plain AP and lateral radiographs typically appear normal. Note that the calcaneal apophysis normally appears dense and irregular; therefore, this finding should not be assumed as the cause of pain. The differential diagnosis includes Sever's disease, tarsal coalition, any inflammatory condition involving the subtalar joint, and benign bone tumors.

Treatment of heel pain is difficult and is generally relieved only with rest until the pain subsides, followed by gradual resumption of activity. Most athletes are unwilling to do this. If the Achilles tendon is tight, it should be stretched (**Figure 39.11**). Padding the heel with a heel cup or a shock-absorbing heel cushion may be helpful. Elevating the heel may provide some pain relief, as this transfers more weight onto the metatarsal heads. The athlete may have to stop wearing cleated shoes, particularly ones with only two cleats over the heel as these concentrate the force. Oral inflammatory agents can be tried, but steroid injection is contraindicated because steroids cause atrophy of the fat pad in the heel.

Sever's Disease

Sever's disease affects both girls and boys, approximately ages 8 to 11 years, and is characterized by bilateral heel pain that becomes worse with activity and, frequently, with wearing cleats. Physical examination reveals local tenderness with mediolateral compression of the calcaneal apophysis and often, heel cord contracture and weakness of the ankle dorsiflexors. Palpation of the plantar surface of the heel or the plantar fascia does not elicit pain. Radiographs are not indicted unless the child does not respond well to treatment. Radiographic evidence of fragmentation and sclerosis of the calcaneal apophysis is normal; it does not confirm the diagnosis (**Figure 39.12**). The heel cord should be stretched if it is tight. Treatment is the same as that for heel pain.

Kohler's Disease

Kohler's disease begins with unilateral foot pain and resolves spontaneously. Typically, symptoms appear in children between ages 2 to 9 years. Physical examination reveals local tenderness on palpation over the tarsal navicular. No other signs of inflammation are present, and pain is worse with weight-bearing. Radiographs of the foot reveal a decrease in the width of the navicular with increased bone density (**Figure 39.13**). Irregular ossification of the navicular, possibly a normal variant, has been seen in 30% of boys

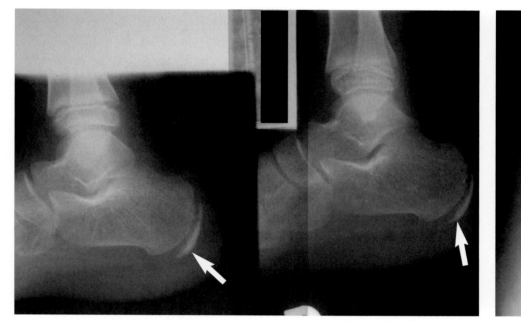

Figure 39.12 Radiographs of a patient referred for Sever's disease of the right heel. While the calcaneal apophysis is sclerotic, so was the apophysis of the left asymptomatic heel.

Figure 39.13 AP radiograph of the foot demonstrating fragmentation of the navicular (Kohler's disease).

and 20% of girls. Pain resolves gradually, and foot anatomy returns to normal, as seen on radiographs. When significant pain interferes with walking, immobilization in a short leg walking cast for an average of 6 weeks may be indicated.

Pump Bump

A pump bump, also called Haglund's deformity, is characterized by a bursa and large palpable prominence of the calcaneus. This condition is primarily a problem of shoe wear, and should respond to changing shoes, or in extreme cases, excision of the bony prominence.

Figure 39.14 Lateral radiograph of a cavus foot. Note increased heighth of the longitundinal arch.

Cavus Foot

A cavus foot is characterized by an arch that is elevated above normal. With a true cavus foot, the heel is often also in varus, and the first metatarsal is plantarflexed (**Figure 39.14**). Athletes with a cavus foot report pain and abnormal shoe wear and are often unable to participate in sports. The exact etiology of cavus foot is not known, but many patients have an underlying neuromuscular condition, which should be diligently investigated. Because of the possible underlying pathology, evaluation by a neurologist, an orthopaedist, or a specialist with expertise in neuromuscular disorders is recommended.

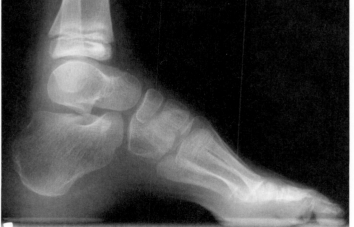

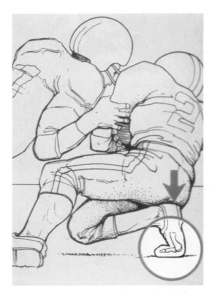

Figure 39.14 Turf toe is characterized by a dorsiflexion injury of the first metatarsophalangeal joint that damages the plantar structures.

Ingrown Toenails

Ingrown toenails generally do not occur until adolescence. Most often, the great toe is involved because of improper trimming of the nails or pressure from shoe wear. The nail edge thickens and overgrows the medial and lateral nail grooves. Granulation tissue forms secondary to infection in the skin fold.

Management consists of patient education on proper nail trimming and shoe wear. The foot should be soaked and cleaned several times a day, and when the nails are trimmed, the nail edges should be elevated with a small wooden stick and cotton. Trimming of the excess granulation tissue and, at times, the nail is required. Surgical treatment is indicated if nonoperative management fails.

Turf Toe

Turf toe typically develops in association with high-velocity sports that are played on either turf or a hard court, such as soccer and football. It is characterized by a dorsiflexion injury of the first metatarsophalangeal joint that damages the plantar structures (**Figure 39.14**). The plantar capsule, the flexor tendons, and the sesamoids can be involved as well. Management presents a challenge because protecting the first metatarsophalangeal joint is difficult, and compliance is challenging. A protective orthosis that extends out along the great toe can be used, as can taping in mild cases. Wearing protective shoes with a rigid dorsal toe box to prevent direct injury or a rigid sole to prevent hyperdorsiflexion can be beneficial as well.

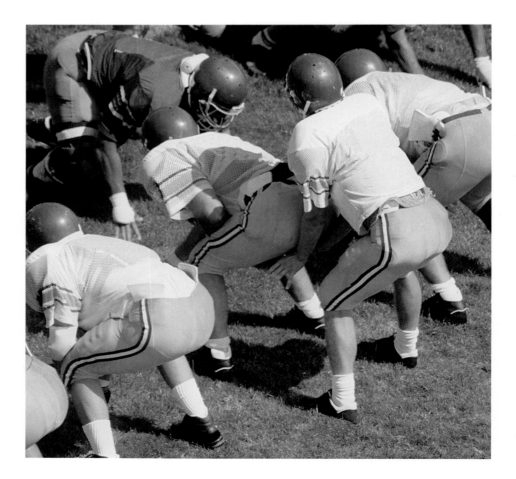

Reflex Sympathetic Dystrophy

Reflex sympathetic dystrophy (RSD) is a condition of unknown etiology, characterized by swelling, discoloration, and excessive perspiration or coolness. The hallmark symptom is pain out of proportion to the original injury. While rare, RSD can affect children, but is more common in adolescents. RSD usually develops after a fracture or sprain of the ankle or foot. Other findings on physical examination can include erythema, warmth, cold, clamminess, hypersensitivity to touch, and dermographia, which is an exaggerated response to scratching a letter on the skin. Patients often have a wheal and erythema that persists longer that normal. Findings should always be compared with the opposite, unaffected foot.

Initial management consists of physical therapy with range of motion and desensitization. Transcutaneous nerve stimulation can be attempted under the supervision of a physical therapist. If these measures fail, tricyclic antidepressants can be used. Lumbar sympathetic blocks can be used in refractory cases but these usually are not necessary.

Return to Play Guidelines

Return to play after foot fractures follows the general outline for return to play criteria under ankle sprains. After immobilization, the athlete must return to activities gradually. Strengthening, range of motion, and proprioceptive exercises are important. In general, walking must precede jogging, which must precede cutting activities. The athlete should have a full range of motion without pain prior to returning to play.

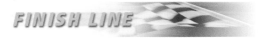

FINISH LINE

Most fractures of the foot in children heal uneventfully and without sequelae in 4 to 6 weeks. All fractures of the physis require careful evaluation to determine prognosis. Fractures that disrupt the physis and the articular surface of the joint need to be anatomically fixed in most instances. The fractures that are most rare are also often the most troublesome, including those that disrupt the physeal line and articular cartilage, fractures of the talus, fractures of the calcaneus, and a diaphyseal fracture of the fifth metatarsal.

For More Information

1. Carrol N: Fractures and dislocations of the tarsal bones, in Letts RM (ed): *Management of Pediatric Fractures.* New York, NY, Churchill Livingstone, 1994, pp 751–766.

2. Baxter MP: Fractures and dislocations of the metatarsals and phalanges of the foot, in Letts RM (ed): *The Management of Pediatric Fractures.* New York, NY, Churchill Livingstone, 1994, 767–788.

3. Sullivan JA: Ankle and foot in the pediatric athlete, in Stanitski CL, DeLee JC, Drez DD, Jr (ed): *Pediatric Orthopaedic Sports Medicine.* Philadelphia, PA, WB Saunders, 1994, pp 441–455.

4. Crawford AH: Fractures and dislocations of the foot and ankle, in Green NE, Swiontkowski MF (eds): *Skeletal Trauma in Children.* Philadelphia, PA, WB Saunders, 1994, vol 3, pp 449–516.

Appendices

This appendix includes official policy statements and recommendations issued by the American Academy of Orthopaedic Surgeons and by the American Academy of Pediatrics. These policy statements formally address many of the issues raised in *Care of the Young Athlete.*

AAOS Policy Statements

AAP Policy Statements

Anabolic Steroids to Enhance Athletic Performance

AMERICAN ACADEMY OF ORTHOPAEDIC SURGEONS

Document Number 1102

The American Academy of Orthopaedic Surgeons recognizes that although anabolic steroids may enhance athletic performance by increasing both the size and strength of athletes, their use can cause serious harmful physiological, pathological, and psychological effects.

The American Academy of Orthopaedic Surgeons believes that anabolic steroids should not be used to enhance performance or appearance, and that they be banned from use in all sports programs. We recommend that sports-governing bodies make every effort to deter and to detect their use. When feasible, the relevant sports medicine bodies should implement aggressive drug testing programs to detect their use and impose harsh penalties for those athletes who use them and those individuals or institutions who facilitate their use.

The Code of Ethics for Orthopaedic Surgeons specifically addresses this issue. It provides in Paragraph VII.B:

> ". . . It is unethical to prescribe controlled substances when they are not medically indicated. It is also unethical to prescribe substances for the sole purpose of enhancing athletic performance."

Use of anabolic steroids has been associated with the following adverse effects: increased risk of benign and malignant tumors of the liver, testes, and prostate; increased risk of serious cardiovascular disease; impaired reproductive functioning in males and females which may be irreversible; tendon weakening and potential ruptures; irreversible closure of bone growth centers in adolescents; menstrual irregularity; and psychological dependence which may lead to withdrawal symptoms and depression upon the cessation of use. Major personality changes may occur, manifested by increasing aggressiveness and intensity, which may lead to intense anti-social or psychotic behavior.

The use of performance-enhancing substances by athletes represents a most serious violation of ethical standards of organized sports activities at all levels, and should not be tolerated.

Recent legislation classifies anabolic steroids as controlled substances, and imposes restrictions on their distribution and use. The Academy strongly supports law enforcement agencies in their efforts to enforce existing legislation to control the distribution and use of anabolic steroids.

Health Care Coverage for Children At Risk

AMERICAN ACADEMY OF ORTHOPAEDIC SURGEONS
Document Number 1141

The American Academy of Orthopaedic Surgeons believes that health care coverage for all children is a mandatory investment in our nation's future.

Equitable access to health care is a social goal that has proved difficult to achieve in the U.S. The existence of substantial barriers in access to health care services for children is cause for particular concern. New initiatives are needed to address both financial and non-financial barriers to care for disenfranchised, "children at risk."[1,2]

The number of uninsured children in the U.S. has increased in the past decade. One in seven children is without health insurance. This is nearly one-fourth of the total uninsured population. When compared to the insured, they are four times more likely to report needing, but not receiving health care.[3]

Uninsured children are less likely to be immunized and less likely to receive care for acute and chronic illnesses and injuries. As a result, many untreated, mild conditions become complicated, costly problems with sometimes permanent impairment.

Uninsured children are most likely to be in low-income, "working poor" families. Most are in two-parent families with at least one working parent.

A growing number of children lack health care coverage because their parents work in the service sector, are self-employed, or are in temporary jobs—most of which fail to offer health insurance. Large and small employers have also tightened their budgets to remain competitive, resulting in reduced benefit packages for employees.[4]

Children with insurance fare better, but they can also face obstacles in accessing appropriate health care.

The costs of anemia, child abuse, preventable injuries, developmental delays and unattended malnutrition are critical health care expenditures. They also fall heavily on society's ledger in the form of social services, education or correctional systems.[5]

The American Academy of Orthopaedic Surgeons believes that the following principles should be the foundation of all children's health insurance programs:

1. All children should receive timely, appropriate health care coverage.

2. Children should be viewed as a population with unique health care needs. They should not be treated uniformly as small adults.

3. Basic health care coverage for all children should include well-child care, early detection programs, and treatment of chronic conditions.

4. Health insurance programs must address children with special needs, including those with heart disease, asthma, epilepsy, juvenile diabetes, cerebral palsy, and many other chronic illnesses.

Too often insurance plans do not recognize children with special needs and they are denied coverage for appropriate outpatient services and assistive devices.

Children with special musculoskeletal needs include those with spina bifida, club foot, dysplastic hip, scoliosis, congenital deformities, spinal cord injury, infections of bones and joints, osteogenesis imperfecta, muscular dystrophy, limb deficiency, limb deformity, juvenile arthritis, and musculoskeletal trauma.

5. The promotion of healthy lifestyles is critical for our nation's children, particularly adolescents.

Health problems that can be reduced through behavioral change must be addressed, including smoking, drug and alcohol use, violence, abuse, and neglect.

6. All health insurance programs for children should include these essential features:

- Coverage for all children

- Pediatric guidelines specific to children's health problems. Adult guidelines should not be applied uniformly to children

- Program oversight to ensure that the funds accomplish what they are intended to accomplish

- Pediatric quality assurance criteria against which to measure and evaluate program achievements

- Education programs for the public, as well as health and medical professionals, on the unique health care requirements of children

- Health education and health promotion programs for parents and children that promote healthy lifestyles and quality of life for children

7. Children's access to care must not be blocked by inadequate insurance or finances, nor by funding that is restricted to particular, or limited, diagnostic categories.

Among the most significant obstacles are financial barriers, including lack of adequate health insurance and inadequate funding for low-income children, and those with special health care needs. Other non-financial barriers arise due to the categorical nature for addressing children's health care needs.[6]

The American Academy of Orthopaedic Surgeons believes that additional measures must be taken to strengthen the public and private health care financing and delivery infrastructure in a manner that will ensure the highest quality of life for all children.

References

1. Newacheck PW, Hughes DC, Stoddard J: Children's Access to Primary Care: Differences by Race, Income and Insurance Status. *Pediatrics* 1996;97:26–32.

2. Freeman HE, Blendon RJ, Aiken LH, et al: Americans Report on their Access to Health Care. Health Affairs (Millwood). 1987;6:6–18.

3. Donelan K, Blendon R, Hill C, et al: Whatever Happened to the Health Insurance Crisis in the United States? *JAMA* 1996;276:1346–1350.

4. Hardy Havens DM, Hannan C: Children first. expanding health insurance coverage for children. *J Pediatr Health Care* 1997;11(2):85–88.

5. Eaton AP: Improving the Health Status of Children, American Academy of Pediatrics, National Association of Children's Hospitals, Testimony before the U.S. Senate, Committee on Labor and Human Resources. April 18, 1997.

6. Hughes DC, Halfon N, Brindis CD, et al: Improving Children's Access to Health Care: the Role of Decategorization. *Bull NY Acad Med* 1996;73:237–254.

Helmet Use by Motorcycle Drivers and Passengers, and Bicyclists

AMERICAN ACADEMY OF ORTHOPAEDIC SURGEONS
Document Number 1110

The American Academy of Orthopaedic Surgeons endorses laws mandating the use of helmets by motorcycle drivers and passengers, and bicyclists.

Orthopaedic surgeons, the medical specialists most often called upon to treat injuries to motorcyclists, believe a significant reduction in fatalities and head injuries could be effected through the implementation of laws mandating the use of helmets by all motorcycle and bicycle drivers and passengers. The American Academy of Orthopaedic Surgeons strongly endorses such mandatory helmet laws.

Numerous studies in various parts of the United States have shown that helmet use reduces the severity and cost associated with injuries to motorcycle riders. Federal efforts beginning with the Highway Safety Act of 1966 achieved the passage of state laws mandating helmet use and by 1975, 47 states had enacted such laws. With the Highway Safety Act of 1977, however, Section 208 of which relaxed the pressure on states to have helmet laws, the federal government created the opportunity to measure the effectiveness of helmet use when 27 states repealed their helmet laws in the following three years.

In 1991, the U.S. Congress attached a provision to its federal highway legislation dictating that states lacking mandatory comprehensive motorcycle helmet laws after September 30, 1993, will have 1.5 percent of their federal highway construction funds for the following fiscal year reallocated to safety programs. If a state still does not have the mandatory laws in place by September 30, 1994, the safety program reallocation will rise to 3 percent. In the mid 1980s, Congress used a similar provision to force all states to raise their legal drinking age to 21. Congressional opponents of the bill have attempted to introduce other legislation that would repeal this provision.

Objective analysis of data from the mid 70s (when helmet laws were widespread) and the late 70s (when more than half the states had repealed such laws) shows clearly that head injuries and fatalities of motorcycle riders are reduced when motorcyclists wear helmets. Moreover, the costs associated with treating motorcycle riders' head injuries have been demonstrated to be significantly reduced—up to 80 percent in one university study—when helmet laws are in effect.

The American Academy of Orthopaedic Surgeons believes that issues of personal freedom should be seen in the context of the fact that the public at large incurs a major part of the cost for injuries to motorcycle riders.

The repeal of helmet laws in many states was based on issues involving some motorcyclists' claims that mandatory use laws infringed on their right to personal freedom. While it can be argued that the states' laws mandating that motorcyclists be licensed to operate the vehicle are a similar infringement, the more important issue is the cost borne by society when a motorcyclist is injured in an accident. Numerous studies have shown that in cases involving motorcyclists who were not wearing helmets, head injuries were more severe, requiring longer, more expensive hospitalization and rehabilitation. Moreover, it has been shown that the public at large bears a major portion of these increased costs, both in the cases where the injured patients' insurance does not cover all the costs associated with care and through the increasing cost of medical insurance premiums. Society must evaluate the claim of infringement on freedom versus the funding of these costs.

The American Academy of Orthopaedic Surgeons believes that the current diversity of state helmet laws provides too little protection for motorcycle riders and for society at large.

Currently, 25 states have comprehensive motorcycle helmet laws in place. Another 22 have partial requirements for minors, student drivers, or passengers. Three states—Illinois, Iowa, and Colorado—have no helmet requirements at all. With federal statistics showing that a motorcycle driver or passenger is twice as likely to receive a head injury in an accident if he or she is not wearing a helmet, such inconsistencies in state laws seem an egregious lack of responsibility by the legislatures in many states.

The American Academy of Orthopaedic Surgeons believes that mandatory helmet laws should be expanded to cover bicyclists as well as motorcycle riders.

In the past several years, thousands of Americans of all ages have taken up bicycling for fun, health and fitness benefits, and as a mode of transportation. With this increase in popularity, however, has come an increase in bicycle-related injury and death.

Each year almost 1,200 bicyclists are killed, 75 percent of those are in collisions between bicycles and motor vehicles. In addition, more than one million bicycle-related injuries are treated each year.

Too few bicycle enthusiasts protect themselves from injury with safety helmets. Three-fourths of bicycle-related deaths and one-third of the injuries involve injury to the head or face. Although studies show that bicycle helmets can reduce head injuries by up to 95 percent, the U.S. Centers for Disease Control and Prevention reports that fewer than 10 percent of all cyclists wear protective helmets, and fewer than 2 percent of those under the age of 15 wear them.

Because one-third of bicycle-related deaths and two-thirds of the injuries involve children under the age of 15, most bicycle safety programs in the United States have been targeted at children. Five states and several more counties currently require the use of bicycle helmets, generally for children under age 16. There are two national safety standards for bicycle helmets sold in this country. Only helmets labeled as meeting the safety requirements of the Snell Memorial Foundation of the American National Standards Institute (ANSI) should be purchased and worn. Bicycle safety programs must also focus on wearing the proper clothing, proper maintenance of the bicycle, and understanding and following the rules of the road.

Injuries from In-Line Skating

AMERICAN ACADEMY OF ORTHOPAEDIC SURGEONS
Document Number 1127

The American Academy of Orthopaedic Surgeons believes that the public should be informed of the dangers and injuries that can occur in the recreational sport called in-line skating and strongly urges proper precautions to prevent and minimize those injuries.

More than 12 million Americans have taken up the new sport of in-line skating, which combines roller skating with ice skating by aligning rollers in the shape of a single blade. In-line skaters may easily reach speeds of more than 25 mph. Whether skating fast or standing still, many in-line skaters have sustained injuries that are preventable.

The number of injuries due to in-line skating is rapidly increasing. Hospital emergency rooms reported 75,922 in-line skating injuries in 1994. More than 40% of these injuries were a fracture or dislocation, 24% were injuries of the wrist, and 5% were injuries of the head. Although head injuries are relatively less common, they can be life threatening, very expensive, and cause long-term disability. The estimated yearly cost of emergency room treatment due to in-line skating injuries is $346 million. This does not include injuries treated in physicians' offices or bruises and scrapes that were never seen or treated.

To reduce the risk of serious injury, the American Academy of Orthopaedic Surgeons strongly urges in-line skaters to follow these safety measures:

- learn the basic skills of the sport, particularly how to stop properly, before venturing into vehicular or pedestrian traffic

- wear a helmet, wrist protectors, and knee and elbow pads

- always put on protective gear before putting on your skates

- perform warm-up exercises before and after skating

- obey traffic signals, stay at the right side of the road and don't weave in and out of lanes

- avoid skating in crowded walkways

Skate boots must fit properly to avoid irritation. The following tips should be considered.

- Don't buy boots that put too much pressure on any area of your foot; the pressure can cause blisters.

- Choose the boot size at the end of the day or after training, when feet will be at their largest.

- When selecting the size of the boot, wear the same type of sock that will be worn when skating.

- Kick both feet into the back of the boots before buckling and skating.

- Be certain the heel doesn't move up and down in the boot during skating.

School Screening Programs for the Early Detection of Scoliosis

AMERICAN ACADEMY OF ORTHOPAEDIC SURGEONS

Document Number 1122

Prevention of severe scoliosis is a major commitment of orthopaedic surgeons. In August 1984, the American Academy of Orthopaedic Surgeons issued a position statement strongly endorsing the concept of school screening for the early detection of scoliosis in children. Scoliosis is a spine deformity characterized by lateral and rotational curvature of the spine. The deformity usually develops during the preadolescent years. In most patients the cause is still unknown and thus the deformity is labeled "idiopathic." In those patients in whom a cause can be identified, neuromuscular disease or congenital abnormality of the spine are the most common findings. The number of adults affected with a significant scoliotic deformity is estimated to be several hundred thousand.

The purpose of school screening is to detect scoliosis at an early stage when the deformity is mild and likely to otherwise go unnoticed. It is at this early stage that bracing programs may be effective in halting progression of the deformity and thus prevent the need for surgical treatment. In addition, the children with more significant scoliosis, who often have no other symptoms, may be detected at a time when surgical treatment is more effective.

The American Academy of Orthopaedic Surgeons and the Scoliosis Research Society continue to support the principle of school screening for scoliosis.

Although its predictive value has not been established to the satisfaction of all, scoliosis screening has been an important factor in improving knowledge about this spinal deformity. Refinements in screening techniques have been made since 1984 and, as knowledge about scoliosis is gained, additional modifications may be necessary.

School screening for scoliosis has expanded rapidly during the past decade and has been important in improving the understanding of this incompletely understood spine deformity. As a result, it is now possible to target more precisely the age at which screening is most beneficial. Because girls achieve adolescence about two years before boys and because girls are afflicted with a magnitude of scoliosis requiring treatment about three to four times more frequently than boys, different screening guidelines are emerging for girls and boys. While the optimum age for screening has not been established with certainty, a reasonable approach would be to screen girls twice, at 10 and 12 (grades 5 and 7), and boys once, at age 13 or 14 (grades 8 or 9).

The American Academy of Orthopaedic Surgeons and the Scoliosis Research Society believe that school screening personnel should be educated in the detection of spinal deformity.

Screening should always include the forward bending test, the most specific test for true scoliosis, but no single test is completely reliable for screening. Therefore, considerable judgment on the part of the screener is necessary to achieve an appropriate referral rate and to avoid unnecessary referrals. To meet the objective of the screening program, the American Academy of Orthopaedic Surgeons and the Scoliosis Research Society recognize the need to keep the referral of students to a minimum.

The American Academy of Orthopaedic Surgeons and the Scoliosis Research Society maintain their commitment to avoid the inappropriate use of spine x-rays.

Not all children referred as a result of screening require x-rays. If x-rays are needed, physicians should take necessary precautions to limit the patient's exposure to radiation.

Educational materials which provide more specific guidelines for conducting school screening programs for scoliosis are available to physicians and school authorities. Further information may be obtained from the Academy and the Scoliosis Research Society.

Sledding Safety

AMERICAN ACADEMY OF ORTHOPAEDIC SURGEONS
Document Number 1137

Every year, thousands of youths and adults are injured sledding down hills in city parks, streets, and resort areas. In 1995, hospital emergency rooms treated 54,727 injuries related to sleds, toboggans, and inflated or plastic tubes and disks used in sledding, according to the National Electronic Injury Surveillance System of the U.S. Consumer Product Safety Commission. The medical, legal, and insurance costs were $365 million. Half of all emergency visits were for injuries to arms and legs; 17 percent, spine; 15 percent, head; and 11 percent facial injuries.

Two-thirds of the injuries were sustained by youths age 14 and younger. Younger children have proportionally larger heads and higher centers of gravity than do older children and adolescents. When the injuries to youths and young adults age 15-24 are included, the 0-24 age group accounts for 85 percent of the total injuries and more than 80 percent of the total cost. From 1991 through 1995, there were 250,361 injuries related to sledding treated in hospital emergency rooms. The economic impact was $1.79 billion.

The American Academy of Orthopaedic Surgeons recommends the following safety guidelines to improve sledding safety:

Essential

- Sled only in designated areas free of fixed objects such as trees, posts, and fences.

- Children in these areas must be supervised by parents or adults.

- All participants must sit in a forward-facing position, steering with their feet or a rope tied to the steering handles of the sled. No one should sled head-first down a slope.

- Do not sled on slopes that end in a street, drop off, parking lot, river, or pond.

Preferred

- Children under 12 years old should sled wearing a helmet.

- Wear layers of clothing for protection from injuries.

- Do not sit/slide on plastic sheets or other materials that can be pierced by objects on the ground.

- Use a sled with runners and a steering mechanism, which is safer than toboggans or snow disks.

- Sled in well-lighted areas when choosing evening activities.

Copyright © 1997, American Academy of Orthopaedic Surgeons

Support of Sports and Recreational Programs for Physically Disabled People

AMERICAN ACADEMY OF ORTHOPAEDIC SURGEONS
Document Number 1123

The American Academy of Orthopaedic Surgeons strongly supports the expressed interests of people with physical disabilities of all ages who want to participate in sports and recreational programs.

Participation in such activities can be fulfilling, increase physical fitness, and enhance personal image. Having the ability to set and achieve goals and the capability to deal with success and failure in the competitive arena are important accomplishments.

The American Academy of Orthopaedic Surgeons believes there should be continued attempts to organize efforts among existing sports and recreational groups to foster communication and improve programs.

Sports and recreational programs for people with physical disabilities, as they exist today, have developed largely through the efforts of a multitude of organizations and individuals, both lay and professional. The full potential of these efforts has not yet been fully realized because no central organizing body exists.

Recreational programs have originated in the home, school, community, and camp. Sports competitions for people with physical disabilities exist at the local, state, national, and international levels within separate organizations whose activities may focus on a specific kind of disability. There is presently no central organizing body that coordinates these efforts.

The American Academy of Orthopaedic Surgeons urges further coordination of efforts to increase the availability of sports and recreation programs for people with physical disabilities. The American Academy of Orthopaedic Surgeons suggests there is a need for public education on the subject.

There are almost 9 million injuries annually that require medical attention, and more than 300,000 of those injuries caused either permanent partial or permanent total disability. In addition, there is a significant number of people with either congenital or non-traumatic acquired disability. Spurred by the pioneer efforts of the original wheelchair athletes, these millions of people have developed a deep interest in recreational and competitive sports activities. When they decide to participate however, they often face additional handicaps. Special education and physical education teachers, counselors, administrators, some physicians, and the general public often are unaware of available resources and the potential of people with physical disabilities.

Sports and recreation activities for people with physical disabilities are beneficial provided the necessary precautions are taken. However, some people with physical disabilities do have special considerations, including insensitive skin, joint deformities, difficulties in balance and coordination, and temperature regulation. Most sports and recreational activities can be adapted for them. Physicians involved with disabled athletes have a role to play in assessing the medical needs limitations. Medical precautions should be appropriate without needless restrictions.

The American Academy of Orthopaedic Surgeons recognizes a need for ongoing research among groups involved in athletic programs for people with physical disabilities.

The American Academy of Orthopaedic Surgeons is committed to the further advancement of sports and recreational activities for people with physical disabilities. The American Academy of Orthopaedic Surgeons recognizes the need for continued research to enhance the ability of people with disabilities to participate in both competitive and recreational sports.

The Need for Daily Physical Activity

AMERICAN ACADEMY OF ORTHOPAEDIC SURGEONS

Document Number 1138

Medical research has proven that people can substantially improve their health and quality of life with moderate physical activity. However, 25 percent of American adults report they don't engage in any physical activity in their leisure time, and 60 percent don't engage in vigorous activity. This is a problem of national concern because of the aging population and evidence that adults exercise less as they get older. By the year 2030, one in five people will be 65 or older and 12 percent of the elderly will be 85 or older.

Some people may not exercise because they don't like vigorous activity, don't have the time, or are worried that it will aggravate a medical condition. However, researchers have found that moderate physical activity at least 30 minutes a day will provide significant health benefits. Even people with chronic conditions such as osteoarthritis and osteoporosis, can improve their health and quality of life with regular, moderate amounts of physical activity.

The American Academy of Orthopaedic Surgeons and the American Geriatrics Society recommend that adults engage in moderate physical activity at least 30 minutes a day on a regular basis.

Regular physical activity slows the loss of muscle mass, strengthens bones and reduces joint and muscle pain. Physical activity also improves mobility, balance, and sleep. These factors all reduce the risk of falling and sustaining a serious injury such as a hip fracture.

Physical activity is safe and beneficial for people with arthritis, high blood pressure, osteoporosis, and other chronic conditions. In fact, the lack of activity can make the condition worse or, at least, make it difficult to live with.

The American Academy of Orthopaedic Surgeons and American Geriatrics Society recommend that adults engage in a variety of daily activities to ensure continued interest and participation.

While some people may enjoy participating in a regularly-scheduled exercise class, other adults can achieve healthful benefits from daily activities such as brisk walking, bicycle riding, swimming, dancing, housework, and gardening.

Adults are encouraged to do different physical activities on different days, and even in short intervals of 15 minutes in the morning and 15 minutes in the afternoon. The healthful benefits of physical activity are cumulative; however, the benefits diminish quickly when physical activity ceases.

The Use of Knee Braces

AMERICAN ACADEMY OF ORTHOPAEDIC SURGEONS
Document Number 1124

Orthopaedists are the medical specialists most often called upon to diagnose and treat injuries to the knee joint. Through the American Academy of Orthopaedic Surgeons, orthopaedists have undertaken the continuing review of the effectiveness of knee braces in the prevention and treatment of knee injuries. The Academy's goal has been to provide physicians and others in the medical community with an informed assessment of the state of the art of knee bracing and to provide guidance to physicians and others in the use of knee braces.

The Academy's 1984 *Knee Braces Seminar Report* classified existing knee braces into three groups:

- **prophylactic knee braces** which are designed to prevent or reduce the severity of knee injuries

- **rehabilitative knee braces** which are designed to allow protected motion of injured knees or knees that have been treated operatively

- **functional knee braces** which are designed to provide stability for the unstable knee.

The 1984 seminar has been followed by continuing examination of the developments in knee bracing and of the published literature in the field. Based on this examination by individual physicians, faculty at continuing medical education programs and by relevant Academy committees, the Academy has adopted the following statement.

AAOS believes that the routine use of prophylactic knee braces currently available has not been proven effective in reducing the number or severity of knee injuries. In some circumstances, such braces may even have the potential to be a contributing factor to injury.

Because knee injuries are common in many sports, particularly contact sports such as football, there is a widespread concern about their impact on players and teams. Non-contact stresses in many other sports also can produce significant knee injuries. Tears of the ligaments and menisci and damage to the articular cartilage of the knee may result in lost playing time and may lead to permanent disability. Most players, coaches, athletic trainers and physicians would welcome a device such as a brace that would reduce the incidence and/or the severity of injuries to the knee. Current prophylactic knee braces are intended to and may mistakenly be believed to meet those goals.

Scientific studies undertaken to demonstrate the effectiveness of prophylactic knee braces in reducing the frequency and severity of knee injuries have failed to show consistent findings regarding the braces that are currently available. Moreover, few studies in this field have included objective data collected over a significant period of time. Injuries to the medial collateral ligament have been the most studied, and no consistent reduction in these injuries attributable to the use of a particular brace has been demonstrated. No reduction in injuries to the anterior cruciate ligament or the menisci have been demonstrated. In some studies there has been increased severity of certain injuries.

AAOS believes that to require players to use knee braces "just in case they might help" is not supported by the studies that have examined the effectiveness of such braces.

The intent of this statement is not to argue that prophylactic knee braces do not work and never will. Instead it is to state that medical science has not demonstrated that, as currently constructed and used, they are effective today. There is no credible, long-term, scientifically conducted study that supports using knee braces on otherwise healthy players. The Academy is concerned that significant amounts of money are being expended in schools in the United States for equipment that is, at best, only hoped to be effective in reducing the frequency or severity of knee injuries.

In regard to other categories of braces, AAOS believes that rehabilitative knee braces and functional knee braces can be effective in many treatment programs, and that this efficacy has been demonstrated by long-term scientifically conducted studies.

Types of braces other than prophylactic knee braces have different structural designs and have been developed to help treat specific problems stemming from injury or disease. *Rehabilitative knee braces* have been designed to provide a compromise between protection and motion. That is, they allow the knee to move, but within specific limits, which has been shown to be beneficial to the injured knee. Rehabilitative knee braces generally are more effective in protecting against excessive flexion and extension than in protecting against anterior and posterior motion.

Functional knee braces aid in the control of unstable knees. Studies have shown that some of the currently available braces are very effective in controlling abnormal motions under low load conditions but not under high loading conditions that occur during many athletic activities. Most studies designed to test whether functional knee braces protect against the knee "giving way" have demonstrated some beneficial effect of the brace. However, the patient and the physician must guard against a false sense of security evoked by the use of such a brace; bio-mechanical studies show that functional knee braces do not restore normal knee stability under high forces related to certain activities. However, when it is properly fitted, used in conjunction with a knee rehabilitation program, and the patient modifies his or her activities appropriately, a functional knee brace can provide an important adjunct in the treatment of knee instability.

Trampolines and Trampoline Safety

AMERICAN ACADEMY OF ORTHOPAEDIC SURGEONS
Document Number 1135

The number and severity of injuries resulting from the use of trampolines is significant and increasing. Hospital emergency rooms treated 52,103 trampoline injuries sustained by children under age 15 in 1995. The estimated cost of medical, legal, insurance, and disability costs and other expenses in 1995 was $272.6 million. Even very young children ages 5 to 9 are at risk; 19,454 injuries related to trampolines were treated in emergency rooms at a cost of $99.8 million. The most common injuries are sprains and fractures, often severe, which usually result from a fall through the trampoline or an uncontrolled maneuver. Although severe or life-threatening injuries are not common, they do occur and can result in paralysis or, rarely, death. Use of the trampoline by more than one child further increases the risk of injury through collisions among jumpers or the catapulting of jumpers off the trampoline.

In an effort to reduce the number and severity of injuries resulting from the use of trampolines, the American Academy of Orthopaedic Surgeons recommends routine observation of the following guidelines:

- Use of trampolines for physical education, competitive gymnastics, diving training, and other similar activities requires careful adult supervision and proper safety measures.

- Trampolines should not be used for unsupervised recreational activity.

- Competent adult supervision and instruction is needed for children at all times.

- Only one participant should use a trampoline at any time.

- Spotters should be present when participants are jumping.

- Somersaults or high risk maneuvers should be avoided without proper supervision and instruction; these maneuvers should be done only with proper use of protective equipment, such as a harness.

- The trampoline jumping surface should be placed at ground level.

- The supporting bars, strings, and surrounding landing surfaces should have adequate protective padding.

A Self-Appraisal Checklist of Health Supervision in Scholastic Athletic Programs

AMERICAN ACADEMY OF PEDIATRICS

Introduction

This checklist has been developed for use by school boards, superintendents, principals, athletic directors, coaches, trainers, and team physicians who are dedicated to providing excellent medical supervision for high school and collegiate athletic programs. Sports medicine program staff may include one to several team physicians, school nurses, and athletic trainers.

The checklist consists of criteria for evaluation of the health aspects of scholastic athletic programs. Use of the checklist will help in evaluating the strengths of the sports medicine program and in defining areas that need improvement. The checklist is designed to be a permanent reference source in each school. Evaluations should be performed annually to ensure continued optimal supervision of school sports and to provide for the safety and protection of athletes.

The checklist is organized into four major categories (I. Organization, Administration, and Staffing; II. Facilities and Equipment; III. Event Coverage; IV. Education) that represent the essential aspects of a sports medicine program. The checklist, therefore, can be useful to personnel in surveying and assessing the existing program and comparing it to an ideal program as identified by the checklist items.

How to Use the Checklist

The Self-Appraisal Checklist for Health Supervision in Scholastic Athletic Programs contains 47 items. Each item represents a criterion against which a sports medicine program can be judged. Evaluative criteria are presented in the form of statements that describe attributes of health supervision of athletes. Each statement sets forth a condition deemed highly desirable for an exemplary program. The evaluator should respond as objectively as possible to each statement as it describes the local program and should record the appraisal by circling:

3 if the evaluator determines that the statement *always* describes the program

2 if the evaluator determines that the statement *sometimes* describes the program

1 if the evaluator determines that the statement *seldom* describes the program

0 if the evaluator determines that the statement *never* describes the program.

A total "possible" score is given for each category, based upon a 3 rating for each statement. The actual score is the total of the ratings given by the evaluator. When the checklist has been completed, program areas needing improvement may be identified on the basis of discrepancies between actual and possible scores.

COMMITTEE ON SPORTS MEDICINE AND FITNESS, 1992–1993

William L. Risser, MD, Chair

Steven J. Anderson, MD

Stephen P. Bolduc, MD

Sally S. Harris, MD

Gregory L. Landry, MD

David M. Orenstein, MD

Angela D. Smith, MD

Liaison Representatives

Kathryn Keely, MD

Canadian Paediatric Society

Richard Malacrea

National Athletic Trainers' Association

Judith C. Young, MD

National Association for Sport and Physical Education

AAP Section Representatives

Arthur M. Pappas, MD

Section on Orthopaedics

Reginald L. Washington, MD

Section on Cardiology

Consultant

Oded Bar-Or, MD

Canadian Paediatric Society

Circle appropriate response as it relates to your program

3 = Always   1 = Seldom

2 = Sometimes   0 = Never

I. Organization, Administration, and Staffing

Possible score - 39 points   Actual score _____ points

1. The organization and function of the school's sports medicine program is under direction of a licensed physician with competence in sports medicine	3	2	1	0
2. Written job descriptions outlining duties and responsibilities for each member of the sports medicine staff are available.	3	2	1	0
3. The medical care staff in the sports medicine program is involved in protecting the health of all athletes, is on call during practices, and attends all sports events that have high injury rates.	3	2	1	0
4. An athletic trainer, certified by the National Athletic Trainers' Association, is responsible for the daily operation of the sports medicine program.	3	2	1	0
5. The primary responsibility of the athletic trainer is to reduce the risk of sports injuries, and, if a physician is not present, initiate their evaluation, treatment, and rehabilitation. Teaching, coaching, or other department functions should not interfere with these responsibilities.	3	2	1	0
6. School administrators and coaches support and follow recommendations of the sports medicine staff regarding treatment, rehabilitation, and the necessity to exclude certain athletes from participation for medical reasons.	3	2	1	0
7. A preparticipation evaluation including history and a medical examination is performed on each prospective competitor at least every 2 years.	3	2	1	0
8. There is a file, accessible to the sports medicine staff, of individual health evaluation reports and explanations of major injuries including test results and consultants' reports.	3	2	1	0
9. There is an ongoing method for maintaining records of weight, injuries, illnesses, and other pertinent medical information regarding the athlete.	3	2	1	0
10. Parents' or guardians' consent for emergency medical treatment is on file with the school health personnel and is available to the sports medicine staff.	3	2	1	0
11. A comprehensive insurance program for care of injuries to athletes is required.	3	2	1	0
12. A regular systematic evaluation is used to review the effectiveness of the total program.	3	2	1	0
13. Equal access to the sports medicine program is provided to all athletes.	3	2	1	0

I. Facilities and Equipment

Possible score - 51 points   Actual score _____ points

1. Adequate funding is allocated to the sports medicine program for:				
a. expendable supplies	3	2	1	0
b. capital improvements	3	2	1	0
c. continuing education	3	2	1	0
d. repairs and maintenance	3	2	1	0

2. There is adequate space to handle the flow and routine care of the
    athletic population:
    a. conditioning and reconditioning programs   3   2   1   0
    b. prophylactic taping, wrapping, and padding   3   2   1   0
    c. privacy for physical examinations   3   2   1   0
    d. office space or station for record keeping   3   2   1   0

3. There is an adequate supply of emergency equipment readily   3   2   1   0
    available, ie:
    a. crutches   b. cervical collar
    c. icepacks   d. knee immobilizers
    e. equipment for maintaining an airway   f. neck immobilization devices
    g. slings   h. spine board
    i. splints   j. stretcher
    k. rubber gloves

4. An adequate supply of first aid supplies is readily available.   3   2   1   0

5. There is an adequate and readily available communication system between the athletic
    participation areas and medical or paramedical assistance.   3   2   1   0

6. There is a written plan for the transportation of injured athletes in practice
    and in contests.   3   2   1   0

7. Physical treatment modalities to provide heat and cold to body parts are available.   3   2   1   0

8. An ample supply of ice and water is readily available.   3   2   1   0

9. The electrical supply in the sports medicine treatment area is controlled by ground
    fault interrupters at the outlet or control panel.   3   2   1   0

10. The sports medicine facility is available for the use of the athletic trainers from all
    competing teams.   3   2   1   0

III. Event Coverage

Possible score - 24 points   Actual score _____ points

1. All coaches and sports medicine personnel are trained in CPR, emergency manage-
    ment of life-threatening injuries, and universal precaution techniques.   3   2   1   0

2. An effective communication system is available to permit immediate access to a
    medical emergency unit.   3   2   1   0

3. A suitable vehicle and designated driver are available for immediate transportation
    of the injured athlete to a designated medical resource that has already been alerted.   3   2   1   0

4. The playing area is surveyed before each event to identify and correct hazards.   3   2   1   0

5. Emergency first aid supplies and equipment are readily available to all
    competing teams.   3   2   1   0

6. Visiting teams have ready access to facilities for care of an injured athlete.   3   2   1   0

7. Environmental conditions are monitored by sling psychrometer or other means
    during hot, and/or humid, weather and appropriate measures are taken to protect
    the athlete from heat-related illness.   3   2   1   0

8. An ample supply of drinking water and ice is available at all times.   3   2   1   0

IV. Education

Possible score - 27 points   Actual score _____ points

1. The sports medicine staff conducts the following educational sessions for all athletes, covering the following:
   a. heat-related illness   3 2 1 0
   b. nutrition   3 2 1 0
   c. harmful effects of all drugs, including alcohol, tobacco, and performance-enhancing products   3 2 1 0
   d. general hygiene for the athlete   3 2 1 0
   e. rehabilitation of injury   3 2 1 0
   f. body weight management/control and eating disorders   3 2 1 0

2. The school makes available, for selected students, an elective course for athletic trainer aides.   3 2 1 0

3. Development activities and continuing education for sports medicine staff are encouraged and funded.   3   2 1 0

4. Aides to the certified staff personnel in the sports program have had training in first aid, basic life support, CPR, and universal precaution techniques.   3 2 1 0

Summary of Scores

	Possible Score	Actual Score	%
Part I. Organization, Administration, and Staffing	39		
Part II. Facilities and Equipment	51		
Part III. Event Coverage	24		
Part IV. Education	27		
Totals	141		

A total "possible" score is given for each category, based upon a 3 rating for each statement. The actual score is the total of the ratings given by the evaluator. When the checklist has been completed, program areas needing improvement may be identified on the basis of discrepancies between actual and possible scores.

This publication has been approved by the Council on Child and Adolescent Health.

The recommendations in this publication do not indicate an exclusive course of treatment or serve as a standard of medical care. Variations, taking into account individual circumstances, may be appropriate.

For additional copies of *A Self-Appraisal Checklist for Health Supervision in Scholastic Athletic Programs,* send pre-paid orders to:

American Academy of Pediatrics, Department of Publications, PO Box 927, Elk Grove Village, IL 60007

Price: $2.95 each

SM0001

For information on quantity discounts, call the Publications Department at the American Academy of Pediatrics, 800/433-7905, ext 7905.

Copyright ©1993

Adolescents and Anabolic Steroids: A Subject Review (RE9720)

AMERICAN ACADEMY OF PEDIATRICS
Committee on Sports Medicine and Fitness
Volume 99, Number 6
June 1997

ABSTRACT. *This revision of a previous statement by the American Academy of Pediatrics provides current information on anabolic steroid use by young athletes. It provides the information needed to enable pediatricians to discuss the benefits and risks of anabolic steroids in a well-informed, nonjudgmental fashion.*

Definition of the Problem

The use of a variety of substances has long accompanied efforts to enhance athletic performance. [1] Such use is not limited to professional and Olympic athletes. Studies focusing on anabolic steroids have shown a continuing and significant increase of use among adolescent athletes and nonathletes alike (Table 1). [2–5] In response to the alarming high rate of use of anabolic steroids and the attendant medical risks, policy statements were issued by the American Academy of Pediatrics in 1989 and the American College of Sports Medicine in 1977 and 1984. [6–8] These statements condemn the use of anabolic steroids but acknowledge that they may enhance strength. It has become evident that prohibitions against anabolic steroid use and

Table 1 *Prevalence of Androgenic Anabolic Steroid Abuse**

Population	Average Age of Users	Number of Respondents	Prevalence (%)	Ref.
Bodybuilders				31
Men	27 years	108	54.6	
Women	24 years	68	10.3	
College students (age not reported)				32
Athletes	1970		15	
	1976		20	
	1980		20	
	1984		20	
Nonathletes	1984		1	
Male bodybuilders	25 years	138	38.4	33
12th-grade male students	17.2 years	3403	6.6	3
11th-grade male (age not reported) students		853	11.1	4
High school students				2
Male	16 years	462	5.0	
Female		439	1.4	
High school students				
2113 total (sic)				
534 grade 9				
496 grade 10				
518 grade 11				
542 grade 12				
Male		1028	6.5	
Female		1085	2.5	

* Adapted from Smith and Perry.15

claims that steroids lack efficacy or produce harm have been insufficient to curtail their use. [9–11]

The American Academy of Pediatrics continues to condemn the use of anabolic steroids for body building or enhancement of sports performance. However, many users, their parents, and their coaches feel that anabolic steroids are useful and even necessary for optimal performance. The Academy's strong opposition to anabolic steroid use may be offset by societies' high rewards for success in sports and a "win at all costs" attitude. Adolescents must interpret mixed messages about the appropriateness of anabolic steroid use as well as ambiguous messages about the benefits and risks of using anabolic steroids. There is a clear need for input that is objective, rational, nonbiased, and readily available to the adolescent. If pediatricians and other pediatric health care advocates are to serve as a much needed "voice of reason," they must be familiar with current information on the risks and benefits of anabolic steroids, use patterns, and the incentives and disincentives for use.

Background

Nonmedical use of anabolic steroids was initially reported in weight lifters and other "strength" athletes in the 1950s. [13] The purported benefit to these athletes was a gain in strength and muscle size beyond that which could be achieved with rigorous training and diet alone. The strength gains and performance-enhancing benefits from anabolic steroids were challenged and often discounted by early medical studies. In 1984, Haupt and Rovere [14] thoroughly reviewed published studies on the efficacy of anabolic steroids. Gains in muscle strength and size do occur, and have been most consistent among subjects using anabolic steroids in conjunction with an adequate dietary nitrogen supply and an adequate strength-training program. The benefit of increased muscle size and strength on sports performance appears to vary with the physical demands of the sport. The benefit is potentially more significant in strength-dependent sports such as weight lifting, shot put throwing, and football (linemen). Increased muscle size and bulk have fewer potential benefits for participation in sports that require speed, agility, flexibility, and/or endurance.

Administration and Mechanisms of Action

Anabolic steroids may be administered orally or by intramuscular injection. [15] Some of the common orally administered anabolic steroids include oxymetholone (Anadrol), oxandrolone (Anavar), methandrostenolone (Dianabol), and stanozolol (Winstrol). Some of the injectable steroids include nandrolone decanoate (Deca-Durabolin), nandrolone phenpropionate (Durabolin), testosterone cypionate (Depo-Testosterone), and boldenone undecylenate (Equipoise).

Individuals using anabolic steroids typically use a combination of oral and injectable drugs during 6- to 12-week cycles. The injectable forms are favored by users because they are less hepatotoxic than oral preparations. However, the oral preparations tend to be cleared more rapidly from the system and may be preferred when drug testing is anticipated.

The simultaneous use of multiple steroid preparations is called "stacking," and the pattern of increasing a dose through a cycle is referred to as "pyramiding." Pyramiding may lead to doses of 10 to 40 times greater than those used for medical indications. Stacking and pyramiding are intended to maximize steroid receptor binding and minimize toxic side effects. The fact that these benefits have not been substantiated scientifically has not appreciably influenced dosing patterns.

Anabolic steroids are believed to exert their effects by binding to androgen receptors at the cellular level, stimulating production of RNA, and ultimately increasing protein synthesis. The various clinical effects are determined by the type and concentrations of androgen receptors and enzymes controlling steroid metabolism in a given organ. The structure of androgen receptors appears to be identical in muscle and other organs.

Anabolic steroids have been shown to have an anti-catabolic effect by improving utilization of protein and by inhibiting the catabolic effect of glucocorticoids. [14, 16] In addition, anabolic steroids may lead to gains in strength by increasing the athlete's aggressiveness, producing euphoria, or decreasing the athlete's sense of fatigue during training. These psychological effects may allow a higher intensity and longer duration of training. A summary of the desired effects of anabolic steroids in sports competitors appears in Table 2.

Side Effects

Many excellent reviews on the adverse effects of anabolic steroids are available (Table 3). [14–21] Because clinical trials are not feasible, much of the information on adverse reactions is anecdotal, or is assumed from known problems associated with therapeutic use of these agents.

Table 2 *Desired Effects of Anabolic Steroids as Perceived by Sports Competitors**

Increased muscle mass

Increased strength

Decreased recovery time

Increased aggression

Promote healing of injuries

Maintain same "advantage" as one's opponent

Obtaining a winning edge

* Adapted from Hough. [15]

Elevations in levels of liver enzymes (aspartate aminotransferase, alanine aminotransferase, and lactate dehydrogenase) are common, whereas the more severe hepatic complications are rare. In men, steroid use depresses levels of luteinizing hormone and follicle-stimulating hormones, which leads to decreased endogenous testosterone production, decreased spermatogenesis, and testicular atrophy. Gynecomastia may result from the peripheral conversion of androgens to estradiol and estrone. The masculinizing effects of anabolic steroids in women include hirsutism, acne, deepening of the voice, clitoral hypertrophy, and male-pattern baldness. These androgenic effects may be irreversible.

Anabolic steroids may adversely affect the serum lipid profile, but their long-term effects on the development of coronary artery disease have not been determined. Thrombotic phenomena associated with anabolic steroid use include strokes, myocardial infarctions, and limb loss. [22, 23]

Some individuals may experience mental status and behavioral changes with anabolic steroid use, including irritability, aggressiveness, euphoria, depression, mood swings, altered libido, and even psychosis. [24] Anabolic steroid withdrawal and dependency disorders have also been reported. [25] Acute anabolic steroid withdrawal may produce symptoms of central nonadrenergic hyperactivity including anxiety, irritability, insomnia, hot flashes, sweats, chills, anorexia, myalgia, nausea, vomiting, piloerection, tachycardia, and hypertension. Depression and anabolic steroid craving may also occur with withdrawal. [25]

Of particular concern is premature physeal closure in any child/adolescent, which results in a decrease in adult height.

Table 3 *Possible Adverse Effects of Anabolic Steroids**

Liver
Hepatocellular damage
Cholestasis
Peliosis hepatis
Hepatoadenoma
Hepatocarcinoma

Reproductive
Males
Testicular atrophy
Oglio- or azoospermia
Impotence
Prostatic hypertrophy
Prostatic carcinoma
Gynecomastia
Females
Amenorrhea
Clitoromegaly
Uterine atrophy
Breast atrophy
Teratogenicity

Musculoskeletal
Early closure of physes in children
(shorter adult height)
Increased rate of muscle strains/ruptures

Endocrine (other than reproductive)
Decreased glucose tolerance

Integument
Acne
Striae
Hirsutism
Male pattern baldness
Edema

Larynx
Deepening of the voice

Cardiovascular
Increased cholesterol
Decreased HDL cholesterol
Increased blood pressure
Thrombosis

Urinary
Wilm's tumor

Psychologic
Mood swings
Aggressiveness
Depression
Psychosis
Addiction

Immunologic (infectious)
Decreased IgA levels
Hepatitis B or C; HIV infection
(if needles are shared)

Withdrawal and Dependency Disorders

* Adapted from Landry and Primos. [20]

Patterns of Anabolic Steroid Use

Surveys on the prevalence of anabolic steroid use in various populations continue to be published (Table 1). [15] The prevalence of self-reported use of anabolic steroids in adolescents has ranged from 5% to 11% of males [2–4] and up to 2.5% of females. [5] Athletes in nonschool sports as well as nonathletes have been shown to represent a significant portion of the user population. [12]

Combined drug use patterns are seen when anabolic steroid users take additional nonsteroidal substances such as human growth hormone [26] or clenbuterol [27] for performance enhancement or anabolic effect. Durant et al [28] showed that anabolic steroid use in adolescents was significantly associated with previous use of cocaine, injectable drugs, alcohol, marijuana, shared needles, and smokeless tobacco. An 18-year-old male who used injectable anabolic steroids has been reported to have acquired immunodeficiency virus infection from sharing needles and syringes. [29]

Summary of Emerging Data

New reports of previously unrecognized patterns of use, side effects, or complications of anabolic steroids continue to emerge. Perhaps the most compelling aspect of the "new literature" is what is not reported. To our knowledge, no study has identified an adolescent population without the temptation and risks of anabolic steroid use. Furthermore, no study has been published showing a decrease in the prevalence of anabolic steroid use over time (though a recent American Medical Association report suggests that this may be occurring) or in response to educational programs. Educational programs directed toward potential users of anabolic steroids have been advocated with the hope that greater knowledge of medical risk would discourage use. [6] Unfortunately, greater knowledge does not clearly change attitudes or behaviors. [10] Educational programs that are biased toward presenting negative side effects (scare tactics) tend to widen the credibility gap between anabolic steroid users and health professionals. [9] Even if the potential benefits of anabolic steroids are acknowledged, many health professionals are concerned that admitting to such benefits may inadvertently condone their use.

Drug-testing programs at the collegiate and Olympic level do not appear to deter anabolic steroid use in aspiring adolescent athletes. In fact, public reporting of drug use violations may paradoxically serve to promote the perceived performance-enhancing benefits of anabolic steroids. [9] Drug testing for these agents at the high school or youth sport levels is impractical and unlikely to occur. Furthermore, sanctions against anabolic steroid users are not enforceable without direct proof of drug use.

Conclusions

Pediatric practitioners cannot depend on community education programs or drug testing to curb the use of anabolic steroids in adolescents. Without evidence to show a significant and consistent decline in use or increasing safety of anabolic steroids, a passive approach to the problem is difficult to justify. The medical community is united in its belief that the use of anabolic steroids and other performance-enhancing substances is unacceptable, therefore, health care providers are obligated to provide sound guidance for those who seek advice.

Pediatricians have an opportunity to fulfill a positive role in the recognition and management of anabolic steroid abuse in adolescents. Recognition begins with an appreciation of the at-risk population. Potential anabolic steroid users have been and will continue to be involved in sports where strength and muscle mass are at a premium. Endurance athletes, female athletes, and nonathletes seeking to add strength, bulk, muscle definition, or to improve their self-image must also be considered to be at risk. It is appropriate for pediatricians to inquire about anabolic steroid use during routine health maintenance visits because of the general health risks and the general distribution of the population at risk.

Because recognition of the anabolic steroid user is unlikely to result from drug testing or disclosure by patients or by the supplier of the drug, physicians must recognize clinical signs that suggest use. Any of the adverse effects in Table 3 may occur, but the pediatrician is most likely to note changes such as otherwise improbable gains in lean body mass, gains in muscle bulk and definition, and behavioral changes such as increased aggressiveness and/or emotional lability. The adolescent anabolic steroid user may also show advanced stages of acne on the chest and back, gynecomastia, early male-pattern baldness, jaundice, and/or testicular atrophy. Blood pressure elevations are common, as are elevated levels of total cholesterol and depressed levels of high-density lipoprotein cholesterol.

If use of anabolic steroids or other performance-enhancing substances is suspected, clinicians must respond in a manner that does not alienate the patient. Responses that are confrontational, judgmental, or in violation of doctor-patient confidentiality will quickly eliminate any opportunity to influence the patient's decision making. It is also important to understand the anabolic steroid user's perspective that the rewards for excellence in sports or a muscular body outweigh the penalties and risks associated with anabolic steroid use. [30, 33] A balanced, informed discussion about the benefits and risks of anabolic steroids is preferable to scare tactics or a one-sided discourse on the inconsistencies and inadequacies of the available medical literature.

The credibility gap between anabolic steroid users and medical personnel can be narrowed by honest acknowledgment that anabolic steroids can have physical effects deemed desirable and even necessary by the user. It may be helpful to distinguish common, non-life-threatening side effects (acne, gynecomastia, balding) from the more rare and potentially fatal complications such as malignancies or thrombotic phenomena.

Anabolic steroid users and potential users should be aware that many of the adverse effects of anabolic steroids may be present without obvious warning signs. Examination of the patient for hypertension, cholesterol and lipid abnormalities, and/or hepatocellular damage, even if none of these are found, can impart a strong message that anabolic steroids can have serious side effects. Testing or laboratory determination for these side effects should include a disclaimer that testing does not condone use and that a negative test does not guarantee freedom from complications.

Medical issues related to anabolic steroid use are only part of the decision-making process. Some anabolic steroid users believe that, regardless of medical consequences, steroids are necessary to be competitive. Other athletes believe that steroid use precludes fair competition and that any success an athlete achieves while using steroids is tainted. Coaches are often influential in an athlete's decision-making process about whether to use anabolic steroids but may give ambiguous messages about what is necessary for success and what is fair in competition.

Part of drug-prevention counseling is providing a healthy alternative to drug use. Most athletes will find a way to meet their sports goals without using anabolic steroids. Athletes may need to be reminded that the health, fitness, and social benefits of sports participation can be readily met without use of performance-enhancing substances. For the athlete who is convinced that steroids are essential for success, it may be helpful to point out role models in the sports community whose success did not depend on the use of drugs.

Current clinical experience and scientific evidence support an approach to the anabolic steroid issue that minimizes preconceptions about the users, recognizes the potential benefits as well as risks of use, and maximizes informed, balanced, and open interaction with patients. There is ample need and justification for pediatric health care practitioners to be increasingly involved in the care of individuals who are using or considering use of these substances.

COMMITTEE ON SPORTS MEDICINE AND FITNESS, 1996 to 1997

Steven J. Anderson, MD, Chair

Stephen P. Bolduc, MD

Elizabeth Coryllos, MD

Bernard Griesemer, MD

Larry McLain, MD

Thomas W. Rowland, MD

Suzanne M. Tanner, MD

Liaison Representatives

Kathryn Keely, MD

Canadian Paediatric Society

Richard Malacrea,

ATC National Athletic Trainers Association

Judith C. Young, PhD

National Association for Sport and Physical Education

AAP Section Liaisons

Reginald L. Washington, MD

Section on Cardiology

Frederick E. Reed, MD

Section on Orthopaedics

Consultants

Oded Bar-Or, MD

Canadian Paediatric Society

William L. Risser, MD, PhD

References

1. Wagner JC. Abuse of drugs used to enhance athletic performance. *Am J Hosp Pharm.* 1989; 46:2059–2067

2. Windsor RE, Dumitru D. Prevalence of anabolic steroid use by male and female adolescents. *Med Sci Sports Exerc.* 1989; 21:494–497

3. Buckley WE, Yesalis CE III, Friedl KE, Anderson WA, Streit AL, Wright JE. Estimated prevalence of anabolic steroid use among male high school seniors. *JAMA.* 1988; 260:3441–3445

4. Johnson MD, Jay MS, Shoup B, Rickert VI. Anabolic steroid use by male adolescents. *Pediatrics.* 1989; 83:921–924

5. Terney R, McLain LG. The use of anabolic steroids in high school students. *AJDC.* 1990; 144:99–103

6. American Academy of Pediatrics, Committee on Sports Medicine. Anabolic steroids and the adolescent athlete. *Pediatrics.* 1989; 83:127–128

7. American College of Sports Medicine. Position statement on the use and abuse of anabolic-androgenic steroids in sports. *Med Sci Sports Exerc.* 1977; 9:xi–xii

8. American College of Sports Medicine. Position stand on anabolic-androgenic steroids. *Med Sci Sports Exerc.* 1987; 19:534–539

9. Marshall E. The drug of champions. *Science.* 1988; 242:183–184

10. Goldberg L, Bosworth EE, Bents RT, Trevisan L. Effect of an anabolic steroid education program on knowledge and attitudes of high school football players. *J Adolesc Health Care.* 1990; 11:210–214

11. Wade N. Anabolic steroids: doctors denounce them, but athletes aren't listening. *Science.* 1973; 176:1399–1401

12. Salva PS, Bacon GE. Anabolic steroids: interest among parents and nonathletes. *South Med J.* 1991; 84:552–556

13. Wilson JD. Androgen abuse by athletes. *Endocr Rev.* 1988; 9:181–199

14. Haupt HA, Rovere GE. Anabolic steroids: a review of the literature. *Am J Sports Med.* 1984; 12:469–484

15. Smith DA, Perry PJ. The efficacy of ergogenic agents in athletic competition. Part I: androgenic-anabolic steroids. *Ann Pharmacother.* 1992; 26:520–528

16. Lamb DR. Anabolic steroids in athletics: how well do they work and how dangerous are they? *Am J Sports Med.* 1984; 12:31–38

17. Kibble MW, Ross MB. Adverse effects of anabolic steroids in athletes. *Clin Pharm.* 1987; 6:686–692

18. Windsor RE, Dumitru D. Anabolic steroid use by athletes: how serious are the health hazards? *Postgrad Med.* 1988; 84:37–38, 41–43, 47–49

19. Hough DO. Anabolic steroids and ergogenic aids. *Am Fam Phys.* 1990; 41:1157–1164

20. Landry GL, Primos WA Jr. Anabolic steroid abuse. *Adv Pediatr.* 1990; 37:185–205

21. Rogol AD, Yesalis CE. Anabolic-androgenic steroids and the adolescent. *Pediatr Ann.* 1992; 21:175–188

22. Ferenchick GS. Are androgenic steroids thrombo-genic? *N Engl J Med.* 1990; 322:476

23. Ferenchick GS, Adelman S. Myocardial infarction associated with anabolic steroid use in a previously healthy 37-year-old weight lifter. *Am Heart J.* 1992; 124:507–508

24. Bahrke MS, Yesalis CE, Wright JE. Psychological and behavioural effects of endogenous testosterone levels and anabolic-androgenic steroids among males: a review. *Sports Med.* 1990; 10:303–337

25. Kashkin KB, Kleber HD. Hooked on hormones? An anabolic steroid addiction hypothesis. *JAMA*. 1989; 262:3166–3170

26. Rickert VI, Pawlak-Morello C, Sheppard V, Jay MS. Human growth hormone: a new substance of abuse among adolescents? *Clin Pediatr*. 1992; 31:723–726

27. Beckett AH. Clenbuterol and sport. *Lancet*. 1992; 340:1165

28. Durant RH, Rickert VI, Ashworth CS, Newman C, Slavens G. Use of multiple drugs among adolescents who use anabolic steroids. *N Engl J Med*. 1993; 328:922–926

29. Sklarek HM, Mantovani RP, Erens E, Heisler D, Niederman MS, Fein AM. AIDS in a body builder using anabolic steroids. *N Engl J Med*. 1984; 311:1701

30. Komoroski EM, Rickert VI. Adolescent body image and attitudes to anabolic steroid use. *AJDC*. 1992; 146:823–828

31. Tricker R, O'Neill MR, Cook D. The incidence of anabolic steroid use among competitive bodybuilders. *J Drug Educ*. 1989; 19:313–325

32. Dezelsky TL, Toohey JV, Shaw RS. Non-medical drug use behaviour at five United States universities: a 15-year study. *Bull Narc*. 1985; 37:49–53

33. Lindstrom M, Nilsson AL, Katzman PL, Janzon L, Dymling JF. Use of anabolic-androgenic steroids among bodybuilders: frequency and attitudes. *J Intern Med*. 1990; 227:407–411

This subject review has been approved by the Council on Child and Adolescent Health.

The recommendations in this statement do not indicate an exclusive course of treatment or serve as a standard of medical care. Variations, taking into account individual circumstances, may be appropriate.

Amenorrhea in Adolescent Athletes (RE9163)

AMERICAN ACADEMY OF PEDIATRICS

Committee on Sports Medicine

Volume 84, Number 2

August 1989, p 394–395

A minority of female athletes participating in ballet, gymnastics, distance running, rowing, and cycling, as well as other sports activities, occasionally experience menstrual and associated physiologic changes. Women competing in the sports of ballet and gymnastics have been reported to have a particularly increased incidence of primary and secondary amenorrhea, decreased bone density, stress fractures, and symptoms of anorexia nervosa. [1–4] Results of several studies have indicated decreased levels of circulating estrogen as well as other metabolic changes. [1, 3–7]

Research designed to determine the etiology of the amenorrhea and the associated changes has shown mixed results.

Low body fat cannot be linked in a causative fashion to hormonal changes or decreased levels of circulating estrogen. Early studies linking minimum body fat and menarche, as well as maintenance of regular menstrual cycles, have not been replicated. [8] However, measurement of percentage of body fat may be helpful in assessing the nutritional status of athletes.

Ballet and gymnastics are perceived by some to be activities that are stressful psychologically. Although stress has been shown to cause amenorrhea, studies to date have not demonstrated the presence of significantly increased levels compared with age-matched girls not participating in ballet and gymnastics. [9]

Some authors have postulated that tall, thin athletes who may be genetically at risk for delayed maturation are naturally attracted to these sports. [10] Some of the delays may relate to preselection. However, no evidence currently exists proving a definite relationship between preselection and the physiologic changes in these athletes.

There is an increased emphasis by athletes, coaches, judges, and spectators on a slender physique for female gymnasts and ballet dancers. Several investigators have shown dietary intakes of adolescent ballerinas that are inadequate in calories, nutritional components, vitamins, and minerals. [2, 6] The most common findings demonstrated in amenorrheic athletes are high intensity of exercise combined with poor nutritional status. Fasting and purging may be encouraged and anorexia nervosa or bulimia hidden in all athletic populations. Coaches need to be educated regarding the seriousness of these behaviors.

Recommendations for dealing with sports-related amenorrhea in adult women have included thorough physical examinations (including pelvic examinations) and endocrine evaluations, as well as estrogen and calcium supplementation. [11] Some of those recommendations are probably appropriate for adolescent athletes. Endocrine evaluation including studies of follicle-stimulating hormone, luteinizing hormone, thyroxine, prolactin, and estradiol should be performed if the athlete has menarche delayed greater than 1 year beyond the age of onset of menses of other female family members or if menses cease for 6 or more months after regular menses have been established. Pregnancy should always be ruled out early in the course of amenorrhea. In situations in which family history is not available, primary amenorrhea should be considered if menarche has not occurred by age 16 years and prompt evaluation initiated. Most adolescent athletes make adequate amounts of estrogen and will have withdrawal bleeding following progestin challenge. The use of supplemental estrogen in the young amenorrheic girl should not be routinely implemented. These young athletes should be encouraged to decrease the intensity of their exercise and to improve their nutritional intake. However, older athletes may be appropriately supplemented with estrogen.

The following recommendations are appropriate.

1. Preparticipation evaluations should include a focus on menstrual function and dietary practices.

2. Education and counseling should be provided to athletes, parents, and coaches regarding adequate intake of nutrients to maintain normal growth and development. [12]

3. During the active season, routine monitoring of menstrual function, growth velocity, dietary changes, weight changes, and, when possible, skin fold thickness should be performed.

4. The possibility of anorexia nervosa should be explored and when diagnosed treated in the same manner as anorexia nervosa in nonathletes.

5. Athletes whose diets provide less than 1200 mg/d of calcium should be supplemented to maintain an intake of 1200 to 1500 mg/d.

6. Amenorrheic athletes within 3 years of menarche should be counseled to decrease the intensity of exercise and improve their nutritional intake, especially protein. The use of hormonal therapy for these younger girls is generally not advised.

7. Because pregnancy continues to be a risk in amenorrheic athletes who are sexually active, the possibility of pregnancy should always be assessed as part of the evaluation.

8. The mature amenorrheic athlete (generally greater than 3 years past menarche or age 16 years), if found to be hypoestrogenemic, may benefit by receiving estrogen supplementation. Optimal therapy has yet to be determined, but supplementation with low-dose oral contraceptives (< 50 mug of estrogen per day) is reasonable.

COMMITTEE ON SPORTS MEDICINE, 1986 to 1989

Michael A. Nelson, MD, Chairman, 1988-1989

Paul G. Dyment, MD, Chairman, 1986-1988

Barry Goldberg, MD

Suzanne B. Haefele, MD

Gregory L. Landry, MD

John J. Murray, MD

William L. Risser, MD

Liaison Representatives

Oded Bar-Or, MD, Canadian Paediatric Society

Richard Malacrea, National Athletic Trainers Association

AAP Section Liaison

David M. Orenstein, MD, Section on Diseases of the Chest

Arthur M. Pappas, MD, Section on Orthopaedics

References

1. Athletic women, amenorrhea, and skeletal integrity, editorial. *Ann Intern Med.* 1985; 102:258–260

2. Benson J, Gillien DM, Bourdet RD, et al. Inadequate nutrition and chronic calorie restriction in adolescent ballerinas. *Physician Sports Med.* 1985; 13:79–90

3. Drinkwater BL, Nilson K, et al. Bone mineral content of amenorrheic and eumenorrheic athletes. *N Engl J Med.* 1984; 311:277–281

4. Warren MP, Brooks-Gunn J, Hamilton LH, et al. Scoliosis and fractures in young ballet dancers: relation to delayed menarche and secondary amenorrhea. *N Engl J Med.* 1986; 314:1348–1353

5. Loucks AB, Horvath SM. Athletic amenorrhea: a review. *Med Sci Sports Exer.* 1985; 17:56–72

6. Braisted JR, Mellin L, Gong EJ, et al. The adolescent ballet dancer: nutritional practices and characteristics associated with anorexia nervosa. *J Adolesc Health Care.* 1985; 6:365–371

7. Wilson C, Emans J, et al. The relationships of calculated percent body, sports participation, age and place of residence on menstrual patterns in healthy adolescent girls at an independent New England high school. *J Adolesc Health Care.* 1984; 5:248–253

8. Frisch RE. Body fat, puberty and fertility. *Biol Rev.* 1984; 59:161–188

9. Warren M. The effects of exercise on pubertal progression and reproduction function in girls. *J Clin Endocrinol Metab.* 1980; 51:1150–1157

10. Malina RM. Menarche in athletes: a synthesis and hypothesis. *Ann Hum Biol.* 1983; 10:1–24

11. Shangold MM. Causes, evaluation and management of athletic oligo-amenorrhea. *Med Clin North Am.* 1985; 69:83–95

12. American Academy of Pediatrics, Committee on Nutrition. *Pediatric Nutrition Handbook.* 2nd ed. Elk Grove Village, IL: American Academy of Pediatrics; 1985. Reaffirmed 10/92.

The recommendations in this statement do not indicate an exclusive course of treatment or serve as a standard of medical care. Variations, taking into account individual circumstances, may be appropriate.

Athletic Participation by Children and Adolescents Who Have Systemic Hypertension (RE9715)

AMERICAN ACADEMY OF PEDIATRICS

Committee on Sports Medicine and Fitness

Volume 99, Number 4

April 1997, p 637–638

ABSTRACT. *Children and adolescents who have systemic hypertension may be at risk for complications when exercise causes their blood pressures to rise even higher. The purpose of this statement is to make recommendations concerning the athletic participation of individuals with hypertension using the 26th Bethesda conference on heart disease and athletic participation and of the second task force on blood pressure control in children as a basis.*

Hypertension is the most common cardiovascular condition seen in people who engage in competitive athletics. [1] Recently, the national institutes of health convened the 26th Bethesda conference to make recommendations concerning the participation of athletes who have heart disease. One of the panels considered hypertension. [1] In 1987, the second task force on blood pressure control in children also briefly addressed exercise for hypertensive youth. [2] This policy statement summarizes the recommendations of these two groups of experts and makes these guidelines more available to pediatricians.

Table 1 presents the classification of hypertension of the second task force [2] and includes some values from the 26th Bethesda conference. [1] All values given in the table apply to patients who are not taking antihypertensive drugs and who are not acutely ill. When the systolic and diastolic blood pressures fall into different categories, the higher category should be

Table 1 Classification of Hypertension [2]

Age, y	High Normal, mm Hg*	Significant Hypertension, mm Hg†	Severe Hypertension, mm Hg¥
6–9			
Systolic	111–121	122–129	>129(129)§
Diastolic	70–77	70–85	>85(84)
10–12			
Systolic	117–125	126–133	>133(134)
Diastolic	75–81	82–89	>89(89)
13–15			
Systolic	124–135	136–143	>143(149)
Diastolic	77–85	86–91	>91(94)
16–18			
Systolic	127–141	142–149	>149(159)
Diastolic	80–91	92–97	>97(99)
>18			
Systolic	Not given	[140–179]¶	>(179)
Diastolic		[90–109]	>(109)

* 90th to 94th percentile for age, boys and girls combined.
† 95th to 98th percentile for age, boys and girls combined.
¥ 99th percentile for age, boys and girls combined.
§ The values in parentheses are those used for the classification of severe hypertension by the 26th Bethesda Conference on cardiovascular disease and athletic participation.
[1] See text for explanation.
¶ Because the Second Task Force did not discuss youth older than 18 years, the values in brackets are those for mild and moderate hypertension given by the 26th Bethesda Conference. [1]

selected to classify the patient's blood pressure status.

Care must be taken to obtain reliable blood pressure recordings. [1, 2] Some athletes have exceedingly large biceps or triceps, and others have long extremities. The width of the blood pressure bladder must be adequate to cover at least 66% [1] or 75% [2] of the individual's upper arm measured between the top of the shoulder and the olecranon and should be of adequate length to encircle the arm completely, [2] which may require the use of a thigh cuff. The athlete should be seated, at rest, and the arm should be supported at heart level. [2] Only after several elevated readings are obtained on separate occasions should the diagnosis of systemic hypertension be made. Further details concerning the measurement of blood pressure are available. [1, 2]

Once the diagnosis of systemic hypertension is confirmed, an evaluation including a history, thorough physical examination, and appropriate laboratory testing should be performed, as outlined in the report of the second task force on blood pressure control in children. [2]

Reports of cerebrovascular accidents during maximal exercise have raised concerns that the rise in blood pressure accompanying strenuous activity may cause harm. [1] The following guidelines recommend temporary restriction for those athletes who have severe hypertension, but the available data do not indicate that strenuous dynamic exercise places these athletes at risk of acute complications of hypertension during exercise or of worsening of their baseline blood pressure values. [1] In dynamic exercise, intramuscular force is not greatly increased as muscles lengthen and contract and joints move through their range of motion. There is a sizable increase in systolic blood pressure, a moderate increase in mean arterial pressure, and a fall in diastolic pressure and total peripheral resistance. In static exercise, relatively large intramuscular forces develop without much change in muscle length or joint motion. Systolic, mean arterial, and diastolic blood pressures rise significantly, and total peripheral resistance remains essentially unchanged. It is the acute increase in diastolic pressure that particularly concerns the experts, as well as the possible increases in muscle mass that may elevate resting blood pressure. Although the limited evidence shows no greater risk with highly static exercise [1], experts are more cautious about allowing athletes with severe hypertension to participate in this type of activity.

Most physical activities and sports have both static and dynamic components. Guidelines for restricting participation should be based on the cardiovascular demands of the activity and the demands of the prac-

tice, training, and/or preparation for that activity.

The experts from the 26th Bethesda conference [1] and those from the Second Task Force on Blood Pressure Control in Children [2] agree on temporary restriction of athletes who have severe hypertension. However, the definition of severe hypertension of the 26th Bethesda conference is more liberal for youth greater than 12 years old than is that of the second task force (Table 1, last column). We recommend the use of the values of the second task force because this group of experts was more pediatric oriented. Since the second task force did not define severe hypertension in youth older than 18 years, only the values of the 26th Bethesda conference are given for this age group (Table 1).

Recommendations

The American Academy of Pediatrics recommends:

- The presence of significant (Table 1) hypertension in the absence of target organ damage or concomitant heart disease should not limit a person's eligibility for competitive athletics. Athletes with significant hypertension should have their blood pressure measured regularly (every 2 months at the physician's office) to monitor the impact of exercise on blood pressure.

- Youth who have severe (Table 1) hypertension need to be restricted from competitive sports and highly static (isometric) activities (Table 2) until their hypertension is under adequate control and they have no evidence of target organ damage. Since cardiovascular conditioning may be less strenuous than competitive athletics, complete restriction of exercise may not be necessary for those with severe hypertension.

- When hypertension and other cardiovascular diseases coexist, eligibility for participation in competitive athletics is usually based on the type and severity of the other cardiovascular disease. [1]

- The young athlete with hypertension, regardless of the degree of severity, should be strongly encouraged to adopt healthy lifestyle behaviors, including the avoidance of exogenous androgens, growth hormone, drugs of abuse (especially cocaine), alcohol, use of tobacco (by all routes), and high sodium intake. [1] In addition, the athlete should be advised that the use of diuretic drugs and ß blockers has been prohibited by some athletic governing bodies. In these instances, other types of medication may need to be considered.

Table 2	*Sports That Have a High Static Component**

Low Dynamic	Moderate Dynamic	High Dynamic
Bobsledding	Body building	Boxing†
Field events (throwing)	Downhill skiing	Canoeing/kayaking
Gymnastics	Wrestling	Cycling
Karate/judo		Decathlon
Luge		Rowing
Sailing		Speeding skating
Rock climbing		
Waterskiing		
Weight lifting		
Windsurfing		

* Adapted from Mitchell et al [3] with permission.
† The American Academy of Pediatrics recommends that youth not participate in boxing.

Addendum

An update to the 1987 task force report on high blood pressure [2] has recently appeared (*Pediatrics*. 1996; 98:649–658). It provides new data on the 90th and 95th percentile values for blood pressure categorized by age, sex, and height and mentions new information on the diagnosis, treatment, and prevention of hypertension in youth. It does not address sports participation for hypertensive patients other than to say that hypertension is "usually not" a contraindication. Members of the working group that developed the update indicate that the 1987 report's recommendations concerning severe hypertension still stand (Stephen R. Daniels, Jennifer M. H. Logie, personal communication).

COMMITTEE ON SPORTS MEDICINE AND FITNESS,1995 to 1996

William L. Risser, MD, PhD, Chair

Steven J. Anderson, MD

Stephen P. Bolduc, MD

Elizabeth Coryllos, MD

Bernard Griesemer, MD

Larry McLain, MD

Suzanne M. Tanner, MD

Liaison Representatives

Kathryn Keely, MD, Canadian Paediatric Society

Richard Malacrea, ATC, National Athletic Trainers Association

Judith C. Young, PhD, National Association For Sport and Physical Education

AAP Section Liaisons

Reginald L. Washington, MD, Section on Cardiology

Frederick E. Reed, MD, Section on Orthopaedics

References

1. Kaplan NM, Deveraux RB, Miller HS Jr. Task Force 4: systemic hypertension. *J Am Coll Cardiol.* 1994; 24:885–888

2. American Academy of Pediatrics, Task Force on Blood Pressure Control in Children. Report of the Second Task Force on Blood Pressure Control in Children—1987. *Pediatrics.* 1987; 79:1–25

3. Mitchell JH, Haskell WL, Raven PB. Classification of sports. *J Am Coll Cardiol.* 1994; 24:864–866

The recommendations in this statement do not indicate an exclusive course of treatment or serve as a standard of medical care. Variations, taking into account individual circumstances, may be appropriate.

Atlantoaxial Instability in Down Syndrome: A Subject Review (RE9528)

AMERICAN ACADEMY OF PEDIATRICS

Committee on Sports Medicine and Fitness

Volume 96, Number 1

July 1995, p 151–154

Definition of the Problem

In 1984, the American Academy of Pediatrics (AAP) published a position statement on screening for atlantoaxial instability (AAI) in youth with Down syndrome. [1] In that statement, the AAP supported the requirement introduced by the Special Olympics in 1983 that lateral neck radiographs be obtained for individuals with Down syndrome before they participate in the Special Olympics' nationwide competitive program for developmentally disabled persons. Those participants with radiologic evidence of instability are banned from certain activities that may be associated with increased risk of injury to the cervical spine. This policy seemed to be prudent in light of the information available at that time. However, the AAP Committee on Sports Medicine and Fitness recently has reviewed the data on which this recommendation was based and has decided that uncertainty exists concerning the value of cervical spine radiographs in screening for possible catastrophic neck injury in athletes with Down syndrome. The 1984 statement therefore has been retired. This review discusses the available research data on this subject.

Background

AAI, also called atlantoaxial subluxation, denotes increased mobility at the articulation of the first and second cervical vertebrae (atlantoaxial joint). This condition is found not only in patients who have Down syndrome but also in some patients who have rheumatoid arthritis, abnormalities of the odontoid process of the axis, and various forms of dwarfism. [1] The causes of AAI are not well understood but may include abnormalities of the ligaments that maintain the integrity of the C-1 and C-2 articulation, bony abnormalities of C-1 or C-2, or both. [1–11]

In its mildest form, AAI is asymptomatic and is diagnosed using radiography. The instability is recognized through lateral neck radiographs in which the excessive mobility of C-2 in relation to C-1 results in an abnormally large distance between the odontoid process of the axis and the anterior arch of the atlas. Symptomatic AAI results from subluxation that is severe enough to injure the spinal cord, or from dislocation at the atlantoaxial joint.

Approximately 15% of individuals in the pediatric age group (< 21 years old) who have Down syndrome also have AAI. [2] Almost all of the persons affected are asymptomatic. Some asymptomatic individuals with Down syndrome who have normal radiographs initially will have abnormal radiographs obtained later, and others with initially abnormal radiographs will have normal follow-up radiographs; the latter change is apparently more common. In one study, 7 of 95 (7.4%) patients with normal radiographs initially had abnormal radiographs 3 to 6 years later in follow-up, and 19 of 95 (20%) patients with abnormal radiographs initially had normal second radiographs. [2] In another longitudinal study of 141 patients, [3] 130 (92%) had changes in the atlantoaxial interval (of less than 1.5 mm) that were judged clinically insignificant. Eleven patients (8%) had changes that ranged from 2 to 4 mm. Nine of these patients with abnormal radiographs had subsequent radiographs that were normal, whereas the two patients with normal radiographs had abnormal radiographs on follow-up.

The neurologic manifestations of symptomatic AAI include easy fatigability, difficulties in walking, abnormal gait, neck pain, limited neck mobility, torticollis or head tilt, incoordination and clumsiness, sensory deficits, spasticity, hyperreflexia, clonus, extensor-plantar reflex, and other upper motor neuron and posterior column signs and symptoms. [1–11] Such symptoms and signs often remain relatively stable for months or years; occasionally they progress, rarely even to paraplegia, hemiplegia, quadriplegia, or death. [1–11] Trauma rarely causes the initial appearance or the progression of these symptoms. [1–11] Nearly all of the individuals who have experienced catastrophic injury to the spinal cord have had weeks to years of preceding, less severe neurologic abnormalities. [1–11]

The Special Olympics' radiologic screening program to prevent catastrophic spinal cord injury has the following characteristics. Lateral spinal cord radiographs are used to screen for asymptomatic AAI, which is thought to be a risk factor for symptomatic AAI. Asymptomatic individuals are banned from participating in several activities that are thought to have a particularly high risk of spinal cord injury—in particular, gymnastics, diving, the pentathlon, the butterfly stroke and diving starts in swimming, the high jump, soccer, and certain warm-up exercises.

For this or any screening program to be worthwhile, several criteria must be met. [12] The target disease, symptomatic AAI, must be sufficiently common and severe enough to justify the work and expense of its detection in the asymptomatic phase. The screening test must have excellent sensitivity and specificity for identifying those with asymptomatic AAI, and asymptomatic AAI must be a proven risk factor for symptomatic AAI. An effective intervention must be available to prevent the progression from asymptomatic to symptomatic disease. The following discussion evaluates how well a radiologic screening program for AAI meets these criteria.

Most importantly, symptomatic AAI is apparently rare in individuals with Down syndrome. In the pediatric age group, only 41 well-documented cases have been described in the published literature. [2, 5–11] New case series or reports on such patients are not likely to be published, however, because symptomatic AAI is no longer remarkable.

One study has shown that the reproducibility of the radiologic test results for AAI is relatively poor. [4] Of 19 children who were evaluated twice within a 10-minute interval, 6 had evidence of AAI. This instability was demonstrated in the first set of films in 5 patients and in the second set in 4 patients. Only 3 of 6 patients had abnormalities on both sets of radiographs. As described previously, other studies have shown that an individual's radiologic status can change over time, most often from abnormal to normal. [2, 3] These changes occur either because of the lack of reproducibility of the test [4] or because of actual variations in atlantoaxial stability over time. [2, 3]

Asymptomatic AAI, which is common, has not been proven to be a significant risk factor for symptomatic AAI, which is rare. In prospective studies of 952 and 1413 individuals with Down syndrome and AAI, one asymptomatic patient became symptomatic during 3 or more years of follow-up after an injury. [3]

In the 41 reported pediatric cases with symptomatic AAI, [2, 5–11] only one patient had had radiographs obtained before neurologic problems developed, [2, 5–11] making it impossible to know whether the other 40 had asymptomatic AAI before they became symptomatic. This individual [5] had a normal radiograph at 6 years of age but became quadriplegic after a tumbling accident at 18 years of age. A radiograph obtained after the injury demonstrated AAI.

The efficacy of the intervention to prevent symptomatic AAI has never been tested. Sports trauma has not been an important cause of symptomatic AAI in the rare patients with this disorder; only 3 of the 41 reported pediatric patients had initial symptoms of AAI or worsening of symptoms after trauma during organized sports participation. [2, 5–11] Members of the Medical Advisory Committee of the Special Olympics think that more such sports-related injuries occur but that they are being overlooked because of a lack of information about the association of AAI and spinal cord injury among health care providers. [13] This claim has not been substantiated with published research.

The arguments for continued screening of patients with Down syndrome include the theoretical possibility of preventing the rare occurrence of sports-related catastrophic spinal cord injury among individuals with asymptomatic AAI. Another purpose is to identify the very rare previously unrecognized patient with symptomatic AAI. Arguments against screening include the rarity of symptomatic AAI, inaccuracy in the screening test, the possibility that patients with abnormal radiographs initially will have normal radiographs later on, and the absence of evidence that the screening program is effective in preventing symptomatic disease. Screening is also expensive. The expense may prevent at least some individuals from participating in the Special Olympics, and the labeling of patients as having AAI may lead to anxiety and to unnecessary medical intervention, although no research has evaluated these possibilities.

The case reports [2, 5–11] indicate that many patients with symptomatic AAI have symptoms and signs of cervical spinal cord compression for weeks or years before they are recognized as having neurologic disease. Current evidence suggests that the presence of these neurologic abnormalities may be more predictive of potential progression of injury than are abnormalities on radiographs in the asymptomatic patient. [2, 5–11] Therefore, despite the difficulties in obtaining good medical histories and physical and neurologic examinations for individuals with Down syndrome, it is clearly important that they receive these evaluations before participation in sports. If possible, these patients should be examined by physicians who have provided their care longitudinally and know their baseline status. In addition, their families must be made aware of the manifestations of symptomatic AAI and instructed to contact their physician immediately if any symptoms appear.

Summary of New or Emerging Data

No recent studies have provided significant new information on the recognition of those asymptomatic patients with Down syndrome and AAI who are at increased risk for spinal cord injury. Research has clarified that computed tomography, as expected, gives more detailed information about bony anomalies and spinal cord compression than do plain radiographs. [14] Other reports have emphasized that other abnormalities of the cervical spine, in particular atlanto-occipital instability, occur in patients with Down syndrome. [15] One study found that children with Down syndrome and asymptomatic AAI who were allowed to play all sports had no serious spinal cord injuries or evidence of neurologic deterioration. [16] The number of subjects was too small, and the duration of follow-up was too brief for this to be conclusive evidence of a lack of risk. In a community study of adults with Down syndrome, those with AAI shown on radiographs were not more likely to have neurologic symptoms suggesting spinal cord injury than those without evidence of AAI. [17] Studies have continued to explore the effect of technique on the measurement of atlantoaxial distance. [14, 18]

Tentative Conclusions

From the available scientific evidence, it is reasonable to conclude that lateral plain radiographs of the cervical spine are of potential but unproven value in detecting patients at risk for developing spinal cord injury during sports participation. It seems that identification of those patients who already have or who later have complaints or physical findings consistent with symptomatic spinal cord injury is a greater priority than obtaining radiographs. Recognition of these symptomatic patients is challenging and requires frequent interval histories and physical examinations, including evaluations before participation in sports, preferably by physicians who have cared for these patients longitudinally. Their parents must learn the symptoms of AAI that indicate the need to seek immediate medical care.

The Special Olympics does not plan to remove its requirement that all athletes with Down syndrome receive radiographs of the cervical spine. Pediatricians therefore will continue to be called on to order these tests. The information in this review can be used to interpret the results for family members.

Clearly, we need better research to determine what combination of symptoms, signs, and findings from imaging studies best identifies those individuals with Down syndrome who are at increased risk of a catastrophic injury to the spinal cord during sports participation. The Special Olympics and the regional centers that care for large numbers of children and adolescents with Down syndrome are in a favorable position to study this problem prospectively in a multicenter study and perhaps by establishing a national injury registry.

COMMITTEE ON SPORTS MEDICINE AND FITNESS, 1994 TO 1995

William L. Risser, MD, PhD, Chair

Steven J. Anderson, MD

Stephen P. Bolduc, MD

Bernard Griesemer, MD

Sally S. Harris, MD, MPH

Larry McLain, MD

Suzanne M. Tanner, MD

Liaison Representatives

Kathryn Keely, MD, Canadian Paediatric Society

Richard Malacrea, ATC, National Athletic Trainers Association

Judith C. Young, PhD, National Association for Sport and Physical Education

AAP Section Liaisons

Arthur M. Pappas, MD, Section on Orthopaedics

Reginald L. Washington, MD, Section on Cardiology

Consultant

Oded Bar-Or, MD, Canadian Paediatric Society

References

1. American Academy of Pediatrics, Committee on Sports Medicine. Atlantoaxial instability in Down syndrome. *Pediatrics.* 1984; 74:152–154

2. Peuschel SM, Scola FH. Atlantoaxial instability in individuals with Down syndrome: epidemiologic, radiographic, and clinical studies. *Pediatrics.* 1987; 80:555–560

3. Pueschel SM, Scola FH, Pezzullo JC. A longitudinal study of atlanto-dens relationships in asymptomatic individuals with Down syndrome. *Pediatrics.* 1992; 89:1194–1198

4. Selby KA, Newton RW, Gupta S, Hunt L. Clinical predictors and radiologic reliability in atlantoaxial subluxation in Down's syndrome. *Arch Dis Child.* 1991; 66:876–878

5. Davidson RG. Atlantoaxial instability in individuals with Down syndrome: a fresh look at the evidence. *Pediatrics.* 1988; 81:857–865

6. Shikata J, Yamamuro T, Mikawa Y, et al. Surgical treatment of symptomatic atlantoaxial subluxation in Down's syndrome. *Clin Orthop.* 1987; 220:111–118

7. Nordt JC, Stauffer ES. Sequelae of atlantoaxial stabilization in two patients with Down's syndrome. *Spine.* 1981; 6:437–440

8. Chaudry V, Sturgeon C, Gates AJ, Myers G. Symptomatic atlantoaxial dislocation in Down's syndrome. *Ann Neurol.* 1987; 21:606–609

9. Williams JP, Somerville GM, Miner ME, Reilly D. Atlanto-axial subluxation and Trisomy-21: another perioperative complication. *Anesthesiology.* 1987; 67:253–254

10. Moore RA, McNicholas KW, Warran SP. Atlantoaxial subluxation with symptomatic spinal cord compression in a child with Down's syndrome. *Anesth Analg.* 1987; 66:89–90

11. Msall ME, Reese ME, DiGaudio K, Griswold K, Granger CV, Cooke RE. Symptomatic atlantoaxial instability associated with medical and rehabilitative procedures in children with Down syndrome. *Pediatrics.* 1990; 85:447–449

12. Sackett DL, Haynes RB, Guyatt GH, Tugwell P. *Clinical Epidemiology: A Basic Science for Clinical Medicine,* 2nd ed. Boston: Little, Brown, and Co; 1991:153–170

13. Peuschel SM. Atlantoaxial instability and Down syndrome. *Pediatrics.* 1988;81:879–880

14. Pueschel SM, Moon AC, Scola FH. Computerized tomography in persons with Down syndrome and atlantoaxial instability. *Spine.* 1992; 17:735–737

15. Stein SM, Kirchner SG, Horev G, Hernanz-Schulman M. Atlanto-axial subluxation in Down syndrome. *Pediatr Radiol.* 1991; 21:121–124

16. Cremers MJ, Bol E, de Roos F, van Gijn J. Risk of sports activities in children with Down syndrome and atlantoaxial instability. *Lancet.* 1993; 342:511–514

17. Roy M, Baxter M, Roy A. Atlantoaxial instability in Down syndrome-guidelines for screening and detection. *J R Soc Med.* 1990; 83:433–435

18. Cremers MJ, Ramos L, Bol E, van Gijn J. Radiological assessment of the atlantoaxial distance in Down syndrome. *Arch Dis Child.* 1993; 69:347–350

This subject review has been approved by the Council on Child and Adolescent Health.

Subject reviews are a category of American Academy of Pediatrics' policy that provide a comprehensive review of the scientific literature and develop tentative conclusions about the significance and impact of emerging or new data. The subject review is designed to inform members of the issues surrounding a particular topic and highlight new or emerging data without stating a position or making specific recommendations.

Cardiac Dysrhythmias and Sports (RE9525)

AMERICAN ACADEMY OF PEDIATRICS
Committee on Sports Medicine and Fitness
Volume 95, Number 5
May 1995, p 786–788

Sudden unexpected death during athletic participation is the overriding consideration in advising individuals with dysrhythmias about participation in sports. The incidence of sudden death is 1 to 2 per 200 000 athletes per year and approximately 12 per year in US high school athletes. [1] Between 5 and 22% of these deaths occur during sports or physical activities that include basketball, racquetball, jogging, football, soccer, and golf. [2] The remainder occur during sedentary activities. [2] Another potential risk for the athlete with a dysrhythmia is injury to self or others from syncope or near syncope while playing sports.

The leading cause of sudden unexpected cardiac death is hypertrophic cardiomyopathy. [1] A dysrhythmia of ventricular or supraventricular origin may be a significant factor in the sudden unexpected death of these individuals. [1] Myocarditis is also a cause of sudden cardiac death. Severe dysrhythmia may be a prominent feature of myocarditis even in the absence of significant cardiac dysfunction. [1] This diagnosis should be considered in an individual who has a recent sudden onset of a symptomatic dysrhythmia. [3] Ventricular dysrhythmias with exercise are a potential cause of death in individuals with arrhythmogenic right ventricular dysplasia (a rare muscle disorder of the right ventricle). [1]

Sudden death resulting from dysrhythmia can occur with exertion or excitement in individuals who have hereditary syndromes that include prolongation of the QTc interval. [3] Sudden death has also been associated with mitral valve prolapse (rarely) and with Wolff-Parkinson-White syndrome. [3]

Medical History

The patient's medical history is of critical importance. Dysrhythmias may be episodic and not apparent at the time of physical examination. Some disorders, such as the prolonged QTc interval syndrome, may be familial, and a family history of dysrhythmias or sudden death sometimes provides a clue to their presence. It is also imperative to distinguish between dysrhythmias occurring in a patient with a structurally normal heart and those occurring in a patient with congenital heart disease, including one who has had cardiac surgery, because the prognosis in the latter group may be less favorable as a result of progression of the lesion. Certain medications or drugs of abuse (eg, tricyclic antidepressants, inhalants, or cocaine) can cause dysrhythmias. [4] Anorexia nervosa can cause a prolonged QTc interval or significant bradycardia. Specific information should be obtained regarding a history of syncope or near syncope, dizziness or light-headedness, seizures, palpitations, chest pain, pallor, previously diagnosed dysrhythmias or heart disease, or use of medications. [2] It is important to determine whether any family members have died suddenly or unexpectedly or have had any of the following conditions: syncope; dysrhythmia; mitral valve prolapse; prolonged QTc syndrome; or hypertrophic cardiomyopathy. [2] Further diagnostic studies and cardiac consultation are indicated if abnormalities are suggested from the history or physical examination.

Testing

The most common dysrhythmias in school-aged children are sinus dysrhythmias and premature atrial contractions. [3] These dysrhythmias are benign if the heart is structurally normal. An electrocardiogram demonstrates sinus dysrhythmia or premature atrial contractions. No other cardiac studies are necessary.

Further evaluation is indicated for ventricular ectopic beats or more complex dysrhythmias. Formal exercise electrocardiography (exercise test) is a useful technique for both the evaluation and documentation of dysrhythmias because exercise may provoke, modify, or suppress the dysrhythmia. The sinus tachycardia that normally occurs during exercise may suppress the dysrhythmia by increasing the sinoatrial node frequency and inhibiting the ectopic focus before it reaches its threshold potential. The sinus rate that usually suppresses this focus is about 150 beats per minute in the asymptomatic patient. If the premature ventricular contractions disappear when the cardiac rate reaches 140 to 150 beats per minute, the ectopic beats are benign and do not require further evaluation. [3] This exercise test may be ordered by a pediatrician or a pediatric cardiologist.

Referral

The presence of a symptomatic dysrhythmia requires exclusion from physical activity until this problem can be adequately evaluated by a cardiologist and controlled. Graded exercise electrocardiographic testing, 24-hour electrocardiographic (Holter) monitoring, transient dysrhythmia monitoring or event monitoring, and echocardiography are often utilized in this evaluation. During both exercise testing and ambulatory monitoring, the patient's activities should be as similar as possible to those experienced during sports participation.

Recommendations

The recommendations of the American Academy of Pediatrics are in agreement with those of the 26th Bethesda Conference on Cardiovascular Abnormalities in the Athlete. [4]

The American Academy of Pediatrics recommends that athletes with dysrhythmias be evaluated. [4] Athletes who are suspected of having structural heart disease or significant conduction defects (eg, the presence of a heart murmur or an abnormal chest radiograph, electrocardiogram, or echocardiogram) or are symptomatic (ie, they experience syncope, near syncope, pallor, chest pain, or other symptoms of dysrhythmia) require consultation with, or referral to, a cardiologist before permission to participate in sports can be granted.

Disturbance of Sinus Node Function

Patients with a structurally normal heart whose dysrhythmia produces no symptoms and does not worsen with increased activity may participate in all sports.

1. Patients with syncope, near syncope, or other symptoms of dysrhythmia must not participate in sports until the cause of their condition has been determined and treated.

2. Patients whose symptoms clearly are attributable to a dysrhythmia should be treated and, if they remain asymptomatic for 3 to 6 months, may participate in all sports after re-evaluation by a cardiologist.

3. Patients treated with a pacemaker must not engage in sports without the approval of a cardiologist.

Premature Atrial Complexes

Patients with premature atrial complexes may participate in all sports.

Atrial Flutter and/or Fibrillation

Patients with atrial flutter, fibrillation, or both must be evaluated by a cardiologist before clearance is given for participation in sports.

Premature Atrioventricular Junctional Complexes

Patients who have a structurally normal heart without evidence of sustained tachycardia and with a normal heart rate response to activity may participate in all sports. Patients with an abnormal heart, depending on the type and extent of heart disease as determined by a cardiologist, may participate in low-intensity sports as described by the 26th Bethesda Conference on Cardiovascular Abnormalities in the Athlete.[5]

Supraventricular Tachycardia

Patients with prior supraventricular tachycardia who have had no recurrences on therapy during the previous 6 months demonstrated by testing may participate in all sports. Patients who do not have any exercise-induced supraventricular tachycardia but experience rare, brief recurrences should have an attempt at prevention but may participate in low-intensity sports as outlined by the 26th Bethesda Conference.[5] Patients with obstructive heart disease, syncope, near syncope, or other symptoms of dysrhythmia must not participate in any competitive sports until they have been adequately treated and have had no recurrence of symptoms or documented dysrhythmia for at least 6 months (by history, exercise electrocardiography, and Holter monitoring).

Ventricular Preexcitation, or Wolff-Parkinson-White Syndrome

Evaluation by a cardiologist is warranted before participation. Patients without structural heart disease or a history of palpitations or tachycardia may participate in most sports. An in-depth evaluation is recommended before participation in moderate or high-intensity sports or competitive situations.[5]

Premature Ventricular Complexes

Patients with no structural heart disease, in whom premature ventricular complexes disappear during exercise at a heart rate of approximately 150 beats per minute, may participate in all sports if the premature ventricular contractions are uniform. All other patients with premature ventricular contractions must be evaluated by a cardiologist before participation is approved. This includes patients in whom premature ventricular complexes increase in frequency or occur in pairs or runs during exercise. Patients with structural heart disease who have premature ventricular contractions must be excluded from high- or moderate-intensity competitive sports, with or without treatment. [5] Patients with premature ventricular complexes and prolongation of the QTc interval must not participate in competitive athletics.

Ventricular Tachycardia

All patients with ventricular tachycardia should be evaluated by a cardiologist. Patients who have unsustained ventricular tachycardia with QRS complexes of uniform configuration at a rate of <150 beats per minute, and who have no structural heart disease or symptoms of dysrhythmia such as syncope or near syncope, may participate in all sports after clearance from a cardiologist. Patients who have structural heart disease; a history of syncope, near syncope, or other symptoms of dysrhythmia; ventricular tachycardia during exertion; or a prolonged QTc interval syndrome must not engage in any competitive sports.

COMMITTEE ON SPORTS MEDICINE AND FITNESS, 1994 to 1995

William L. Risser, MD, PhD, Chair

Steven J. Anderson, MD

Stephen P. Bolduc, MD

Bernard Griesemer, MD

Sally S. Harris, MD, MPH

Larry McLain, MD

Suzanne M. Tanner, MD

Liaison Representatives

Kathryn Keely, MD, Canadian Paediatric Society

Richard Malacrea, ATC, National Athletic Trainers Association

Judith C. Young, PhD, National Association for Sport and Physical Education

AAP Section Liaisons

Arthur M. Pappas, MD, Section on Orthopaedics

Reginald L. Washington, MD, Section on Cardiology

Consultant

Oded Bar-Or, MD, Canadian Paediatric Society

References

1. McCaffrey FM, Braden DS, Strong WB. Sudden cardiac death in athletes: a review. *Am J Dis Child.* 1991; 145:177–183

2. Driscoll DJ. Cardiovascular evaluation of the child and adolescent before participation in sports. *Mayo Clin Proc.* 1985; 60:867–873

3. Bricker JT, Ross B. Arrhythmias in sports. In: Gilette PC, Garson A, eds. *Pediatric Dysrhythmias: Electrophysiology and Pacing.* Philadelphia, PA: WB Saunders Company; 1990:617–629

4. Zipes DP, Garson A. Task Force VI: Arrhythmias. *J Am Coll Cardiol.* 1994; 24:892–899

5. The 26th Bethesda Conference. Recommendations for determining eligibility for competition in athletes with cardiovascular abnormalities. *J Am Coll Cardiol.* 1994; 24:845–899

This statement has been approved by the Council on Child and Adolescent Health.

The recommendations in this statement do not indicate an exclusive course of treatment or serve as a standard of medical care. Variations, taking into account individual circumstances, may be appropriate.

Climatic Heat Stress and the Exercising Child (RE2217)

AMERICAN ACADEMY OF PEDIATRICS

Committee on Sports Medicine

Volume 69, Number 6

June 1982

Heat-induced illness is preventable. Physicians, teachers, coaches, and parents must be made aware of the potential hazards of high-intensity exercise in hot climates and of the measures needed to prevent heat-related illness in preadolescents.

Because of the following morphologic and functional differences, exercising children do not adapt to extremes of temperature as effectively as adults when exposed to a high-climatic heat stress. [1]

1. Children have a greater surface area-mass ratio than adults, which induces a greater heat transfer between the environment and the body.

2. Children produce more metabolic heat per mass unit than adults when walking or running. [2]

3. Sweating capacity is not as great in children as in adults. [3,4]

4. The capacity to convey heat by blood from the body core to the skin is reduced in the exercising child. [4,5]

The foregoing characteristics do not interfere with the ability of the exercising child to dissipate heat effectively in a neutral or mildly warm climate. However, when air temperature exceeds skin temperature, children have less tolerance to exercise than do adults. The greater the temperature gradient between the air and the skin, the greater the effect on the child. [4, 6, 7]

Upon transition to a warmer climate, any exercising individual must allow time for conditioning for heat (acclimatization). Intense and prolonged exercise undertaken before acclimatization may be detrimental to health and might even lead to fatal heat stroke. [8] Although children can acclimatize to exercise in the heat, [6, 9] the rate of their acclimatization is slower than that of adults. [1] Therefore, a child will need more exposures to the new climate to sufficiently acclimatize.

Children frequently do not instinctively drink enough liquids to replenish fluid loss during prolonged exercise and may become gravely dehydrated. [10] A major consequence of dehydration is an excessive increase in body temperature during exercise. For a given level of dehydration, children are subject to a greater increase in core temperature than are adults. [10] Clinically, the dehydrated child is more prone to heat-related illness than the fully hydrated one. [11, 12]

Children with the following conditions are at a potentially greater risk of heat stress: obesity, febrile state, cystic fibrosis, gastrointestinal infection, diabetes insipidus, diabetes mellitus, chronic heart failure, caloric malnutrition, anorexia nervosa, sweating insufficiency syndrome, and mental deficiency.

Based on the foregoing responses of children to exercise in hot climates, the Committee recommends:

1. The intensity of activities that last 30 minutes or more should be reduced whenever relative humidity and air temperature are above critical levels. Information concerning relative humidity may be obtained from a nearby US Weather Bureau or by use of a sling psychrometer (School Health Supplies, PO Box 409, 300 Lombard Rd, Addison, IL 60101; approximate cost $30) to compare dry bulb and wet bulb temperature levels.

2. At the beginning of a strenuous exercise program or after traveling to a warmer climate, the intensity and duration of exercise should be restrained initially and then gradually increased over a period of ten to 14 days to accomplish acclimatization to the effects of heat.

3. Prior to prolonged physical activity, the child should be fully hydrated. During the activity, periodic drinking (eg, 150 ml of cold tap water each 30 minutes for a child weighing 40 kg) should be enforced.

4. Clothing should be lightweight, limited to one layer of absorbent material in order to facilitate evaporation of sweat and expose as much skin as possible. Sweat-saturated garments should be replaced by dry ones. Rubberized sweat suits should never be used to produce loss of weight.

Proper health habits can be learned. The child athlete who may be exposed to a hot climate must be educated to observe the foregoing principles. Emphasis should be given to heat acclimatization, fluid intake, proper clothing, air temperature, and humidity.

COMMITTEE ON SPORTS MEDICINE, 1979 to 1981

Thomas E. Shaffer, MD, Chairman (1981-)

Thomas G. Flynn, MD, Chairman (1978-1980)

Elizabeth Coryllos, MD

Paul G. Dyment, MD

John H. Kennell, MD

Eugene F. Luckstead, MD

Robert N. McLeod, Jr, MD

Nathan J. Smith, MD

William B. Strong, MD

Melvin L. Thornton, MD

Clemens W. Van Rooy, MD

John Murray, MD

Liaison Representatives

Frederick W. Baker, MD, Canadian Paediatric Society

Lucille Burkett, American Alliance for Health, Physical Education and Recreation

Oded Bar-Or, MD, American College of Sports Medicine

Henry Levison, MD, Section on Diseases of the Chest

Richard Malacrea, National Athletic Trainers Association

James Moller, MD, Section on Cardiology

References

1. Bar-Or O: Climate and the exercising child— A review. *Int J Sports Med.* 1980;1:53

2. Aastrand PO: *Experimental Studies of Physical Working Capacity in Relation to Sex and Age.* Copenhagen, Munksgaard, 1952

3. Haymes EM, McCormick RJ, Buskirk ER: Heat tolerance of exercising lean and obese prepubertal boys. *J Appl Physiol.* 1975; 39:457

4. Drinkwater BL, Kupprat IC, Denton JE, et al: Response of prepubertal girls and college women to work in the heat. *J Appl Physiol.* 1977; 43:1046

5. Drinkwater BL, Horvath SM: Heat tolerance and aging. *Med Sci Sports.* 1979; 11:49

6. Wagner JA, Robinson S, Tzankoff SP, et al. Heat tolerance and acclimatization to work in the heat in relation to age. *J Appl Physiol.* 1972; 33:616

7. Haymes EM, Buskirk ER, Hodgson JL, et al: Heat tolerance of exercising lean and heavy prepubertal girls. *J Appl Physiol.* 1974; 36:566

8. Fox EL, Mathews DK, Kaufman WS, et al: Effects of football equipment on thermal balance and energy cost during exercise. *Res Q Am Assoc Health Phys Educ Recreat.* 1966; 37:332

9. Inbar O: Acclimatization to Dry and Hot Environment in Young Adults and Children 8–10 Years Old, dissertation, Columbia University, New York, 1978

10. Bar-or O, Dotan R, Inbar O, et al: Voluntary hypohydration in 10- to 12-year-old boys. *J Appl Physiol.* 1980; 48:104

11. Danks DM, Webb DW, Allen J: Heat illness in infants and young children: A study of 47 cases. *Br Med J.* 1962; 2:287

12. Taj-Eldin S, Falaki N: Heat illness in infants and small children in desert climates. *J Trop Med Hyg.* 1968; 71:100

13. American College of Sports Medicine: Position statement on prevention of heat injuries during distance running. *Med Sci Sports.* 1975; 7:7

This statement has been approved by the Council on Child and Adolescent Health.

The recommendations in this statement do not indicate an exclusive course of treatment or serve as a standard of medical care. Variations, taking into account individual circumstances, may be appropriate.

PEDIATRICS (ISSN 0031 4005). Copyright © 1982 by the American Academy of Pediatrics.

No part of this statement may be reproduced in any form or by any means without prior written permission from the American Academy of Pediatrics except for one copy for personal use.

Fitness, Activity, and Sports Participation in the Preschool Child (RE9265)

AMERICAN ACADEMY OF PEDIATRICS

Committee on Sports Medicine and Fitness

Volume 90, Number 6

December 1992, p 1002–1004

A sedentary lifestyle has been linked to the development of coronary artery disease, hypertension, diabetes mellitus, obesity, and other chronic diseases of adulthood. Although these conditions are predominantly diseases of adulthood, they are thought to be lifelong processes with their origins in childhood. The promotion of physical activity in early childhood may be important as the initial step in developing lifelong habits that may help forestall future chronic illness. Although some children may be too sedentary, others are participating in training programs and competitive sports that are inappropriate for the preschool age group. Guidelines for fitness and sports participation for preschool children younger than 6 years must be based on a careful consideration of the physical fitness needs as well as the unique developmental requirements and limitations of this age group.

Levels of Childhood Fitness

The results of recent national physical fitness testing of school-aged children have raised the concern that we are in the midst of a youth fitness crisis. It is clear from these studies that school-aged children have more body fat and weight than children had 20 years ago. [1, 2] However, because of the lack of comparable physical fitness tests done in the past, it has been difficult to determine if there has been a decline in physical fitness. Although national surveys, such as the National Children and Youth Fitness Study, have determined norms for field test measures of physical fitness in school-aged children, no such data exist for children younger than 6 years. In addition, it is unknown whether there has been any change in the level of physical fitness of preschool children in recent years.

The type and amount of exercise for optimal functional capacity and health in preschool and school-aged children in general have not been determined. Most preschool children are inherently active and experience a strong drive for motor activity. Motor activity is the means by which preschoolers explore their environments, achieve physical closeness, and communicate with others, and it is an essential component for their physical and cognitive development. It is likely that most preschool children achieve adequate levels of physical fitness when allowed to express their innate curiosity and natural propensity for active exploration in a safe environment. Under these circumstances, specific intervention to improve the physical fitness of preschool children is usually unnecessary.

Childhood obesity affects a significant subset of preschool children. Studies of young children suggest that a low physical activity level is a primary factor contributing to excessive fat accumulation. [3] The large amount of time that many children spend watching television has been linked to an increase in childhood obesity. [4] Children aged 2 to 5 years are estimated to watch 25.5 hours of television per week, which cuts significantly into time available for more vigorous activities. [5] Obese children and those with a strong genetic predisposition for obesity may benefit from interventions designed to encourage daily physical activity.

Motor Development

There is no evidence that children's motor development can be accelerated or their subsequent sports performance influenced by physical training during the preschool years. For example, there is no proof that special training can groom a preschooler to become a future champion. Most children follow the same sequence of acquisition of motor skills. This appears to be an innate process that occurs independent of gender. The rate at which children master motor skills, however, is variable and cannot be predicted for an individual child. [6] During the preschool years, children learn to perform tasks such as throwing, kicking, running, hopping, jumping, and catching. Among 4-year-old children, only 20% are proficient at throwing and 30% at catching. [7] A number of skills are not yet fully developed in preschool-aged children. It is this lack of maturity rather than poor motor coordination that limits a child's ability to perform certain tasks. During the preschool years, motor skills are best learned in an unstructured, noncompetitive setting in which a child can experiment and learn by trial and error on an individual basis. Specific skills can be refined through repetitive practice only after the relevant level of motor development has been reached.

Organized Sports Participation

A preschool child's readiness to participate in organized sports or structured exercise sessions depends on a combination of factors: (1) neurodevelopmental level (motor skills acquisition); (2) social development (interaction with coaches and teammates); and (3) cognitive level (ability to understand instructions). [8] "Sports readiness" will occur at different rates for individual children and is best determined by the child's eagerness to participate and subsequent enjoyment of the activity.

Organized sports sessions should be tailored to match the developmental level of the preschool child. Preschool children characteristically have short attention spans and are easily distracted. Therefore, exercise sessions should be short and emphasize playfulness, experimentation, and exploration of a wide variety of movement experiences. A reasonable format would consist of no longer than 15 to 20 minutes of structured activity combined with 30 minutes of free play. Concentration will be maximized if instructional sessions take place in a setting with minimal distractions or variations. Modifications of equipment and rules can be made to suit the developmental level and attention span of the participants. Such modifications are changes in the size of balls, softer balls, smaller fields, shorter duration of games and practices, reduced number of participants playing at the same time, frequent changing of positions, and not keeping score. Instruction should follow a "show and tell" format that emphasizes physical demonstration rather than verbal instruction since preschoolers need visual cues in addition to simple auditory cues for full comprehension of instructional material. [9] Competition with others requires rapid decision making that may be beyond the cognitive capabilities of preschoolers and may also interfere with the learning of fundamental skills. Competition offers no advantage and should be minimized. Rather, the focus should be on varied movement experiences. Factors such as fun, success, variety, freedom, family participation, peer support, and enthusiastic leadership encourage and maintain participation, whereas others such as failure, embarrassment, competition, boredom, regimentation, and injuries discourage subsequent participation. [10] Structured exercise sessions should be supervised by adults knowledgeable about the specific needs and limitations of the preschool age group.

Role of the Pediatrician

Pediatricians have a unique opportunity to encourage appropriate physical activity habits during the preschool years as a basis for establishing lifelong behavior important for general well-being and prevention of subsequent disease. All preschool children should be encouraged to participate regularly in a form of physical activity appropriate for their developmental level. Pediatricians should incorporate an assessment of physical activity into well-child visits when taking histories by addressing topics such as the following: interest and participation in active as opposed to sedentary hobbies; time spent watching television; activity level relative to peers; participation in organized physical activity programs; and exercise habits of family members. Pediatricians can educate parents, teachers, and coaches regarding the developmental progression and limitations of preschool children as they relate to physical activities and the appropriate structure, goals, and safety issues pertaining to exercise sessions for this age group.

American Academy of Pediatrics Recommendations

1. All preschool children should participate regularly in a form of physical activity appropriate for their developmental level and physical health status.

2. Emphasis should be placed on promotion of physical activity as a natural and lifelong activity of healthy living. Goals of accelerating motor development to maximize subsequent sports ability are inappropriate and futile, and should be discouraged.

3. Free play designed to provide opportunities for each child to develop fundamental motor skills and to reach his or her potential at his or her own rate is preferable to structured sessions.

4. Readiness to participate in organized sports should be determined individually, based on the child's (not the parent's) eagerness to participate and subsequent enjoyment of the activity. Children are unlikely to be ready before age 6 years.

5. In structured sports programs, goals of participation and enjoyment should be emphasized rather than those of competition and victory. Sessions should be supervised by adults knowledgeable about the specific needs and limitations of preschool children. Setting, format, rules, and equipment should be modified accordingly.

6. Pediatricians should assess preschoolers' physical activity level and time spent in passive activities, such as television watching, by incorporating relevant questions into the medical history during health assessment visits. Appropriate physical activity should be promoted by counseling parents, teachers, and coaches.

7. Parents and other family members should be encouraged to serve as role models for their children by participating in regular physical activity programs themselves. In addition, physical activities that parents can do with young children should be encouraged.

COMMITTEE ON SPORTS MEDICINE AND FITNESS, 1991 to 1992

Michael A. Nelson, MD, Chair

Barry Goldberg, MD

Sally S. Harris, MD

Gregory L. Landry, MD

David M. Orenstein, MD

William L. Risser, MD

Liaison Representatives

Kathryn Keely, MD, Canadian Paediatric Society

Richard Malacrea, National Athletic Trainers Association

Judith C. Young, PhD, National Association for Sport and Physical Education

AAP Section Liaison

Arthur M. Pappas, MD, Section on Orthopaedics

Reginald L. Washington, MD, Section on Cardiology

Consultant

Oded Bar-Or, MD, Canadian Paediatric Society

References

1. Ross JG, Gilbert GG. The national children and youth fitness study: a summary of findings. *J Phys Educ Recreation Dance.* 1985; 56:45–50

2. Ross JG, Gilbert GG. The national children and youth fitness study, II: a summary of findings. *J Phys Educ Recreation Dance.* 1987; 58:51–56

3. Griffiths M, Payne PR. Energy expenditure in small children of obese and non-obese parents. *Nature.* 1976; 260:698–700

4. Dietz WH, Jr, Gortmaker SL. Do we fatten our children at the television set? Obesity and television viewing in childhood and adolescents. *Pediatrics.* 1985; 75:807–812

5. A. C. Nielsen Company. *1988 Report on Television.* Northbrook, IL: A. C. Nielsen Company; 1988:8–9

6. Seefeldt V, Haubenstricker J. Patterns, phases or stages. An analytical model for the study of developmental movement. In: Kelso JS, Clark JE, eds. *The Development of Movement Control and Coordination.* New York, NY: John Wiley; 1982:309–318

7. Guttendge MA. A study of motor achievements of young children. *Arch Psychol.* 1939; 244:1–178

8. Dyment PG. Neurodevelopmental milestones: when is a child ready for sports participation? In: Sullivan JA, Grana WA, eds. *The Pediatric Athlete.* Park Ridge, IL: American Academy of Orthopaedic Surgeons; 1990:27–29

9. Weiss MR, Klint KA. Show and tell in the gymnasium: an investigation of developmental differences in modeling and verbal rehearsal of motor skills. *Res Q Exerc Sport.* 1987; 58:234–241

10. Rowland TW. Clinical approaches to the sedentary child. In: *Exercise and Children's Health.* Champaign, IL: Human Kinetics Books; 1990:259–274

This statement has been approved by the Council on Child and Adolescent Health.

The recommendations in this statement do not indicate an exclusive course of treatment or serve as a standard of medical care. Variations, taking into account individual circumstances, may be appropriate.

Human Immunodeficiency Virus [Acquired Immunodeficiency Syndrome (AIDS) Virus] in the Athletic Setting (RE9220)

AMERICAN ACADEMY OF PEDIATRICS

Committee on Sports Medicine and Fitness

Volume 88, Number 3

September 1991, p 640–641

Because athletes may bleed following trauma, they represent a theoretical risk to others if they are infected with the human immuno-deficiency virus [HIV, acquired immunodeficiency syndrome (AIDS) virus]. Two questions have concerned coaches, athletic trainers, and school administrators: Should an athlete known to be infected with HIV be allowed to participate in competitive sports, and should the universal precautions recommended for health care workers [1] be used when handling athletes' blood and body fluids?

The risk of infection from skin exposure to the blood of a child or adolescent infected with HIV is unknown, but it is apparently minute and is much less than the risk of HIV infection by needlesticks from infected patients of approximately 1:250. [2] Although it is theoretically possible that transmission of HIV could occur in sports such as wrestling and football in which bleeding and skin abrasions are common, no such transmission has been reported in these sports. There is one report of possible transmission of HIV involving a collision between soccer players. [3] However, this report from Italy remains undocumented.

If an HIV-infected athlete would choose to pursue another sport, this possible risk to others would be avoided; but, in the absence of any proven risk, involuntary restriction of an infected athlete is not justified. Informing others of the athlete's status would probably lead to his or her exclusion due to inappropriate fear and prejudice and therefore should also be avoided. This advice must be reconsidered if transmission of HIV is found to occur in the sports setting. Athletes should also be made aware of the hazards of needle sharing for illicit drug use, including steroids.

Universal precautions adapted for the athletic setting are provided in Recommendation 6. Risk of exposure to a variety of infectious diseases is greater for coaches and trainers because of their interaction with many athletes. Competitors have extraordinarily low exposure rates. Coaches and athletic trainers should use these precautions if they are exposed repetitively to athletes' blood, because a rare athlete may have an HIV infection and because the athletic staff may not know

this (as a result of the current practice of nondisclosure or because HIV-infected individuals may be asymptomatic and unaware of their infection).

The American Academy of Pediatrics recommends:

1. Athletes infected with HIV should be allowed to participate in all competitive sports. This advice must be reconsidered if transmission of HIV is found to occur in the sports setting.

2. A physician counseling a known HIV-infected athlete in a sport involving blood exposure, such as wrestling or football, should inform him of the theoretical risk of contagion to others and strongly encourage him to consider another sport.

3. The physician should respect a HIV-infected athlete's right to confidentiality. This includes not disclosing the patient's status of infection to the participants or the staff of athletic programs.

4. All athletes should be made aware that the athletic program is operating under the policies in Recommendations 1 and 3.

5. Routine testing of athletes for HIV infection is not indicated.

6. The following precautions should be adopted:

    a. Skin exposed to blood or other body fluids visibly contaminated with blood should be cleaned as promptly as is practical, preferably with soap and warm water. Skin antiseptics (eg, alcohol) or moist towelettes may be used if soap and water are not available.

    b. Even though good hand-washing is an adequate precaution, [4] water-impervious gloves (latex, vinyl, etc) should be available for staff to use if desired when handling blood or other body fluids visibly contaminated with blood. Gloves should be worn by individuals with nonintact skin. Hands should be washed after glove removal.

    c. If blood or other body fluids visibly contaminated with blood are present on a surface, the object should be cleaned with fresh household bleach solution made for immediate use as follows: 1 part bleach in 100 parts of water, or 1 tablespoon bleach to 1 quart water (hereafter called "fresh bleach solution"). For example, athletic equipment (eg, wrestling mats) visibly contaminated with blood should be wiped clean with fresh bleach solution and allowed to dry before reusing.

d. Emergency care should not be delayed because gloves or other protective equipment are not available.

e. If the care giver wishes to wear gloves and none are readily available, a bulky towel may be used to cover the wound until an off-the-field location is reached where gloves can be used during more definitive treatment.

f. Each coach and athletic trainer should receive training in first aid and emergency care and be provided with the necessary supplies to treat open wounds.

g. For those sports with direct body contact and other sports where bleeding may be expected to occur [5]
   1. If a skin lesion is observed, it should be cleansed immediately with a suitable antiseptic and covered securely [5].
   2. If a bleeding wound occurs, the individual's participation should be interrupted until the bleeding has been stopped and the wound is both cleansed with antiseptic and covered securely or occluded. [5]

h. Saliva does not transmit HIV. However, because of potential fear on the part of those providing cardiopulmonary resuscitation, breathing (Ambu) bags and oral airways for use during cardiopulmonary resuscitation should be available in athletic settings for those who prefer not to give mouth-to-mouth resuscitation.

i. Coaches and athletic trainers should receive training in prevention of HIV transmission in the athletic setting; they should then help implement the recommendations suggested above.

COMMITTEE ON SPORTS MEDICINE AND FITNESS, 1990 to 1991

Michael A. Nelson, MD, Chairman

Barry Goldberg, MD

Sally S. Harris, MD

Gregory L. Landry, MD

David M. Orenstein, MD

William L. Risser, MD

Liaison Representatives

Kathryn Keely, MD, Canadian Paediatric Society

Richard Malacrea, National Athletic Trainers Association

Judith C. Young, PhD, National Association for Sport and Physical Education

AAP Section Liaison

Arthur M. Pappas, MD, Section on Orthopaedics

References

1. Centers for Disease Control. Update: recommendations for prevention of HIV transmission in health-care settings. *MMWR.* 1987; 36(suppl 1):1–18

2. Henderson DK, Saah AJ, Zak BJ, et al. Risk of nosocomial infection with human T-cell lymphotropic virus type III/lymphadenopathy-associated virus in a large cohort of intensively exposed health care workers. *Ann Intern Med.* 1986; 104:644–647

3. Torre D, Sampietro C, Ferraro G, Zeroli C, Speranza F. Transmission of HIV-1 infection via sports injury. *Lancet.* 1990; 335:1105

4. Task Force on Pediatric AIDS, American Academy of Pediatrics. Pediatric guidelines for infection control of human immunodeficiency virus (acquired immunodeficiency virus) in hospitals, medical offices, schools, and other settings. *Pediatrics.* 1988; 82:801–807

5. World Health Organization in collaboration with the International Federation of Sports Medicine. Consensus Statement from Consultation on AIDS and Sports. Geneva, Switzerland: January 16, 1989

This statement has been approved by the Council on Child and Adolescent Health.

The recommendations in this statement do not indicate an exclusive course of treatment or serve as a standard of medical care. Variations, taking into account individual circumstances, may be appropriate.

In-line Skating Injuries in Children and Adolescents (RE9739)

AMERICAN ACADEMY OF PEDIATRICS
Committee on Injury and Poison Prevention and Committee on Sports Medicine and Fitness
Volume 101, Number 4
April 1998, p 720–722

ABSTRACT. *In-line skating has become one of the fastest-growing recreational sports in the United States. Recent studies emphasize the value of protective gear in reducing the incidence of injuries. Recommendations are provided for parents and pediatricians, with special emphasis on the novice or inexperienced skater.*

Since its introduction in 1980, in-line skating has become one of the fastest growing recreational sports for children and teenagers in the United States. An estimated 17.7 million people younger than 18 years participated in this sport in 1996, a 24% increase over the previous year.[1] The sport offers the benefits of aerobic fitness,[2] independent transportation for younger children, the opportunity to play roller hockey or cross-train for other sports, and venues for competition in artistic, speed skating, and endurance events. Entry-level skates now cost less than $20 per pair, a 10-fold decrease in the past decade. The low cost and multiple benefits of participation have allowed the sport to thrive beyond the limits of a "fad," as evidenced by the existence of a professional roller hockey league, in-line speed skating competition at the Pan American Games, trick-skating competition at the Entertainment and Sports Programming Network (ESPN) Extreme Games, several periodicals for enthusiasts, an international skaters association, a formal training program for instructors,[3] and summer training camps.

As the sport has grown, so has the number of participants injured. In 1996, an estimated 76,000 children and teenagers younger than 21 years were injured sufficiently while in-line skating to require emergency department care, compared with about 415,000 bicyclists. The most common reasons cited for injuries during in-line skating were losing one's balance because of a road defect or debris, being unable to stop, out-of-control speeding, or doing a trick.[4] In one study, novice skaters incurred 14% of all injuries requiring treatment.[4] The wrist is the most common site of injury (37% of all injuries), and two thirds of wrist injuries are fractures. Few skaters die. Of a total of 36 who died since 1992, the US Consumer Product Safety Commission Clearinghouse reported that 31 had collided with a motor vehicle.

Wearing proper gear is essential for safe skating. This includes a helmet, wrist guards, knee pads, and elbow pads. Wrist guards are designed to prevent wrist injuries by preventing sudden extreme hyperextension, absorbing some shock of impact, dissipating kinetic forces by forward sliding on their hard volar plates, and preventing local gravel burns. A helmet, elbow pads, and knee pads are recommended for shock absorption.[5–9] Recent research[4] has evaluated the effectiveness of such gear and indicates that wearing wrist guards could reduce the number of wrist injuries by 87%, wearing elbow pads could reduce the number of elbow injuries by 82%, and wearing knee pads could reduce the number of knee injuries by 32%. Although in this study the number of in-line skaters who sustained a head injury was not sufficient to determine the degree of protection afforded by helmets, others[10] have reported that a bicycle helmet or similar approved sports helmet[11] is strongly protective against the occurrence of a head injury to bicyclists in the same physical environment to which a skater is exposed. Helmet use by child and adolescent skaters is required by law in New York and Oregon. Skaters who participate in roller hockey or perform tricks should wear heavy-duty protective gear, including well-constructed wrist guards, knee pads, elbow pads, and a full-head helmet that covers the ears.

"Truck-surfing" or "skitching" refers to skating behind or alongside a vehicle while the skater holds on to the vehicle. This enables a skater to travel at the same velocity as the vehicle. However, it can be very dangerous because the skater cannot slow down fast enough to prevent colliding with the vehicle or being thrown into oncoming traffic or the roadbed if the vehicle suddenly slows, stops, or turns. If the skater falls, his or her enhanced momentum will likely result in a greater force of impact, and consequently, a more severe injury. Several deaths have been caused by skitching.

The design of the skates should match the ability of the skater. Three- or four-wheeled skates are suitable for novice- or intermediate-level skaters, depending on the child's foot size. Five-wheeled skates are high-performance, extremely low-friction skates that should be used only by competitive or long-distance skaters. Skates should fit snugly to allow good, responsive control. Skates, whether rented or owned, should be well maintained: the brake pads should not be worn down, the wheels should be worn symmetrically and turn freely. Skates with expandable shells or interchangeable liners are now available to accommodate the child's growing foot.

Skating skill is not acquired easily or quickly. Good balance and speed control are essential skills to learn. In the past, children acquired skating skills on traditional "quad" skates, rather than in-line skates, but that pattern appears to be changing. The age at which children are ready to use in-line skates safely is not known with certainty because a combination of factors are involved: physical factors (foot size and body strength); skill factors (general athletic ability and large-muscle coordination); and behavioral factors (vigilance in watching the surface for debris and defects, sufficient attention to traffic, judgment). Although most 7- and 8-year-olds can acquire the skills needed to in-line skate, some children may acquire these skills earlier or later. Judgment and ability to avoid obstacles, including bicyclists, pedestrians, and other skaters, are needed. Training may help the novice learn the sport; more than 2000 certified instructors now teach in the United States.

With either type of skate, the novice should preferably learn indoors at a skating rink, where surface conditions, speed, and lighting are controlled without the presence of motor vehicle traffic or other obstacles. Novices particularly need a flat, smooth surface free of debris.

Once a skater can control speed and direction on an indoor rink, he or she is ready to skate on a path or open lot. Hills (even small ones) should be avoided at first. The path selected should be isolated from motor vehicle, bicycle, and pedestrian traffic to the greatest extent possible until the skater is competent enough to avoid such obstacles. Separate trails are advisable where possible. Trail designs have been published, including recommendations for design speed, surface composition, drainage, trail width, and sight distances.[8] Trails should be kept free of sand, dirt, leaves, and twigs, which can become trapped between the wheels and cause a sudden change in velocity with loss of balance. Good drainage is needed so that puddles do not form—water changes the coefficient of friction and results in a sudden change in velocity. Trails should also flatten for at least 30 ft before intersections.[8]

Recommendations

The American Academy of Pediatrics recommends that pediatricians provide the following advice to patients and families concerned with this activity:

Parents need to understand both the benefits and risks of in-line skating. Children and their parents should appreciate that injuries are particularly common in novice skaters, roller hockey players, and those performing tricks.

Full protective gear needs to be used at all times, including a helmet, wrist guards, knee pads, and elbow pads. The helmet should be certified by the American National Standards Institute (ANSI), the American Society for Testing and Materials (ASTM), the Snell Memorial Foundation, or the Consumer Product Safety Commission. Skaters performing tricks need special heavy-duty protective gear.

If skating takes place on the streets, pediatricians should strongly encourage parents, children, and adolescents to use streets that are blocked off or closed to through traffic (eg, dead-end streets or cul-de-sacs).

Special attention should be paid to the needs of novice skaters to avoid injuries. They should skate on an indoor or outdoor rink, rather than on a path or street. Inexperienced children should not attempt to do tricks.

"Truck-surfing" or "skitching" should be prohibited for all skaters under any circumstance.

The type and fit of the skates should be carefully considered when they are purchased or rented and should be appropriate for the child's size, ability, and purpose.

Skaters should vigilantly watch for road debris and defects, which may precipitate a loss of balance. They should be trained to react appropriately to these and other rapidly occurring and unpredictable circumstances by learning to stop quickly and fall safely and by avoiding traffic. Instruction in skating by a teacher certified by the International In-Line Skating Association is recommended.

Children with large-muscle motor skill or balance problems and those with any uncorrected hearing or vision deficit should skate only in a protected environment. Appropriate areas include a skating rink or outdoor area where the skater is either alone or where no motor vehicle or bicycle traffic occurs and where all other skaters and pedestrians travel in same direction.

State legislation that requires helmet use while skating should be encouraged.

COMMITTEE ON INJURY AND POISON PREVENTION, 1997 to 1998

Murray L. Katcher, MD, PhD, Chairperson

Phyllis Agran, MD, MPH

Danielle Laraque, MD

Susan H. Pollack, MD

Barbara L. Smith, MD

Gary A. Smith, MD, DrPh

Howard R. Spivak, MD

Susan B. Tully, MD

Liaison Representatives

Ruth A. Brenner, MD, National Institute of Child Health and Human Development

Stephanie Bryn, MPH, Maternal and Child Health Bureau

William P. Tully, MD, Pediatric Orthopaedic Society of North America

Cheryl Neverman, US Dept of Transportation

Richard A. Schieber, MD, MPH, Centers for Disease Control and Prevention

Richard Stanwick, MD, Canadian Paediatric Society

Deborah Tinsworth, US Consumer Product Safety Commission

Section Liaisons

Marilyn Bull, MD, MPH, Section on Injury and Poison Prevention

Victor Garcia, MD, Section on Surgery

COMMITTEE ON SPORTS MEDICINE AND FITNESS, 1997 to 1998

Steven J. Anderson, MD, Chairperson

Stephen P. Bolduc, MD

Bernard Griesemer, MD

Miriam D. Johnson, MD

Larry G. McLain, MD

Thomas W. Rowland, MD

Eric Small, MD

Liaison Representatives

Kathryn Keely, MD, Canadian Paediatric Society

Richard Malacrea, ATC, National Athletic Trainers Association

Judith C. Young, PhD, National Association for Sport and Physical Education

Section Liaisons

Reginald L. Washington, MD, Section on Cardiology

Frederick E. Reed, MD, Section on Orthopaedics

References

1. American Sports Data, Inc. *American Sports Analysis: Summary Report.* Hartsdale, NY: American Sports Data, Inc; 1996

2. Snyder AC, O'Hagan KP, Clifford PS, Hoffman MD, Foster C. Exercise responses to in-line skating: comparisons to running and cycling. *Int J Sports Med.* 1993; 14:38–42

3. International In-Line Skating Association. *Level I Certified Instructor Manual.* Minneapolis, MN: International In-line Skating Association; 1993

4. Schieber R, Branche-Dorsey CM, Ryan GW, Rutherford GW, Stevens JA, O'Neil J. Risk factors for injuries from in-line skating and the effectiveness of safety gear. *N Engl J Med.* 1996; 335:1630–1635

5. Schieber RA, Branche-Dorsey CM, Ryan GW. Comparison of in-line skating injuries with roller-skating and skateboarding injuries. *JAMA.* 1994; 271:1856–1858

6. Calle SC. In-line skating injuries, 1987 through 1992. *Am J Public Health.* 1994; 84:675

7. Heller D. Rollerblading injuries. *Hazard.* 1993; 15:11–13

8. International In-line Skating Association. *Guidelines for Establishing In-line Skate Trails in Parks and Recreational Areas.* Minneapolis, MN: International In-line Skating Association; 1992

9. US Consumer Product Safety Commission. *Safety Commission Warns About Hazards With In-line Roller Skates: Safety Alert.* Bethesda, MD: US Consumer Product Safety Commission; August 1991

10. Sacks JJ, Holmgreen P, Smith SM, Sosin DM. Bicycle-associated head injuries and deaths in the United States from 1984 through 1988: how many are preventable? *JAMA.* 1991; 266:3016–3018

11. Centers for Disease Control and Prevention. Injury-control recommendations: bicycle helmets. *MMWR.* 1995; 44(RR-1):1–17

Knee Brace Use by Athletes (RE9175)

AMERICAN ACADEMY OF PEDIATRICS
Committee on Sports Medicine
Volume 85, Number 2
February 1990

The knee is the most frequently injured joint during athletic events, and the medial collateral ligament is one of the most frequently injured ligamentous structures of the knee. The medial collateral ligament is a prime stabilizer of the medial side of the knee. The most frequent cause of injury to this ligament is a blow from the lateral side of the knee or thigh with or without a rotatory force, which causes a valgus stress. In the growing child, similar forces to the lateral side of the knee may result in a femoral fracture due to displacement of the distal epiphysis.

It has become a goal of sports medicine enthusiasts to decrease the number of knee injuries and, specifically, the medial knee injury. The most readily apparent method to protect the knee is to provide additional external support. The lateral unidirectional articulated knee brace, strapped to the thigh and the calf, was developed in an attempt to reduce knee injuries. These lateral knee-stabilizing braces, the so-called "prophylactic knee braces," have become widely used by football players at all levels of skill. A number of early reports provided mixed conclusions as to the value of these braces. [1] Two recent comprehensive studies both concluded that so-called preventive braces are not preventive and may, in fact, be harmful. [2, 3]

Based on current evidence, the American Academy of Pediatrics recommends that lateral unidirectional knee braces not be considered standard equipment for football players because of lack of efficacy and the potential of actually causing harm.

COMMITTEE ON SPORTS MEDICINE, 1989 to 1990

Michael A. Nelson, MD, Chairman
Barry Goldberg, MD
Sally S. Harris, MD
Gregory L. Landry, MD
William L. Risser, MD

Liaison Representatives

Oded Bar-Or, MD, Canadian Paediatric Society
Richard Malacrea, National Athletic Trainers Association
Roswell Merrick, National Association for Sport and Physical Education

AAP Section Liaison

David M. Orenstein, MD, Section on Diseases of the Chest
Arthur M. Pappas, MD, Section on Orthopaedics

References

1. France EP, Paulos LE, Jayaraman G, Rosenberg TD. Biomechanics of lateral knee bracing, II: impact response of the braced knee. *Am J Sports Med.* 1987; 15:430–438

2. Teitz CC, Hermanson BK, Kronmal RA, et al. Evaluation of the use of braces to prevent injury to the knee in collegiate football players. *J Bone Joint Surg Am.* 1987; 69:2–9

3. Grace TG, Skipper BJ, Newberry JC, et al. Prophylactic knee braces and injury to the lower extremity. *J Bone Joint Surg Am.* 1988; 70:422–427

This statement has been approved by the Council on Child and Adolescent Health.

The recommendations in this statement do not indicate an exclusive course of treatment or serve as a standard of medical care. Variations, taking into account individual circumstances, may be appropriate.

Reprint requests to Publications Dept, American Academy of Pediatrics, 141 Northwest Point Blvd, PO Box 927, Elk Grove Village, IL 60009-0927.

Medical Conditions Affecting Sports Participation (RE9432)

AMERICAN ACADEMY OF PEDIATRICS
Committee on Sports Medicine and Fitness
Volume 94, Number 5
November 1994, p 757–760

In 1988 the American Academy of Pediatrics (AAP) published an analysis of medical conditions affecting sports participation. [1] This statement was endorsed by the American Medical Association, replacing their own recommendations. [2] A further modification of this analysis is presented here, with additions and changes that attempt to increase its accuracy and completeness and to include current information.

In Table 1, sports are categorized by their probability for collision or contact. In "collision" sports (eg, boxing, ice hockey, football, or rodeo), athletes purposely hit or collide with each other or inanimate objects, including the ground, with great force. In "contact" sports (eg, basketball and soccer), athletes routinely make contact with each other or inanimate objects, but usually with less force than in collision sports. Table 1 does not separate collision and contact sports because there is no clear dividing line between them. In "limited contact" sports such as softball and squash, contact with other athletes or inanimate objects is either occasional or inadvertent.

Sports with limited contact, for example downhill skiing and gymnastics, can be as dangerous as the contact or collision activities. Even in noncontact sports serious injuries can occur, such as in power lifting. Overuse injuries are not related to contact or collision. For all these reasons, the categorization of sports in Table 1 reflects imperfectly their relative risk of causing injury. The categorization does, however, give an idea of the comparative likelihood that participation in different sports results in acute traumatic injuries from blows to the body.

We assessed the medical conditions listed in Table 2 to determine whether participation would create an increased risk of injury or adversely affect the medical condition. This table is of value when physicians examine an athlete with one of the listed problems. Decisions about sports participation are often complex, and the usefulness of this table is limited by the frequency with which it recommends individual assessment when a "Qualified Yes" or a "Qualified No" appears. For the majority of chronic health conditions, however, current evidence supports the participation of children and adolescents in most athletic activities.

The physician's clinical judgment is essential in applying these recommendations to a specific patient. This judgment involves the available published information on the risks of participation; the advice of knowledgeable experts; the current health status of the athlete; the level of competition; the position played; the sport in which the athlete participates; the maturity of the competitor; the availability of effective protective equipment that is acceptable to the athlete; the availability and efficacy of treatment; whether treatment, for example rehabilitation of an injury, has been completed; whether the sport can be modified to allow safer participation; and the ability of the athlete and parents to understand and accept risks involved in participation. Potential dangers of associated training activities also need to be considered. For example, strength training is now a part of conditioning for many sports.

Unfortunately, adequate data on the risks of a particular sport for an athlete with a medical problem are often limited or lacking, and an estimate of risk becomes a necessary part of decision making. If restriction from a sport is believed to be necessary, the physician should counsel the athlete and family concerning safe alternative activities.

The strenuousness of a sport is an additional characteristic relevant to athletes with cardiovascular or pulmonary disease. A strenuous sport can place dynamic (volume) or static (pressure) demands on the cardiovascular system, or both. These demands vary not only with the activities of the sport, but also with such factors as its associated training activities and the level of emotional arousal and fitness of the competitors. Table 3 lists sports by their strenuousness as classified by experts. [3] The authors of the table state that the classification "may be of theoretical interest, but its practical value is unknown because our current knowledge regarding the relative risks of these two types of exercise (dynamic and static) for various cardiovascular abnormalities is limited." [3]

Physicians making decisions about sports participation for patients who have more than mild congenital

Table 1 — *Classification of Sports by Contact*

Contact/Collision	Limited Contact	Noncontact
Basketball	Baseball	Archery
Boxing*	Bicycling	Badminton
Diving	Cheerleading	Body building
Field hockey	Canoeing/kayaking(white water)	Bowling
Football	Fencing	Canoeing/kayaking (flat water)
Ice hockey	Field	Crew/rowing
Lacrosse	High jump	Curling
Martial arts	Pole vault	Dancing
Rodeos	Floor hockey	Field
Rugby	Gymnastics	Discus
Ski jumping	Handball	Javelin
Soccer	Horseback riding	Shot put
Team handball	Racquetball	Golf
Water polo	Skating	Orienteering
Wrestling	Skiing (country)	Power lifting
	Softball	Race walking
	Squash	Riflery
	Ultimate Frisbee	Rope jumping
	Volleyball	Running
	Weight lifting	Sailing
		Scuba diving
		Strength training
		Swimming
		Table tennis
		Tennis
		Track

* Participation not recommended.

heart disease or who have cardiac dysrhythmias are encouraged to consider consulting a cardiologist and to review Ref. 3. (Reference 3 is under revision; the report of the 17th Bethesda Conference will be published soon in The Journal of the American College of Cardiology.) Information on sports participation for patients with hypertension is also available. [4] Primary hypertension must be severe before exclusion from sports is indicated. [4]

In recent legal decisions, athletes have been permitted to participate in sports despite known medical risks. When an athlete's family disregards medical advice against participation, the physician should ask all family members to sign written informed consent statements indicating that they have been advised of the potential dangers of participation and understand them.

Information on the impact of medical problems on risk of injury during sports participation is available in the second edition of the AAP's manual on sports medicine. [5] In addition, several position statements of the Academy have relevant material. All but the most recent [6–8] of these statements are included as appendices in the manual. Statements on mitral valve prolapse, cardiac dysrhythmias, and eye protection are in preparation.

Table 2 *Medical Conditions and Sports Participation*

This table is designed to be understood by medical and nonmedical personnel. In the "Explanation" section below, "needs evaluation" means that a physician with appropriate knowledge and experience should assess the safety of a given sport for an athlete with the listed medical condition. Unless otherwise noted, this is because of the variability of the severity of the disease or of the risk of injury among the specific sports in Table 1, or both.

Condition	May Participate?
Atlantoaxial instability (instability of the joint between cervical vertebrae 1 and 2) *Explanation:* Athlete needs evaluation to assess risk of spinal cord injury during sports participation.	Qualified Yes
Bleeding disorder *Explanation:* Athlete needs evaluation.	Qualified Yes
Cardiovascular diseases	
Carditis (inflammation of the heart) *Explanation:* Carditis may result in sudden death with exertion.	No
Hypertension (high blood pressure) *Explanation:* Those with significant essential (unexplained) hypertension should avoid weight and power lifting, body building, and strength training. Those with secondary hypertension (hypertension caused by a previously identified disease), or severe essential hypertension, need evaluation. Reference 4 defines significant and severe hypertension.	Qualified Yes
Congenital heart disease (structural heart defects present at birth) *Explanation:* Those with mild forms may participate fully; those with moderate or severe forms, or who have undergone surgery, need evaluation. Reference 3 defines mild, moderate, and severe disease for the common cardiac lesions.	Qualified Yes
Dysrhythmia (irregular heart rhythm) *Explanation:* Athlete needs evaluation because some types require therapy or make certain sports dangerous, or both. [3]	Qualified Yes
Mitral valve prolapse (abnormal heart valve) *Explanation:* Those with symptoms (chest pain, symptoms of possible dysrhythmia) or evidence of mitral regurgitation (leaking) on physical examination need evaluation. All others may participate fully. [3]	Qualified Yes
Heart murmur *Explanation:* If the murmur is innocent (does not indicate heart disease), full participation is permitted. Otherwise the athlete needs evaluation (see congenital heart disease and mitral valve prolapse above).	Qualified Yes
Cerebral palsy *Explanation:* Athlete needs evaluation.	Qualified Yes
Diabetes mellitus *Explanation:* All sports can be played with proper attention to diet hydration, and insulin therapy. Particular attention is needed for activities that last 30 minutes or more.	Yes
Diarrhea *Explanation:* Unless disease is mild, no participation is permitted, because diarrhea may increase the risk of dehydration and heat illness. See "Fever" below	Qualified No
Eating disorders Anorexia nervosa Bulimia nervosa *Explanation:* These patients need both medical and psychiatric assessment before participation.	Qualified Yes

Table 2 *Medical Conditions and Sports Participation—cont'd.*

Condition	May Participate?
Eyes	
Functionally one-eyed athlete	Qualified Yes

Loss of an eye
Detached retina
Previous eye surgery or serious eye injury
Explanation: A functionally one-eyed athlete has a best corrected visual acuity of <20/40 in the worse eye. These athletes would suffer significant disability if the better eye was seriously injured as would those with loss of an eye. Some athletes who have previously undergone eye surgery or had a serious eye injury may have an increased risk of injury because of weakened eye tissue. Availability of eye guards approved by the American Society for Testing Materials (ASTM) and other protective equipment may allow participation in most sports, but this must be judged on an individual basis. [9, 10]

Fever	No

Explanation: Fever can increase cardiopulmonary effort, reduce maximum exercise capacity, make heat illness more likely, and increase orthostatic hypotension during exercise. Fever may rarely accompany myocarditis or other infections that may make exercise dangerous.

Heat illness, history of	Qualified Yes

Explanation: Because of the increased likelihood of recurrence, the athlete needs individual assessment to determine the presence of predisposing conditions and to arrange a prevention strategy.

HIV infection	Yes

Explanation: Because of the apparent minimal risk to others, all sports may be played that the state of health allows. In all athletes, skin lesions should be properly covered, and athletic personnel should use universal precautions when handling blood or body fluids with visible blood. [6]

Kidney: absence of one	Qualified Yes

Explanation: Athlete needs individual assessment for contact/collision and limited contact sports.

Liver: enlarged	Qualified Yes

Explanation: If the liver is acutely enlarged, participation should be avoided because of risk of rupture. If the liver is chronically enlarged, individual assessment is needed before collision/contact or limited contact sports are played.

Malignancy	Qualified Yes

Explanation: Athlete needs individual assessment.

Musculoskeletal disorders	Qualified Yes

Explanation: Athlete needs individual assessment.

Neurologic

History of serious head or spine trauma, severe or repeated concussions, or craniotomy. [5, 11]	Qualified Yes

Explanation: Athlete needs individual assessment for collision/contact or limited contact sports, and also for noncontact sports if there are deficits in judgment or cognition. Recent research supports a conservative approach to management of concussion.

Convulsive disorder, well controlled	Yes

Explanation: Risk of convulsion during participation is minimal.

Table 2 *Medical Conditions and Sports Participation—cont'd.*

Condition	May Participate?
Convulsive disorder, poorly controlled *Explanation:* Athlete needs individual assessment for collision/contact or limited contact sports. Avoid the following noncontact sports: archery, riflery, swimming, weight or power lifting, strength training, or sports involving heights. In these sports, occurrence of a convulsion may be a risk to self or others.	Qualified Yes
Obesity *Explanation:* Because of the risk of heat illness, obese persons need careful acclimatization and hydration.	Qualified Yes
Organ transplant recipient *Explanation:* Athlete needs individual assessment.	Qualified Yes
Ovary: absence of one *Explanation:* Risk of severe injury to the remaining ovary is minimal.	Yes
Respiratory	
Pulmonary compromise including cystic fibrosis *Explanation:* Athlete needs individual assessment, but generally all sports may be played if oxygenation remains satisfactory during a graded exercise test. Patients with cystic fibrosis need acclimatization and good hydration to reduce the risk of heat illness.	Qualified Yes
Asthma *Explanation:* With proper medication and education, only athletes with the most severe asthma will have to modify their participation.	Yes
Acute upper respiratory infection *Explanation:* Upper respiratory obstruction may affect pulmonary function. Athlete needs individual assessment for all but mild disease. See "Fever" above.	Qualified Yes
Sickle cell disease *Explanation:* Athlete needs individual assessment. In general, if status of the illness permits, all but high exertion, collision/contact sports may be played. Overheating, dehydration, and chilling must be avoided.	Qualified Yes
Sickle cell trait *Explanation:* It is unlikely that individuals with sickle cell trait (AS) have an increased risk of sudden death or other medical problems during athletic participation except under the most extreme conditions of heat, humidity, and possibly increased altitude. [I2] These individuals, like all athletes, should be carefully conditioned, acclimatized, and hydrated to reduce any possible risk.	Yes
Skin: boils, herpes simplex, impetigo, scabies, molluscum contagiosum *Explanation:* While the patient is contagious, participation in gymnastics with mats, martial arts, wrestling, or other collision/contact or limited contact sports is not allowed. Herpes simplex virus probably is not transmitted via mats.	Qualified Yes
Spleen, enlarged *Explanation:* Patients with acutely enlarged spleens should avoid all sports because of risk of rupture. Those with chronically enlarged spleens need individual assessment before playing collision/contact or limited contact sports.	Qualified Yes
Testicle absent or undescended *Explanation:* Certain sports may require a protective cup	Yes

Table 3   *Classification of Sports by Strenuousness [3]*

High to Moderate Intensity

High to Moderate Dynamic and Static Demands	High to Moderate Dynamic and Low Static Demands	High to Moderate Static and Low Dynamic Demands
Boxing*	Badminton	Archery
Crew/rowing	Baseball	Auto racing
Cross-country skiing	Basketball	Diving
Cycling	Field hockey	Equestrian
Downhill skiing	Lacrosse	Field events (jumping)
Fencing	Orienteering	Field events (throwing)
Football	Ping-pong	Gymnastics
Ice hockey	Race walking	Karate or judo
Rugby	Racquetball	Motorcycling
Running (sprint)	Soccer	Rodeoing
Speed skating	Squash	Sailing
Water polo	Swimming	Ski jumping
Wrestling	Tennis	Water skiing
	Volleyball	Weight lifting

Low Intensity (Low Dynamic and Low Static Demands)

Bowling

Cricket

Curling

Golf

Riflery

* Participation not recommended.

COMMITTEE ON SPORTS MEDICINE AND FITNESS, 1993 to 1994

William L. Risser, MD, PhD, Chair

Steven J. Anderson, MD

Stephen P. Bolduc, MD

Sally S. Harris, MD

Gregory L. Landry, MD

David M. Orenstein, MD

Suzanne M. Tanner, MD

Liaison Representatives

Kathryn Keely, MD, Canadian Paediatric Society

Richard Malacrea, National Athletic Trainers' Association

Judith C. Young, PhD, National Association for Sport and Physical Education

AAP Section Liaisons

Arthur M. Pappas, MD, Section on Orthopedics

Regionald L. Washington, MD, Section on Cardiology

Consultant

Oded Bar-Or, MD

Rainer Martens, PhD

References

1. American Academy of Pediatrics, Committee on Sports Medicine. Recommendations for participation in competitive sports. *Pediatrics.* 1988; 81:737–739

2. American Medical Association. *Medical Evaluation of the Athlete: A Guide.* Chicago: American Medical Association; 1976

3. Sixteenth Bethesda Conference. Cardiovascular abnormalities in the athlete: recommendations regarding eligibility for competition. *J Am Coll Cardiol.* 1985; 6:1189–1190

4. National Heart, Lung, Blood Institute. Report of the Second Task Force on Blood Pressure Control in Children—1987. *Pediatrics.* 1987; 79:1–25

5. Dyment PG, ed. *Sports Medicine: Health Care for Young Athletes.* 2nd ed. Elk Grove Village, IL: American Academy of Pediatrics; 1991

6. American Academy of Pediatrics, Committee on Sports Medicine Fitness. Human immunodeficiency virus [acquired immunodeficiency syndrome (AIDS) virus] in the athletic setting. *Pediatrics.* 1991; 88:640–641

7. American Academy of Pediatrics, Committee on Sports Medicine Fitness. Horseback riding and head injuries. *Pediatrics.* 1992; 89:512

8. American Academy of Pediatrics, Committee on Sports Medicine and Fitness. Risk of injury from baseball and softball in children 5 to 14 years of age. *Pediatrics.* 1994; 93:690–692

9. Dorsen PJ. Should athletes with one eye, kidney, or testicle play contact sports? *Phys Sportsmed.* 1986; 14:130–133, 137–138

10. Vinger PF. The one-eyed athlete. *Phys Sportsmed.* 1987; 15:48–52

11. The Sports Medicine Committee, Colorado Medical Society. *Guidelines for management of concussion in sports.* Denver: Colorado Medical Society; 1990

12. Pearson HA. Sickle cell trait and competitive athletics: is there a risk? *Pediatrics.* 1989; 83:613–614

This statement has been approved by the Council on Child and Adolescent Health.

The recommendations in this statement do not indicate an exclusive course of treatment or serve as a standard of medical care. Variations, taking into account individual circumstances, may be appropriate.

Mitral Valve Prolapse and Athletic Participation in Children and Adolescents (RE9523)

AMERICAN ACADEMY OF PEDIATRICS
Committee on Sports Medicine and Fitness
Volume 95, Number 5
May 1995, p 789–790

Mitral valve prolapse (MVP) is generally a benign condition characterized by the protrusion of the mitral valve leaflets into the left atrium during systole. The prevalence of MVP in individuals under the age of 18 years is estimated to be 5% but is higher in those with Marfan's syndrome and other collagen vascular disorders. [1] A midsystolic nonejection click with or without a late systolic murmur is the auscultatory hallmark of this syndrome. The diagnosis of MVP in children and adolescents should be based primarily on auscultatory findings and not on minor echocardiographic findings. [1]

The prognosis in children and adolescents with isolated MVP appears to be excellent and complications are rare. In 553 children, aged 15 days to 18 years, who were involved in studies with a follow-up period of 6 to 9 years, the following were reported: subacute bacterial endocarditis (one case), cerebral vascular accidents (two cases), migraine headaches (four cases), and chest pain (12 cases). [2, 3] Only four cases of sudden death have been reported in patients younger than 20 years of age. [1–4]

In a study of 103 patients with MVP, 16% were found to have premature ventricular beats during exercise electrocardiography (ECG) (exercise test). [3] Thirty-eight percent were found to have premature ventricular contractions (PVCs) on 24-hour ECG (Holter) monitoring. This study, however, does not report the true prevalence of dysrhythmias because all these subjects had been referred to a pediatric cardiologist for evaluation. It is likely that these reported numbers are high because asymptomatic patients are less often referred.

In patients suspected of having MVP, a thorough medical history should include questions regarding the occurrence of near syncope, syncope, palpitations, or chest pain. Family history should be evaluated for the presence of sudden death or MVP in the family.

Patients suspected of having MVP should be examined sitting, standing, squatting, and supine to elicit the changes in the auscultatory findings with different body positions. Maneuvers such as squatting or hand-grip exercise tend to increase left ventricular volume and decrease the degree of MVP and mitral regurgitation. (The click will move toward the second heart sound and the murmur will become softer.) Conversely, any maneuver that decreases left ventricular volume such as the Valsalva maneuver, sudden change from supine to sitting or sitting to standing, or inspiration, will increase the degree of MVP. (The click will move toward the first heart sound and the murmur will become louder and longer.)

If the patient is symptomatic (chest pain, dysrhythmias, palpitations, syncope, near syncope) or if the presence of mitral insufficiency is suspected (systolic murmur), the patient's condition should be evaluated further with a resting ECG, an echocardiogram, a 24-hour ECG (Holter) monitor, and an exercise ECG (exercise test). This evaluation may require referral to a cardiologist.

When the pediatrician diagnoses MVP in an asymptomatic child, it is important to explain to the parents and the patient that the finding is benign and in the majority of cases not associated with any problems or complications. This reassurance and education at the time that the diagnosis is made will prevent the common iatrogenic phenomenon of "cardiac non-disease."

Recommendations

The American Academy of Pediatrics recommends the following:

1. All asymptomatic patients with MVP in the absence of mitral insufficiency or a family history of sudden death associated with MVP may engage in all activities.

2. Patients with MVP who are symptomatic (chest pain, palpitations, dysrhythmias, near syncope, syncope) or who have mitral regurgitation should have their conditions further evaluated before they are cleared for athletic competition. This evaluation should include a resting ECG, an echocardiogram, a 24-hour ECG (Holter) monitor, and an exercise ECG (exercise test). [5] Evaluation by a cardiologist is suggested.

COMMITTEE ON SPORTS MEDICINE AND FITNESS, 1994 to 1995

William L. Risser, MD, PhD, Chair

Steven J. Anderson, MD

Stephen P. Bolduc, MD

Bernard Griesemer, MD

Sally S. Harris, MD, MPH

Larry McLain, MD

Suzanne M. Tanner, MD

Liaison Representatives

Kathryn Keely, MD, Canadian Paediatric Society

Richard Malacrea, ATC, National Athletic Trainers Association

Judith C. Young, PhD, National Association for Sport and Physical Education

AAP Section Liaisons

Arthur M. Pappas, MD, Section on Orthopaedics

Reginald L. Washington, MD, Section on Cardiology

Consultant

Oded Bar-Or, MD, Canadian Paediatric Society

References

1. Warth DC, King ME, Cohen JM, Tesoriero VL, Marcus E, Weyman AE. Prevalence of mitral valve prolapse in normal children. *J Am Coll Cardiol.* 1985; 5:1173–1177

2. Bisset GS, Schwartz DC, Meyer RA, James FW, Kaplan S. Clinical spectrum and long-term follow-up of isolated mitral valve prolapse in 119 children. *Circulation.* 1980; 62:423–429

3. Kavey RE, Blackman MS, Sondheimer HM, Byrum CJ. Ventricular arrhythmias and mitral valve prolapse in childhood. *J Pediatr.* 1984; 105:885–890

4. Jeresaty RM. Mitral valve prolapse: definition and implications in athletes. *J Am Coll Cardiol.* 1986; 7:231–236

5. Maron BJ, Isner JM, McKenna WJ. Task force 3: hypertrophic cardiomyopathy, myocarditis, and other myopericardial diseases and mitral valve prolapse. 26th Bethesda Conference. Recommendations for determining eligibility for competition in athletes with cardiovascular abnormalities. *J Am Coll Cardiol.* 1994; 24:880–885

This statement has been approved by the Council on Child and Adolescent Health.

The recommendations in this statement do not indicate an exclusive course of treatment or serve as a standard of medical care. Variations, taking into account individual circumstances, may be appropriate.

Organized Athletics for Preadolescent Children (RE9165)

AMERICAN ACADEMY OF PEDIATRICS
Committee on Sports Medicine and Committee on School Health
Volume 84, Number 3
September 1989

Each year in the United States, millions of preadolescent children participate in organized athletics. Some organized athletic programs are community based; others are school sponsored, either as extracurricula programs or as part of physical education classes. Most coaches in community-based programs are volunteers who have no formal training or expertise in coaching. The credentials and training of grade school coaches are highly variable. Therefore, many US preadolescents are involved in athletics without the benefit of specific program goals aimed at ensuring the most beneficial physical, psychologic, and recreational outcomes.

Coaches, officials, parents, and program designers all play critical roles in shaping the child's early athletic experience and the child's self-esteem. The goals of the program and the behavior of all of the adults involved should focus upon assisting the child to develop: (1) an enjoyment of sports and fitness that will be sustained through adulthood, (2) physical fitness, [1] (3) basic motor skills, (4) a positive self-image, (5) a balanced perspective on sports in relation to the child's school and community life, and (6) a commitment to the values of teamwork, fair play, and sportsmanship. In addition, efforts must be made to make the sport as safe as possible.

Enjoyment of sports and fitness in childhood will increase the likelihood of a child pursuing these activities through adulthood. Children should be allowed to try a variety of sports and to choose sports that appeal to them. If children require more than gentle encouragement, then they are not ready for involvement. Unstructured free play should be encouraged to enhance enjoyment of sports, as well as to promote spontaneity and creativity.

Coaches, officials, parents, and program designers should view the preadolescent years as a time for teaching fundamental motor skills; developing fitness in a practical, safe, and gradual manner; and promoting desired attitudes and values. Practice sessions should incorporate these elements and allow time for unstructured play. The actual game or sporting event should also be managed in a manner that stresses these goals more than winning. To the extent possible, each child should receive equal playing time. Game rules should be modified to accommodate the child's need to learn or be adapted to age-appropriate skills or fitness. If possible, the child participants should be grouped according to size, skill, and maturational level rather than age. This is especially true at ages 11 to 14 years when some children are prepubertal and others are well into puberty.

The important objective for parents, coaches, and officials should be to enhance the child's self-image. Mastery of the sport (the athlete's performance within the activity) should be emphasized, instead of winning or pleasing others. Coaches and parents should assist children in setting realistic goals. Good effort should be praised, and mistakes should be met with encouragement and corrective instruction. Adults must clearly show that the child's worth is unrelated to the outcome of the game. Unconditional approval should be given for participating and having fun. Athletic programs should deemphasize playoffs and avoid all-star contests, excessive publicity, and elaborate recognition ceremonies that single out individuals. Ceremonies should recognize all participants.

Children may need assistance in maintaining a proper balance between sports and other life activities. Practice and game schedules should not interfere with school responsibilities, and family life should not revolve around the "child athlete" to the exclusion of other family members or needs.

The most effective means of instilling desirable attitudes and values is by role modeling. Coaches, officials, and parents must continuously monitor their own behavior to be sure it reflects the sharing, cooperation, honesty, and restraint they wish to see in the children. Coaches' lifestyle and behavior should reflect the health values they want to encourage in the children (weight control, fitness, good nutrition, and avoidance of alcohol, tobacco, and drugs).

Every program should provide adequate safeguards by requiring: (1) preparticipation physical examinations at least every 2 years; (2) warm-up procedures; (3) the availability of a medically trained person who is competent in recognizing significant injuries during practices and games of contact sports; (4) the establishment of policies for first-aid, referral of injured participants, treatment, rehabilitation, and certification for return to participation [2, 3]; (5) suitable and well-maintained sports facilities; (6) appropriate protective equipment; (7) strict enforcement of rules concerning safety; and (8) a formal surveillance method to ensure that goals are met.

All coaches, whether paid or volunteer, should be required to review the guidelines and goals described above. In addition they should complete a coaching certification program that covers teaching techniques, basic sports skills, fitness, first-aid, sportsmanship, self-image enhancement, and motivation. Available certification programs for coaches include: (1) National Youth Sports Coaches Association, 2611 Old Okeechobee Rd, West Palm Beach, FL 33409 and (2) American Coaching Effectiveness Program, Human Kinetics Publishers, Inc, Box 5076, Champaign, IL 61820.

The pediatrician's role is to advise parents, schools, and community groups regarding these recommendations and to discuss these issues with parents as part of regular anticipatory guidance.

COMMITTEE ON SPORTS MEDICINE, 1988 to 1989

Michael A. Nelson, MD, Chairman

Barry Goldberg, MD

Suzanne B. Haefele, MD

Gregory L. Landry, MD

William L. Risser, MD

Liaison Representatives

Oded Bar-Or, MD, Canadian Paediatric Society

Richard Malacrea, National Athletic Trainers Association

AAP Section Liaison

David M. Orenstein, MD, Section on Diseases of the Chest

Arthur M. Pappas, MD, Section on Orthopaedics

COMMITTEE ON SCHOOL HEALTH, 1988 to 1989

Martin C. Ushkow, MD, Chairman

Beverley J. Bayes, MD

Philip R. Nader, MD

Jerry Newton, MD

Steven R. Poole, MD

Martin W. Sklaire, MD

Liaison Representatives

Jeffrey L. Black, MD, American School Health Association

Janice M. Fleszar, American Medical Association

Vivian Haines, National Association of School Nurses

Paul W. Jung, EdD, American Association of School Administrators

Patricia Lachelt, MS, National Association of Pediatric Nurse Associates and Practitioners

James H. Williams, National Education Association

Charles Zimont, MD, American Academy of Family Physicians

References

1. American Academy of Pediatrics, Committees on Sports Medicine and School Health. Physical fitness and the schools. *Pediatrics.* 1987; 80:449–450

2. American Academy of Pediatrics, Committee on Sports Medicine. *Sports Medicine: Health Care for Young Athletes.* Elk Grove Village, IL: American Academy of Pediatrics; 1983

3. American Academy of Pediatrics, Committee on School Health. *School Health: A Guide for Health Professionals.* Elk Grove Village, IL: American Academy of Pediatrics; 1987:182

The recommendations in this statement do not indicate an exclusive course of treatment or serve as a standard of medical care. Variations, taking into account individual circumstances, may be appropriate.

This statement has been approved by the Council on Child and Adolescent Health. Reprint requests to Publications Department, American Academy of Pediatrics, 141 Northwest Point Blvd, PO Box 927, Elk Grove Village, IL 60009-0927.

Participation in Boxing by Children, Adolescents, and Young Adults (RE9703)

AMERICAN ACADEMY OF PEDIATRICS

Committee on Sports Medicine and Fitness

Volume 99, Number 1

January 1997, p 134–135

ABSTRACT. *Because boxing may result in serious brain and eye injuries, the American Academy of Pediatrics opposes this sport. This policy statement summarizes the reasons.*

The American Academy of Pediatrics opposes the sport of boxing for children, adolescents, and young adults. Amateur boxing is a collision sport in which winning is based on the number and force of punches successfully landed on an opponent's head and/or body. This deliberately exposes boxing participants to potentially devastating neurologic and ocular injuries. [1, 2] Despite these potential dangers, thousands of boys and girls continue to participate in amateur boxing.

Supporters of amateur boxing suggest that it teaches self-defense, discipline, strength, and agility while building self-confidence, character, and courage. [3] For some youth, boxing may provide a supervised, structured, goal-oriented alternative to the streets. Impoverished youth may see professional boxing as a means of financial gain—without regard to attendant medical risks. [2]

The overall risk of injury in amateur boxing is actually lower than in some other collision sports such as football, rugby, and ice hockey. However, as opponents of boxing have emphasized, boxing is the only sport where direct blows to the head are rewarded and the ultimate victory may be to render the opponent senseless. Participants in boxing are at risk for dementia pugilistica, a chronic encephalopathy caused by the cumulative effects of multiple subconcussive blows to the head. Numerous studies of professional boxers document this hazard and its potentially devastating consequences on long-term health. [2, 4–6] Because amateur fights last only three rounds, compared to as many as 15 rounds in professional boxing, it is reasonable to expect that amateur boxers receive fewer blows to the head and thus, suffer fewer brain injuries. However, recent studies have shown that amateur boxers still are at risk for acquiring cognitive abnormalities and/or focal neurologic deficits. [7–11] Although other studies have not confirmed these findings, the "safety" of amateur boxing remains unproven. [12, 13]

Prophylactic measures with helmets, unlimited lengths of hand bandage, and heavier gloves have not decreased the frequency of matches that are stopped for neurologic reasons. [5, 14] Ocular injuries are a risk, [15–17] even for amateur boxers, and may account for more hospitalizations than neurologic injuries. [1]

Despite abundant evidence of the medical risks of boxing and clear opposition from medical associations in the United States, boxing is likely to remain as a sporting option for interested youth. Pediatricians can help young people make more informed choices about participation in boxing and hopefully direct their patients toward safer activities.

Recommendations

The American Academy of Pediatrics recommends that pediatricians:

1. Vigorously oppose boxing as a sport for any child, adolescent, or young adult;

2. Educate "at risk" patients about the medical risks of boxing and provide information that supports the Academy's opposition to the sport; and

3. Encourage young athletes to participate in sports in which intentional head injury is not the primary objective.

COMMITTEE ON SPORTS MEDICINE AND FITNESS, 1994 to 1995

William L. Risser, MD, PhD, Chair

Steven J. Anderson, MD

Stephen P. Bolduc, MD

Bernard Griesemer, MD

Sally S. Harris, MD, MPH

Larry McLain, MD

Suzanne M. Tanner, MD

Liaison Representatives

Kathryn Keely, MD
Canadian Paediatric Society
Richard Malacrea, ATC
National Athletic Trainers Association
Judith C. Young, PhD
National Association for Sport and Physical Education

AAP Section Liaison

Reginald L. Washington, MD
Section on Cardiology

References

1. Enzenauer RW, Mauldin WM. Boxing-related ocular injuries in the United States Army, 1980 to 1985. *South Med J.* 1989; 82:547–549

2. Casson IR, Siegel O, Sham R, Campbell EA, Tarlau M, DiDomenico A. Brain damage in modern boxers. *JAMA.* 1984; 251:2663–2667

3. Enzenauer RW, Montrey JS, Enzenauer RJ, Mauldin WM. Boxing-related injuries in the US Army, 1980 through 1985. *JAMA.* 1989; 261:1463–1466

4. Drew RH, Templer DI, Schuyler BA, Newell TG, Cannon WG. Neuropsychological deficits in active licensed professional boxers. *J Clin Psychol.* 1986; 42:520–525

5. Kaste M, Kuurne T, Vilkki J, Katevuo K, Sainio K, Meurala H. Is chronic brain damage in boxing a hazard of the past? *Lancet.* 1982; 2:1186–1188

6. Jordan BD, Jahre C, Hauser WA, et al. CT of 338 active professional boxers. *Radiology.* 1992; 185:509–512

7. Haglund Y, Persson HE. Does Swedish amateur boxing lead to chronic brain damage? A retrospective clinical neurophysiological study. *Acta Neurol Scand.* 1990; 82:353–360

8. Heilbronner RL, Henry GK, Carson-Brewer M. Neuropsychologic test performance in amateur boxers. *Am J Sports Med.* 1991; 91:376–380

9. Haglund Y, Eriksson E. Does amateur boxing lead to chronic brain damage? A review of some recent investigations. *Am J Sports Med.* 1993; 21:97–109

10. Holzgraefe MD, Lemme W, Funke W, Felix R, Felten R. The significance of diagnostic imaging in acute and chronic brain damage in boxing: a prospective study in amateur boxing using magnetic resonance imaging (MRI). *Int J Sports Med.* 1992; 13:616–620

11. McLatchie G, Brooks N, Galbraith S, et al. Clinical neurological examination, neuropsychology, electroencephalography and computed tomographic head scanning in active amateur boxers. *J Neurol Neurosurg Psychiatry.* 1987; 50:96–99

12. Haglund Y, Edman G, Murelius O, Oreland L, Sachs C. Does Swedish amateur boxing lead to chronic brain damage? A retrospective medical, neurological and personality trait study. *Acta Neurol Scand.* 1990; 82:245–252

13. Jordan BD, Zimmerman RD. Magnetic resonance imaging in amateur boxers. *Arch Neurol.* 1988; 45:1207–1208

14. Schmidt-Olsen S, Jensen SK, Mortensen V. Amateur boxing in Denmark: the effect of some preventive measures. *Am J Sports Med.* 1990; 18:98–100

15. Giovinazzo VJ, Yannuzzi LA, Sorenson JA, Delrowe DJ, Campbell EA. The ocular complications of boxing. *Ophthalmology.* 1987; 94:587–596

16. Wedrich A, Velikay M, Binder S, Radax U, Stolba U, Datlinger P. Ocular findings in asymptomatic amateur boxers. *Retina.* 1993; 13:114–119

17. Jones NP. Eye injury in sport. *Sports Med.* 1989; 7:163–181

This statement has been approved by the Council on Child and Adolescent Health.

The recommendations in this statement do not indicate an exclusive course of treatment or serve as a standard of medical care. Variations, taking into account individual circumstances, may be appropriate.

Physical Fitness and the Schools (RE7097)

AMERICAN ACADEMY OF PEDIATRICS
Committee on Sports Medicine, and Committee on School Health
Volume 80, Number 3
September 1987

During the last decade our concept of what "physical fitness" means has undergone a major change. Traditionally the "physically fit" child was one who had obvious motor (or athletic) abilities, ordinarily defined by such parameters as muscle strength, agility, speed, and power. But the high levels of power, speed, and agility necessary for success in most competitive sports have little or no relevance in the daily lives of most adults. Today, the words "physical fitness" imply optimal functioning of all physiologic systems of the body, particularly the cardiovascular, pulmonary, and musculoskeletal systems. [1]

Defining Physical Fitness

Physical fitness is now considered to include five components: muscle strength and endurance, flexibility, body composition (ie, degree of fatness), and cardiorespiratory endurance. Good cardiorespiratory endurance may be associated with a lessened chance of disability or death due to cardiovascular disease. Schools in the United States have traditionally emphasized sports such as football and baseball, both of which require agility and skill but are not particularly fitness enhancing. Aerobic activities (eg, activities requiring maintenance of 75% of maximal heart rate for 20 to 25 minutes), if performed at least three times a week, can lead to enhanced cardiorespiratory endurance. This improvement in fitness can be achieved by swimming, running, bicycling, field hockey, aerobic dancing, fast walking, etc.

School Programs

Unfortunately, just as the understanding of the importance of health-related physical fitness has become widespread, our ability to direct youth activities toward fitness is being countered by several new pressures: (1) Financial strains may lead public school systems to reduce physical education budgets. (2) Widespread disenchantment with the results of several decades of "progressive education experiments" has resulted in pressures on school administrators to do away with "frills" and to return to the "basics"; this might lead to deemphasis of physical education classes. (3) Children and adolescents are lured to watch television in their spare time. (4) Finally, most aerobic activities (eg, running, swimming laps) are not perceived to be pleasurable, and it is extremely difficult to motivate children to begin a lifelong habit of maintaining a high degree of physical fitness if this involves repeated endurance physical activities.

American children do not perform well on standardized tests of fitness. [2, 3] In one 1985 study, 40% of boys 6 to 12 years of age could not do more than one pull-up, nor could 70% of girls of all ages. [2] In this 1985 study, general levels of physical fitness were compared with levels found in a 1975 study of randomly selected students; in general, there had been no improvement in physical fitness levels. The National Children and Youth Fitness Study of the US Department of Health and Human Services compared body composition values for children in 1985 with values for a group of children tested in the 1960s; it was concluded that on the average children are fatter now. [3]

Role of Pediatrician

Because financial support for fitness programs in the schools is unlikely to increase in the foreseeable future, and television is unlikely to become less attractive, we must anticipate the probability that our children's degree of physical fitness will decline. Pediatricians must acquaint themselves with this problem and appeal to their local school boards to maintain, if not increase, the school's physical education program of physical fitness. School programs should emphasize the so-called lifetime athletic activities such as cycling, swimming, and tennis. Schools should decrease time spent teaching the skills used in team sports such as football, basketball, and baseball. Physical fitness activities at school should promote a lifelong habit of aerobic exercise. During anticipatory guidance sessions, pediatricians should encourage parents to see that all family members are involved in fitness-enhancing physical activities, so that these activities become an integral part of the family's lifestyle.

COMMITTEE ON SPORTS MEDICINE, 1986 to 1987

Paul G. Dyment, MD, Chairman

Barry Goldberg, MD

Suzanne B. Haefele, MD

John J. Murray, MD

Michael A. Nelson, MD

Liaison Representatives

Oded Bar-Or, MD, Canadian Paediatric Society

Richard Malacrea, MD, National Athletic Trainers Association

AAP Section Liaison

David M. Orenstein, MD, Section on Diseases of the Chest

Arthur M. Pappas, MD, Section on Orthopaedics

COMMITTEE ON SCHOOL HEALTH, 1986 to 1987

Joseph R. Zanga, MD, Chairman

Michael A. Donlan, MD

Jerry Newton, MD

Maxine M. Sehring, MD

Martin W. Sklaire, MD

Martin C. Ushkow, MD

Liaison Representatives

Jeffrey L. Black, MD, American School Health Association

Patricia Lachelt, National Association of Pediatric Nurse Associates and Practitioners

Nick Staresinic, PhD, American Association of School Administrators

Bonnie Wilford, PhD, American Medical Association

Charles Zimont, MD, American Academy of Family Physicians

References

1. Pate RR: A new definition of youth fitness. *Phys Sports Med.* 1983; 11:77–83

2. Reiff GG, Dixon WR, Jacoby D, et al: *Youth Physical Fitness in 1985.* Washington, DC, President's Council on Physical Fitness and Sports, 1985

3. US Department of Health and Human Services: The National Children and Youth Fitness Study. *J Phys Educ Recreation Dance.* January 1985, pp 44–90

Promotion of Healthy Weight Control Practices in Young Athletes (RE9615)

AMERICAN ACADEMY OF PEDIATRICS
Committee on Sports Medicine and Fitness
Volume 97, Number 5
May 1996, p 752–753

Many athletes engage in unhealthy weight-control practices. This new policy statement urges pediatricians to attempt to identify and help these athletes and provides information about how to support sound nutritional behavior.

Athletes may engage in unhealthy weight-control practices, particularly in sports in which thinness or "making weight" is judged important to success, such as body building, cheerleading, dancing (especially ballet), distance running, diving, figure skating, gymnastics, horse racing, rowing, swimming, weight-class football, and wrestling. [1–3] Some athletes may use extreme weight-loss practices that include overexercising; prolonged fasting; vomiting; using laxatives, diuretics, diet pills, other licit or illicit drugs, and/or nicotine; and use of rubber suits, steam baths, and/or saunas. The majority of these disordered eating behaviors do not meet *Diagnostic and Statistical Manual of Mental Disorders,* 4th ed, criteria [4] for anorexia nervosa or bulimia nervosa.

In two surveys of 208 female collegiate athletes, 32% and 62% practiced at least one of the following unhealthy weight-control behaviors: self-induced vomiting, binge eating more than twice weekly, and using laxatives, diet pills, and/or diuretics. [5, 6] Of 713 high school wrestlers in Wisconsin, 257 (36%) demonstrated two or more behaviors related to bulimia nervosa. [7] In a survey of 171 collegiate Indiana wrestlers concerning their behaviors in high school, 82% had fasted for more than 24 hours, 16% had used diuretics, and 9.4% had induced vomiting at least once a week. [8] Many athletes are secretive about these potentially harmful practices.

Disordered eating may have a negative short-term impact on athletic performance. Athletes who lose weight rapidly by dehydration are probably impairing their athletic performance, especially if it involves strength or endurance, [9] and these strength deficits may persist even after rehydration. [10] The literature on the permanent risks associated with disordered eating is sparse, except for reports on the risk of suboptimal calcium deposition or loss of bone mineral mass among female athletes in whom menstrual disorders develop. [11] The consequences of anorexia nervosa and bulimia nervosa are well documented and can be fatal.

Young athletes are sometimes encouraged to gain weight for sports such as football. These players also need careful guidance so that, if weight gain is appropriate, they increase lean-body and fat mass by appropriate amounts. [12, 13]

Recommendations

1. The goal of athletes, parents, coaches, and clinicians is maintenance of a healthy weight through sound eating behaviors and appropriate exercise.

2. Pediatricians are encouraged to attempt to identify athletes who demonstrate disordered eating or have eating disorders by inquiring about their body image, desired weight, and current eating habits and weight-control practices, as well as inquiring about coaches' and parents' opinions concerning an appropriate weight. Those athletes who cannot control their abnormal behavior should be referred to an appropriate physician (such as an adolescent medicine specialist) for evaluation and treatment.

3. Pediatricians are encouraged to help those who want to lose weight by helping them observe the established principles for healthy weight reduction. [12, 13] These principles are discussed in the manual *Sports Medicine: Health Care for Young Athletes,* [13] published by the American Academy of Pediatrics. The weight goal should be based on appropriate body composition (percentage of body fat) and should consist of a range of values. [13, 14]

4. Pediatricians may need to consult with athletes' coaches, other health care providers, and parents to facilitate a consensus on weight goals. If weight loss is necessary, it should take place during the off-season, so that athletes do not compromise their performance through inadequate energy intake or loss of muscle mass. It is preferable to have a health care provider (pediatrician, athletic trainer, or school nurse) weigh the athlete. Punitive measures should be avoided if young athletes do not lose weight. Similar care should be taken with athletes who want to gain weight.

COMMITTEE ON SPORTS MEDICINE AND FITNESS, 1995 to 1996

William L. Risser, MD, PhD, Chair

Steven J. Anderson, MD

Stephen P. Bolduc, MD

Elizabeth Coryllos, MD

Bernard Griesemer, MD

Larry McLain, MD

Suzanne M. Tanner, MD

Liaison Respresentatives

Kathryn Keely, MD, Canadian Paediatric Society

Richard Malacrea, National Athletic Trainers Association

Judith C. Young, PhD, National Association for Sport and Physical Education

AAP Section Liaisons

Reginald L. Washington, MD, Section on Cardiology

Frederick E. Reed, MD, Section on Orthopaedics

Consultant

Gregory L. Landry, MD

References

1. Garner DM, Garfinkel PE, Rockert W, Olmsted MP. A prospective study of eating disturbances in the ballet. *Psychother Psychosom.* 1987; 48:170–175

2. Drummer GM, Rosen LW, Heusner WW, Roberts PJ, Counsilman JE. Pathogenic weight-control behaviors of young competitive swimmers. *Physician Sportsmed.* 1987; 15:75–86

3. Thompson RA, Sherman RT. Specific sports and eating disorders. In: *Helping Athletes With Eating Disorders.* Champaign, IL: Human Kinetics Publishers; 1993:45–65

4. American Psychiatric Association. *Diagnostic and Statistical Manual of Mental Disorders.* 4th ed. Washington, DC: American Psychiatric Association; 1994

5. Rosen LW, McKeag DB, Hough DO, Curley V. Pathogenic weight-control behavior in female athletes. *Physician Sportsmed.* 1986; 14:79–84

6. Rosen LW, Hough DO. Pathogenic weight-control behaviors of female college gymnasts. *Physician Sportsmed.* 1988; 16:141–144

7. Oppliger RA, Landry GL, Foster SW, Lambrecht AC. Bulimic behaviors among interscholastic wrestlers: a statewide survey. *Pediatrics.* 1993; 91:826–831

8. Stiene HA. A comparison of weight-loss methods in high school and collegiate wrestlers. *Clin J Sport Med.* 1993; 3:95–100

9. Saltin B. Aerobic and anaerobic work capacity after dehydration. *J Appl Physiol.* 1964; 19:1114–1118

10. Costill DL, Sparks KE. Rapid fluid replacement following thermal dehydration. *J Appl Physiol.* 1973; 34:299–303

11. Skolnick AA. "Female athlete triad" risk for women. *JAMA.* 1993; 270:921–923

12. Clark N. How to lose weight and maintain energy. In: *Nancy Clark's Sports Nutrition Guidebook.* Champaign, IL: Leisure Press; 1990:186–196

13. American Academy of Pediatrics, Committee on Sports Medicine and Fitness. Weight control in athletes. In: *Sports Medicine: Health Care for Young Athletes.* 2nd ed. Elk Grove Village, IL: American Academy of Pediatrics; 1991:137–145

14. American Academy of Pediatrics, Committee on Sports Medicine and Fitness. Assessing physical activity and fitness in the office setting. *Pediatrics.* 1994; 3:686–689

Protective Eyewear for Young Athletes (RE9630)

AMERICAN ACADEMY OF PEDIATRICS

American Academy of Pediatrics Committee on Sports Medicine and Fitness and American Academy of Ophthalmology Committee on Eye Safety and Sports Ophthalmology

Volume 98, Number 2

August 1996, p 311–313

The American Academy of Pediatrics and the American Academy of Ophthalmology recommend mandatory protective eyewear for all functionally one-eyed individuals and for athletes who have had eye surgery or trauma and whose ophthalmologists recommend eye protection. Protective eyewear is also strongly recommended for all other athletes.

Background

More than 41 000 sports-related and recreational eye injuries were treated in hospital emergency departments in 1993. [1] Seventy-one percent of the injuries occurred in individuals younger than 25 years; 41% occurred in individuals younger than 15 years; and 6% occurred in children younger than 5 years. Children and adolescents are particularly susceptible to injuries because of their fearless manner of play and their athletic immaturity. [2–4]

Ten sports or sports groupings are highlighted in this statement based on their popularity and the high incidence of eye injuries (see Table 1). [1] Baseball and basketball are associated with the most eye injuries in athletes 5 to 24 years old. [5] Participation rates and information on the severity of the injuries are unavailable, however; therefore, the relative risk of significant injuries cannot be determined for various sports.

The high frequency of sports-related eye injuries in young athletes indicates the need for an awareness among athletes and their parents of the risks of participation and of the availability of a variety of approved sports eye protectors. When properly fitted, appropriate eye protectors have been found to reduce the risk of significant eye injury by at least 90%. [4, 6, 7]

Table 1 *Estimated Sports and Recreational Eye Injuries: 1993**

Sport/Recreation Activity	Estimated Injuries	Age Group		
		5 yrs	5-14 yrs	15-24 yrs
Basketball	8521	112	2241	3413
Baseball	6136	363	3150	1407
Swimming and pool sports	3439	43	1608	729
Racquet and court sports	3183	34	668	1064
Football	2197	0	1097	998
Ball sports (unspecified)	1749	194	743	320
Soccer	1319	0	731	365
Golf	969	43	486	112
Hockey (all types)	946	19	342	515
Volleyball	821	0	180	263
Total selected sports	29280	808	11246	9186
Other sports and recreational activities	11751	1457	3483	2977
Total	41031	2265	14729	12163

* Reprinted with permission from Prevent Blindness America (formerly National Society to Prevent Blindness), 1993 Sports and Recreational

Evaluation

It would be ideal if all children and adolescents wore appropriate eye protection for all sports and recreational activities. All youth involved in organized sports should be encouraged to wear appropriate eye protection.

Physicians must strongly recommend that athletes who are functionally one-eyed wear appropriate eye protection during all sports and recreational activities. (Functionally one-eyed athletes are those with a best-corrected visual acuity of worse than 20/40 in the poorer-seeing eye, assuming that adequate amblyopia [lazy eye] therapy has been accomplished.) [4, 5, 8]

If the better eye is severely injured, functionally monocular athletes will be severely handicapped. In many states, they cannot obtain drivers' licenses. [9]

Athletes who have had eye surgery or trauma to the eye may have weakened eye tissue that is more susceptible to injury. [10] These athletes may need eye protection and should be evaluated and counseled by an ophthalmologist.

Various kinds of eye protection are described below and in the Glossary. Different brands of sports goggles vary significantly in the way they fit. An experienced ophthalmologist, optometrist, or optician can help an athlete select appropriate goggles that fit well.

Indigent athletes may have trouble affording eye evaluations or protective eyewear. Sports programs may have to assist these athletes in the evaluation process and in obtaining protective eyewear.

Recommendations

To implement the policy, we recommend the following specific interventions:

1. Appropriate protective eyewear for low-eye risk sports (see Table 2) consists of an approved street-wear frame that meets American National Standards Institute (ANSI) standard Z87.1 with polycarbonate or CR-39 lenses. A strap must secure the frame to the head. These glasses must be fitted by an experienced ophthalmologist, optometrist, or optician.

2. Appropriate protective eyewear for high-eye risk sports is itemized in Table 2. The sports goggles must have lenses made of polycarbonate, which is stronger than CR-39 plastic. An experienced ophthalmologist, optometrist, or optician must fit these goggles. Because some children have narrow facial features, they may be unable to wear even the smallest sports goggles. These children must be fitted with approved street-wear frames described for low-eye risk sports. Athletes with a high range of refractive error cannot use lenses made of polycar-

bonate. They may wear contact lenses (high power) protected by sports goggles with polycarbonate plano (nonprescription) lenses. For sports in which face masks or helmets with eye protectors or shields must be worn, we strongly recommend that functionally one-eyed athletes also wear sports goggles with polycarbonate lenses to ensure protection. The helmet must fit properly and have a chin strap for optimal protection.

3. Contact lenses offer no protection; therefore, we strongly recommend that athletes who wear contact lenses also wear appropriate polycarbonate eye protection over the lenses. Polycarbonate (plano) non-prescription lenses should be used in street-wear frames for low-eye risk sports or in sports goggles for high-eye risk sports.

4. Athletes must replace sports eye protectors that are damaged or yellowed with age, because they may have become weakened.

5. Functionally one-eyed athletes and those who have had eye injuries or surgery must not participate in boxing, wrestling, and full-contact martial arts. Eye protection is not practical in boxing or wrestling and is not allowed in martial arts.

COMMITTEE ON SPORTS MEDICINE AND FITNESS, 1995 to 1996

William L. Risser, MD, PhD, Chair
Steven J. Anderson, MD
Stephen P. Bolduc, MD
Elizabeth Coryllos, MD
Bernard Griesemer, MD
Larry McLain, MD
Suzanne M. Tanner, MD

Liaison Representatives

Kathryn Keely, MD, Canadian Paediatric Society
Richard Malacrea, ATC, National Athletic Trainers Association
Judith C. Young, PhD, National Association for Sport and Physical Education

AAP Section Liaison

Reginald L. Washington, MD, Section on Cardiology

Consultants

Oded Bar-Or, MD
Jack Jeffers, MD
Rainer Martens, PhD
Michael Nelson, MD

Table 2 *Sports With High Risk of Eye Injury With Appropriate Eye Protectors*

Sport	Eye Protection*
Badminton	Sports goggles with polycarbonate lenses
Baseball	Polycarbonate face guard or other certified safe protection attached to helmet for batting and base running; sports goggles with polycarbonate lenses for fielding
Basketball	Sports goggles with polycarbonate lenses
Bicycling (LER)†	Sturdy street-wear frames with polycarbonate or CR-39 lenses
Boxing	None is available
Fencing	Full face cage
Field hockey (both sexes)	Goalie, full face mask; all others, sports goggles with polycarbonate lenses
Football	Polycarbonate shield on helmet
Full-contact martial arts	Not allowed
Handball†	Sports goggles with polycarbonate lenses
Ice hockey	Helmet and full face protection
Lacrosse (male)	Helmet and full face protection required
Lacrosse (female)	Should at least wear sports goggles with polycarbonate lenses and have option to wear helmet and full face protection
Racquetball†	Sports goggles with polycarbonate lenses
Soccer	Sports goggles with polycarbonate lenses
Softball	Polycarbonate face guard or other certified safe protection attached to helmet for batting and base running; sports goggles with polycarbonate lenses for fielding
Squash¥	Sports goggles with polycarbonate lenses
Street hockey	Sports goggles with polycarbonate lenses; goalie, full face cage§
Swimming and pool sports	Swim goggles recommended
Tennis, doubles	Sports goggles with polycarbonate lenses
Tennis, singles	Sturdy street-wear frames with polycarbonate lenses
Track and field (LER)	Sturdy street-wear frames with polycarbonate or CR-39 lenses
Water polo	Swim goggles with polycarbonate lenses
Wrestling	None is available

* For sports in which face masks or helmets with eye protection are worn, functionally one-eyed athletes and those with previous eye trauma or surgery for whom their ophthalmologists recommend eye protection must also wear sports goggles with polycarbonate lenses to ensure protection.
† LER indicates low eye risk.
¥ Goggles without lenses are not effective.
§ A street hockey ball can penetrate into a molded goalie mask and injure an eye.

AMERICAN ACADEMY OF OPHTHALMOLOGY

Committee on Eye Safety and Sports Ophthalmology

John Jeffers, MD, Chair
M. Bowes Hamill, MD

Francis G. La Piana, MD
Monica L. Monica, MD
John O'Neill, MD
William G. Squires, MD
C. Douglas Witherspoon, MD

Glossary

CR-39 lenses. Lenses made of an allyl-resin plastic (CR-39 is a registered trademark of PPC Industrial) with a center thickness of 3 mm that meet or exceed ANSI standard Z87.1. They are used for strong prescriptions (above -8.00 sphere and -4.00 cylinder) for which polycarbonate is not suitable. Lenses made from this plastic are not as strong as those made with polycarbonate and should not be used in sports goggles for high-eye risk sports.

Polycarbonate lenses. Prescription or nonprescription lenses made of polycarbonate material with a center thickness of at least 2 mm that meet or exceed ANSI standard Z87.1. These are designed to fit in street-wear frames as well as sports goggles.

Polycarbonate shields and face guards. Molded protective shields and face guards designed to be a part of, or to be attached to, various sports helmets.

Sports goggles. Unhinged protective eyewear with a molded frame and temple with prescription or nonprescription polycarbonate lenses with a center thickness of 3 mm. An elastic band secures the goggles to the athlete's head.

Street-wear frames. Sturdy daily wear frames with a posterior lip to prevent inward displacement of the lenses. They should meet ANSI standard Z87.1.

Resources

American Academy of Ophthalmology, Department ESC, Attention: Inquiry Clerk, PO Box 7424, San Francisco, CA 94120-7424 (Eye Safety for Children brochure, include a self-addressed, stamped, legal-size envelope with each request); and Prevent Blindness America (formerly National Society to Prevent Blindness), 500 E Remington Rd, Schaumburg, IL 60173.

Standards: American National Standards Institute, 11 West 42nd St, New York, NY 10036 (Practice for Occupational and Educational Eye Face Protection [ANSI standard Z87.1]); American Society for Testing and Materials, 100 Barr Harbour Dr, West Conshohocken, PA 19428 (Face Guards for Youth [ASTM standard F910-86] and Specifications for Eye Protectors for Use by Players of Racquet Sports [ASTM standard F803-88]); and American Hockey Association of the United States, Canadian Amateur Hockey Association, and Canadian Standards Association (Hockey Helmets and Face Guards).

References

1. Prevent Blindness America. *1993 Sports and Recreational Eye Injuries.* Schaumburg, IL: Prevent Blindness America; 1994

2. Nelson LB, Wilson TW, Jeffers JB. Eye injuries in childhood: demography, etiology, and prevention. *Pediatrics.* 1989; 84:438–441

3. Grin TR, Nelson LB, Jeffers JB. Eye injuries in childhood. *Pediatrics.* 1987; 80:13–17

4. Jeffers JB. An on-going tragedy: pediatric sports-related eye injuries. *Semin Ophthalmol.* 1990; 5:216–223

5. Erie JC. Eye injuries: prevention, evaluation, and treatment. *Phys Sports Med.* 1991; 19(11):108–122

6. Larrison WI, Hersh PS, Kunzweiler T, Shingleton BJ. Sport-related ocular trauma. *Ophthalmology.* 1990; 97:1265–1269

7. Strahlman E, Sommer A. The epidemiology of sports-related ocular trauma. *Int Ophthalmol Clin.* 1988; 28:199–202

8. Wichmann S, Martin DR. Single-organ patients: balancing sports with safety. *Phys Sports Med.* 1992; 20(2):176–182

9. Federal Highway Administration. *Manual on Uniform Traffic Control Devices for Streets and Highways.* Washington, DC: Department of Transportation; 1988

10. Vinger PF. The eye and sports medicine. In: Tasman W, ed. *Duane's Clinical Ophthalmology.* 1994; 5:chap 45

The recommendations in this statement do not indicate an exclusive course of treatment or serve as a standard of medical care. Variations, taking into account individual circumstances, may be appropriate.

Risk of Injury from Baseball and Softball in Children 5 to 14 Years of Age (RE9409)

AMERICAN ACADEMY OF PEDIATRICS
Committee on Sports Medicine and Fitness
Volume 93, Number 4
April 1994, p 690–692

Baseball is one of the most popular sports in the United States, with estimates of 4.8 million children 5 to 14 years of age participating annually in organized and recreational baseball and softball. Interest in and fascination with the sport have grown since the beginning of the 20th century, but it was not until 1965 that the issue of "Little League elbow" raised concern about the safety of the game. Recently, highly publicized catastrophic impact injuries from contact with a ball or bat have raised new safety concerns. These injuries provided the impetus for this review of the safety of baseball for 5- to 14-year-old participants. The discussion focuses principally on baseball, but softball is considered in accord with the availability of relevant literature. This statement mainly concerns injuries during practices and games in organized settings; players and bystanders also can be injured in casual play.

The term Little League elbow was used in 1965 to denote radiologic evidence of fragmentation of the medial epicondylar apophysis and osteochondrosis of the head of the radius and capitellum. [1, 2] Subsequent studies of children 12 years old and younger [3, 4] have found a substantially lower incidence of abnormalities than originally described. [1, 2] Early detection and intervention seem to permit the complete resolution of symptoms and underlying structural abnormalities. [5] More serious abnormalities become more common after the age of 13 years. [6–8] The role that repetitive throwing in 5- to 14-year-old children may play in the evolution of elbow overuse injuries at an older age remains to be determined. In response to concern about Little League elbow, many youth leagues have attempted to limit the stress placed on young pitching arms. For example, Little League Baseball, Inc limits pitchers to a maximum of six innings of pitching per week and requires mandatory rest periods between pitching appearances.[9] Instruction in proper pitching mechanics is another way to prevent serious overuse throwing injuries. [5, 10]

The overall incidence of injury in baseball ranges between 2% and 8% of participants per year. Most injuries are minor soft tissue trauma, usually to the face and upper extremity. [11, 12] Sliding is the cause of one third of the injuries to the lower extremity. In softball and baseball, the Velcro-stabilized breakaway base significantly reduces this risk. [13, 14]

Recently, concern has been raised about injuries to the eye. [15–17] Baseball seems to be the leading cause of sports-related eye injuries in children, and the highest incidence occurs in those 5 to 14 years of age. Approximately one third of baseball-related eye injuries result from being struck by a pitched ball. As a result, in this age group, the Sports Eye Safety Committee of the National Society to Prevent Blindness has recommended the use of batting helmets with polycarbonate faceguards that meet Standard F910 of the American Society for Testing and Materials. [18] These cover the lower part of the face from the tip of the nose to below the chin; they also protect against injuries to the teeth and facial bones. Functionally one-eyed athletes (those with best corrected vision in the worst eye of <20/50) must use these faceguards; they also must protect their eyes when fielding by using polycarbonate sports goggles. Eye protection also may be particularly important for young athletes who have had previous surgery or serious eye injury.

Recently the potential of catastrophic injury resulting from direct contact with a bat, baseball, or softball has received publicity. Deaths have occurred from impact to the head resulting in intracranial bleeding and from nonpenetrating blunt chest impact probably causing ventricular fibrillation or asystole. [19-21] Statistics compiled by the US Consumer Product Safety Commission [11, 22, 23] indicate that in the 8-year period from 1973 to 1980, 40 baseball- or softball-related deaths were reported in children 5 to 14 years of age. Of these deaths, 21 resulted from head and neck injuries, 17 from nonpenetrating impact to the chest, and 2 from other causes, an average of 5 deaths per year. In the 5-year period of 1986 through 1990, 16 baseball- or softball-related deaths were recorded, an average of 3.3 per year. Eight deaths were due to head and neck injuries, seven were caused by chest impact, and one was due to other causes. It would seem that there has been no significant recent change in impact-related deaths in baseball and softball, but conclusions must be tempered by differences in the sources for data surveillance for the two periods studied. [11, 22, 23]

Direct contact by the ball is the most frequent cause of death and serious injury in baseball. Children 5 to 14 years of age seem to be uniquely vulnerable to blunt chest impact, because their thoraces may be more elastic and more easily compressed. [24, 25] Preventive measures to protect young players from direct ball contact include utilization of batting helmets and face protectors while at bat and on base; utilization of the catcher's helmet, mask, and chest and neck protectors; the elimination of the on-deck circle; and the protective screening of dugouts and benches. Future equipment may include chest protectors for batters and pitchers if this equipment can be developed in an efficacious and acceptable manner. Modifications in the hardness and compressibility of softballs and baseballs have been developed for use by children of different ages, with the intent of reducing the force of impact while maintaining performance characteristics. The National Operating Committee on Standards for Athletic Equipment (NOCSAE) has developed standards for these softer baseballs. [26] Studies evaluating their playing characteristics and capacity to reduce injury are in progress; but, at the time this review was completed, it was not yet clear whether these balls offer an advantage in injury prevention.

Compared with older players, children less than 10 years of age often have less coordination, slower reaction times, a reduced ability to pitch accurately, and a greater fear of being struck by the ball. Some developmentally appropriate rule modifications are therefore advisable for this age group, including the use of an adult pitcher, a pitching machine, or a batting tee; the avoidance of head-first sliding; and perhaps the use of softer balls, if they are proven to be safer than standard ones.

There have been anecdotal reports of rare but serious cervical spine injuries occurring when a player slides head-first, hitting an opponent with the top of the helmet. This injury is similar to that caused by spearing in football. If further injury surveillance confirms the need, such sliding may need to be banned in players older than 10 years.

Much of the injury research has concerned baseball, or has not differentiated between baseball and softball. Injury risks seem to be similar in softball, except that softball players are less likely to incur overuse injuries of the pitching arm. Therefore, the same recommendations for injury prevention in baseball apply to softball, except for limitation on pitching.

Recommendations

The American Academy of Pediatrics recommends:

1. Pediatricians may be supportive of the desire of 5- to 14-year-old children to participate in baseball and softball. Catastrophic and chronically disabling injuries are rare and do not seem to have been increasing in frequency in the past decade. Surveillance of baseball and softball injuries should be continued.

2. All preventive measures should be employed to protect young baseball pitchers from disabling throwing injuries. These measures include a restriction on the amount of pitching, in both organized and informal settings; instruction in proper biomechanics; and education of parents, coaches, and children to permit early diagnosis and treatment of overuse pitching injuries.

3. All preventive measures that can reduce serious and catastrophic injuries should be employed in both baseball and softball. These include the use of approved batting helmets; the catcher's helmet, mask, and chest and neck protectors; and rubber spikes. The elimination of the on-deck circle, the protective fencing of dugouts and benches, and the use of breakaway bases are also recommended. Protective equipment should always be sized properly and well maintained. These preventive measures should be employed in both games and practices and in organized and informal participation. Developmentally appropriate rule modifications such as alternative pitching techniques and the avoidance of head-first sliding should be implemented for children less than 10 years of age.

4. Baseball and softball players should be encouraged to reduce the risk of eye injury by wearing polycarbonate eye protectors on their batting helmets. These should be required for the functionally one-eyed athlete (best corrected vision in the worst eye of <20/50) or for athletes with previous eye surgery or severe eye injuries, if their ophthalmologists judge them to be at increased risk of eye injury. The latter two groups should also protect their eyes when fielding by using polycarbonate sports goggles.

5. Consideration should be given to utilizing low-impact NOCSAE-approved baseballs and softballs for children 5 to 14 years of age, if these balls demonstrate satisfactory playing characteristics and reduce injury risk. Children younger than 10 years of age should be particularly encouraged to use the lowest impact NOCSAE-approved balls because these children tend to be less skilled and coordinated. A variety of studies should be undertaken to determine the efficacy of low-impact balls in reducing serious impact injuries. Research should be continued to develop other new, improved, and efficacious safety equipment.

COMMITTEE ON SPORTS MEDICINE AND FITNESS, 1992 to 1993

William L. Risser, MD, Chair
Steven J. Anderson, MD
Stephen P. Bolduc, MD
Sally S. Harris, MD
Gregory L. Landry, MD
David M. Orenstein, MD
Angela D. Smith, MD

Liaison Representatives

Kathryn Keely, MD, Canadian Paediatric Society
Richard Malacrea, National Athletic Trainers Association
Judith C. Young, PhD, National Association for Sport and Physical Education

AAP Section Liaisons

Arthur M. Pappas, MD, Section on Orthopaedics
Reginald L. Washington, MD, Section on Cardiology

Consultants

Oded Bar-Or, MD, Hamilton, Ontario, Canada
Barry Goldberg, MD, New Haven, CT

References

1. Brodgon BG, Crow NE. Little leaguer's elbow. *Am J Roentgenol.* 1960; 83:671–675
2. Adams JE. Injury to the throwing arm: a study of traumatic changes in the elbow joints of boy baseball players. *Calif Med.* 1965; 102:127–132
3. Gugenheim JJ, Stanley RF, Woods GW, Tullos HS. Little league survey: the Houston study. *Am J Sports Med.* 1976; 4:189–200
4. Larson RL, Singer KM, Bergstrom R, Thomas S. Little league survey: the Eugene study. *Am J Sports Med.* 1976; 4:201–208
5. Pappas AM. Elbow problems associated with baseball during childhood and adolescence. *Clin Orthop.* 1982; 164:30–41
6. Barnes DA, Tullos HS. An analysis of 100 symptomatic baseball players. *Am J Sports Med.* 1978; 6:62–67
7. Grana WA, Rashkin A. Pitcher's elbow in adolescents. *Am J Sports Med.* 1980; 8:333–336
8. Jobe FW, Nuber G. Throwing injuries of the elbow. *Clin Sports Med.* 1986; 5:621–636
9. Official Regulations and Playing Rules of Little League Baseball. Williams-port, PA: Little League Baseball Incorporated; 1991:13
10. Albright JA, Jokl P, Shaw R, Albright JP. Clinical study of baseball pitchers: correlation of injury to the throwing arm with method of delivery. *Am J Sports Med.* 1978; 6:15–21
11. Rutherford GW, Miles RB, Brown VR, MacDonald B. *Overview of Sports-Related Injuries to Persons 5–14 Years of Age.* Washington, DC: US Consumer Product Safety Commission; 1981
12. Hale CJ. Protective equipment for baseball. *Phys Sports Med.* 1979; 7:59–63
13. Janda DH, Wojtys EM, Hankin FM, Benedict ME, Hensinger RN. A three-phase analysis of the prevention of recreational softball injuries. *Am J Sports Med.* 1990; 18:632–635
14. Centers for Disease Control Prevention. Sliding-associated injuries in college professional baseball. *MMWR.* 1993; 42:223, 229–230

15. Grin TR, Nelson LB, Jeffers JB. Eye injuries in childhood. *Pediatrics.* 1987; 80:13–17

16. Caveness LS. Ocular and facial injuries in baseball. *Int Ophthalmol Clin.* 1988; 28:238–241

17. Nelson LB, Wilson TW, Jeffers JB. Eye injuries in childhood: demography, etiology, and prevention. *Pediatrics.* 1989; 84:438–441

18. *Specification for Face Guards for Youth Baseball,* F910. Philadelphia, PA: American Society for Testing Materials; 1986

19. Doty DB, Anderson AE, Rose EF, Go RT, Chiu CL, Ehrenhaft JL. Cardiac trauma: clinical and experimental correlations of myocardial contusion. *Ann Surg.* 1974; 180:452–460

20. Langer JC, Winthrop AL, Wesson DE, et al. Diagnosis and incidence of cardiac injury in children with blunt thoracic trauma. *J Pediatr Surg.* 1989; 24:1091–1094

21. Ildstad ST, Tollerud DJ, Weiss RG, Cox JA, Martin LW. Cardiac contusion in pediatric patients with blunt thoracic trauma. *J Pediatr Surg.* 1990; 25:287–289

22. Rutherford GW, Kennedy J, McGhee L. *Hazard Analysis: Baseball and Softball Related Injuries to Children 5–14 Years of Age.* Washington, DC: US Consumer Product Safety Commission; June 1984

23. *Baseball-Deaths-Calendar Year 1986 to Present: Reported Incidents.* Washington, DC: US Consumer Product Safety Commission National Injury Information Clearinghouse; October 30, 1990

24. Snyder RG, Spencer NL, Schneider LW, Owings CL. *Physical Characteristics of Children as Related to Death and Injury for Consumer Product Design and Use.* Ann Arbor, MI: Highway Safety Research Institute, University of Michigan; 1975. UM-HSRI-BI-75-5

25. King AI, Viano DC. *Baseball Related Chest Impact: Final Report to Consumer Product Safety Commission.* July 15, 1986

26. National Operating Committee on Standards for Athletic Equipment Baseball Helmet Task Force. *Standard Method of Impact Test Performance Requirements for Baseball/Softball Batters' Helmets, Baseballs, and Softballs.* Kansas City, MO: National Operating Committee on Standards for Athletic Equipment; 1991

This statement has been approved by the Council on Child and Adolescent Health.

The recommendations in this statement do not indicate an exclusive course of treatment or serve as a standard of medical care. Variations, taking into account individual circumstances, may be appropriate.

Strength Training, Weight and Power Lifting, and Body Building by Children and Adolescents (RE9196)

AMERICAN ACADEMY OF PEDIATRICS

Committee on Sports Medicine

Volume 86, Number 5

November 1990, p 801–803

Some children and many adolescents use weights to increase strength or enlarge muscles. A smaller number compete in the sports of weight lifting, power lifting, and body building.

Definitions

Free weights are dumbbells and barbells that are used without the external support of a machine.

Major lifts are lifts used in the sports of weight and power lifting. Also used are the power clean and the incline and overhead presses. These lifts involve the use of free weights lifted through the extremes of joint motion in a ballistic rather than a controlled fashion. They have significant potential to cause injury. [1–3] In the clean and jerk, the athlete lifts the barbell in a two-step movement from the floor to the chest and then over the head; the snatch involves the same movement of the barbell performed without interruption with a different technique. The power clean requires raising the barbell from the floor to the shoulders in a two-part maneuver. The dead lift is accomplished by raising the barbell from the floor by straightening the flexed knees. In the squat lift, the athlete holds the barbell behind the head on the shoulders, squats until the thighs are parallel with the floor, and then straightens the legs. In the bench press, the athlete lies supine on a bench, holds the barbell over the chest with the arms extended, lowers the weight to the chest, and then raises it again. The incline press is similar, except that the bench is at a 30 degrees angle. In the overhead press, the lifter stands and raises the barbell from in front of the chest to over the head by extending the arms.

Strength training ("weight training," "resistance training") is the use of a variety of methods, including exercises with free weights and weight machines, to increase muscular strength, endurance, and/or power for sports participation or fitness enhancement.

Weight lifting and power lifting are competitive sports in which an athlete attempts to lift a maximal amount of free weight in specific lifts. In weight lifting, the lifts performed are the clean and jerk and the snatch. In power lifting, they are the squat lift, dead lift, and bench press.

Body building is a competitive sport in which the participant uses several resistance training methods, including free weights, to develop muscle size, symmetry, and definition.

Strength Training in the Prepubescent Athlete

Recent research has shown that short-term programs in which prepubescent athletes are trained and supervised by knowledgeable adults can increase strength without significant injury risk. [4–6] These studies did not evaluate the relationship between improved strength, injury prevention, or enhanced athletic performance. No data exist defining risks of injury in less well-organized programs.

Strength Training in the Prepubescent and Postpubescent Athlete

Interscholastic athletic programs in secondary schools are increasingly emphasizing strength training as a conditioning method for participants in male and female sports. The major lifts are often used.

Although the incidence is unknown, strength training in adolescence occasionally produces significant musculoskeletal injury, eg, epiphyseal fractures, ruptured intervertebral disks, and low back bony disruptions, especially during use of the major lifts. [1–3] Safety requires careful planning of several aspects of a program. This includes devising a program for the intensity, duration, frequency, and rate of progression of weight use, as well as selection of sport-specific exercises appropriate for the physical maturity of the individual. Proper supervision should be provided during training sessions. [7–9]

Weight Lifting, Power Lifting, and Body Building

More than 600 teenagers are registered with the United States Weight Lifting Federation, and more than 3000 with the United States Power Lifting Federation. The limited available data indicate that these sports have a significant risk of injury. Brown and Kimball [3] determined that 71 adolescent power lifters with a mean age of 16 years and a mean duration of 17 months participation sustained 98 musculoskeletal injuries, causing discontinuance of training for a total of 1126 days. Body building, with at least 8500 adolescent participants, uses some of the same exercises and presumably is associated with the same risks.

Lifting Maximal Amounts of Weight

Because very little data are available on the relative rate of injury at different ages, controversy exists concerning when young athletes should be allowed to lift maximal amounts of weight. The United States Weight and Power Lifting Federations recommend the age of 14 years. Other experts suggest an older age, for example 16 years. [7] Given the widely varying tempo of pubertal development among adolescents, a more appropriate guideline is one based on physical maturation. If male and female athletes have reached Tanner stage 5 in the development of their secondary sexual characteristics, they will have passed their period of maximal velocity of height growth, [10, 11] during which the epiphyses appear to be especially vulnerable to injury. [12] This level of developmental maturity is reached at a mean age of approximately 15 years in both sexes, with much individual variation. [10, 11]

Training for Coaches

It is essential that coaches have training in supervising strength training programs. Adequate instruction may be obtained in collegiate or graduate school programs or from continuing education courses offered by college strength training instructors. A convenient training program of high quality is offered by the National Strength and Conditioning Association, [8] with home study of written materials and videotapes followed by a certification examination.

Recommendations

The American Academy of Pediatrics recommends:

1. Strength training programs for prepubescent, pubescent, and postpubescent athletes should be permitted only if conducted by well-trained adults. The adults should be qualified to plan programs appropriate to the athlete's stage of maturation, which should be assessed objectively by medical personnel.

2. Unless good data become available that demonstrate safety, children and adolescents should avoid the practice of weight lifting, power lifting, and body building, as well as the repetitive use of maximal amounts of weight in strength training programs, until they have reached Tanner stage 5 level of developmental maturity.

COMMITTEE ON SPORTS MEDICINE, 1989 to 1990

Michael A. Nelson, MD, Chairman

Barry Goldberg, MD

Sally S. Harris, MD

Gregory L. Landry, MD

William L. Risser, MD

Liaison Representatives

Oded Bar-Or, MD, Canadian Paediatric Society

Richard Malacrea, National Athletic Trainers Association

Roswell Merrick, National Association for Sport and Physical Education

AAP Section Liaison

David M. Orenstein, MD, Section on Diseases of the Chest

Arthur M. Pappas, MD, Section on Orthopaedics

References

1. Brady TA, Cahill BR, Bodnar LM. Weight training-related injuries in the high school athlete. *Am J Sports Med.* 1982; 10:1–5

2. Gumbs VL, Segal D, Halligan JB, et al. Bilateral distal radius and ulnar fractures in adolescent weight lifters. *Am J Sports Med.* 1982; 10:375–379

3. Brown EW, Kimball RG. Medical history associated with adolescent powerlifting. *Pediatrics.* 1983; 72:636–644

4. Sewal L, Micheli LJ. Strength training for children. *J Pediatr Orthop.* 1986; 6:143–146

5. Rians CB, Weltman A, Cahill BR, et al. Strength training for prepubescent males: is it safe? *Am J Sports Med.* 1987; 15:483–489

6. Servedio FJ, Bartels RL, Hamlin RL, et al. The effects of weight training using Olympic lifts on various physiological variables in pre-pubescent boys. *Med Sci Sports Exerc.* 1985; 17:288

7. Fleck SJ, Kraemer WJ. *Designing Resistance Training Programs.* Champaign, IL: Human Kinetics Books; 1987

8. *How to Build a Strength and Conditioning Program in Your High School.* National Strength and Conditioning Association. PO Box 81410, Lincoln, NE 68501. Tel. 402-472-3000

9. Cahill BR, ed. *Proceedings of the Conference on Strength Training in the Prepubescent;* 1988; Chicago. American Orthopaedic Society for Sports Medicine, 70 West Hubbard St, Suite 202, Chicago, IL 60610

10. Marshall WA, Tanner JM. Variations in the pattern of pubertal changes in girls. *Arch Dis Child.* 1969; 44:291–303

11. Marshall WA, Tanner JM. Variations in the pattern of pubertal changes in boys. *Arch Dis Child.* 1970; 45:13–23

12. Smith NJ, Stanitski CL. *Sports Medicine.* Philadelphia, PA: WB Saunders Co; 1987:33

This statement has been approved by the Council on Child and Adolescent Health.

The recommendations in this statement do not indicate an exclusive course of treatment or serve as a standard of medical care. Variations, taking into account individual circumstances, may be appropriate.

Triathlon Participation by Children and Adolescents (RE9635)

AMERICAN ACADEMY OF PEDIATRICS
Committee on Sports Medicine and Fitness
Volume 98, Number 3
September 1996, p 511–512

ABSTRACT. *Triathlon is a sport combining swimming, cycling, and running in one continuous event. It is a relatively new sport for children and adolescents, and participation is growing rapidly. The purpose of this statement is to provide pediatricians and others with information on the participation in triathlons by young athletes. A list of triathlon events is given in the "Resources" section at the end of this statement.*

Triathlons specifically for children and adolescents began in 1985 with the formation of the Ironkids Bread Race Series. Participation is growing steadily. In 1994, a total of 18 events, 3 regional championships and 1 national championship, involving more than 5000 youth were held. Approximately 70% of the participants are boys, with increasing participation by girls. Although other independent triathlons for young athletes are held, the Ironkids events continue to be the only structured series. Distances required for the swimming, biking, and running components are relatively short, and there are two levels of participation based on age. Athletes usually participate individually but can also join a three-person relay team.

Adolescents aged 15 to 19 years compete at the Olympic distance in the junior category in events sanctioned by the sport's national governing body, Tri/Fed USA. The Junior National Team was started in 1991 for elite athletes in this age group. International competitions, including an annual world championship, are held. Ultradistance triathlons restrict participation to athletes 18 years or older. Adolescents also compete in sprint distance triathlons that are approximately half the Olympic distance and are the most popular triathlon distance.

No reports in the medical literature address the safety or injury characteristics of young athletes training for or participating in triathlons. In a previous statement, the American Academy of Pediatrics considered the risks of distance running for children and found no reason for restriction of activity. [1] No fatalities or known permanent morbidity have occurred during the Ironkids events. The duration of triathlons for athletes younger than 15 years is typically under 1 hour for most participants and is therefore not longer than a variety of other endurance sports activities. The training of an elite young triathlete is unlikely to be more rigorous than that of young athletes in other sports. In fact, most participants do not engage in lengthy training. Those who do, however, may be at risk for associated overuse injuries and other problems associated with strenuous training, eg, secondary amenorrhea with its associated risk of loss of bone mass.[2]

Recommendations

The American Academy of Pediatrics recommends that:

1. Triathlons for children and adolescents should be specifically designed for their participation, with emphasis on safety, fun, and fitness rather than competition. Currently available information indicates that triathlon participation is safe for young athletes.

2. Appropriate safety precautions for triathlons include, but are not limited to: 1) consideration of the need to shorten or cancel the event depending on the weather conditions (assessment of the risk of hypothermia or heat illness); 2) a pre-event swimming test, in which each participant is required to swim the event distance; 3) the presence of an appropriate number of lifeguards during the swimming portion; 4) swimming in pools with appropriate water temperature rather than in open water; 5) a bicycle course that is closed to motor vehicle use; 6) mandatory use of bicycle helmets; 7) provision of fluids during the running and bicycling parts of the race and at the end of the race; 8) a plan to deal with medical problems, including emergencies; and 9) medical screening before participation is allowed.

Table 1 *Triathlon Distance and Duration*

Type	Distance, Swim/Bike/Run	1994 Top Finish Times	
		Male	**Female**
Ironkids juniors (ages 7–10 y)	100 m/5 K/1 K	0:18:19	0:19:30*
Ironkids seniors (ages 11–15 y)	200 m/10 K/2 K	0:29:31	0:31:36*
Olympic distance			
Juniors (ages 15–19)		2:04:15	2:22:06†
Adults (ages ≥ 20 y)	1500 m/40 K/10 K	1:54:18	2:12:29†
Ironman (ages ≥ 18 y)	2.4 mi/112 mi/26.2 mi	8:20:27	9:20:14¥

* Ironkids National Championship, Nashville, TN, September 10, 1994.
† Tri/Fed USA National Amateur Championship, Columbia, MD, August 14, 1994.
¥ Ironman Triathlon World Championship, Kailua-Kona, HI, October 15, 1994.

COMMITTEE ON SPORTS MEDICINE AND FITNESS, 1995 to 1996

William L. Risser, MD, PhD, Chairperson

Steven J. Anderson, MD

Stephen P. Bolduc, MD

Elizabeth Coryllos, MD

Bernard Griesemer, MD

Larry McLain, MD

Suzanne M. Tanner, MD

Liaison Representatives

Kathryn Keely, MD, Canadian Paediatric Society

Richard Malacrea, ATC, National Athletic Trainers Association

Judith C. Young, PhD, National Association for Sport and Physical Education

AAP Section Liaison

Reginald L. Washington, MD, Section on Cardiology

Consultant

Sally S. Harris, MD, MPH

References

1. American Academy of Pediatrics, Committee on Sports Medicine and Fitness. Risks in distance running for children. *Pediatrics.* 1990; 86:799–800

2. American Academy of Pediatrics, Committee on Sports Medicine and Fitness. Amenorrhea in adolescent athletes. *Pediatrics.* 1989; 84:394–395

Resources

Gatorade Triathlon Series. Exclusive Sports Marketing, Inc, 1060 Holland Dr, Suite 3L, Boca Raton, FL 33427; (407) 241-3801

Ironman Mainland Office. World Triathlon Corporation, 1570 US Hwy 19N, Tarpon Springs, FL 34689; (813) 942-4767

Ironkids Bread Race Series. Campbell-Taggart, Inc, PO Box 1830, St Louis, MO 63118-0830; (314) 259-7279

Tri/Fed USA. National Office, 3595 E. Fountain Blvd, PO Box 1010, Colorado Springs, CO 80901; (719) 597-9090

This statement has been approved by the Council on Child and Adolescent Health.

The recommendations in this statement do not indicate an exclusive course of treatment or serve as a standard of medical care. Variations, taking into account individual circumstances, may be appropriate.

Glossary of Orthopaedic Terms

Arthrodesis The surgical process of promoting bone growth across a joint to eliminate the joint and stop motion. The usual purpose is relief of pain or stabilization of an undependable joint.

Capsule A complex ligamentous structure surrounding a joint like a sleeve. It is a composite of ligaments, tendon expansions, and tendon attachments. The capsule allows motion of joints while stabilizing them, especially in rotation.

Cartilage A cellular tissue that, in the adult, is specific to joints, but in children forms a template for bone formation and growth. Hyaline cartilage is a low-friction cellular tissue that coats joint surfaces. Fibrocartilage is tough with high collagen content, such as found in the meniscus of the knee, or the annulus fibrosus portion of the intervertebral disk.

Closed fracture A fracture in which the integrity of the surrounding skin is intact.

Closed reduction A procedure in which normal relationships are restored to a fractured bone or dislocated joint; no incision is needed.

Condyle The knobby portion of the end of a long bone that articulates with another bone through a joint and serves as a point of attachment for tendons and ligaments.

Cox-, Coxa (Hip) Coxa vara is a varus, or adduction, deformity of the hip.

Cubitus (Elbow) Cubitus varus is a bow or adduction deformity of the elbow.

Delayed union A delay in normal fracture healing; not necessarily a pathologic process.

Diaphysis The shaft of a bone; the portion between the metaphyses at either end.

Dislocation A disruption in the relationship of two bones forming a joint in which the bones have (at least momentarily) completely moved out of their normal positions. Usually, bones lie alongside one another, locked in that position until replaced by a closed or open reduction.

Epiphysis The end of a bone; the portion that articulates with an adjacent bone to form a joint.

Extensor Relating to the extensor side of a limb, usually the posterior surface, but is anterior on the leg from embryonic limb rotation.

External fixation Surgical insertion of pins through the skin that are then attached to an external frame to stabilize a fracture or joint.

Flexor Relating to the flexor side of a limb, usually the anterior surface, but is posterior on the leg from embryonic limb rotation.

Fracture A disruption in the integrity of a bone.

Fracture-dislocation A fracture of bone associated with a dislocation of its adjacent joint.

Fusion (Arthrodesis) A biologic "welding" process in which adjacent joint surfaces are excised to facilitate bony growth from one side of the joint to the other and stop painful joint motion. In the spine, bone graft material "welds" two vertebral bodies to create a single bone and stop motion of the adjacent vertebrae.

Genu (Knee) Genu valgum is a knock-knee deformity; genu varum is a bowleg deformity.

Internal fixation Surgical insertion of a device that stops motion across a fracture or joint to encourage bony healing or fusion.

Kyphosis A deformity of the spine in which the spine bends forward.

Ligament A collagenous tissue that either binds together two bones to form a joint, or acts to suspend a structure in a certain position.

Lordosis A deformity of the spine in which the spine sways, or extends backwards.

Malunion Healing of a fracture in an unacceptable position. Malunions are worst when they angulate the bone away from the plane of motion of the adjacent joints.

Meniscus A fibrocartilage structure in the knee, interposed between the femur and tibia on the medial and lateral sides.

Metaphysis The broad portion of the bone adjacent to a joint.

Myelopathy An abnormal condition of the spinal cord, whether through disease or compression. The usual consequences are spasticity, impairment of sensation, and impairment of bowel and bladder function.

Neuropathy An abnormal condition involving a peripheral nerve.

Nonunion Failure of a fracture to heal. With continued motion through a nonunion, a pseudarthrosis will form.

Open fracture A fracture that communicates with air through a disruption of the skin.

Open reduction An open surgical procedure in which normal or near-normal relationships are restored to a fractured bone or dislocated joint.

Osteomyelitis Infection of bone, either bacterial or mycotic. These infections may be lifelong and are difficult to treat.

Osteonecrosis Literally, death of bone. This term is also known as aseptic necrosis, or death of bone in the absence of infection. In children, it occurs in Legg-Calvé-Perthes disease, and in adults may occur in the femoral head (in association with alcoholism) or in the medial tibial plateau. Removing dead bone and laying down new bone is an incredibly slow process; the surrounding bony architecture usually collapses before the process occurs, leaving irreversible bony deformity and arthritis.

Osteosynthesis The process of bony union, as in fracture healing. It is a biologic welding process that is sometimes facilitated with grafts of bone from the iliac crest and insertion of fixation devices.

Palmar The anterior surface of the forearm, wrist, and hand.

Percutaneous pinning Insertion of pins into bone through small puncture wounds in the skin for stabilization of a fracture or a dislocated joint that was realigned by closed reduction.

Physis The growth plate. It is interposed between the metaphysis and epiphysis and is cartilaginous in structure.

Plantar The sole, or flexor surface of the foot.

Pseudarthrosis A false joint produced when a fracture fails to heal. It develops a pseudocapsule and synovial-like fluid.

Scoliosis A deformity of the spine in which the spine bends to the right or left. With double curves, one may be to the right and the other to the left. Curves to the left in the thoracic region may be from an intraspinal tumor.

Septic arthritis Infection of a joint, either bacterial or mycotic.

Spondylolisthesis A slippage or subluxation of one vertebral body on the one below; the slippage can be anterior, posterior, or to either the right or left side. The common causes are degenerative changes in the disk and facet structures in adults, and a specific defect in the lamina called spondylolysis, which appears at or before early adolescence and creates a deformity that persists throughout life.

Subluxation An incomplete disruption in the relationship of two bones forming a joint. The joint surfaces are still related to one another, but are not perfectly aligned.

Synovium The lining of a joint that produces synovial fluid for joint lubrication.

Tendon A highly collagenous tissue attached to muscle at one end and to a bone at the other. It transmits forces of muscular contraction to cause motion across a joint.

Tenosynovium The sheath within which a tendon glides as it transmits muscle forces across joints.

Trochlea A groove in a bone that articulates with another bone, or serves as a channel for a tendon to track in.

Valgus Abduction of a distal bone in relation to its proximal partner. Valgus of the knee is a knock-knee deformity, with abduction of the tibia in relation to the femur.

Varus Adduction of a distal bone in relation to its proximal partner. Varus of the knee is a bowleg deformity, with adduction of the tibia in relation to the femur.

Volar The anterior surface of the forearm, wrist, and hand.

Index

DATE DUE

HIGHSMITH #45230

Printed
in USA